Master Dentistry

Master Dentistry

Volume 2: Restorative Dentistry, Paediatric Dentistry and Orthodontics

FOURTH EDITION

Giles McCracken, BDS, PhD, FDSRCPS(Glasg), FDS(Rest Dent), PGCAP FHEA

Professor of Restorative Dentistry
School of Dental Sciences
Newcastle University/Newcastle upon Tyne Hospitals NHS Foundation Trust
Newcastle upon Tyne
United Kingdom

For additional online content visit ExpertConsult.com

Elsevier

London   New York   Oxford Philadelphia   St Louis   Sydney   2021

Notices

Practitioners and researchers must always rely on their own experience and knowledge in evaluating and using any information, methods, compounds or experiments described herein. Because of rapid advances in the medical sciences, in particular, independent verification of diagnoses and drug dosages should be made. To the fullest extent of the law, no responsibility is assumed by Elsevier, authors, editors or contributors for any injury and/or damage to persons or property as a matter of products liability, negligence or otherwise, or from any use or operation of any methods, products, instructions, or ideas contained in the material herein.

Previous editions copyrighted 2013, 2008, and 2003.

ISBN: 978-0-7020-8144-6

Content Strategist: Alexandra Mortimer
Publication Service Manager: Deepthi Unni
Project Manager: Radjan Lourde Selvanadin
Design: Bridget Hoette
Illustrator: GW Inc.
Illustration Manager: Narayanan Ramakrishnan
Marketing Manager: Allison Kieffer

Printed in India

Last digit is the print number: 9 8 7 6 5 4 3 2 1

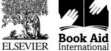

Contents

Preface

The philosophy behind this textbook remains unchanged from that of my predecessor editor Peter Heasman and the chapter authors of all three editions. The emphasis remains on supporting the reader's understanding, learning and self-assessment so that they are able to explore their own level of knowledge, identify their strengths and, perhaps more importantly, weaknesses or gaps in their knowledge base, which can then be addressed. Basically, this book comprises 12 chapters on key aspects of restorative dentistry, sedation, paediatric dentistry, orthodontics and professionalism.

Feedback from undergraduate dental students continues to confirm that they value the structure of the book, especially the sections on assessment. The popularity of various assessment methods, however, continues to change on a regular basis and those assessment methods presented in this textbook have been reviewed to ensure that they remain in touch with contemporary education philosophy. This edition has 'single best answer' format questions introduced in most chapters.

I should like to record my sincere thanks to Peter who brought me in as a chapter author initially and suggested I step forward as editor. The foundations of this book are strong, I hope that the modifications and additions to the work of you and the previous chapter authors adds further value to our readers.

I am grateful and thank my colleagues Dr Hawa Fathi and Mr Khaleel Shazada for sharing and discussing their knowledge and insights into Equality, Diversity and Inclusion in education, the wider world and how it relates to the themes and topics in this book.

Finally, I am deeply indebted to the hard work, patience and talents of the contributing authors. They are experts in their respective specialties and have worked diligently to revise and update this fourth edition of *Master Dentistry Volume 2*. Thank you all!

GIM
Newcastle-upon-Tyne
2020

Using This Book

Philosophy of the Book

Most students need a textbook that will provide all the basic facts within a discipline and that also facilitates understanding of the subject. This textbook achieves these objectives and also provides test questions for the student to explore their level of knowledge. It is also important for students to achieve a 'feel for the subject' and learn communication skills.

The book is designed to provide basic information necessary to pass an undergraduate examination in restorative, paediatric and orthodontic dentistry. It also expands on the core curriculum to allow the motivated student an opportunity to pursue the subject in greater detail. The information is presented in such a way as to aid recall for examination purposes and also to facilitate understanding of the subject. Key facts are highlighted, and principles of diagnosis and management emphasised. It is hoped that the book will also be a satisfactory basis for postgraduate practice and studies.

Do not think though that this book offers a 'syllabus'. It is impossible to draw boundaries around the scientific basis and clinical practice of dentistry. Learning is, therefore, a continuous process carried out throughout your career. This book includes all that you *must* know, most of what you *should* know and some of what you *might* already know.

We assume that you are working towards one or more examinations, probably in order to qualify. Our purpose is to show you how to overcome this barrier. As we feel strongly that learning is not simply for the purpose of passing examinations, the book aims to help you to pass but also to develop *useful* knowledge and understanding.

This introductory chapter aims to help you:

- to understand how the emphasis on self-assessment can make learning easier and more enjoyable
- to use this book to increase your understanding as well as knowledge
- to plan your learning.

LAYOUT AND CONTENTS

Each chapter begins with a brief overview of the content and a number of learning objectives are listed at the start of each subsection. The main part of the text in each chapter describes important topics in major subject areas. We have tried to provide the essential information in a logical order with explanations and links. In order to help you, we have used lists to set out frameworks and to make it easier for you to put facts in a rational sequence. Tables are used to link quite complex and more detailed information. Techniques used in various procedures are listed in boxes.

You have to be sure that you are reaching the required standards, so the final section of each chapter is there to help you to check your knowledge and understanding. The self-assessment is in the form of multiple choice questions, extended matching items questions, case histories, short notes, data interpretation, possible viva questions and picture questions. Questions are designed to integrate knowledge across different chapters and to focus on the decisions you will have to take in a given clinical situation. Detailed answers are given with reference to relevant sections of the text; the answers also contain information and explanations that you will not find elsewhere, so you have to do the assessments to get the most out of this book.

How to Use This Book

If you are using this book as part of your examination preparations, we suggest that your first task should be to map out on a sheet of paper three lists dividing the major subjects (corresponding to the chapter headings) into your strong, reasonable and weak areas. This will give you a rough outline of your revision schedule, which you must then fit in with the time available. Clearly, if your examinations are looming, you will have to be ruthless in the time allocated to your strong areas. The major subjects should be further classified into individual topics. Encouragement to store information and to test your ongoing improvement is by the use of the self-assessment sections – you must not just read passively. It is important to keep checking your current level of knowledge, both strengths and weaknesses. This should be assessed objectively – self-rating in the absence of testing can be misleading. You may consider yourself strong in a particular area whereas it is more a reflection on how much you enjoy and are stimulated by the subject. Conversely, you may be weaker in a subject than you would expect simply because the topic does not appeal to you.

It is a good idea to discuss topics and problems with colleagues/friends; the areas that you understand least well will soon become apparent when you try to explain them to someone else.

Effective Learning

You may have wondered why an approach to learning that was so successful in secondary school does not always work at university. One of the key differences between your studies at school and your current learning task is that you are now given more responsibility for setting your own learning objectives. While your aims are undoubtedly to pass examinations, you should also aim to develop learning skills that will serve you throughout your career. That means taking full responsibility for self-directed learning. The earlier you start, the more likely you are to develop the learning skills you will need to keep up with changes in clinical practice.

We know that students learn in all sorts of different ways, and differ in their learning patterns at different stages in a given course. You may intend to do as little work as you can get away with, or you may do the least that will guarantee to get you through the examinations; however, the students who gain most are usually those who take a deep and sustained interest in the subject. It will be worth the effort to start out this way, even if good intentions flag a little towards the end.

You will also get more out of your course by participating actively. Handouts, if given, may help, but they are rarely a satisfactory substitute for your own lecture notes. Remember that timetabled teaching sessions are not the only opportunities for effective learning. It is safer to regard lectures, practicals and tutorials as a guide to the core material that you are expected to master. Greater depth and breadth to this core knowledge must be achieved by reference to more detailed texts. Well-organised departments will provide a set of learning objectives and a reading list early in the course. Many lecturers will give more detailed learning objectives, either in their handouts or verbally at the start of a lecture. If not, paragraph headings can be used as a rough guide to the teacher's expectations. An active approach to learning does not necessarily mean being highly individualistic or overcompetitive. Many students gain a broader and deeper understanding of the subject by working in small informal groups. This may be particularly helpful when it comes to revision.

The final run up to examinations should require little more than a tying up of loose ends and a filling of learning gaps. An effective way of doing this is to work through a steady stream of self-assessment questions and to keep a daily note of points that need clearing up. In other words, concentrate on what you do not know and strengthen the links with what you already know. By this time, the value of pigeonholing factual information within a framework should be self-evident.

APPROACHING THE EXAMINATIONS

The discipline of learning is closely linked to preparation for examinations. Many of us opt for a process of superficial learning that is directed towards retention of facts and recall under examination conditions because full understanding is often not required. It is much better if you try to acquire a deeper knowledge and understanding, combining the necessity of passing examinations with longer-term needs, particularly with the prospect of continuing professional development after qualification.

First you need to know how you will be examined. Does the examination involve clinical assessment such as history taking and clinical examination? If you are sitting a written examination, what are the length and types of questions? How many must you answer and how much choice will you have?

Now you have to choose what sources you are going to use for your learning and revision. Textbooks come in different forms. At one extreme, there is the large reference book. This type of book should be avoided at this stage of revision and only used (if at all) for reference, when answers to questions cannot be found in smaller books. At the other end of the spectrum is the condensed 'lecture note' format, which often relies heavily on lists. Facts of this nature on their own are difficult to remember if they are not supported by

understanding. In the middle of the range are the medium-sized textbooks. These are often valuable irrespective of whether you are approaching final university examinations or the first part of professional examinations. Our advice is to choose one of the several medium-sized books on offer on the basis of which you find the most readable. The best approach is to combine your lecture notes, textbooks (appropriate to the level of study) and past examination papers as a framework for your preparation.

Armed with information about the format of the examinations, a rough syllabus, your own lecture notes and some books that you feel comfortable in using, your next step is to map out the time available for preparation. You must be realistic, allow time for breaks and work *steadily*, not cramming. If you do attempt to cram, you have to realise that only a certain amount of information can be retained in your short-term memory. Cramming simply retains facts. If the examination requires understanding, you will undoubtedly have problems.

It is often a good idea to begin by outlining the topics to be covered and then attempting to summarise your knowledge about each in note form. In this way, your existing knowledge will be activated and any gaps will become apparent. Self-assessment also helps to determine the time to be allocated to each subject for examination preparation. If you are consistently scoring excellent marks in a particular subject, it is not very effective to spend a lot of time trying to achieve the 'perfect' mark.

In an essay, it is many times easier to obtain the first 50% of the marks than the last. You should also try to decide on the amount of time to assign to each subject based on the likelihood of it appearing in the examination.

THE MAIN TYPES OF EXAMINATION

Multiple Choice Questions

Most multiple choice questions test recall of information. The aim is to gain the maximum marks from what you can remember. The common form consists of a stem with several different phrases that complete the statement. Each statement is to be considered in isolation from the rest and you have to decide whether it is 'True' or 'False'. There is no need for 'Trues' and 'Falses' to balance out for statements based on the same stem; they may all be 'True' or all 'False'. The stem must be read with great care and, if it is long with several lines of text or data, you should try and summarise it by extracting the essential elements. Make sure you look out for the 'little' words in the stem such as *only, rarely, usually, never* and *always*. Negatives such as *not, unusual* and *unsuccessful* often cause marks to be lost. *May occur* has entirely different connotations to *characteristic*. The latter generally indicates a feature that is normally observed, the absence of which would represent an exception to a general rule, e.g. regular elections are a characteristic of a democratic society. Regular (if dubious) elections may occur in a dictatorship but they are not characteristic.

Remember to check the marking method before starting. Some still employ a negative system in which marks are lost for incorrect answers. The temptation is to adopt a cautious approach in answering a relatively small number of questions. This can lead to problems, however, as we all make simple mistakes or even disagree vehemently with the answer favoured by the examiner! Caution may lead you to answer too few questions to pass after the marks have been deducted for incorrect answers.

Extended Matching Items (EMIs)

The extended matching items questions are becoming more popular for dental assessments and lend themselves well to clinical dental situations. You are usually presented with an overarching theme for the question set and then a list of 10–15 options from which you have to choose your answers. There is then a short lead-in statement followed by the stems; a set of questions, often clinical vignettes, for which you are asked to select, in your opinion, the one best response from the aforementioned list. For example, the list may be causes of dental pain (Necrotising Gingivitis, reversible pulpitis, irreversible pulpitis, and so on), and the clinical vignettes describe signs and symptoms for which there is ONE BEST ANSWER to select from the list. Occasionally, you may be asked to select two answers from the list or more than one answer may be appropriate for one question. As with any type of assessment, it is crucial that you read the instructions for the question before attempting to answer so that you know exactly what you are being asked to do. EMIs are notoriously time-consuming and difficult to write and are usually as challenging for the examiners to write as they are for the candidates to answer! One of the more common pitfalls when writing these questions is for the list of potential options to comprise heterogeneous, unrelated items, for example five causes of dental pain, three partial denture components, two drugs used for sedation and two periodontal diagnoses. If the vignette is based on dental sedation then you only have to choose from the two drugs rather than the other options that are simply irrelevant. These questions tend not to be negatively marked so you would then have a 50–50 chance of being right should you need to guess!

Essays

Essays are not negatively marked. Relevant facts will receive marks as will a logical development of the argument or theme. Conversely, good marks will not be obtained for an essay that is a set of unconnected statements. Length matters little if there is no cohesion. Relevant graphs and diagrams should also be included but must be properly labelled.

Most people are aware of the need to 'plan' their answer; yet few do this. Make sure that what you put in your plan is relevant to the question asked, as irrelevant material is, at best, a waste of valuable time and, at worst, causes the examiner to doubt your understanding. It is especially important in an examination based on essays that time is managed and all questions are given equal weight, unless guided otherwise in the instructions. A brilliant answer in one essay will not compensate for not attempting another because of time. Nobody can get more than 100% (usually 70–80%, tops) on a single answer! It may even be useful to begin with the questions about which you feel you have

least to say so that any time left over can be safely devoted to your areas of strength at the end.

Short Notes

Short notes are not negatively marked. The system is usually for a 'marking template' to be devised that gives a mark(s) for each important fact (also called criterion marking). Nothing is gained for style or superfluous information. The aim is to set out your knowledge in an ordered, concise manner. The major faults of students are, first, devoting too much time to a single question thereby neglecting the rest, and, second, not limiting their answer to the question asked. For example, in a question about the treatment of periodontal disease, all facts about periodontal disease should not be listed, only those relevant to its treatment.

Picture Questions

Pattern recognition is the first step in a picture quiz. This should be coupled with a systematic approach looking for, and listing, abnormalities. For example, the general appearance of the facial skeleton as well as the local appearance of the individual bones and any soft tissue shadows can be examined in any radiograph. Make an attempt to describe what you see even if you are in doubt. Use any additional statements or data that accompany the radiographs as they will give a clue to the answer required.

Case History Questions

A more sophisticated form of examination question is an evolving case history with information being presented sequentially; you are asked to give a response at each stage. They are constructed so that a wrong response in the first part of the question still means that you can obtain marks from the subsequent parts. Patient management problems are designed to test the recall and application of knowledge through an understanding of the principles involved. You should always give answers unless the instructions indicate the presence of negative marking.

Viva/Oral Examination

The viva or oral examination can be a nerve-wracking experience. You are normally faced with two examiners (perhaps including an external examiner) who may react with irritation, boredom or indifference to what you say. You should try and strike a balance between saying too little and too much. It is important to try not to go off the topic. Aim to keep your answers short and to the point. It is worthwhile pausing for a few seconds to collect your thoughts before launching into an answer. Do not be afraid to say 'I don't know'; most examiners will want to change tack to see what you do know.

In some centres, oral examinations are only offered to candidates who have either distinguished themselves or who are in danger of failing. Interviews for the two types of candidate vary considerably. In the 'distinction' setting, the examiner may try to discover what the candidate does *not* know and may also be looking for evidence of knowledge of the current literature. A small number of topics will usually be considered in depth. In the pass/fail setting, the examiner will try to cover many topics, often quite superficially. She/he will try to establish whether the candidate did badly in the written examination because of ignorance in just a couple of areas, or whether ignorance is wide ranging.

Remember also that the examiners may have your written paper in front of them; if you have done particularly badly in one topic, they may well take this up in the oral examination. This is not an attempt to be unpleasant, but a chance for you to redeem yourself somewhat, so be prepared.

CONCLUSIONS

You should amend your framework for using this book according to your own needs and the examinations you are facing. Whatever approach you adopt, your aim should be for an understanding of the principles involved rather than rote learning of a large number of poorly connected facts.

List of Contributors

The editor(s) would like to acknowledge and offer grateful thanks for the input of all previous editions' contributors, without whom this new edition would not have been possible.

Oliver Bailey, BDS(Hons), MFDS RCSEd, PG Cert Clin Implant Dent, FHEA, MDTFEd
Clinical Fellow in Restorative Dentistry
School of Dental Sciences
Newcastle University/Newcastle upon Tyne Hospitals NHS
   Foundation Trust
Newcastle upon Tyne
United Kingdom

Heidi Bateman, PhD, BDS, LLM, PgCME, PgDipDPH, SFHEA, FDTFEd, FAcadMEd
Clinical Trainer in Restorative Dentistry/Honorary Clinical Senior Lecturer
School of Dental Sciences
Newcastle University/Newcastle upon Tyne Hospitals NHS
   Foundation Trust
Newcastle upon Tyne
United Kingdom

Alison Cairns, PhD, MSc, BDS, MFDS, M Paed Dent, FDS (Paed Dent) RCPSG, PGDAP, FHEA
Senior Lecturer/Honorary Consultant
Paediatric Dentistry
Glasgow Dental Hospital and School, Glasgow
United Kingdom

Ian Ellis, BDS, SFHEA
Clinical Trainer in Restorative Dentistry/Clinical and Academic Lead in Removable Prosthodontics
School of Dental Sciences
Newcastle University/Newcastle upon Tyne Hospitals NHS
   Foundation Trust
Newcastle upon Tyne
United Kingdom

Janice Ellis, PhD, BDS(Hons), FDS RCS (Rest Dent), FDS RCSEd, FHEA, PGCE
Professor of Dental Education/Director of Dental Education
School of Dental Sciences
Newcastle University/Newcastle upon Tyne Hospitals NHS
   Foundation Trust
Newcastle upon Tyne
United Kingdom

Richard Holliday, PhD, BDS (Hons), MFDS RCSEd, MFDS an eundem RCSEng, MClinRes, M Perio RCSEd
Senior Clinical Lecturer/ Honorary Consultant in Restorative Dentistry
School of Dental Sciences
Newcastle University/Newcastle upon Tyne Hospitals NHS
   Foundation Trust
Newcastle upon Tyne
United Kingdom

Douglas Lovelock, MSc, BDS, MDS, FDSRCS, DDRRCR
Retired Consultant & Honorary Senior Lecturer
Radiology & Oral Surgery
School of Dental Sciences
Newcastle University/Newcastle upon Tyne Hospitals NHS
   Foundation Trust
Newcastle upon Tyne
United Kingdom

Catherine Theresa McCann, BDS, MFDS, MPaed Dent, FDS (Paed Dent) RCPSG, PgCert
Specialty Dentist in Paediatric Dentistry
Royal Belfast Hospital for Sick Children, Belfast
United Kingdom

Giles McCracken, PhD, BDS, FDS RCPSG, FDS(Rest Dent), PGCAP FHEA
Professor of Restorative Dentistry
School of Dental Sciences
Newcastle University/Newcastle upon Tyne Hospitals NHS
   Foundation Trust
Newcastle upon Tyne
United Kingdom

Declan Millett, BDSc, DDS, FDSRCPS(Glasg), FDSRCS(Eng), DOrthRCS(Eng), MOrthRCS(Eng), FHEA
Professor of Orthodontics/Consultant Orthodontist
Dental School
University College Cork, Cork
Ireland

Francis Nohl, MBBS, BDS, MSc, MRD,
FDS(Rest Dent), DDS
Consultant in Restorative Dentistry/Honorary
   Clinical Senior Lecturer
School of Dental Sciences
Newcastle University/Newcastle upon Tyne Hospitals NHS
   Foundation Trust
Newcastle upon Tyne
United Kingdom

Jillian Phillips, BDS (Hons), MFDS, MPaed Dent,
MClin Dent (Paediatric Dentistry)
Post CCST Trainee in Paediatric Dentistry
Paediatric Dental Department
Glasgow Dental Hospital and School Glasgow
United Kingdom

Nigel Douglas Robb, TD, PhD, BDS, FDSRCSEd,
FDS(Rest Dent), FDSRCPS(Glasg), FDTF RCSEd, FHEA
Professor
School of Dentistry and Oral Health
Griffith University, Southport
Queensland
Australia

Simon Stone, PhD, BDS, MFDS RCSEd, MEndo RCSEd,
FDTFEd, FHEA
Senior Clinical Lecturer/Honorary Consultant
   (Endodontics)
School of Dental Sciences
Newcastle University/Newcastle upon Tyne Hospitals NHS
   Foundation Trust
Newcastle upon Tyne
United Kingdom

Phillip Tomson, PhD, BDS, MFDS RCSEd, RCSEng, FDS
(Rest Dent) RCSEd
Senior Clinical Lecturer and Honorary Consultant
   in Restorative Dentistry
School of Dentistry
Institute of Clinical Sciences, University of Birmingham
   Birmingham
Birmingham
United Kingdom

1 *Periodontology*

Overview

A healthy or a stable periodontium is an important prerequisite both for the maintenance of a functional dentition and to ensure a long-term, successful outcome of restorative dental treatment. In view of the high prevalence of gingivitis and periodontitis in the population, all dental patients should undergo periodontal screening, although more thorough clinical and radiographic examinations are essential before a definitive periodontal diagnosis is confirmed and a treatment plan formulated. These examinations, together with medical, dental and social histories, may also reveal predisposing and risk factors that increase an individual's susceptibility to, and the subsequent rate of progression of, periodontal disease.

The intensive oral hygiene phase of treatment and the patient's compliance with a personalised plaque-control regimen are of major importance in stabilising the disease and improving the long-term prognosis for an affected dentition. Scaling and root surface instrumentation (RSI) are frequently indicated to disrupt the subgingival biofilm and remove calculus. Recognising predisposing local factors, modifying systemic factors and modifying environmental factors that determine periodontal health has become increasingly important for the dental team. Additional adjunctive treatments that may be indicated are periodontal surgery, guided tissue regeneration (GTR), systemic or locally delivered antimicrobials and the management of localised problems such as furcation defects, mucogingival problems, endodontic–periodontal lesions and loss of attachment (LOA) that has been exacerbated by occlusal trauma.

In 2017 the classification of periodontal and peri-implant diseases changed and therefore this affects the diagnoses we arrive at for patients attending our practices. This chapter seeks to begin to align to the new terminology that is establishing itself around the world. Readers are encouraged to engage with the extensive publications from the 2017 World Workshop and to review the interpretations by specialist organisations such as the British Society of Periodontology, European Federation of Periodontology and American Academy of Periodontology on how to implement this change into your clinical practice.

The new classification is summarised as follows (Caton et al., 2018):

- Periodontal Health, Gingival Diseases and Conditions
  - Periodontal health and gingival health
  - Gingivitis: Dental Biofilm-Induced
  - Gingival diseases: non–dental biofilm-induced
- Forms of Periodontitis
  - Necrotising periodontal diseases
  - Periodontitis as a manifestation of systemic diseases
  - Periodontitis
- Other Conditions Affecting the Periodontium
  - Systemic diseases or conditions affecting the periodontal supporting tissues
  - Periodontal abscesses and endodontic–periodontal lesions
  - Mucogingival deformities and conditions
  - Traumatic occlusal forces
  - Tooth- and prosthesis-related factors

1.1 Healthy Periodontium

LEARNING OBJECTIVES

You should:
- know the clinical and radiographic features of healthy periodontal tissues in adults and in children
- be familiar with the histological structures of the periodontium.

The diagnostic skills required to identify periodontal diseases, particularly in the early stages, are based upon a sound knowledge of the clinical appearance of healthy tissues.

Within the 2017 classification of periodontal and gingival health, the following categories are considered:

- Clinical gingival health on an intact periodontium
- Clinical gingival health on a reduced periodontium
    - Stable periodontitis patient
    - Non-periodontitis patient

The 2017 consensus defined periodontal health. Two states of health are proposed: pristine periodontal health in cases where there is an absence of inflammation clinically (no bleeding on probing) and clinically healthy cases having limited levels of clinical markers of inflammation (<10% bleeding on probing). The gingiva is pink, firm in texture and extends from the free gingival margin to the mucogingival line. The interdental papillae are pyramidal in shape and occupy the interdental spaces beneath the contact points of the teeth. Gingiva is keratinised and stippling is frequently present. The gingiva comprises the free and the attached portions.

The *free gingiva* is the most coronal band of unattached tissue demarcated by the free gingival groove, which can sometimes be detected clinically. The depth of the gingival sulcus ranges from 0.5 to 3.0 mm.

The *attached gingiva* is firmly bound to underlying cementum and alveolar bone and extends apically from the free gingival groove to the mucogingival junction. The width of attached gingiva varies considerably throughout the mouth. It is usually narrower on the lingual aspect of the mandibular incisors and labially, adjacent to the canines and first premolars. In the absence of inflammation, the width of the attached gingiva *increases* with age.

The *mucogingival line* is often indistinct. It defines the junction between the keratinised, attached gingiva and the oral mucosa. Oral mucosa is non-keratinised and, therefore, appears redder than the adjacent gingiva. The tissues can be distinguished by staining with Schiller's iodine solution; keratinised gingiva stains orange and non-keratinised mucosa stains purple–blue. This can be used to determine clinically the width of keratinised tissue that remains (e.g. in areas of gingival recession).

RADIOGRAPHIC FEATURES

The crest of the interdental alveolar bone is well defined and lies approximately 0.5–1.5 mm apical to the cemento-enamel junction (CEJ; Fig. 1.1). The periodontal membrane space, often identifiable on intraoral radiographs taken using a paralleling technique, is approximately 0.1–0.2 mm wide. This accounts for the slight tooth mobility that is sometimes observed when lateral pressure is applied to a tooth with a healthy periodontium.

HISTOLOGY

Epithelial components include:

- junctional epithelium (JE) cells: non-keratinised and attached to the tooth surface by a basal lamina and hemidesmosomes
- sulcular epithelium: non-keratinised and lines the gingival crevice

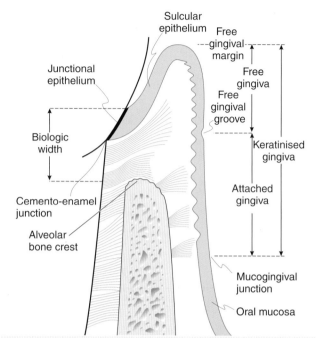

Fig. 1.1 Diagrammatic representation of the epithelial and connective tissue attachments of the gingiva.

- oral epithelium: keratinised and extends from the free gingival margin to the mucogingival line.

Gingival connective tissue core contains ground substance, blood vessels and lymphatics, nerves, fibroblasts and bundles of gingival collagen fibres (dentogingival, alveologingival, circular and trans-septal). The combined epithelial and gingival fibre attachment to the tooth surface is the *biologic width* (2017 classification system recommended this is now called '*supracrestal tissue attachment*'), which is typically 2 mm, not including the sulcus depth (see Fig. 1.1).

Periodontal connective tissues comprise alveolar bone, periodontal ligament, principal and oxytalan fibres, cells, ground substance, nerves, blood vessels and lymphatics, and cementum.

PERIODONTAL TISSUES IN CHILDREN

The gingiva in children may appear red and inflamed. Compared with mature tissue, there is a thinner epithelium that is less keratinised, greater vascularity of connective tissues and less variation in the width of the attached gingiva.

During tooth eruption, the gingival sulcus depths may reach 5 mm and gingival margins will be at different levels on adjacent teeth. Following tooth eruption, a persistent hyperaemia can lead to swollen and rounded interproximal papillae, thus giving an appearance of gingivitis.

Radiographic Features

In the primary dentition, the radiographic distance between the cementoenamel junction (CEJ) and the alveolar crest is 0–2 mm. Greater variation (0–4 mm) is observed at sites adjacent to erupting permanent teeth and exfoliating primary teeth. The periodontal membrane space is wider in children because of the thinner cementum, immature alveolar bone and a more vascular periodontal ligament.

GINGIVAL CREVICULAR FLUID

Gingival crevicular fluid (GCF) is a serum exudate that is derived from the microvasculature of the gingiva and periodontal ligament. The 'preinflammatory' flow of GCF may be mediated by bacterial products from subgingival plaque that diffuse intercellularly and accumulate adjacent to the basement membrane of the junctional epithelium. This creates an osmotic gradient; consequently, GCF flow can be regarded as a transudate rather than an inflammatory exudate in patients who may be described as having pristine periodontal health. The condition of pristine periodontal health is unlikely to be seen in practice, with the definition of being a clinically healthy case more likely. Therefore GCF in patients who have clinical periodontal health, in some ways, is similar to serum but also contains components from microbial sources, interstitial fluid and locally produced inflammatory and immune products of host origin. The proportions of these components are dependent upon:

- the presence and composition of subgingival plaque
- the rate of turnover of gingival connective tissue
- the permeability of epithelia
- the degree of inflammation.

Several techniques have been developed for collecting GCF from the gingival sulcus:

- absorbent paper strips
- microcapillary tubes
- gingival washing.

The fluid can then be analysed for specific mediators of the immunoinflammatory response (e.g. cytokines) and breakdown products of connective tissues, both of which have been associated with ongoing periodontal destruction.

CLINICAL GINGIVAL HEALTH ON A REDUCED PERIODONTIUM

The 2017 classification now recognises that gingival health is present after treatment that has stabilised periodontitis where loss of periodontal attachment has occurred; it also recognises there is also a situation where there is gingival health on a reduced periodontium after crown lengthening surgery and gingival recession.

1.2 History and Examination

LEARNING OBJECTIVES

You should:
- understand the importance of obtaining thorough histories (medical, social and presenting complaint) from patients who attend for treatment
- know those medical conditions that impact periodontal diseases and therapy
- be familiar with the diagnostic procedures and special tests to be used when evaluating patients with periodontitis.

From the periodontal viewpoint, the aims of history taking and the clinical examination are to establish the extent of periodontal destruction and to evaluate the effects of disease on the remaining dentition. It is also important to evaluate the individual patient's susceptibility to periodontal disease and, as far as possible, identify the sites that appear to be associated with active or ongoing destruction and need to be considered a priority for treatment.

PRESENTING COMPLAINT

One of the principal features of periodontal diseases is that their onset and progression occur often in the absence of pain. This means that the onus for detection rests firmly with the clinician, and the importance of regular examinations must be impressed upon the patient, with emphasis placed on prevention to stabilise rather than cure. The well-informed patient who is a regular dental attender should be able to detect some of the signs or symptoms that are associated with the early stages of plaque accumulation. Unfortunately, many patients are irregular dental attenders and only present with complaints that are the consequence of oral neglect. When gingivitis and periodontal inflammation do cause symptoms, the chief complaints are usually 'bleeding gums', 'bad taste or breath', 'localised pain' and teeth that have 'changed position' or 'become loose'. Details of when such problems started, the frequency of pain or discomfort and any associated symptoms should be recorded. The expectations of the patient with regard to the outcome of treatment should also be discussed at this stage.

Gingival Bleeding

Bleeding gums is perhaps the most common complaint of patients with periodontal disease. The bleeding is usually noticed during, or following, toothbrushing or eating. When bleeding occurs spontaneously, a patient may complain of tasting blood on awakening in the morning. The severity of the haemorrhage does not necessarily relate to the severity of disease, as a marginal gingivitis can be associated with quite profuse bleeding. Gingival bleeding is exacerbated by the use of certain drugs (anticoagulants, antithrombotics and fibrinolytic agents). Symptoms of relatively recent and sudden onset should be investigated thoroughly when taking the medical history.

Drifting of Teeth

Drifting of anterior teeth and the appearance of spaces between teeth are often the first signs of an underlying periodontal problem. When teeth begin to drift, it is because their periodontal support has been compromised to such an extent that the teeth are no longer in equilibrium with forces from occlusion and the adjacent soft tissues. In some instances, this position of equilibrium is so finely balanced that the destruction of only crestal bone and the coronal periodontal fibre groups will precipitate changes in tooth position. Furthermore, the pressures exerted on the teeth by gingiva that are swollen through oedematous or fibrous change can also induce tooth movement. Drifting of anterior teeth may also be a consequence of an occlusal interference in the posterior segments, which leads to a forward slide of the mandible during its arc of movement from the retruded contact position to the intercuspal position.

Loose Teeth

When periodontal disease remains untreated, attachment loss is progressive and teeth become increasingly mobile. The degree of mobility that some patients accept before attending for treatment is remarkable and many patients still believe that increasing tooth mobility and, ultimately, tooth loss is a natural consequence of the ageing process. An increase in mobility also occurs when a tooth is subject to traumatic occlusal forces, particularly those of a 'jiggling' nature. Mobility may be the first signs of an advanced stage of periodontitis or perhaps a rapid type of disease.

Bad Taste and Halitosis

Altered sensation of taste can accompany the halitosis that is associated with:

- necrotising periodontal diseases (necrotising gingivitis/periodontitis/stomatitis)
- purulent exudate from a periodontal abscess
- poor oral hygiene/accumulated food debris from packing beneath open contact points, in furcations, beneath overhanging or leaking restorations and associated with dentures
- excessive bacterial growth on the dorsal surface of the tongue.

Pain

Acute and often quite severe pain is a feature of necrotising periodontal diseases and herpetic gingivostomatitis. Pain, particularly on eating, is also a symptom of an acute periodontal abscess and/or an endodontic–periodontal lesion. Gingival recession with exposure of root surfaces can also precipitate pain if dentine is exposed as a result of toothbrush abrasion. This pain is characterised as sharp and transient, with a sudden onset that is precipitated by extremes of temperature. Pain is not typically a feature of gingivitis or periodontitis, however.

DENTAL HISTORY

The dental history provides an indication of the patient's overall attitude to dental care. Lengthy intervals between appointments and attendance for only symptomatic treatment suggest a low priority on dental health and a patient who is unlikely to appreciate and comply with comprehensive periodontal care.

The reasons for previous loss of teeth should be established and a record made of previous and recent dental treatment. Information (including radiographs) relating to previous dental treatment should, whenever possible, be sought by written request from a previous dentist, and the written response incorporated in the patient's notes. Another criterion sometimes used to assess dental behaviour is the frequency with which a patient brushes (or claims to brush!) their teeth. It is more important to assess the efficiency of the method of toothbrushing rather than to place too much emphasis on frequency. An individual who brushes once a day for 4–5 minutes is often able to maintain a superior standard of plaque control (oral hygiene) than a patient who brushes several times a day, but ineffectively and for only short periods of time.

In young patients in particular, a note should be made of previous orthodontic treatment. Extended periods of fixed appliance therapy can cause loss of crestal alveolar bone partly from tooth movements and partly from the periodontal inflammation that is a consequence of limited access to cleaning interproximally and subgingivally. More importantly from the diagnostic viewpoint, teeth that have been tipped rather than moved bodily through bone often have an angular alveolar crest on the mesial and distal surfaces. Such topography can give the appearance of the lesions often seen in localised periodontitis.

SOCIAL HISTORY

Details of the patient's occupation, diet and consumption of alcohol and tobacco should be noted. When an occupation involves considerable social contact, there may be a greater awareness of small changes of tooth position and appearance.

Stress induced by life events (e.g. examinations, divorce or change of employment) should also be noted as they may promote bruxism and aggravate existing tooth mobility from periodontal disease. Psychological stress has been shown to be associated with delayed wound healing of connective tissue and bone, necrotising periodontal diseases and periodontitis. As most patients have some element of stress in their lives, the potential influence of this on periodontal diseases should be appreciated. High levels of unmanaged stress, and particularly financial strain, has been implicated as a specific risk factor in periodontal disease.

Smoking is a known risk factor for periodontal disease and is considered in Section 1.6. The frequency and duration of smoking should be established and the detrimental effects of smoking on periodontal, oral and general health must be conveyed to the patient before any treatment is started.

It should now be apparent that much of the information that can be derived from a thorough personal and dental history has a bearing on establishing the susceptibility of an individual to periodontal diseases. When potential systemic and environmental factors are established, it is often not possible to determine their individual effects on the disease process because many of the factors are inter-related. For example, an individual who has job insecurity and is under financial strain may be also a smoker and a poor dental attender.

MEDICAL HISTORY

A thorough medical history must be recorded and updated at each visit. The patient's perception of their present health status is also a valuable indicator of their psychological make-up and potential compliance with treatment.

A patient with a history of rheumatic fever, congenital cardiac defects or prosthetic heart valves does not automatically require antibiotic prophylaxis before periodontal probing and treatment. Similarly, patients who have received prosthetic joint implants do not routinely require antibiotic prophylaxis. Ultrasonic scalers can be used in patients with cardiac pacemakers in accordance with the manufacturers' guidance, which normally recommends that the ultrasonic handpiece and cables should be kept at least 15 cm away from the pacemaker device.

Patients with diabetes are at particular risk of periodontal breakdown, especially when poorly controlled. A positive family history should be noted and vigilant periodontal monitoring undertaken sometimes engaging with their diabetes care team. The patient who is HIV-positive is also at risk of extensive and increased periodontal breakdown.

Patients with particular food fads or unusual diets should be questioned as part of an overall dietary analysis to evaluate their vitamin and protein intake. Nutritional deficiencies may modify the severity and extent of periodontal diseases by altering the host resistance and potential for repair, although such deficiencies are rare in developed countries.

Gastric hyperacidity and reflux from hiatus hernia and gastric ulceration predispose to erosion and root caries if there is existing gingival recession. Patients who are pregnant should be monitored carefully during the second and third trimesters as endocrine changes may lead to marked gingival inflammation and the development of epulides. Routine radiographic assessment of periodontal disease should be avoided during pregnancy.

Current medications must be noted, especially dosage and types of medication. When a patient is receiving anticoagulant therapy, the general medical practitioner or patient's physician must be consulted with a view to managing the anticoagulant dosage to coincide with invasive periodontal treatment, thus reducing the risk of postoperative haemorrhage. Some drugs such as phenytoin, ciclosporin and nifedipine can cause gingival enlargement, which may compromise good oral hygiene, leading to aesthetic problems. For patients with a history of or currently taking intravenous bisphosphonates, oral bisphosphonates with immunosuppressants or a previous history of bisphosphonate-related osteonecrosis of the jaw (BRONJ), extractions and periodontal surgery should be carefully considered to manage any risk of BRONJ. Any antimicrobials used in the treatment of periodontal diseases are contraindicated for certain patients for whom the unwanted effects of the drugs may be enhanced, or because of a potential interaction with drugs that the patient is already taking.

EXAMINATION

Extraoral Examination

A careful extraoral examination may reveal important signs that are associated with periodontal problems. A severe periodontal abscess can lead to facial swelling and a regional lymphadenopathy. Prominent maxillary incisors make a lip seal difficult to achieve and this may aggravate an existing gingivitis. The drying effect on exposed gingiva produced by mouth breathing leads to enlarged and erythematous gingiva, particularly in the maxillary anterior region. Mouth breathing does not inevitably lead to increased plaque accumulation and gingivitis but should be regarded as a predisposing factor in a susceptible patient.

Intraoral Examination

A record should be made of local factors that predispose to the accumulation of plaque (e.g. restorations with overhanging margins, poorly contoured and deficient restorations and partial dentures).

A quick and simple method of assessing the level of oral hygiene is to score, after disclosing, the number of plaque-covered smooth tooth surfaces as a percentage of all smooth surfaces. On each surface, plaque is recorded as being either present or absent (a dichotomous scoring method). Patients are informed of their scores and realistic targets can be set for the patient to achieve at future visits. This method gives a useful overall assessment of plaque control as well as identifying tooth surfaces that are difficult to clean. These occur typically at interproximal sites and on the lingual smooth surfaces of mandibular molars.

In epidemiological studies, it is easier and quicker to select six teeth per subject to be broadly representative of the entire dentition. These so-called Ramfjord teeth are: $\frac{6/14}{41/6}$

A number of indices have been used for scoring plaque, oral debris and calculus on a quantitative basis (Table 1.1). Periodontal diseases and gingivitis occur in all patients regardless of age. Periodontitis is prevalent in adults and gingivitis is extremely common in children. Furthermore, some children and young adults are also at risk from the more severe, rapid progressing periodontal diseases. It is, therefore, imperative that all dental patients undergo a screening examination to provide a rapid, basic assessment of periodontal status. The Basic Periodontal Examination (BPE) has evolved from the Community Periodontal Index of Treatment Needs (CPITN) and is a quick method for assessing a patient's periodontal status. The examination involves the use of a specially designed periodontal probe with a 0.5-mm diameter ball end and a coloured band extending 3.5–5.5 mm from the tip (Fig. 1.2). The dentition is divided into sextants; each tooth is probed circumferentially and only the highest score in each sextant is recorded. The score codes are used as a guide to determine the need for periodontal treatment (Table 1.2). A BPE score of 3 means that full probing depths (six sites per tooth) around all the teeth in that sextant should be recorded. A score of 4 in any sextant means that probing depths should be recorded throughout the entire dentition.

Gingiva

Visual examination of the gingiva may reveal colour changes of the tissues, gingival swelling (generalised or localised), ulceration, suppuration and gingival recession. Where there is gingival enlargement, the tissues should be probed gently to assess consistency and texture. Oedematous tissues are soft and may have a tendency to bleed spontaneously or following pressure and gentle manipulation. Conversely, fibrous tissue is usually quite firm and resistant to pressure.

The width of attached gingiva should be assessed and measured as the distance from the free gingival margin to the mucogingival line minus the depth of the gingival crevice (in health) or periodontal pocket (when disease is present). Sites with minimal or no apparent attached gingiva should be noted together with the inflammatory condition of the associated marginal tissues. At such sites, the attached gingiva can be dyed with Schiller's iodine solution so that the border between the keratinised (orange) and nonkeratinised (dark blue) epithelium (mucogingival junction)

Table 1.1 Indices for Scoring Oral Debris, Plaque and Calculus.

Index	Deposit	Scoring System	Score
Plaque index (Silness and Löe 1964)	Plaque	0 no plaque 1 film of plaque seen with disclosing solution or by running probe along surface 2 moderate accumulation seen with naked eye 3 abundance of plaque in pocket and on tooth surface	Record on six surfaces of tooth Divide total by number of surfaces scored
Plaque index (Quigley and Hein 1962)	Plaque	0 no plaque 1 separate flecks at cervical margin 2 continuous band of plaque >1 mm wide at cervical margin 3 band of plaque 1 mm wide but covering <1/3 of coronal tooth surface 4 plaque on >1/3 but <2/3 of coronal surface 5 plaque on >2/3 of coronal tooth surface	Record scores on six surfaces of each tooth Divide total by number of surfaces scored
Oral hygiene index (Greene and Vermillion 1960)	Scores debris and calculus as separate components	0 no deposits 1 not covering more than 1/3 of exposed tooth surface 2 coronal deposits >1/3 but <2/3 of tooth surface; individual flecks of subgingival calculus 3 deposits on >2/3 tooth surface; continuous band of subgingival calculus	Scores made on facial and lingual surfaces Record worst score/sextant Index = total scores/number of sextants
Volpe–Manhold index (VMI 1969)	Calculus	The height and width of calculus is measured with a graduated probe along three planes on the lingual surfaces of six lower anterior teeth	Any calculus scores 0.5 mm Index is the sum of the individual measurements divided by the number of scores made

Greene JC, Vermillion JR. The oral hygiene index: a method for classifying oral hygiene status. *J Am Dental Assoc.* 1960;61:172–179; Quigley GA, Hein JW. Comparative cleaning efficiency of manual and power brushing. *J Am Dental Assoc.* 1962;65:26–29; Silness J, Löe H. Periodontal disease in pregnancy. II. Correlation between oral hygiene and periodontal condition. *Acta Odont Scand.* 1964;24:747–759 and Volpe AR, Manhold JH. A method of evaluating the effectiveness of potential calculus inhibiting agents. *N Y State Dental J.* 1962;28:289–290.

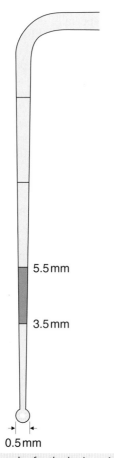

5.5 mm

3.5 mm

0.5 mm

Fig. 1.2 Colour-coded probe for the basic periodontal examination. (World Health Organization *(WHO)* probe.)

Table 1.2 The Basic Periodontal Examination (BPE).

Code*	Probing	Treatment Needs
0	Coloured area of the probe is completely visible; no calculus detected; no gingival bleeding on probing	No need for periodontal treatment
1	Coloured area is completely visible; no calculus detected; bleeding on probing	Oral hygiene instruction (OHI)
2	Coloured area is completely visible; supra- or subgingival calculus detected, or overhanging restorations	OHI; elimination of plaque-retentive areas; scaling and RSI
3	Coloured area is partly visible, indicating probing depth of greater than 3.5 mm but less than 5.5 mm	OHI; elimination of plaque-retentive areas; RSI
4	Coloured area completely disappears, indicating probing depth of greater than 5.5 mm	Assess the need for more complex treatment in addition to OHI and RSI; referral to a specialist may be necessary

The symbol (*) should be added to score where furcation involvement is evident.
RSI, Root surface instrumentation.
Reproduced by kind permission of the British Society of Periodontology and Implant Dentistry.

is seen and the actual width of keratinised tissue becomes more readily apparent. Sites of gingival recession are recorded by measuring from the CEJ to the free gingival margin of the affected site. Sensitivity of associated exposed root surfaces should also be recorded.

The presence of a prominent labial frenum may effectively reduce the width of attached gingiva, although the precise role of a frenal attachment as a predisposing factor to gingival recession is disputed. A prominent frenum can, however, reduce sulcus depth and restrict access for tooth brushing; it can thus lead to the development of local periodontal problems.

Periodontal Probing

Periodontal probing should be undertaken systematically on each tooth to determine the probing depth, the presence of bleeding after probing and the extent of attachment loss. The probe should be moved gently around the sulcus to avoid trauma. A force of approximately 0.25 N is recommended, but this is difficult to achieve consistently without the use of a pressure-sensitive probe. An attempt should be made to probe along the contour of the root surface although, interproximally, it is necessary to angle the probe slightly to reach the site directly beneath the contact area. This site should be probed from the buccal and the lingual aspects since deep pockets frequently develop here.

A number of factors may lead to errors in measuring probing depths:

- thickness of the probe
- contour of the tooth surface
- angulation of probing
- pressure applied
- presence of calculus deposits.

The extent of inflammation is also important. A probe will more easily penetrate the pocket epithelium and the adjacent connective tissues when the tissues are inflamed. A probing depth measurement is influenced by the position of the gingival margin and the integrity of the tissues at the base of the pocket, and these factors are dependent upon the extent of inflammation in the tissues. Attempts have been made to reduce probing errors by using constant pressure probes and electronic probes. In addition, computer-assisted probes have been developed for automatic recording of probe measurements or to allow voice-activated data entry. These probes have a high degree of resolution, measuring with a precision of 0.1–0.2 mm, but their accuracy and repeatability still depends upon angulation and positioning of the probe by the operator.

A more precise assessment of the degree of periodontal destruction is made by measuring from the CEJ to the base of the pocket. This gives an approximation of the loss of connective tissue attachment to the root surface. The loss of attachment is easier to measure when there has been gingival recession and the CEJ is visible. When patients are being monitored longitudinally before and after treatment, sequential attachment level measurements can be made relative to a fixed point (e.g. an incisal edge or cusp tip). The differences between successive measurements then give an estimate of the *change* in attachment level, which is often used to assess the success or failure of a particular treatment.

About 20–30 seconds after probing, each site is re-evaluated to determine the presence or absence of bleeding from the base of the pocket. Bleeding is simply a consequence of the trauma caused by probing the epithelial pocket lining and connective tissue. Bleeding on probing has been implicated as an *indicator* of active disease. Longitudinal clinical trials, however, suggest that bleeding has a low sensitivity for disease progression. Conversely, absence of bleeding is a good indicator of periodontal health or inactivity. Any site with a probing depth of less than 4 mm that does not exhibit bleeding on probing is not likely to require treatment beyond root surface instrumentation leading to biofilm disruption and polishing.

Furcation Involvement

A curved explorer is used to determine the topography of the furcation lesion in multirooted teeth, allowing accurate classification into three groups.

Class I has initial involvement. The tissue destruction does not exceed more than 3 mm (or not more than one-third of the tooth width) into the furcation.
Class II includes cul-de-sac involvement. The tissue destruction extends deeper than 3 mm (or more than one-third of the tooth width) into the furcation but does not completely pass through the furcation.
Class III has through-and-through involvement. The lesion extends across the entire width of the furcation; consequently, an instrument can be passed between the roots to emerge on the other side of the tooth.

Tooth Mobility

Mobility is assessed by applying a labiolingual, horizontal force to each tooth in turn using the handles of dental mirrors. Movement is scored according to a simple index, such as:

0 normal, physiological mobility (<0.3 mm)
1 horizontal mobility up to 1.0 mm
2 moderate horizontal mobility of 1.0–2.0 mm
3 severe mobility >2.0 mm in horizontal plane or vertical movements

RADIOGRAPHIC EVALUATION

Radiographic selection criteria for periodontal disease should take into account the diagnosis made from the clinical examination and the overall state of the patient's dentition. The panoramic radiograph, particularly if obtained using modern machines, is an alternative to full mouth periapical radiography on the basis of diagnostic yield of clinically unsuspected patterns of bone loss. In the posterior segments, vertical bitewings are often a useful supplement if a panoramic view suggests bone loss localised to this region.

Radiographic features that can be identified include:

- pattern of bone loss: horizontal/vertical, localised/generalised
- furcation involvement
- variation in root anatomy
- subgingival calculus
- widening of the periodontal membrane space
- periapical infection (periodontal–endodontic lesions)
- overhanging restorations.

A decreased alveolar bone height on a radiograph is only a historical record of previous periodontal involvement and gives little, if any, information on recent, current or future activity.

1.3 Gingivitis

You should:
- know the differential diagnosis of the various forms of gingivitis and gingival diseases
- be able to provide appropriate therapy.

In this section, we describe the clinical features of gingivitis that is dental biofilm-induced and gingival diseases that are non-dental biofilm-induced. The treatment of gingivitis and periodontitis is discussed in Section 1.12 although specific aspects of treatment are also noted in this section (and Section 1.4). The microbiology and pathogenesis of gingivitis are discussed in Section 1.5. The 2017 classification separates these concepts further as follows:

- Gingivitis: Dental Biofilm-Induced
  - Associated with dental biofilm alone
  - Mediated by systemic or local risk factors
  - Drug-influenced gingival enlargement
- Gingival Diseases: Non-Dental Biofilm-Induced
  - Genetic/developmental disorders
  - Specific infections
  - Inflammatory and immune conditions
  - Reactive processes
  - Neoplasms
  - Endocrine, nutritional and metabolic diseases
  - Traumatic lesions
  - Gingival pigmentation

GINGIVITIS: DENTAL BIOFILM-INDUCED

Gingivitis that is dental biofilm-induced alone is an inflammatory lesion of the gingiva. Accumulation of dental plaque in the gingival sulcus initiates the development of an inflammatory lesion (subclinical) that, after 10–20 days, is detected clinically as an established chronic gingivitis.

The Health and Social Care Information Centre reported data from the Children's Dental Health Survey in 2013 covering England, Wales and Northern Ireland. Gum inflammation was recorded in 22% of 5-year-olds, 46% of 8-year-olds, 60% of 12-year-olds and 52% of 15-year-olds. These data suggest a reduction in the prevalence of gingival inflammation in this population of children compared to the 20-year period between 1983 and 2003 (Fig. 1.3), but the statistical significance of these differences in the groups was limited in some cases.

Clinical Features

The gingiva become swollen, shiny and soft or spongy, they can be red but this depends upon pigmentation of the oral soft tissues. Sulcus depths increase (false pockets) as a result of the tissue swelling from inflammatory oedema. Bleeding occurs after gentle probing. The interdental papillae and marginal gingiva are initially involved before inflammation spreads to the attached gingiva.

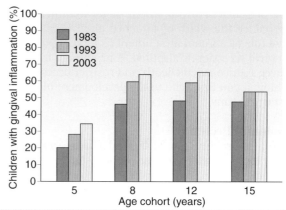

Fig. 1.3 Prevalence of gingival inflammation in UK children aged 5–15 years (1983–2003).

Treatment

- Instruction in toothbrushing.
- Use of interdental cleaning aids.
- Supragingival scaling.
- Elimination of plaque-retentive factors.
- Subgingival scaling and polishing.

Gingivitis: Mediated by Systemic or Local Risk Factors

Gingival inflammation can be further modulated by any systemic conditions a patient has and is now categorised gingivitis mediated by systemic or local risk factors. Systemic factors such as smoking, hyperglycaemia, pharmacological agents, hormones and haematological conditions are grouped under this heading. A number of examples of these conditions are considered in the following text. Examples of local risk factors mediating gingivitis are poorly adapted restorations and oral dryness.

Gingivitis: Mediated by Sex Steroid Hormones

In pregnancy, an increase in circulating levels of oestrogen, progesterone and their metabolites has been shown to aggravate a pre-existing gingivitis. The hormones and their metabolites effect an increase in gingival vasculature and the permeability of the capillary network. A similar increase in the severity of gingivitis may also be seen at, or around, puberty.

Clinical Features

Pregnancy-associated gingivitis is a generalised, marginal, oedematous inflammation. The extent of gingival enlargement is variable but an increase in gingival bleeding is a common complaint. The severity of the gingivitis tends to increase from the second to the eighth month of pregnancy. There is often some resolution during the final trimester and after parturition. A local gingival overgrowth (i.e. pregnancy epulis) may result from chronic irritation or mild trauma to the soft tissues.

Treatment

A preventive regimen is preferred whenever possible. Otherwise a conventional treatment approach including oral hygiene instruction (OHI) and scaling should be undertaken.

GINGIVAL DISEASES: NON-DENTAL-PLAQUE-INDUCED

There are a number of gingival conditions that occur through a mechanism that is not primarily caused by dental plaque. These conditions are often made worse by the presence or build-up of dental plaque altering the severity of the involvement of gingival tissues. Importantly these conditions are not resolved through patients improving their plaque control alone and need interventions other than periodontal management. Some examples from this part of the classification are considered later along with the historical descriptive term of desquamative gingivitis.

Primary Herpetic Gingivostomatitis

Primary herpetic gingivostomatitis is now classed as a gingival disease that is non-dental plaque-induced under specific infections. It is an acute, common and highly infectious disease caused by herpes simplex virus. Most adults have neutralising antibodies to the virus, indicating that an acquired immune response developed in childhood. Circulating maternal antibodies provide immunity in the first 12 months of life. Transmission of the virus is predominantly by droplet infection and the incubation period is about 5–10 days. Primary infection occurs most frequently in young children aged between 2 and 5 years but the disease can affect young adults.

Clinical Features

The clinical features and history are so specific that diagnosis of the disease is not difficult.

Symptoms are fever, pyrexia, headaches, general malaise, mild dysphagia and regional lymphadenopathy.

Signs are of the onset of an aggressive marginal gingivitis and formation of fluid-filled vesicles with a grey membranous covering on the gingiva, tongue, palate and buccal mucosa. The vesicles burst after only a few hours to leave painful, yellow–grey ulcers with red, inflamed margins. The ulcers heal without scarring after about 14 days.

Treatment

Treatment is mainly palliative: bed rest, soft diet and maintain fluid intake. Paracetamol suspension is given for pyrexia and severe disease is treated with aciclovir (please refer to your local guidelines for current dosage recommendations). In young children, plaque can be controlled with chlorhexidine spray two or three times a day.

Complications

In immunocompromised patients, the disease can be severe and run a protracted course. Other complications like aseptic meningitis and encephalitis are rare.

Latent herpes viruses dormant in the host's sensory ganglia are reactivated by exposure to sunlight, stress, nutritional deficiency, malaise or systemic upset. The clinical features are an attenuated presentation of the primary infection. Herpes labialis presents as a 'cold sore' at the mucocutaneous borders or commissures of the lips. The cold sores may be managed with topical aciclovir cream (5%), five times a day, for 5–7 days.

Plasma Cell Gingivitis

Plasma cell gingivitis is now classed as a gingival disease that is non-dental plaque-induced under inflammatory and immune conditions. It is uncommon and thought to be contact hypersensitivity reaction frequently attributed to the use of cinnamon-flavoured chewing gum. Cinnamon-, mint- and herbal-flavoured toothpastes are also implicated. Microscopically, the epithelium is atrophic and there is a massive infiltrate of plasma cells in the connective tissues.

Clinical Features

In plasma cell gingivitis, the gingiva appear fiery-red in appearance with varying degrees of swelling. The lesion extends to involve the entire width of attached gingiva. The reaction may affect other areas such as the tongue, palate and cheeks. Lips can be dry and desquamative with an angular cheilitis. The principal symptom is extreme soreness of the affected areas.

Treatment

Treatment involves identification and withdrawal of the causative allergen. If toothbrushing is painful during the acute stage, chlorhexidine mouthrinse can be given for chemical plaque control.

Desquamative Gingivitis

Desquamative gingivitis is not a discrete clinical entity, and therefore not included in the 2017 classification, but rather a term that has been used to describe a gingival manifestation common to this part of the new classification including the following disorders:
- benign mucous membrane pemphigoid
- lichen planus
- pemphigus vulgaris.

Clinical Features

The fiery-red, desquamative lesions affect the entire width of keratinised gingiva and may be localised or generalised throughout the mouth.

Treatment

A joint management approach by specialists in oral medicine and periodontics is warranted. A biopsy of the affected region may be indicated to confirm the specific diagnosis. Oral hygiene instruction and scaling to remove hard deposits which may act as irritants should be undertaken. See Volume 1 for the pharmacological management of mucocutaneous lesions.

1.4 Periodontal Diseases

The terminology in the 2017 classification has three forms of periodontitis identified.
- Necrotising periodontal disease
- Periodontitis as manifestation of systemic diseases
- Periodontitis

A significant change is the loss of the terms aggressive and chronic periodontitis with these entities now covered by periodontitis as one pathophysiology. Periodontitis as a diagnosis is described further through a framework of Staging into four levels of severity and Grading into three rates of progression.

NECROTISING PERIODONTAL DISEASES

These conditions, considered to be a distinct entity through the current understanding of the pathophysiology, are separated into three forms based on differences in extent of the lesion(s). Necrotising gingivitis (NG) remains within the gingival tissues, necrotising periodontitis (NP) extends into the periodontium and necrotising stomatitis (NS) involves the periodontium and oral cavity. This group of conditions is characterised by their clinical presentation of the underlying inflammatory response to a spirochetal/bacterial infection and necrosis of tissues. NP is strongly associated with impairment of a patient's immune system, either as a chronic condition as with AIDS or severe malnutrition or temporarily in patients who smoke or are under stress.

NG is an acute condition that has a tendency to recur. In Europe and the United States, the incidence is highest in the 16- to 30-year-old age group. In African countries, a more severe extensive form of NS, also known as noma or cancrum oris, is found in children as young as 1–2 years.

Clinical Features

'Punched out' ulcers occur covered with a yellow–grey pseudomembranous slough. The tips of interdental papillae are affected first, but spread to the labial and lingual marginal gingiva can be rapid. This condition is painful and accompanied by a distinctive halitosis. A pre-existing or longstanding chronic gingivitis is usually present.

Aetiology

A fusiform–spirochaetal complex is traditionally associated with necrotising periodontal diseases being first demonstrated at the end of the 1800s. Culture studies and more contemporary microbiological research strengthen the link to genera and species such as *Prevotella intermedia*, *Treponema*, *Selenomonas* and *Fusobacterium* in this group of conditions.

Pathology

Ulceration of the gingival epithelium occurs with necrosis of connective tissues. Superficially, deposits of fibrin are intermeshed with large numbers of dead and dying cells: epithelial cells, neutrophils and bacteria. Deeper tissues demonstrate a dense infiltrate of neutrophils characteristic of non-specific inflammation.

It is possible that all of the predisposing factors act through the common pathway of lowering the patient's cell-mediated immune response. The nature of the disease and the likelihood of recurrence with incomplete treatment must be explained carefully to the patient.

Risk Factors

Pre-existing gingivitis confirms a poor standard of plaque control.

Smoking favours the development of an anaerobic Gram-negative flora and depresses the chemotactic response of neutrophils.

Physiological stress, producing high plasma levels of corticosteroids, predisposes to NG and is a possible explanation for epidemics in college students or army personnel.

Malnutrition and debilitation predispose to infection and severe NG in underdeveloped countries.

HIV infection also predisposes to an NG that may progress to an NP.

Treatment

Reduce cigarette consumption. Oral hygiene instruction and ultrasonic scaling. A soft, multitufted brush should be recommended if a medium (or hard) textured brush is too painful to use. If mechanical therapy is painful, then a 3-day course of systemic metronidazole 200 mg, three times a day, is indicated. Oxygenating mouthrinses (hydrogen peroxide, sodium hydroxyperborate) cleanse necrotic tissues. Subgingival scaling and prophylaxis are essential to prevent recurrence. Incomplete treatment leads inevitably to recurrence and loss of gingival contour. A longstanding necrotising gingivitis may progress to a chronic necrotising periodontitis.

PERIODONTITIS

Periodontitis is a chronic bacterially induced inflammation of the periodontium that leads to its destruction. National survey data from the United Kingdom suggest approximately 45% of adults have some 4-mm pockets present and 8% have pockets of 6 mm or greater (Health and Social Care Information Centre 2011).

Clinical Features

Pocket Formation

Periodontal pocket formation is one of the most important clinical signs of periodontitis. A pocket is defined as a pathologically deepened gingival sulcus. Pockets can be classified as *true* pockets, which result from apical migration of the junctional epithelium following loss of connective tissue attachment to the root surface, or *false* pockets, which result from gingival enlargement with no alteration in the position of the junctional epithelium. Additionally, pockets can be *suprabony*, in which case the junctional epithelium remains entirely coronal to the alveolar crest, or *infrabony*, in which case the junctional epithelium extends apically beyond the alveolar crest (Fig. 1.4).

Bleeding

Bleeding on probing occurs at inflamed sites where thin and ulcerated junctional and pocket epithelia are traumatised by the probe tip.

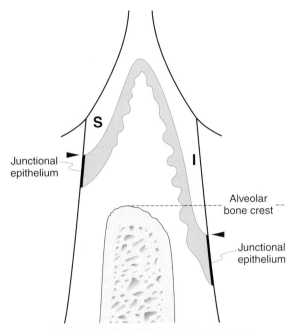

Fig. 1.4 Supra- *(S)* and infrabony *(I)* pockets.

Alveolar Bone Resorption

Alveolar bone resorption occurs concurrently with attachment loss and pocket formation. Two distinct patterns of bone destruction are recognised radiographically. *Horizontal* bone loss occurs when the entire width of interdental bone is resorbed. *Vertical* bone defects are produced when the interdental bone adjacent to the root surface is more rapidly resorbed, leaving an angular, uneven morphology. Frequently, both patterns of bone resorption are seen at different sites in the same patient. Infrabony defects are also classified according to the number of remaining base walls: one-, two- or three-walled defects (Fig. 1.5). Such observations are ususally confirmed by direct vision during flap surgery.

Tooth Mobility

Tooth mobility can be either physiological or pathological.

Physiological mobility allows slight movements of a tooth within the socket to accommodate masticatory forces, without injury to the tooth or its supporting tissues.

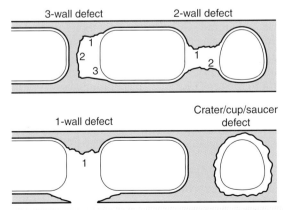

Fig. 1.5 Diagrammatic representation of infrabony defects.

Pathological mobility is increased or increasing mobility as a result of connective tissue attachment loss. Its extent depends upon the quantity of remaining bony support, the degree of inflammation in the periodontal ligament and gingiva, and the magnitude of traumatic occlusal forces (see Section 1.9) that may be acting upon the teeth. A reduction in mobility follows successful treatment and resolution of inflammation. A scale for the assessment of tooth mobility is given in Section 1.2.

Migration of teeth may occur following attachment loss or gingival overgrowth. Frequently, maxillary incisors drift labially, resulting in increased overjet and diastemata. Affected teeth also have a tendency to over-erupt.

Gingival Recession

Gingival recession is localised or generalised.

Localised recession is associated with factors such as toothbrush trauma and factitious injury, superimposed upon anatomical factors such as bony dehiscences or thin alveolar bone plates.

Generalised recession occurs when the gingival margin migrates apically as a result of ongoing periodontal disease or following resolution of gingival inflammation and oedema, as a consequence of successful periodontal treatment.

Furcatio n Lesions

Furcation lesions (see also Section 1.2) arise when attachment loss occurs vertically and horizontally between the roots of multirooted teeth. Lesions are detected using:

- direct visualisation
- a furcation probe
- radiographic examination.

The Classification of Periodontitis

This revised edition of the book has moved to align to the 2017 classification of periodontitis. A fundamental change in the classification is the loss of the separate diagnoses of aggressive periodontitis and chronic periodontitis where a consensus was reached that these terms reflected the same pathophysiology. The 2017 classification now has staging, extent and grading definitions to assign severity, distribution and rate of progress of the disease as follows:

- Stages
  - Stage I — Initial periodontitis
  - Stage II — Moderate periodontitis
  - Stage III — Severe periodontitis with potential for additional tooth loss
  - Stage IV — Severe periodontitis with potential for loss of the dentition
- Extent and distribution
  - Localised – less than 30% teeth affected
  - Generalised – 30% or more teeth affected (Fig. 1.6A)
  - Molar-incisor pattern (see Fig. 1.6B)
- Grades
  - Grade A — Slow rate of progression
  - Grade B — Moderate rate of progression
  - Grade C — Rapid rate of progression

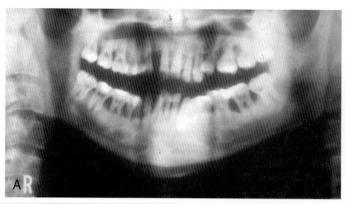
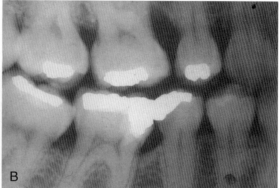

Fig. 1.6 (A) Radiograph showing the irregular bone loss with both vertical and horizontal defects in generalised rapid rate progression periodontitis. (B) Radiograph showing distinctive bone loss around first molar teeth in molar-incisor pattern periodontitis.

1.5 Microbiology and Pathogenesis of Periodontal Diseases

LEARNING OBJECTIVES

You should:
* understand the key steps involved in the accumulation and maturation of dental plaque
* know the microbiology associated with different periodontal conditions and understand why certain specific pathogens are important in periodontitis
* understand the histological changes that occur during the development of gingivitis and periodontitis, and how these changes relate to the clinical signs of disease
* understand the importance of the interactions between plaque bacteria and host defence mechanisms in the pathogenesis of periodontitis
* be familiar with specific destructive mechanisms in periodontal disease progression.

MICROBIOLOGY OF PERIODONTAL DISEASES

Dental Plaque

Dental plaque is an accumulation of bacteria and intercellular matrix that forms the biofilm that adheres to the surfaces of teeth and other oral structures in the absence of effective oral hygiene. Accumulation of plaque and the interaction of this biofilm with the host's immune and inflammatory response that is then modified by environmental factors becomes a key aetiological factor in the pathogenesis of periodontal diseases. Plaque is generally classified as being *supragingival* or *subgingival*.

Supragingival Plaque

Supragingival plaque is located on the clinical crowns of the teeth, at or above the gingival margin. It forms as a soft, yellow–white layer on the tooth surface. It accumulates primarily at the gingival margin and also other regions (grooves, pits, under overhanging restorations) where there is protection from the mechanical cleaning effect of the oral soft tissues. The rate of plaque formation varies among individuals and is influenced by oral hygiene, dietary composition and salivary flow rates. Small amounts of plaque may not be visible to the unaided eye but may be detected by running a periodontal probe or explorer around the gingival margin, or by the use of disclosing solutions.

Subgingival Plaque

Subgingival plaque is found within the gingival sulcus or periodontal pocket, below the gingival margin. It develops from the downgrowth of supragingival plaque into the gingival sulcus or periodontal pocket; it cannot be seen directly unless the overlying gingiva is retracted. The composition of subgingival plaque differs from that of supragingival plaque as a result of the unique conditions that exist in the gingival sulcus, which favour colonisation and growth of anaerobic bacteria. In the sulcus, there is an altered redox potential, protection from cleansing mechanisms within the oral cavity and GCF supplies a ready flow of nutrients, immune and inflammatory products to the biofilm.

Composition and Formation of Plaque

Plaque biofilm consists of micro-organisms (accounting for approximately 75% of the plaque volume) suspended in an extracellular matrix. More than 700 bacterial species have been identified in dental plaque. Some non-bacterial organisms that are also found in plaque include yeasts, *Mycoplasma* spp. and viruses. The extracellular matrix consists of organic and inorganic components derived from plaque bacteria, saliva and GCF. Organic components include extracellular polysaccharides secreted by plaque bacteria (which have storage and anchorage roles), salivary glycoproteins (which are important in the initial adherence of bacteria to the tooth surface), desquamated oral epithelium cells and defence cells. The inorganic component primarily comprises calcium and phosphorus from saliva.

Following professional tooth cleaning, plaque formation occurs in a predictable sequence of events.

1. *Acquired pellicle formation* (immediately after cleaning). Salivary glycoproteins selectively adsorb onto the tooth surface. The acquired pellicle functions as a protective, lubricating layer, but it also allows for biofilm adherence.

2. *Early colonisation* (0–7 days after cleaning). The tooth surface is initially colonised by Gram-positive cocci, predominantly *Streptococcus* spp. Over the next 7 days, the numbers of all bacterial types increase, although their relative proportions alter. Gram-positive rods, particularly *Actinomyces* spp. become more prevalent, as do Gram-negative cocci (e.g. *Veillonella* spp.) and rods (e.g. *Capnocytophaga* spp). As the bulk of the plaque increases, an oxygen-deprived environment develops within the deeper layers of the biofilm and conditions begin to favour the growth of anaerobic organisms like *Fusobacterium* spp (Gram-negative rods) and *P. intermedia*.
3. *Late colonisation and maturation* (>7 days after cleaning). If undisturbed, the biofilm mass matures through further growth of species already present and the appearance of late colonising species. Late colonisers do not attach to clean tooth surfaces and are often virulent organisms that have been implicated as specific periodontal pathogens. *Porphyromonas gingivalis*, motile Gram-negative rods and spirochaetes are important examples of late colonising organisms.

Dental Calculus

Calculus is a hard, mineralised substance that forms on the surfaces of teeth and other solid structures in the oral cavity following the prolonged accumulation of dental plaque. Calculus is plaque that has become mineralised by calcium and phosphate ions from saliva. Inorganic calcium phosphate crystals grow within the plaque matrix and enlarge until the plaque is mineralised. The mixture of inorganic crystals changes as the calculus ages. Brushite ($CaHPO_4.2H_2O$) forms first and is followed by octocalcium phosphate ($Ca_8(HPO_4)_4$). Mature calculus contains predominantly crystals of hydroxyapatite ($Ca_{10}(PO_4)_6.OH_2$) and tricalcium phosphate ($Ca_3(PO_4)_2$). Calculus crystals grow into close contact with the tooth, gaining mechanical retention in surface irregularities. The outer surface of calculus remains covered by a layer of unmineralised biofilm.

Supragingival Calculus

Supragingival calculus forms as yellow–white calcified deposits located at, or just coronal to, the gingival margin and is frequently stained brown by tobacco and certain foods and drinks. The mineralisation of plaque to form calculus is influenced by salivary gland secretions and, consequently, deposits of calculus are found in close proximity to the duct openings of major salivary glands, in particular the buccal surfaces of maxillary molars, and the lingual surfaces of mandibular anterior teeth.

Subgingival Calculus

Subgingival calculus forms apical to the gingival margin, particularly at interproximal sites, as tenacious dark brown–black deposits on the root surface. If the gingival margin is dried, the dark colour of subgingival calculus may be seen through the marginal soft tissues. A fine calculus probe is used to detect deeper subgingival calculus, and interproximal deposits may be seen on radiographs. Direct vision of subgingival calculus may be achieved using a gentle stream of air to reflect the gingival margin or following gingival recession or during periodontal surgery.

Calculus itself is not a cause of periodontitis, but it is plaque retentive and keeps the biofilm in close proximity to the tissues; it also impairs the ability of the patient to remove plaque.

Specific Periodontal Conditions

Periodontal Health

Total recovery of organisms from the gingiva is low and mainly comprises Gram-positive species, particularly streptococci and *Actinomyces* (e.g. *Streptococcus sanguis*, *Streptococcus mitis*, *Actinomyces naeslundii*, *Actinomyces viscosus*). The predominance of these species may exert a protective influence for the host by preventing the colonisation or proliferation of more pathogenic organisms (e.g. *S. sanguis* produces H_2O_2, which is toxic to *Aggregatibacter actinomycetemcomitans*). Pathogenic species may be isolated from healthy sites but probably represent a transient component of maturing plaque.

Plaque-Induced Gingivitis

A more complex bacterial flora develops in chronic gingivitis comprising a mixture of Gram-positive and Gram-negative species, and aerobic and anaerobic organisms (Fig. 1.7). Gram-positive organisms include the *Streptococcus* and *Actinomyces* spp. found in health; Gram-negative organisms include *P. intermedia*, *Fusobacterium nucleatum*, *Eikenella corrodens* and *Capnocytophaga* spp.

Periodontitis

Micro-organisms most often identified in sites exhibiting periodontitis include *P. gingivalis*, *A. actinomycetemcomitans*, *Tannerella forsythia* (previously referred to as *Bacteroides forsythus*), *P. intermedia*, *A. naeslundii*, *Campylobacter rectus*, *E. corrodens*, *F. nucleatum*, *Treponema* and *Eubacterium* spp.

A. actinomycetemcomitans has been strongly hinted in localised more rapidly progressing molar-incisor pattern periodontitis and may comprise more than 90% of cultivable bacteria at affected sites. Other organisms associated with this pattern of periodontitis include *P. gingivalis*, *P. intermedia* and *Capnocytophaga* spp. Generalised more rapidly progressing periodontitis has been thought to be associated with increased prevalence of *P. gingivalis*, *A. actinomycetemcomitans*, *T. forsythia*, *P. intermedia* and *E. corrodens*.

PATHOGENESIS OF PERIODONTAL DISEASES

Pathogenesis is the sequence of events leading to the occurrence of a disease. In periodontology, the pathogenesis of gingivitis and periodontitis is related but tends to be described separately, and although the historical clinical and histological changes that occur are well known, the details of specific pathogenic mechanisms are less clearly defined even in light of new research used in support of the new classification.

Gingivitis

Pathogenesis

As plaque bacteria accumulate at the gingival margin, bacterial products (e.g. metabolic by-products, H_2S, endotoxin, proteases) cross the junctional epithelium and invoke an inflammatory response in the gingival tissues. This response is characterised by increased vascular permeability,

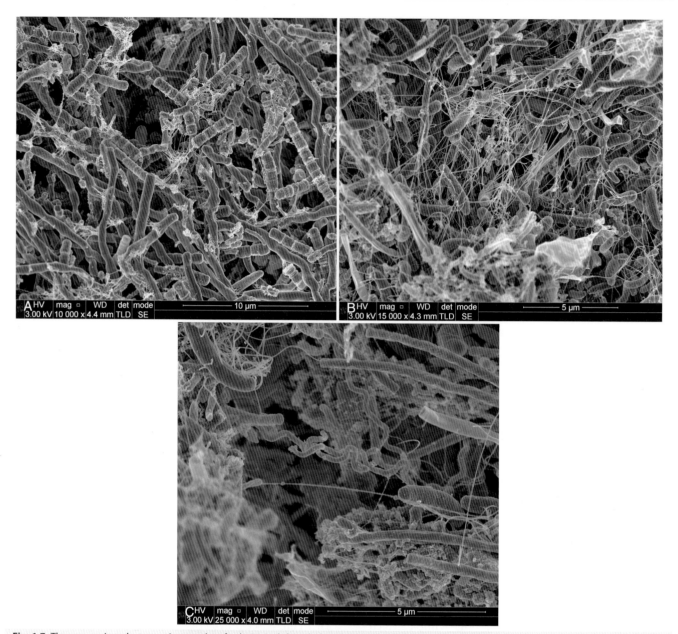

Fig. 1.7 Three scanning electron micrographs of subgingival dental plaque in patients with periodontitis (note the differing levels of magnification A) 10000, B) 15000, C) 25000). The composition and structure with the abundance of extracellular material, diversity of bacteria species and spaces result in a complex three dimensional structure of these biofilms.

vasodilatation and leakage of fluid and inflammatory and immunological products into the tissues and gingival sulcus. This change in the environment leads to a host–microbe interaction in what is described by Meyle and Chapple in 2015 as incipient dysbiosis in their contemporary model of the pathogenesis of periodontitis. Neutrophils migrate from the blood vessels into the tissues and the gingival sulcus. Collagen fibres around blood vessels and apical to the junctional epithelium are degraded. After several days, lymphocytes (particularly T cells) and macrophages accumulate. Fibroblasts show morphological changes and have a reduced ability to form collagen. Ultimately, plasma cells become the predominant inflammatory cell type, collagen depletion continues and the junctional epithelium proliferates. The established clinical

gingivitis inflammatory lesion is confined to the tissues adjacent to the junctional and sulcular epithelia.

Histopathology

For descriptive purposes, the inflammatory changes occurring during the development of gingivitis have been described as the *initial*, *early* and *established* gingival lesions, although there are no clear boundaries between these stages histologically.

The *initial inflammatory lesion* develops after 0–4 days of plaque accumulation and is characterised by:

- vascular dilatation and increased vascular permeability, leading to leakage of fluid from vessels, and increased GCF flow

- migration of neutrophils out of vessels into the tissues, through the junctional and sulcular epithelia, and into the gingival sulcus
- breakdown of collagen fibres around blood vessels.

The *early inflammatory lesion* develops after approximately 4–7 days of plaque accumulation. It is characterised by:

- continued vascular dilatation and increased permeability, with increased fluid exudation, and migration of neutrophils into the tissues
- increased breakdown of collagen subjacent to the junctional epithelium
- accumulation of lymphocytes (particularly T lymphocytes) and macrophages
- cytotoxic changes in fibroblasts, resulting in a reduced capacity for collagen formation
- proliferation of the cells of the junctional epithelium.

The *established inflammatory lesion* is apparent after approximately 14–21 days of undisturbed plaque growth and coincides with the clinical diagnosis of chronic gingivitis. Histopathological changes include:

- further engorgement of blood vessels, leading to venous stasis and the superimposition of a dark blue tinge over the erythematous gingiva
- migration of plasma cells into the gingival connective tissues to become the predominant inflammatory cell type
- continued collagen depletion
- continued proliferation of the junctional epithelium, forming epithelial ridges with widened intercellular spaces.

By definition, the inflammatory changes occurring in gingivitis are confined to the gingiva and do not involve alveolar bone or result in apical migration of the junctional epithelium. The *advanced inflammatory lesion* occurs when the inflammation extends beyond the gingiva. Extension beyond the gingiva is coincident with the clinical diagnosis of periodontitis (see the following text).

Initiation of Gingivitis

Plaque is essential for the initiation of gingivitis. Accumulation of plaque leads to gingivitis; as plaque biofilm matures, the subgingival environment alters to favour the growth of Gram-negative organisms. The inflammatory lesion in the gingiva leads to increased GCF flow, and products from the tissues are utilised as nutrients and interact with pathogenic organisms. The inflammatory changes in the tissues lead to increased permeability of the junctional epithelium, allowing bacterial products to penetrate the tissues more easily. The host responds to the bacterial challenge by continuing to mount an immune inflammatory response, such that neutrophils, lymphocytes and macrophages are activated to combat the growth and spread of bacteria. As a result, a chronic inflammatory state develops in which there is a balance between the host and the bacteria, and there are continued attempts at resolution in the presence of continued inflammation and destruction.

Periodontitis

Pathogenesis

Gingivitis may persist indefinitely, and little is known about the precise factors that influence a shift from gingivitis to destructive periodontitis. An alteration in the balance between the bacteria and the host response leading to a state of dysbiosis may be important in determining disease progression. The acquisition of a more pathogenic biofilm, or an impaired host response (e.g. as a result of altered immune function, psychological stress or smoking), may tip the balance in favour of disease progression.

In this chronically inflamed state, putative periodontal pathogens that possess specific virulence factors which can contribute to destructive processes and/or impair host defences tend to predominate. The host-derived immune inflammatory response also results in the destruction of periodontal hard and soft tissues, leading to the clinically observed signs of periodontitis. There are a number of host-derived mechanisms of destruction.

Neutrophils spill lysosomal enzymes and granule contents (including lysozyme, elastase, collagenase, proteases, myeloperoxidase) during phagocytosis or following cell death, resulting in damage to the surrounding tissues.

Stimulation of neutrophils results in a sudden increase in oxygen consumption by the cells (the 'respiratory burst'), which is utilised to oxidise reduced nicotinamide adenine diphosphate (NADPH), leading to the production of superoxide radical ($\cdot O_2-$), and H_2O_2 (hydrogen peroxide), which in turn is converted by the enzyme myeloperoxidase to hypochlorous acid, all of which are destructive oxidants for both bacteria and host tissues.

Collagenases from neutrophils and fibroblasts destroy connective tissue fibres of the periodontal ligament.

Proliferation of the epithelial cells of the junctional epithelium follows the destruction of collagen fibres in the periodontal ligament; the epithelial cells migrate apically along the root surface, resulting in pocket formation. This allows for downgrowth of subgingival plaque into the altered and protected environment of the periodontal pocket, favouring the growth of pathogenic anaerobes and resulting in a perpetuating cycle of destructive changes.

Osteoclasts are stimulated to resorb alveolar bone by cytokines and inflammatory mediators released by neutrophils and macrophages, including interleukins (ILs) and PGE_2.

ROLE OF IMMUNE CELLS. Neutrophils represent the first cellular host defence mechanism against plaque bacteria and predominate in the gingival sulcus and the junctional epithelium. Neutrophils possess a formidable array of antimicrobial weaponry. Monocytes infiltrate the gingival connective tissues and develop into macrophages, which either digest the antigen completely or present the antigen to lymphocytes. Neutrophils, therefore, are involved in the initial acute response, whereas macrophages and lymphocytes characterise a more longstanding or chronic inflammatory response and are activated in response to deeper penetration of bacteria and their products. Differences in periodontal disease expression between individuals are probably a consequence of different response traits of the immune-inflammatory cells. This model of disease progression requires a pathogenic (dysbiotic) flora to initiate the host response, which has a key role in modulating the severity of disease expression. It is clear that patients with defective defences (e.g. those with neutrophil defects or HIV infection) are at significantly greater risk for periodontal disease than those with an expected immune-inflammatory responses.

Histopathology

The transition from established gingivitis to periodontitis constitutes the development of the *advanced* inflammatory lesion (Fig. 1.8), which is characterised by:

- vascular proliferation and vasodilatation; vessels becoming engorged with blood
- plasma cells and B lymphocytes in the connective tissues
- the pocket epithelium being very thin, frequently ulcerated and permeable to bacterial products, inflammatory mediators and defence cells
- connective tissues exhibiting signs of degeneration and foci of necrosis
- fibres of the periodontal ligament apical to the junctional epithelium being destroyed by collagenases
- the junctional epithelium proliferating in an apical direction
- exposed cementum adsorbing bacterial products and becoming soft and necrotic
- osteoclast bone resorption, driven by plaque and host-derived mediators such as endotoxin, prostaglandins, interleukins and tumour necrosis factor (TNF), becoming evident.

Specific Pathogenic Mechanisms

The tissue destruction observed in periodontitis arises partly from direct injury sustained from factors produced by plaque bacteria, but mostly it arises from the resultant activation of the local inflammatory/immune response and the release of inflammatory mediators.

DIRECT INJURY BY PLAQUE BACTERIA. Many periodontopathogens produce substances that have potentially harmful effects on the periodontal tissues, including enzymes such as proteases, collagenases and hyaluronidase, and metabolic waste products including NH_3, H_2S and butyric acid. Organisms such as *P. gingivalis* and *A. actinomycetemcomitans* also possess virulence factors that have direct cytopathic effects, including the destruction of host tissues and inhibition of defensive mechanisms. Whereas bacteria are essential for the initiation of periodontal diseases, however, the signs of destructive periodontitis result predominantly from the activation of host inflammatory and immune processes in response to the presence of bacterial products in the tissues.

INJURY VIA INFLAMMATION. The host tissues produce certain endogenous mediators during the inflammatory response to bacteria and their products.

Histamine is present mainly in mast cells and basophils, particularly around blood vessels. Mast cells degranulate, releasing histamine, in response to many stimuli, including the binding of complement proteins and binding of antigen to immunoglobulin (Ig)E-sensitised mast cells. Histamine causes changes in the vascular plexus subjacent to the junctional epithelium, vasodilatation and increased vascular permeability.

The *complement system* comprises a series of over 20 proteins that are present in inactive form in serum and are activated in gingival inflammation. The system has three functions: (1) targeting phagocytic cells to micro-organisms (opsonisation); (2) recruiting immune cells to sites of inflammation (chemotaxis); and (3) bacterial destruction. There are two pathways of activation of the complement cascade. The classical pathway is activated by antigen (e.g. a bacterial cell or fragment) binding to IgM or IgG. The alternate pathway is initiated by various substances, including endotoxin. Complement activation causes various pro-inflammatory events, including leukocyte chemotaxis, opsonisation of micro-organisms, stimulation of the respiratory burst ('killing phase') in neutrophils and mast cell degranulation. Activated complement proteins can directly damage bacterial or host cells by binding to cell membranes and causing osmotic lysis.

Kinins are peptides produced as a result of activation of kallikrein in inflammatory conditions. Bradykinin is one such peptide; it causes increased vascular permeability and leukocyte emigration from blood vessels.

Arachidonic acid metabolites include the prostaglandins and leukotrienes. Prostaglandin levels are increased in the gingival tissues at inflamed sites and cause vasodilatation and increased vascular permeability. Prostaglandins also modulate lymphocyte function and stimulate osteoclastic bone resorption. Leukotriene B_4 causes increased vascular permeability and is chemotactic for neutrophils and increases adhesion of neutrophils to endothelial cells.

Oxygen free radicals are produced during the respiratory burst in neutrophils when reduced NADPH traps O_2, reducing it via O_2, H_2O_2 and OH to H_2O. Free radicals are essential for the bactericidal activity of neutrophils but can be spilled into the surrounding tissues during phagocytosis or following cell necrosis. Oxygen radicals not only kill bacteria but also damage host defence cells, fibroblasts, endothelium

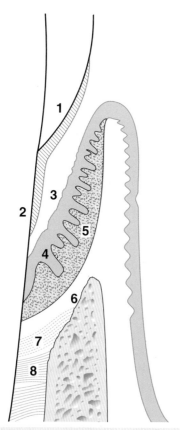

Fig. 1.8 Histopathological development of the advanced inflammatory lesion. *1* = dental plaque; *2* = plaque front; *3* = ulcerated pocket epithelium; *4* = epithelial ridges; *5* = cellular infiltrate (neutrophils, macrophages, plasma cells and invading bacteria); *6* = resorbed alveolar bone; *7* = connective tissue fibre destruction; *8* = intact ligament fibres.

and connective tissue matrix. They also activate latent collagenases present in the extracellular environment.

Matrix metalloproteinases (MMPs) are a family of enzymes capable of degrading extracellular matrix macromolecules including collagens, elastin, fibronectin and proteoglycan core protein. MMPs have a zinc ion at the active site, are secreted in latent form and are activated by proteolytic activity or reactive oxygen radicals once outside the cell. MMPs are produced by neutrophils, macrophages, fibroblasts and keratinocytes. MMP-8 is a collagenase produced by neutrophils; it is rapidly released and is the predominant collagenase in GCF sampled from periodontitis sites.

Cytokines are bioactive polypeptides produced by a variety of cells that function in pro-inflammatory networks in the periodontium. Cytokines include the interleukins, tumour necrosis factors and interferon-γ. Members of the IL-1 cytokine family have a central role in the regulation of immune-inflammatory responses, particularly IL-1β. Macrophages are the predominant source of IL-1β, which has pro-inflammatory effects including enhancement of bone resorption, inhibition of bone formation, stimulation of prostaglandin synthesis, increased collagenase production, proliferation of fibroblasts and potentiation of neutrophil degranulation. TNFα is another example of a potent pro-inflammatory mediator and it induces the formation of collagenase, PGE_2 and interleukins, and also induces bone resorption and inhibits bone formation.

Patterns of Progression of Periodontitis

Early studies investigating the progression of periodontitis concluded that there is continuous, linear loss of attachment over time, although the rate of progression varied according to the population studied. Longitudinal monitoring of patients reveals that many periodontal sites do not change over long periods, and destruction at a site may arrest and progress no further. Periodontitis is thought to progress by *bursts* of destructive activity. The *random burst model* of disease progression states that:

- certain sites remain free of destruction throughout life
- some sites demonstrate a brief burst of destruction that may last an undefined period of time before becoming quiescent
- sites that experienced destruction may never demonstrate an active burst again, or may be subject to one or more bursts later
- the bursts are random with regard to time and previous episodes of destruction.

An extension of this theory is the *asynchronous multiple burst theory*, in which multiple sites show breakdown within a short period of time, with prolonged periods of remission.

1.6 Risk Factors and Predisposing Factors

LEARNING OBJECTIVES

You should:
- know what is meant by the term 'risk factor'
- understand the important risk factors for periodontitis
- be aware of the reasons for the increased risk of progressive periodontitis in patients with uncontrolled diabetes
- understand the problems that iatrogenic plaque-retentive factors can create, and know how to avoid and correct them.

RISK FACTORS

Risk factors can be defined as characteristics, behavioural aspects or environmental exposures that are associated with a specific disease.

Several risk factors have been associated with the onset and/or progression of periodontal disease. These include:

- poor access to dental care
- a history of periodontitis
- stress
- systemic disease (such as diabetes)
- genetic factors
- smoking.

Tobacco Smoking

Smokers have a significantly higher prevalence of periodontal disease (pocket depths, attachment loss, bone loss) than non-smokers and this observation cannot only be explained by lower levels of oral hygiene and/or socioeconomic factors. Observations from numerous clinical studies suggest that smoking increases, in a dose-dependent manner, the risk of:

- periodontal destruction
- tooth loss
- recurrence of periodontitis
- peri-implant disease (see Chapter 5).

Smoking also reduces the magnitude and predictability of the success of periodontal treatment. The rate of progression of periodontitis and the rate of tooth loss are reduced in ex-smokers when compared with current smokers. This, together with the evidence that implicates smoking as a significant risk factor for periodontitis, suggests that:

- an assessment of smoking status must be made during history taking
- the dentist, dental therapists and dental hygienist must take an active part in encouraging all patients who are smokers to quit as part of an oral health care strategy.

Novel nicotine products, such as electronic cigarettes (e-cigarettes), have become popular since their introduction to the market in the late 2000s. Although the evidence base is still developing, it is generally agreed that, although not risk free, they are much safer than tobacco smoking and may be a useful cessation aid. Further research is needed to understand the impacts (positive or negative) of e-cigarettes on oral health, particularly in the context of a tobacco smoker with periodontitis switching to an e-cigarette.

DIABETES MELLITUS

Diabetes mellitus is a metabolic disorder that is associated with inadequate insulin secretion (type 1 diabetes) or decreased responsiveness to insulin (type 2). Both are characterised by elevated blood glucose levels. In type 1 diabetes, there is a sudden onset in predominantly young patients. Type 2 usually has a gradual onset in middle age, associated with obesity and sedentary lifestyles, though there are increasing numbers of cases affecting younger patients. The general symptoms are thirst, hunger, polyuria and weight loss. The incidence of both types combined is about 3–6% in the United Kingdom.

Generally, a person with well-controlled diabetes is not at increased risk for periodontal disease. However, poorly controlled diabetes (HbA$_{1c}$ >8%, 64 mmol/mol) increases the risk of periodontitis two- to three-fold, and multiple periodontal abscesses or suppurating pockets are often a feature.

The subgingival microflora in patients with diabetes is similar to that in people who do not have diabetes. Several factors likely contribute to increased risk of periodontitis in diabetes. Both periodontitis and diabetes are pro-inflammatory conditions, and upregulated cytokine production locally may contribute to increased tissue damage. Impaired neutrophil function includes reduced chemotaxis, phagocytosis and intracellular killing. Hyperglycaemia results in the glycation of structural proteins such as collagen, leading to the formation of advanced glycation end-products (AGEs), which activate inflammatory cells such as macrophages, leading to increased release of tissue-destructive enzymes and pro-inflammatory cytokines.

Extraction of hopelessly involved teeth is followed by conventional non-surgical or surgical therapy. Systemic antimicrobials (amoxicillin and metronidazole) are indicated for persistent or recurrent infections.

PREDISPOSING (PLAQUE-RETENTIVE) FACTORS

Overhanging Restorations

Poor technique when restoring teeth can result in amalgam overhangs; these occur frequently at interproximal sites and are avoided by ensuring that matrix bands are closely adapted to the tooth surface when packing amalgam. Overhangs render interproximal cleaning impossible and result in plaque-induced inflammation, loss of attachment and alveolar bone destruction.

Treatment
It is best to remove any overhang:

- Where access permits, remove overhang with a fine diamond bur.
- Replace restoration if necessary.
- OHI (interproximal cleaning), RSI.

Defective Crown Margins

Supragingival crown margins are easy to clean but may compromise appearance. Subgingival margins are generally indicated at aesthetically important sites, but care must be taken not to compromise the supracrestal tissue attachment (biologic width). Crown margins should not 'interrupt' the normal contour of the tooth surface. A *positive* defect, or ledge, is one in which the crown margin extends beyond the intended margin of the prepared tooth. A *negative* defect finishes short of the margins of the preparation.

Defective margins inevitably result in plaque accumulation even if the overall standard of oral hygiene is high.

Gingival tissues are erythematous and oedematous and bleed readily on probing.

Treatment

- At try-in, reject crowns with defective margins and take new impressions.
- Small positive defects may be corrected with fine diamond burs and polishing stones.
- Replace the defective crown.

Bridge Pontics

Bridge pontics must be carefully designed to facilitate cleaning and minimise plaque accumulation. This is achieved by ensuring the pontics are clear of the gingival tissues. A compromise between aesthetics and cleansibility is usually necessary. Pontics should have smooth surfaces, be convex in all directions and have minimal, light contact on the buccal surface of the edentulous ridge. This allows for self-performed cleaning with superfloss and is aesthetically pleasing. Pontics that impinge on the soft tissues increase plaque accumulation and inflammation. Aesthetics are compromised as a result of poor soft tissue appearance.

Treatment
- Replace bridge.
- OHI (superfloss) and scaling.

Partial Dentures

Removable prostheses encourage plaque accumulation in the absence of effective oral hygiene. Acrylic dentures with interproximal collets ('gum strippers') can increase plaque-induced inflammation, destructive periodontitis and recession of the gingival tissues. Framework components and clasps of cobalt–chrome dentures positioned too close to the gingival margin aggravate plaque-induced inflammation and, occasionally, cause direct trauma.

Prevention
- Utilise tooth support in preference to mucosal support.
- Ensure adequate clearance of the gingival tissues by saddles, major and minor connectors and clasps.
- Avoid interproximal collets.
- Simplify denture design where possible.

Treatment
- Replace poorly designed dentures.
- OHI and denture hygiene (clean denture with a toothbrush and water; leave denture out at night).

Orthodontic Appliances

Fixed and removable appliances encourage plaque accumulation. Fixed appliances require considerable effort to keep brackets, bands, wires, elastics and tooth surfaces plaque free. Removable appliances can be taken from the mouth to be cleaned and allow toothbrushing. Plaque-induced gingivitis in the region of the appliance is likely.

Prevention
- Appliances should not be provided to patients who are unable to practise good oral hygiene.
- Ensure adequate clearance of the gingival tissues.
- Simplify appliance design.

Treatment
- OHI with mini-interdental and interproximal brushes, superfloss.

1.7 Furcation and Periodontal–Endodontic Lesions

LEARNING OBJECTIVES

You should:
- understand the significance of periodontal abscesses, furcation involvements in periodontitis and endodontic–periodontal lesions
- be able to diagnose and classify these conditions
- be familiar with the indications for, and techniques of, treatment of these lesions
- be able to differentiate between the different types of furcation and endodontic–periodontal lesion and plan treatment accordingly.

PERIODONTAL ABSCESSES

Acute periodontal abscess is an acute suppurative inflammatory lesion within the periodontal pocket or gingival sulcus, which usually arises from:

- an acute exacerbation of chronic periodontitis
- trauma to the pocket epithelium (from instrumentation, toothbrush bristles, food impaction)
- orthodontic movement of teeth through untreated, periodontally compromised tissues.

The clinical signs and symptoms of a periodontal abscess are:

- gingival erythema
- swelling of the overlying gingivae
- discharge of pus from the gingival margin
- pain from the affected site made worse by biting
- unpleasant taste
- tenderness to percussion
- acute pain on probing, with discharge of pus and blood.

Treatment

The basic treatment of periodontitis is discussed in detail in Section 1.11 and invariably includes:

- oral hygiene instruction: systematic toothbrushing technique and interproximal cleaning aids (dental floss, mini-interdental brushes, interspace brushes)
- RSI to disrupt biofilm and remove calculus
- re-evaluation to assess the response to treatment, reinforce oral hygiene instruction and provide further instrumentation if necessary.

Treatment of a periodontal abscess:

- Incision if drainage cannot be achieved through the pocket.
- Subgingival instrumentation and irrigation with chlorhexidine.
- Warm saline mouthrinses to encourage further drainage.
- Systemic antimicrobials when there is evidence of spread of infection and involvement of regional lymph nodes: metronidazole 400 mg, three times a day, for 5 days is

effective against anaerobes; penicillins may also be prescribed.
- Re-evaluation to assess response to treatment and prognosis of the affected tooth.

FURCATION LESIONS

The loss of attachment that occurs with periodontitis eventually reaches the furca of multirooted teeth. Attachment loss then continues both in vertical and horizontal directions, frequently giving rise to lesions with complex bone topography. The management of furcation lesions depends, to some extent, upon the severity of the defect at diagnosis. The early detection of incipient lesions improves the long-term prognosis of the tooth involved. A detailed knowledge of furcation anatomy is, therefore, fundamental to the management of teeth with furcation involvement.

Furcation Anatomy

Root Anatomy

There are numerous concavities, convexities and grooves associated with root surfaces (Fig. 1.9). The roots of the mandibular molars are typically broad and flattened mesiodistally. Concavities are found on the furcal aspects of mandibular first molar roots, with those on the distal surfaces of mesial roots being the most accentuated. The roots of the mandibular second and third molars demonstrate similar anatomy, although the roots are closer together and may be fused.

The maxillary first molar usually has three separate roots: mesiobuccal, distobuccal and palatal. The two buccal roots are flattened and the broader, mesiobuccal root has a groove on its distal surface. The palatal root is conical and may be fused to the distobuccal root. The flattened contour of the mesiobuccal root means that the mesiopalatal entrance to the furca of maxillary first molars is accessible to probing. The second and third maxillary molars

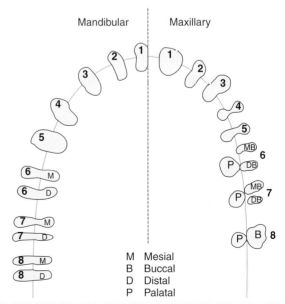

Fig. 1.9 Typical root morphology seen at horizontal cross-sections made at half root lengths.

have the same basic root anatomy as that of the first molar. The roots tend to be less divergent and fused roots are more prevalent. The maxillary first premolar has two roots (buccal and palatal) in about 50% of individuals. The second maxillary premolar may also have two roots, although more commonly the root is single with pronounced grooves on the mesial and distal surfaces. Mandibular incisors, canines and premolars can all have multiple roots, and supplemental roots are common on maxillary and mandibular molars.

Furcation entrance dimensions vary significantly between teeth. On the upper first molar, the mesial and distal furcal entrances are usually sufficiently wide to accommodate periodontal instruments. The buccal entrance is narrower and approximately the width of a Gracey curette. The furcal dimensions on second molars are narrower than the corresponding widths on the first molar. The buccal and distal openings are often accessible to only fine ultrasonic instruments. In the mandible, the buccal and lingual furcal dimensions of molars are virtually identical. Entrances on the second molar are narrower than those on the first and are approximately the same width as the blade of a Gracey curette.

Cervical-enamel projections (CEPs) (Fig. 1.10) or enamel spurs are pointed, extensions of enamel that arise from the cervico-enamel junction and extend apically, towards and occasionally into the furca of molar teeth. Localised periodontal defects are associated with CEPs in about 90% of patients. Periodontal attachment to CEPs is epithelial in nature; consequently, the distance from the base of the gingival crevice to the point of root bifurcation is effectively reduced. Examination of dry skull material often shows early bone loss, some cratering or small notch-like lesions adjacent to CEPs.

Intermediate furcation ridges run mesiodistally, in the midline across the bi- and trifurcations of molars. When situated buccally or lingually, they form an exaggerated arch at the entrance of furca. Furcation ridges have a core of dentine but are composed predominantly of cellular cementum,

which increases in thickness with age. Ridges are natural obstructions to both plaque-control procedures and professional debridement of furcation lesions. Cementum ridges can be recontoured relatively easily during the instrumentation of affected furca.

Accessory root canals are a common finding in the furca of molar teeth. They provide pathways through which inflammation can spread, either from the pulp to the periodontal ligament or, more rarely, from a deep periodontal pocket or abscess to the pulp. Furcation involvement may, therefore, be of pulpal origin, and an assessment of tooth vitality should confirm the diagnosis. When a furcation lesion is of both pulpal and periodontal origin, then complete resolution will only follow combined periodontal and endodontic treatments.

Enamel pearls are isolated 'droplets' of enamel that are found predominantly on the root surfaces of molars and premolars. They form when small islands of Hertwig's epithelial root sheath are retained on dentine during root development. Enamel pearls have no periodontal fibre insertions and occasionally retain a connection with the cementoenamel junction. Pearls are a further potential obstruction to instrumentation of root surfaces.

Distribution of Furcation Lesions

Epidemiological studies show that the prevalence and severity of furcation lesions increase with age, as the severity of periodontal disease increases. In one study of more than 600 molars, furcation lesions were observed much more frequently in maxillary than in mandibular molars. One possible explanation for this is the position of the furcal openings in the upper and lower teeth. Maxillary molars have mesial and distal furcation entrances that, being sited interproximally (from where plaque is more difficult to remove), are at increased risk of periodontal destruction. Mandibular molars have only buccal and lingual entrances to furcation and these sites are more accessible to oral hygiene practices. The third molars in both jaws have less furcation involvement than first or second molars, principally because the roots are smaller, less divergent and often fused to form a single tapering root.

Classification and Diagnosis

The scoring system for assessing furcations is given in Section 1.2. Intraoral, periapical radiographs taken using the paralleling technique are a useful adjunct to furcation diagnosis. In the maxilla, superimposition of palatal roots of molars and premolars on the furcation makes radiographic interpretation of bone levels difficult. A general assessment of the height of alveolar bone, the presence of vertical bone defects and a reduction in radio-opacity of intra-radicular bone may suggest a furcation lesion. The mesial and distal location of roots of mandibular molars usually enables a clear radiographic view of furcation anatomy.

Radiographs of teeth with advanced furcation involvement frequently show vertical bone defects that extend to, or around, a root apex. Vitality testing should be undertaken as an aid to establishing pulpal involvement and to confirm, or exclude, a periodontal–endodontic lesion. The presence of periapical disease is an important factor to take into consideration when assessing the prognosis of a furcation-involved tooth.

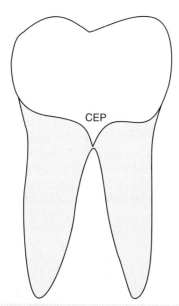

Fig. 1.10 Cervical-enamel projection *(CEP)* or spur.

Treatment

The basic aims of treatment are to eliminate disease, to provide an environment that the patient is able to clean using home care oral hygiene measures and to establish a maintenance regimen to prevent reinfection and disease recurrence over the long term. Better access and direct vision for instrumentation can be achieved by raising flaps, which also facilitates identification of anatomical irregularities. The surgical approach also allows root anatomy to be modified as well as osseous recontouring, and the creation of an improved morphology of the soft tissues.

Traditionally, the more radical and complex methods of treatment have been used for treatment of the more severe defects (Table 1.3). Such a guide is clearly very useful, although it is important to assess each patient carefully before deciding upon a definitive treatment plan.

Plaque Biofilm Control and Preventive Measures

Many aspects of treatment aim to provide improved access for self-performed plaque control oral hygiene. Patients, therefore, require very careful monitoring to ensure that plaque can, and is, being removed from *all* aspects of the treated furcation. For this purpose, certain oral hygiene aids are essential. The single tufted, interspace brush is indicated for cleaning shallow cave entrances of grade 1 lesions, as well as more accessible areas such as those created following root resection. An interdental brush is indicated for cleaning between roots (e.g. in tunnels where the brushes can be used immediately postoperatively to clean subgingivally). Superfloss and floss threaders are also useful in these circumstances. Root caries is a concern at all furcation-treated sites, but particularly at those at which it is difficult to maintain a plaque-free surface. A daily rinse with a sodium fluoride solution should be included in the immediate postsurgical schedule. Thereafter, regular applications of a fluoride varnish to the root and furcation surfaces are advisable as part of a maintenance recall programme.

Root Surface Instrumentation

RSI is often the only treatment required for incipient lesions. Curettes, reciprocating and rotating instruments are not always able to remove calculus from areas such as the furcation roof and the concave distal surfaces of mesial roots. The finer tips of ultrasonic scalers may improve efficacy of instrumentation.

Flap Surgery

With grade 2 and 3 lesions, RSI is likely to be more effective following the elevation of mucoperiosteal flaps. The exact topography of the defect is assessed after the removal of any granulation tissue, and the remaining bone support of individual roots can be evaluated. At this stage, it is useful to compare the actual severity of the lesion with the grade that was given at the initial examination, when, because of the presence of soft tissues, a degree of underestimation of severity is likely. Flaps are replaced and sutured to achieve a gingival architecture that is conducive to effective home care oral hygiene measures. This is not always attainable, however, without undertaking some modification of the tissues within, or adjacent to, the furcation entrance.

Furcoplasty

The aim of furcoplasty is to produce a healthy gingival papilla in the furcation entrance, which should be accessible to self-performed plaque control. In addition to RSI, furcoplasty comprises two tissue modification procedures:

- *Odontoplasty* is the removal of tooth substance to widen a narrow entrance to the furcation. To prevent postoperative dentine sensitivity, only very limited removal of tooth tissue should be carried out.
- *Osteoplasty* is the recontouring of the adjacent bone of the buccal, lingual or palatal alveolar plates that provide no tooth support.

Tunnel preparation

In grade 2 and 3 defects, inter-radicular osteoplasty to create a tunnel through the furcation has been described. This procedure can be undertaken on any multirooted tooth, although mandibular first and second molars, with their long and well-separated mesial and distal roots, are the favoured candidates. Closure of the mucoperiosteal flaps through the furcation is achieved using an inter-radicular suture and the patency of the tunnel in the immediate postoperative period is maintained by placing a small surgical dressing in the tunnel. Nevertheless, proliferation of soft tissues in the tunnel is common, leading to postsurgical pocketing of 2–3 mm. Furthermore, the tunnel that has been created remains a difficult area to achieve meticulous plaque control, and root caries in the furcation is a potential complication. For these reasons, tunnel preparations are now performed rarely.

Bone Regeneration

Regenerative techniques using non-resorbable and resorbable membranes have been applied successfully to the treatment of furcation defects (see Section 1.11).

Root Amputation

In some cases, it is possible to improve the prognosis for a multirooted tooth with furcation involvement by surgically amputating one (or more) of its roots. This procedure effectively eliminates the most periodontally compromised root, with the aim being to make the furcation more accessible for

Table 1.3 Treatment of Furcation Lesions.

Grade	Treatment Options
1	Oral hygiene Scaling, Root surface instrumentation Furcoplasty
2	Oral hygiene Scaling, RSI with or without surgical access Root resection Guided tissue regeneration
3	Oral hygiene Scaling, RSI, with or without surgical access Root resection Hemisection Tunnel preparation Extraction

cleaning. If a single root is amputated from a maxillary molar, the entire crown can be maintained in occlusion but plaque-retentive overhangs must be avoided, and the periodontal support of the remaining roots must be sufficient to support the retained natural crown. When both furcations are affected, it is usually best to divide the roots to assess the precise involvement and mobility of each root separately before deciding which can be retained and which should be removed (with the patient being forewarned that none of the roots may be saved). If the mesial or distal root of a mandibular molar is resected, if there is any doubt whether the single remaining root could support the entire crown of the tooth, then a hemisection is the procedure of choice, removing the involved root and its coronal half of crown. It is then usually necessary to place an indirect restoration (partial or full crown) the remaining part of the tooth.

MAXILLARY MOLARS. Whenever a root amputation is planned, it is always far preferable to place a root filling before the surgical procedure. Thus, the roots which are planned to be retained should be root filled with gutta-percha well in advance of the root resection surgery. For the root which is to be resected, the most appropriate material to fill the coronal part of the root is mineral trioxide aggregate (MTA). This is a mixture of various calcium silicates and other minerals that is supplied as a powder, and when mixed with sterile water creates a grainy, sandy mixture. This should be packed into the canal at the level the planned root resection.

At the time for the root resection (which should be at least 1–2 months after completion of root canal therapy to ensure that no complications arise as a result of the endodontic treatment itself), it may be necessary to raise a flap to visualise the planned location of the resection. Surgical access has the advantages of:

- better vision of the surgical site
- direct evaluation of bone in the remaining furcations
- improved access for recontouring the cut root surface and adjacent part of the crown
- reducing the likelihood of soft tissue trauma
- eliminating soft tissue defects when repositioning flaps.

However, flaps may not be needed if the level of resection is supragingival.

Whether a flap is raised or not, the root is sectioned with burs, and then using burs is effectively 'shaved' smooth so that there are no overhangs (Fig. 1.11). By packing MTA to a sufficient depth above and below the intended point of the resection, there should be no danger of exposing any unfilled aspect of the root canal system. MTA, once set, is insoluble in saliva, and does not result in any unwanted inflammatory lesion in the soft tissues, and is therefore the ideal material to be exposed to the oral environment following the resection.

MANDIBULAR MOLARS. A decision regarding which root to retain and which to resect in mandibular molars should be made prior to surgery. Candidate roots for resection include:

- those with excessively curved root canals that would complicate endodontics
- those that are associated with more extensive bone loss
- those with radiographic evidence of periapical infection.

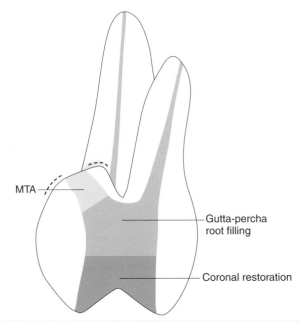

Fig. 1.11 Root resection on a previously root-filled maxillary molar. Note the rounded contours of cut/resected surface (---) *MTA*, Mineral trioxide aggregate.

When a hemisection is indicated on a last standing first (or second) mandibular molar, and there is an intact segment in front of the affected tooth, then if either the mesial or distal roots could justifiably be removed, the mesial half of the hemisected tooth should be retained to maintain an intact occlusal segment without the need to resort to bridges.

A gutta-percha root filling is placed in the root to be retained and an plastic restoration placed in the access cavity down to the level of the planned section. Full-thickness mucoperiosteal flaps are raised to maximise vision and improve access, and the tooth is divided. After extraction of the condemned root, the retained part is examined carefully and any irregular edges, or spicules of enamel, dentine or bone, are removed. Redundant soft tissue is excised, before the mucoperiosteal flaps are repositioned and sutured. Ultimately, a crown will need to be placed on the retained root fragment.

Extraction

Grade 3 furcation involvements of several multirooted teeth are a common finding in patients with advanced periodontal disease. Increased tooth mobilities in both horizontal and vertical directions can severely compromise function, and it may be in the operator's and the patient's best interests to extract teeth with hopeless prognoses so that a concerted effort is targeted to managing the teeth that have a more favourable chance of being retained. If function is not compromised, however, and the patient is free of associated symptoms, then a conservative approach of furcation instrumentation and instruction in oral hygiene measures at regular intervals may slow the progression of disease. In this way, a functional dentition can be maintained intact for many years.

It is essential to evaluate a number of important general criteria before deciding upon whether a tooth with a furcation lesion should be treated and restored, or extracted. The patient must be committed to receiving the proposed treatment and be able to achieve, and maintain, a high standard of oral hygiene. The involved tooth must also be a valued part of the dentition. For example, it may maintain the integrity of the arch or provide an abutment for a proposed bridge or partial denture. Furthermore, the time and the number of visits needed for treatment, and the expense likely to be incurred, should not be overlooked. All should be discussed with the patient before a definitive treatment plan is formulated.

Prognosis

Clearly, the outcome of the procedure is dependent upon the experience of the clinician not only in carrying out the treatment, but also in case selection and determining the most appropriate treatment. Generally, the treatment that is selected depends predominantly upon the degree of furcation involvement at diagnosis. Molars with tunnel preparations have been shown to have a poor prognosis because of their susceptibility to root caries.

Observations suggest that very few failures occur during the first 5 years after root resection. The 10-year follow-up studies of root resections show a success rate of 60–70%. Further, a high proportion of failed cases result from non-periodontal causes such as caries, root fractures and periapical infection, as well as problems with crowns and bridges (recurrent caries, cement washout, loss of retention). The long-term outcome is, therefore, dependent upon the overall restorative management of the patient as well as the standard and selection of periodontal care.

Five- and 10-year studies of buccal class II furcation defects that have been treated using resorbable and non-resorbable membranes confirm that these techniques improve the prognosis for the affected teeth.

ENDODONTIC–PERIODONTAL LESIONS

Endodontic–periodontal lesions are inflammatory reactions originating in either the pulp or the periodontal ligament with the potential to spread from one site to the other via a number of pathways: apical foramina, lateral and furcation accessory root canals, exposed dentinal tubules and root defects caused by caries, fractures or perforations during operative procedures.

There are five types of lesions based on the pathogenic interactions of pulpal–periodontal disease:

1. primary endodontic
2. endodontic with secondary periodontal involvement
3. primary periodontal
4. periodontal with secondary endodontic involvement
5. combined lesions.

In the 2017 classification, Herrera et al. suggest an alternative approach:

- Endodontic–periodontal lesion with root damage
  - Root fracture or cracking/Root canal or pulp perforation/External root resorption
- Endodontic–periodontal lesion without root damage
  - Lesions in periodontitis patients
  - Lesions in non-periodontitis patients

Primary Endodontic Lesions

Infection from a necrotic pulp drains into the periodontium to produce a periapical abscess. This remains localised, drains coronally through the periodontal membrane and gingival sulcus or tracks through the alveolar bone to leave a swelling and a sinus opening in the attached gingiva. There is no periodontal aetiology.

Clinical features involve persistent discomfort rather than frank pain and a negative response of the tooth to a vitality test. Periapical radiolucency can be seen on radiograph, which may show evidence of spread coronally. There is no loss of alveolar bone height on mesial and distal alveolar crest. Furcation bone loss between molar roots suggests spread of infection via accessory furcation canal.

Root canal treatment is indicated.

Endodontic Lesions With Secondary Periodontal Involvement

Untreated or inadequately managed endodontic lesions can become a persistent source of infection to the marginal periodontium (Fig. 1.12A).

Clinical features are similar to those of primary endodontic lesions. Gingival inflammation, increased probing depth, bleeding or pus on probing may be evident. Subgingival plaque and calculus can be detected. Radiographs show periapical radiolucency and some resorption of crestal alveolar bone.

Treatment involves root canal treatment and replacement of a previous, unsatisfactory root filling, OHI, scaling and prophylaxis. Extraction should be considered in the case of an extensive lesion.

Primary Periodontal Lesions

Periodontal infection that spreads to involve the periapical tissues is a primary periodontal lesion. It may be associated with a local anatomical defect such as a radicular groove on a maxillary lateral incisor.

Clinical features include localised, longstanding pain or discomfort and a positive response of the tooth to a vitality test. Gingivitis occurs, and localised deep pocketing is seen, with pus and bleeding following probing or application of pressure to the gingiva. Radiographs show localised bone resorption, which can appear as horizontal, vertical or furcation defects. Anatomical predisposing factors may occasionally be detected.

Treatment includes OHI and RSI. Surgical treatment to improve access for instrumentation or to eliminate anatomical factors may be indicated. Locally delivered antimicrobials can be considered if infection persists. Consider extraction in the case of an extensive lesion.

Periodontal Lesions With Secondary Endodontic Involvement

Secondary endodontic involvement is seen when infection spreads from the periodontium to the pulp, causing pulpitis and necrosis (see Fig. 1.12B).

Clinical features are similar to those of primary periodontal lesions but the tooth gives a negative response to vitality testing. Radiographic appearance may be identical to teeth with periodontal involvement only, although bone loss is generally more extensive. Conversely, narrow, tortuous defects can be associated with grooves on the root surface.

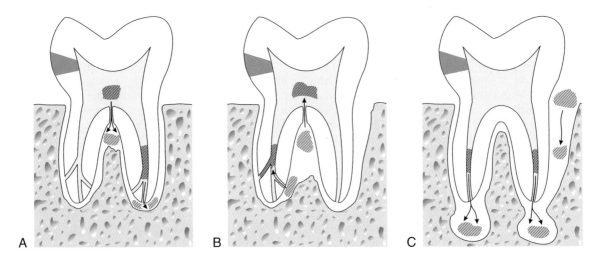

⟶ Spread of inflammation

Fig. 1.12 Endodontic–periodontal lesions. (A) An endodontic lesion with secondary periodontal involvement in the furcation. (B) A periodontal lesion with secondary endodontic involvement. (C) A combined lesion with both primary pulpal and periodontal origins.

Treatment involves root canal therapy, OHI and RSI. Local antimicrobials should be considered if infection persists. Surgery can facilitate access to deeper pockets/anatomical defects or allow regenerative procedures. Extraction should be considered in an extensive lesion.

Combined Lesions

In combined lesions, the periodontal infection 'coalesces' with a periapical lesion of pulpal origin. There are two distinct origins: periodontal and periapical (see Fig. 1.12C).

The clinical features and management of combined lesions are the same as for periodontal lesions with secondary endodontic involvement. The remaining periodontal attachment is often minimal; consequently, tooth mobility is usually quite pronounced. Root amputation or hemisection may be indicated but the prognosis is often poor.

1.8 Gingival Problems

LEARNING OBJECTIVES

You should:
- be aware of the aetiology, clinical relevance and treatment options for gingival recession
- be familiar with the aetiology and treatment options for the various forms of gingival enlargement.

GINGIVAL RECESSION

When gingival recession occurs, the width of attached gingiva is reduced or eliminated. A narrow width of attached gingiva is compatible with health and the width of attached gingiva alone should not be regarded as the only 'risk factor' for gingival recession.

Gingival recession can affect any site in the mouth and, depending upon aetiological factors, may be localised or generalised.

Aetiology

There is often an element of trauma that can be identified as a contributing factor, particularly to localised recession:

- excessive toothbrushing force, incorrect technique or use of a particularly abrasive dentifrice
- traumatic incisor relationships
- habits such as rubbing the gingiva with a fingernail or the end of a pencil.

Generalised recession occurs when the gingival margin migrates apically as a consequence of ongoing periodontal disease or following resolution of inflammation after successful periodontal treatment. Localised or generalised recession may also be a complication of orthodontic treatment when teeth (roots) are moved labially through an existing dehiscence or thin labial alveolar plate.

An exposed root surface on an anterior tooth is often aesthetically unacceptable. Exposure of dentine may cause extreme sensitivity and root surfaces are susceptible to caries. Sibilant speech may result from widened interdental spaces.

Clinical Features

Apical migration of the gingival complex exposes the root surface. Wear cavities on root surfaces are indicative of toothbrush abrasion as an aetiological factor.

Stillman's cleft (Fig. 1.13A) is an incipient lesion, a narrow, deep and slightly curved cleft extending apically from the free gingival margin. As the recession progresses apically, the cleft becomes broader, exposing the cementum of the root surface. When the lesion reaches the mucogingival junction, the apical border of oral mucosa is usually inflamed because of the difficulty in maintaining good plaque control at this site.

McCall's festoon (see Fig. 1.13B) is a rolled, thickened band of gingiva usually seen adjacent to canines when recession approaches the mucogingival junction.

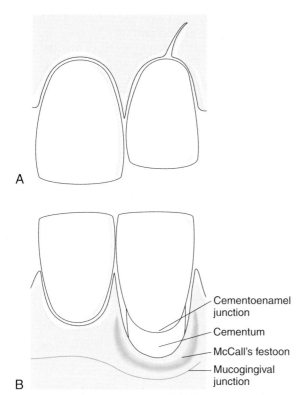

Fig. 1.13 Mucogingival lesions. (A) Stillman's cleft and (B) McCall's festoon in which a rolled, fibrous 'curtain' of gingiva occurs.

Labels in figure:
Cementoenamel junction
Cementum
McCall's festoon
Mucogingival junction

Predisposing Factors

Dehiscences (clefts) or fenestrations (windows) are natural defects in labial alveolar plates that are often, but not exclusively, associated with prominent roots or teeth that are crowded out of the arch. Such defects need not necessarily initiate recession but rather increase its rate of progression once established.

Treatment

- Record the magnitude of recession (clinically or on study models) on a regular basis to assess progression or stability.
- Eliminate aetiological factors.
- OHI.
- Topical desensitising agents/fluoride varnish.
- Gingival veneer to cover exposed roots/embrasure spaces.
- Crown teeth (after diagnostic wax up) but exercise extreme caution to prevent exposure of coronal pulp at level of radicular preparation.
- Mucogingival surgery (see Section 1.11).

GINGIVAL ENLARGEMENT

Gingival enlargement may occasionally be the first presenting sign of an underlying systemic disorder. A full medical history should always be taken, and clinicians must be alert for additional signs and symptoms to confirm the diagnosis. A systematic approach will reveal the medication history, haemorrhagic tendencies, abdominal and gastrointestinal upset or any respiratory problems. Careful extraoral and intraoral examinations are necessary to determine the nature and extent of the lesion, additional signs and predisposing or traumatic factors. Referral to a specialist centre for additional investigations may be appropriate.

Gingival Fibromatosis

Gingival fibromatosis is an uncommon condition with an autosomal dominant inheritance pattern. There is generalised fibrous enlargement of the gingiva as a result of the accumulation of bundles of collagen fibres. It is frequently associated with fibrous enlargement of the maxillary tuberosities.

Treatment is usually not required, unless access for cleaning is impaired or aesthetics are compromised. It tends to recur following surgical excision.

Chronic Hyperplastic Gingivitis

Chronic hyperplastic gingivitis is a historic term that may occur following prolonged accumulation of dental plaque. It is frequently associated with concomitant systemic medications, though predisposing factors may not be identifiable. There is firm gingival enlargement, particularly at interdental sites, although an inflammatory component may also be present. The gingiva may partially cover the crowns of teeth, resulting in aesthetic problems and cleaning difficulties.

Treatment is oral hygiene instruction, scaling and gingivectomy.

Drug-Influenced Gingival Enlargements

Phenytoin, ciclosporin and the calcium-channel blockers (notably nifedipine) are all associated with the unwanted effect of gingival enlargement.

Incidence
The incidence varies between the different drugs; it affects approximately 50% of patients taking phenytoin, 30% taking ciclosporin and 20% taking nifedipine. Prevalence is increased in children and adolescents. It predominantly affects the anterior gingival tissues.

Clinical Features
Enlargement commences within the interdental papillae, which enlarge until they coalesce, involving all of the attached gingivae. Excess tissues extend coronally and may interfere with speech, occlusion and mastication. Aesthetics are severely compromised. The colour varies from pink to deep red–purple, depending on the degree of inflammation in the tissues. Occasionally, it can present in the edentulous.

Histopathology
The epithelium is parakeratinised and acanthotic, often with long, slender, elongated rete ridges. Fibrous tissue forms the bulk of the enlargement, featuring a proliferation of fibroblasts and increased collagen content. Inflamed tissues are highly vascularised and contain collections of inflammatory cells. Plasma cells predominate, although lymphocytes and macrophages are also present.

Pathogenesis
The precise mechanism of enlargement is uncertain and involves complex interactions between the drug, fibroblasts,

plaque-induced inflammation and genetic factors. It has been suggested that subpopulations of fibroblasts synthesise increased quantities of collagen, the relative proportions of which are genetically determined. Plaque-induced inflammation is a prerequisite for enlargement in inflamed tissues, high-activity fibroblasts may become sensitised to the effects of systemic drugs. A drug-related increase in the metabolism of certain hormones (e.g. androgens) by fibroblasts may explain the increased incidence observed in adolescents. Human lymphocyte antigen expression may be associated with fibroblast phenotype and could act as a marker for gingival enlargement.

Treatment

A strict programme of OHI and plaque control must be implemented. Discussion with the patient's physician must be held to consider alternative medications and notification of this event as a side effect of the drug. Persistent enlarged tissues may also be surgically excised.

Crohn's Disease

Crohn's disease is a chronic granulomatous disorder of unknown aetiology affecting any part of the gastrointestinal tract.

Oral manifestations include oedema, hypertrophy and fissuring of the buccal mucosa ('cobblestone appearance'), swelling of the lips and cheeks, mucosal tags, oral ulceration and angular cheilitis. An erythematous granular enlargement of the entire width of the attached gingiva may be evident.

Orofacial Granulomatosis

Orofacial granulomatosis is not a discrete clinical entity but describes the common clinicopathological presentation of a variety of disorders including Crohn's disease and some topical hypersensitivity reactions.

Acute Leukaemia

Malignant proliferation of white blood cells and their precursors results in increased numbers of circulating leukocytes and infiltration of tissues by leukaemic cells giving several periodontal manifestations.

Gingival enlargement results from infiltration of the gingival connective tissues by leukaemic cells. It gives impaired plaque control and further inflammatory oedema.
Gingival bleeding results from the thrombocytopenia that accompanies the leukaemia and may be spontaneous.
Acute periodontal abscesses can develop from an acute exacerbation of pre-existing periodontitis.

Treatment

OHI and effective mechanical plaque control are essential but are impaired by enlarged, bleeding tissues. Chemical antiplaque agents (e.g. chlorhexidine) should be prescribed and acute infections managed with systemic antimicrobials.

Sarcoidosis

Sarcoidosis is a systemic chronic granulomatous disorder of unknown aetiology typically affecting the lungs, lymph nodes, liver, skin and eyes.

Oral lesions are rare, but reported periodontal manifestations include a hyperplastic granulomatous gingivitis. Altered lymphocyte and neutrophil function may (rarely) lead to rapid periodontal destruction.

Wegener's Granulomatosis

Wegener's granulomatosis is a systemic disease characterised by necrotising granulomas of the respiratory system and kidneys, and necrotising vasculitis of small arteries.

There is a characteristic hyperplastic gingivitis with petechiae and an ulcerated 'strawberry' appearance.

Gingival condition improves when systemic drug therapy (prednisolone and cyclophosphamide) is initiated.

Epulides

Epulides are localised hyperplastic lesions arising from the gingiva.

Aetiology

Trauma and chronic irritation from plaque and calculus invoke a chronic inflammatory response in which continued inflammation and attempts at repair proceed concurrently. Excessive production of granulation tissue results, forming the epulis.

Clinical Features

Fibrous epulis is a firm, pink, pedunculated mass that may be ulcerated if traumatised. Histologically, it comprises chronically inflamed, hyperplastic fibrous tissue, which may be richly cellular or densely collagenous. Metaplastic bone and/or foci of dystrophic calcification are common.

Vascular epulis (pyogenic granuloma and pregnancy epulis) is a soft, purple–red swelling, frequently ulcerated, which bleeds readily. Histologically, a proliferation of richly vascular tissue is supported by a fibrous stroma with a thin, often extensively ulcerated epithelium. A pregnancy epulis is a pyogenic granuloma occurring in a pregnant female. Vascular and fibrous epulides probably represent different phases of the same inflammatory process.

Peripheral giant cell granuloma (GCG) presents as a dark reddish–purple, ulcerated swelling, frequently arising interdentally and often extending buccally and lingually. It may cause superficial erosion of crestal alveolar bone. Radiographs are essential to differentiate from a central GCG that has perforated the cortex to present as a peripheral swelling. Histologically, GCG contains multiple foci of osteoclast-like giant cells supported by a richly vascular and cellular stroma.

Treatment

Surgical excision is the treatment of choice. Haemostasis may be problematic when removing pregnancy epulides. These can be left until after parturition as they then tend to reduce in size and become increasingly fibrous. Excision during pregnancy generally results in recurrence.

Iatrogenic Gingival Enlargement

Denture-Induced Enlargement

Chronic trauma from ill-fitting dentures, particularly when associated with poor oral hygiene, can result in hyperplasia of the underlying gingival tissues. Frequently this is associated with prostheses supported by mucosa only, with inadequate gingival clearance and poor stability. The tissues may be oedematous, erythematous and bleed readily; they can become increasingly fibrous over the long term.

Treatment is with OHI, denture hygiene, RSI and replacement of defective prostheses.

Orthodontically Induced Enlargement

Orthodontic movement of teeth occasionally results in the 'heaping-up' of gingival soft tissues in the direction of tooth movement. This occurs more frequently when teeth are repositioned with removal appliances (tipping movement) than when using fixed appliances (bodily movement).

The gingiva 'accumulates' in the direction of tooth movement. It frequently affects the palatal gingiva adjacent to maxillary incisors when these are being retracted. The enlargement tends to resolve on completion of orthodontic treatment.

OHI and appliance hygiene are usually the only treatments needed.

Cystic Lesions

Gingival cysts account for less than 1% of cysts of the jaws. More common in neonates, these tend to resolve spontaneously in early life. In adults, they are generally chance findings in histological sections from gingivectomy specimens and are typically asymptomatic. Cystic lesions are probably odontogenic in origin, arising from remnants of the dental lamina.

Developmental lateral periodontal cysts may present with expansion of alveolar bone, but most are incidental findings on radiographs. They resemble gingival cysts if arising near the alveolar bone crest. Radiographically, they appear as a radiolucency with well-defined bony margins.

Treatment is by surgical excision.

1.9 Trauma and the Periodontium

LEARNING OBJECTIVES

You should:
- be alert to the possibility that certain traumatic injuries to the periodontium may be self-inflicted
- be aware of the potential relationships that exist traumatic occlusal forces and periodontal disease
- be able to classify traumatic incisor relationships.

The periodontium has an inherent capacity to adapt to physiological or traumatic forces that occur during normal function or hyperfunction. In some cases, the trauma exceeds the adaptive nature of the tissues and pathologic change and injury result.

SELF-INFLICTED TRAUMA

Factitious Gingivitis

A minor form of self-inflicted trauma is seen in young children. Food packing or local inflammation provides a locus of irritation and the child picks or rubs the area with a finger nail, pencil or abrasive food such as crisps or nuts. If untreated, ulceration and inflammation persist and gingival recession may ensue. The lesion usually resolves when the habit is corrected.

The lesions of the major form are more severe and widespread both intra- and extraorally. They present as ulcers, abrasions, gingival recession or blisters, which may be blood filled. Trauma can be inflicted subconsciously, or purposely in an attempt to deceive clinicians into diagnosing organic disease. Outlines of lesions provide clues as to the object used to produce them. The lesions are remarkably resistant to conventional treatment and may reflect an underlying psychological problem. Referral to a psychologist/psychiatrist is advised but rarely welcomed by patients.

Oral Hygiene Practices

Used incorrectly and without instruction, toothbrushes and interproximal cleaning aids can cause irreversible trauma to both periodontal tissues and teeth. Injudicious toothbrushing causes gingival abrasions, clefting and recession, which can be localised or generalised. Excessive toothbrushing force also produces typical V-shaped abrasion cavities. Localised defects can be caused by mini-interdental brushes, incorrect use of floss and dental woodpoints.

IATROGENIC TRAUMA

Dental procedures and components of poorly designed restorations or appliances can cause direct local irritation/trauma to the gingiva. Examples include:

- injudicious use of rotary, ultrasonic and scaling instruments
- placement of excessive gingival retraction cord or leaving remnants of material in the gingival sulcus after taking an impression
- spillage of caustic chemicals used in dental treatments
- components of fixed/removable orthodontic appliances
- components of removable partial dentures
- extension of a palatal denture base into the interproximal areas to rest upon the gingival papillae.

In the short term, traumatic lesions of the soft tissues are reversible when the stimulus is removed. More persistent chronic irritation can lead to gingival recession.

TRAUMATIC OCCLUSAL FORCES

Historical Perspective

In 1965, Irving Glickman suggested that, in order to understand fully the role of trauma from occlusion in periodontal disease, the periodontium should be considered as two zones:

1. The zone of irritation comprises the marginal and interdental gingiva, which are susceptible to plaque-induced inflammation.
2. The zone of co-destruction comprises the periodontal ligament, alveolar bone and cementum, which become involved when marginal gingival inflammation spreads in the alveolar crest.

Glickman's hypothesis was that excessive occlusal force, in the presence of gingivitis, acts as a co-destructive factor, altering the pathway of inflammation so that it spreads directly into the periodontal ligament (Fig. 1.14). The presence of inflammation was crucial in reducing the adaptive capacity

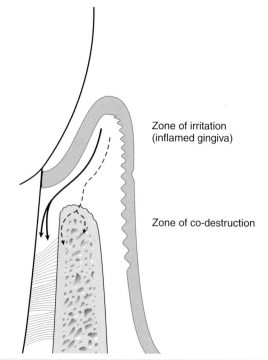

Fig. 1.14 Glickman's occlusal trauma hypothesis. Gingival inflammation in the presence of occlusal trauma spreads into the periodontal ligament *(solid arrows)* to produce a vertical bone defect, rather than through the channels in the alveolar bone *(dotted arrows)*.

Zone of irritation (inflamed gingiva)

Zone of co-destruction

of the healthy periodontium to occlusal forces, the consequence being the development of vertical, infrabony defects around affected teeth. This hypothesis is almost certainly an oversimplification of the interaction between periodontal inflammation and occlusal trauma. Nevertheless, it provided a basis from which subsequent animal model experiments were developed.

Jiggling forces act successively, in opposite directions, thus preventing the tooth from moving orthodontically away from the forces and subjecting the periodontium to alternating phases of pressure and tension. Such forces may originate from the components of removable prostheses or appliances. Observations made from animal experiments suggest that the teeth subjected to jiggling forces show an accelerated progression of experimental periodontitis compared with controls. Tooth mobility increases progressively as affected sites display both horizontal and vertical bone loss, with the latter being similar to that described by Glickman.

These observations have led to the following conclusions:

- Traumatic occlusal forces initiate neither periodontitis nor connective tissue attachment loss in a healthy periodontium, although there may be an increase in tooth mobility due to compensatory widening of the periodontal membrane space.
- Jiggling forces may exacerbate pre-existing periodontitis; both the inflammatory and traumatic components should be managed.

Occlusal Interferences

Occlusal interferences or premature occlusal contacts can arise when the occlusal morphology and/or position of

teeth are altered (e.g. following placement of restorations or after orthodontic therapy).

Clinical Features

Traumatic occlusal forces can give rise to pain, fracture or faceting of cusps, attrition, bruxism, increased tooth mobility and temporomandibular joint symptoms. Widening of the periodontal membrane space can be seen in radiographs and suggests tissue remodelling as an attempt to adapt to the interference. In the presence of periodontal inflammation, a persistent interference with increased occlusal loading can produce localised, infrabony defects.

Treatment

The periodontal inflammation must be resolved and the interference identified. It can be confirmed by mounting study models in retruded contact position on a semi-adjustable articulator. Occlusal adjustment is then undertaken.

TRAUMATIC INCISOR RELATIONSHIPS

The Akerly classification identifies the relationship between the maxillary and mandibular incisors, and the nature of complete overbite (Fig. 1.15).

Class I: lower incisors impinge upon the palatal mucosa.
Class II: lower incisors occlude on the palatal gingival margins of the maxillary teeth.
Class III: a deep, traumatic overbite (class II division 2) exists with shearing of the mandibular labial and maxillary palatal gingiva.
Class IV: lower incisors occlude with the palatal surfaces of upper incisors; evidence of tooth wear owing to attrition can be seen and there is minimal, if any, effect upon supporting tissues.

Aggravating factors include inherent development of a severe, class II division 2 incisor relationship; injudicious orthodontic or restorative treatment; gradual loss of posterior support with distal movement of premolars and canines; and the presence of powerful lip musculature.

Treatment

Interventive treatment is possible for developmental cases in childhood. In adults, it is important to establish periodontal health, to protect tissues temporarily with a soft acrylic splint and to restore posterior dimension. More complex relationships may require orthodontic therapy, orthognathic surgery and segmental or full mouth rehabilitation, with or without the use of Dahl and overlay appliances.

1.10 Periodontal Manifestations of Syndromes and Medical Conditions

LEARNING OBJECTIVES

You should:
- understand the periodontal implications of certain rare, and sometimes life-threatening, systemic conditions.

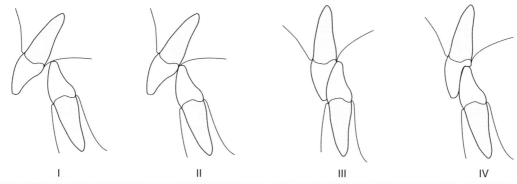

Fig. 1.15 The Akerly classification of traumatic incisor relationships. (I) Palatal trauma. (II) Trauma at the gingival crevice. (III) Shearing trauma of the class II division 2 overbite. (IV) Palatal attrition.

There are many systemic disorders that affect the periodontium through influencing periodontal inflammation. Several of these are associated with extensive periodontal tissue loss. Many of these syndromes are associated with profound abnormalities of neutrophil function, which predispose these patients to their periodontal problems. The following are examples; some occur more often and others very rarely in the population with varying strengths of association to periodontitis.

DOWN SYNDROME

Down syndrome is a common autosomal chromosome abnormality: trisomy of number 21. It occurs in about 1 in 700 births. The incidence increases with age of the mother at childbirth.

Clinical Features

Affected children have increased susceptibility to severe types of periodontitis. Institutionalised patients have a greater prevalence of dental and periodontal problems than those looked after at home. Systemic links to periodontitis are thought to be through intrinsic immune system defects. In addition, local clinical factors that predispose to accumulation of dental plaque and restrict access for its removal include:

- class III malocclusion with crowding
- anterior open bite
- lack of lip seal leading to drying of plaque
- reduced salivary flow
- high frenal attachments
- tongue thrusting.

Treatment

A good standard of plaque control can be difficult to achieve because of lack of dexterity and motivation. Use of antimicrobial mouthrinse may help to reduce plaque deposits between regular visits for scaling and prophylaxis.

PAPILLON–LEFEVRE SYNDROME

Papillon–Lefevre syndrome is a rare condition transmitted as an autosomal recessive trait that results from mutations in the cathepsin C gene, and that has an estimated incidence of 1–4 per million births. A history of consanguinity between parents is found in about 30% of affected individuals.

Clinical Features

The syndrome is characterised by a diffuse palmar–plantar hyperkeratosis and severe rapidly progressing periodontitis, with an onset of about 2 years of age. The child may be edentulous by 5–6 years. Progressive periodontal destruction usually also affects the permanent dentition, with patients becoming edentulous by the age of 20 years. The clinical presentation may show wide variation, and occasionally the skin and periodontal lesions present on their own as distinct clinical entities. Variations in periodontal presentation include those affecting only the primary dentition and a late-onset disorder where the primary dentition remains unaffected. Defects in neutrophil adhesion, chemotaxis and phagocytosis have been observed in some patients.

Treatment

Intensive periodontal therapy includes OHI, chlorhexidine rinses, scaling and prescription of antimicrobials to control acute phases. Severely involved teeth must be extracted. The loss of teeth is almost inevitable, even with a high degree of patient compliance. A more realistic aim is to maintain alveolar bone height to support removable or implant-retained prostheses.

EHLERS–DANLOS SYNDROME

Ehlers–Danlos syndrome is an autosomal dominant or recessive trait with the primary defect being related to the synthesis and extracellular polymerisation of collagen molecules.

Clinical Features

The main features are excessive mobility of joints and increased extensibility of skin, which is also susceptible to bruising and scarring following superficial wounds. The oral soft tissues are prone to bruising and haemorrhage because of defective support of the lamina propria. Gingival bleeding may occur after toothbrushing.

Pathology

Lesions are characterised by massive proliferation of Langerhans cells (resembling histiocytes), with varying numbers of eosinophils and multinucleate giant cells. Histopathological changes of teeth have been detected: enamel hypoplasia, abnormalities of dentine and an increased incidence of pulp stones.

Treatment

Conventional treatment for periodontal disease is undertaken but extreme caution must be taken because of the fragility of the soft tissues and their susceptibility to trauma.

Oral lesions are accessible for biopsy to confirm a diagnosis. Local excision and curettage of bone lesions is often successful, although the prognosis is poor when soft tissues become widely involved. When a patient presents with oral lesions, a complete radiographic screening or bone scan is needed to detect or exclude multifocal involvement.

LEUKOCYTE ADHESION-DEFICIENCY SYNDROME

The leukocyte adhesion-deficiency syndrome is a single gene defect with an autosomal recessive pattern of inheritance.

Clinical Features

Delayed separation of the umbilical cord occurs at birth and there is impaired wound healing and severe, often life-threatening bacterial infections. Severe periodontitis is present with gingivitis, profuse bleeding and suppurating pockets. The permanent dentition is also affected. In mild variants, symptoms can be mild and the disease appears stable over long periods, only for an acute phase to develop and the patient to deteriorate very rapidly. The syndrome is usually fatal by about 30 years.

Pathology

Impaired adhesion of neutrophils to vessel walls occurs as a result of restricted expression of cell surface integrins.

Treatment

Palliative treatment is used for periodontitis, which is of secondary importance to the life-threatening infections which occur.

LANGERHANS CELL HISTIOCYTOSIS

Langerhans cell histiocytosis is a group of conditions characterised by widespread proliferation of foci of histiocytic cells with features of Langerhans cells. The acute form, Letterer–Siwe disease (multifocal, multisystem), is usually fatal in infancy. Eosinophilic granuloma (unifocal) and Hand–Schuller–Christian disease (multifocal, unisystem) are closely related.

Clinical Features

Single or multiple osteolytic lesions involve the pituitary fossa and the frontal, orbital and sphenoid bones of the skull. Progressive involvement may cause diabetes insipidus and exophthalamus (Hand–Schuller–Christian disease). Other bones involved include the ribs, pelvis, clavicle, femur and humerus. Osteolytic involvement of alveolar bone is more common in the mandible and presents as severe periodontitis with a generalised and irregular pattern of bone resorption. Involved bone shows radiolucencies of considerable size. Pain and excessive tooth mobility are common early symptoms. Recurrent acute periodontal abscess formation is also common and the gingiva can be swollen, oedematous, necrotic and ulcerated.

HYPOPHOSPHATASIA

Hypophosphatasia is an inborn error of metabolism with autosomal recessive and dominant patterns of inheritance. There is a deficiency of the liver/kidney/bone isoenzyme of alkaline phosphatase, which is crucial for the mineralisation of hard tissues.

Clinical Features

Juvenile (childhood) hypophosphatasia has an age of onset around 2 years. The bone defects can lead to mild bowing of the legs, proptosis and a delay in closure of the fontanelles. Aplastic or hypoplastic cementum leads to premature loss of the primary dentition through extensive root resorption or bone loss as a result of a weakened periodontal attachment and disuse atrophy. The gingiva can appear quite healthy. In the adult form, which presents during middle age, the periodontal changes are localised to the incisor region.

Treatment

When primary teeth are lost, it is important to maintain space for their permanent successors, which erupt prematurely.

1.11 Treatment of Periodontal Disease

LEARNING OBJECTIVES

You should:
- understand the importance of effective plaque control in determining the success of periodontal therapy
- know how plaque control may be achieved in individual patients
- know the instruments and techniques required to perform RSI
- understand the principal indications for various surgical treatments
- be familiar with the basic procedures involved in periodontal surgery.

MECHANICAL PLAQUE CONTROL

Plaque control refers to the removal of plaque from the tooth surface and gingival tissues, and prevention of new microbial growth. Effective plaque control results in resolution of gingival inflammation and is fundamentally important in all periodontal therapy. Periodontal treatment performed in the absence of plaque control is certain to fail, resulting in disease recurrence. Mechanical plaque control is performed using toothbrushes, toothpaste and other cleaning aids. Plaque-control programmes should be tailored to the requirements of individual patients. Motivation of patients to change their behavioural habits is a great challenge and patients must be encouraged to understand the importance of their contribution to maintaining health and preventing disease.

Powered Toothbrushes

The brushheads of powered (electric) toothbrushes tend to be more compact than those of their manual counterparts; this feature facilitates interproximal brushing and cleaning of the less accessible posterior teeth. Bundles of bristles are arranged in rows (similar to manual brushes) or in a circular pattern mounted in a round head. Some brushes have single, compact tufts, which are specifically designed for interproximal cleaning. The traditional design of brushhead operates with a side-to-side or back-and-forth motion. The circular heads have an oscillating motion and the single tufted heads also operate with a rotary action.

Traditionally, powered toothbrushes have been considered advantageous for people with disabilities, patients with fixed orthodontic appliances and those who are hospitalised or institutionalised and who may need a careworker or nurse to support them with oral hygiene.

Numerous studies have confirmed that, for most patients, powered toothbrushes are slightly more effective than manual brushes. This may be because of better mechanical cleaning *per se*, although the 'novelty effect' of using a powered toothbrush is a likely contributing factor.

Toothbrushes

Toothbrushes vary in design and size, and the type of brush used is a matter of personal preference. Bristles are generally made of nylon, which is relatively flexible, resistant to fracture and does not become saturated with water. Bristles are arranged in tufts, and rounded bristles cause fewer scratches on the gingiva than do flat-ended bristles. Softer bristles have greater flexibility and have been shown to reach further interproximally and subgingivally. Hard bristles are more likely to result in gingival trauma. The technique and the force applied when brushing are more important determinants of plaque-removal capability and likelihood of gingival trauma than the hardness of the bristles themselves. With use, toothbrushes begin to show signs of excessive wear and flattening of bristles; generally, they should be replaced approximately every 3 months.

Toothpastes

Toothpastes are used as aids for cleaning tooth surfaces and contain abrasives (e.g. silica), water, preservatives, flavouring, colouring, detergents and therapeutic agents (e.g. fluoride). Abrasives (approximately 20–40% of the paste) enhance plaque removal but may result in damage to the tooth surface if there is overzealous brushing. Smokers' toothpastes and tooth powders contain significantly higher proportions of abrasives and their use is not recommended. Chemotherapeutic agents (e.g. chlorhexidine) may be added to toothpastes and are discussed in more detail in the following sections.

Toothbrushing Techniques

Powered toothbrushes have specific designs and techniques for use to be effective. It is therefore important to demonstrate the manufacturer's recommended way of using the brush directly with the patient. For manual toothbrushes the majority of patients use a 'horizontal scrub' technique, which frequently does not clean effectively around gingival margins and can lead to tooth wear. When brushing, a systematic approach is essential, and all accessible surfaces of all teeth should be cleaned thoroughly. The Bass technique is useful for the majority of patients with or without periodontal disease. The Charters' technique is useful for gentle gingival cleaning, particularly during healing immediately after periodontal surgery.

Bass Technique
- The toothbrush is placed at the gingival margin, with bristles orientated at 45° to the long axis of the tooth, pointing in an apical direction.
- Short vibratory strokes are applied to the brush so that the bristles are not dislodged (this forces the bristles interproximally and approximately 1 mm subgingivally, resulting in gingival blanching).
- After about 20 strokes, the brush is repositioned to clean the next group of teeth.

Charters' Technique
- The toothbrush is placed on the tooth with the bristles orientated at 45° to the long axis of the tooth, pointing in a coronal direction, such that the sides of the bristles are against the gingiva.
- A short back-and-forth motion is applied so that the sides of the bristles flex against the gingiva.

Interproximal Cleaning Aids

Interproximal areas are particularly susceptible to plaque accumulation. Toothbrushing does not effectively remove plaque from these surfaces and additional cleaning aids are required.

Dental Floss
Floss is usually made from nylon and is available as a twisted or untwisted multifilament, with or without a coating of wax (wax facilitates passage beyond the contact point), as a thread or in tape form. Floss made from expanded polytetrafluoroethylene (Teflon) materials that do not fray is also available. The plaque-removal capabilities of different types of floss do not vary significantly. Floss should be wrapped around the fingers then stretched tightly between the thumbs, or thumb and first finger, of each hand so that it can be eased carefully past the interproximal contact point. The floss should be moved carefully up and down the proximal surface of each tooth, from just below the contact point to just below the gingival margin. Floss holders, which stretch the floss between two plastic arms, may be useful for patients with limited manual dexterity.

Interspace Brushes
Interspace brushes look like toothbrushes that contain just one tuft of bristles. These are especially useful for cleaning:

- interproximal surfaces of teeth when adjacent teeth are absent
- distal surfaces of the most posterior remaining tooth
- the lingual surfaces of mandibular teeth
- around orthodontic appliances

- areas of gingival recession
- areas of crowding with instanding teeth that are missed by a regular toothbrush
- tooth/root concavities and incipient (class I) furcation lesions.

Interdental Brushes

Interdental brushes are conical or tube-like brushes ('bottle brushes') made of bristles mounted on a twisted metal wire handle. They are used by patients with periodontitis to clean:

- interproximally, particularly in locations where there is loss of the interdental papillae and there is sufficient room for the brush to be placed
- in class II and class III furcations
- around implant restorations (wire handle should be plastic coated to prevent scratching of the titanium surface).

CHEMICAL PLAQUE CONTROL

Chemical agents have been incorporated into mouthrinses and toothpastes with the objective of inhibiting the formation of plaque and calculus. Antiplaque agents may also have a significant clinical effect of resolving an established gingivitis. Available products include the cationic agents and phenols.

Cationic Agents

Chlorhexidine Digluconate

Chlorhexidine is available as a mouthrinse (0.2%, 0.12% or 0.06% w/v). The compound can also be applied as a gel and has been incorporated into chewing gum, slow-release devices and periodontal packs.

At low concentrations, chlorhexidine is bacteriostatic; at high concentrations, it is bactericidal. The mode of action of chlorhexidine in killing bacteria is dependent upon the drug having access to cell walls. This is facilitated by electrostatic forces, since chlorhexidine is positively charged, while the phosphate and carboxyl groups of bacterial cell walls carry negative charges. Binding causes disruption of the osmotic barrier and interference with membrane transport.

Rinsing with chlorhexidine reduces the number of bacteria in saliva by between 50% and 90%. A maximum reduction of 95% occurs around 5 days, after which the numbers increase gradually to maintain an overall reduction of 70–80% at 40 days.

An important property of chlorhexidine is its substantivity, that is, the retention in the mouth and subsequent release from oral structures. After a 1-minute oral rinse of 10 mL of chlorhexidine 0.2%, approximately 30% of the drug is retained; within 15 seconds of rinsing, half will have bonded to receptor molecules.

Chlorhexidine mouthrinses and gels are beneficial:

- after periodontal surgery
- in the management of periodontal problems for people with disabilities
- for preventing phenytoin-induced gingival overgrowth
- in the management of gingivitis and periodontitis in patients with HIV
- for patients wearing fixed orthodontic appliances or an intermaxillary fixation device.

The main unwanted effects are staining of the teeth, restorations and the tongue, and taste disturbances. There are increasing levels of hypersensitivity reactions in patients reported.

Quaternary Ammonium Compounds

Quaternary ammonium compounds include cetylpyridinium chloride (often combined with domiphen bromide), benzalkonium chloride and benzethonium chloride. These substances have a net positive charge, which reacts with the negatively charged phosphate groups on bacterial cell walls. The walls are disrupted, resulting in increased permeability and loss of cell contents.

Studies suggest that cetylpyridinium chloride 0.05% (with or without domiphen bromide) and benzethonium chloride cause a reduction in plaque of between 25% and 35%, but with less obvious effects on gingival inflammation. Cetylpyridinium chloride (0.1%) is also marketed as a prebrushing rinse.

Phenols

Phenols exert a non-specific antibacterial action that is dependent upon the ability of the drug, in the non-ionised form, to penetrate the lipid components of bacterial cell walls. Phenolic compounds also exhibit anti-inflammatory properties, which may result from their ability to inhibit neutrophil chemotaxis, the generation of neutrophil superoxide anions and the production of prostaglandin synthetase.

Listerine

An over-the-counter antiplaque agent that contains thymol (0.06%), eucalyptol (0.09%), methyl salicylate (0.06%) and methanol (0.04%) in 16.9% alcohol. (Listerine, Johnston & Johnston, xxxxxx) I can't find a UK address for J&J. Twice daily rinsing with 20 mL of Listerine as a supplement to normal oral hygiene has demonstrated a 35% reduction in plaque and gingivitis. An alcohol-free product is also available.

Triclosan

Triclosan is a bisphenol, non-ionic germicide with a broad spectrum of activity against Gram-positive and Gram-negative bacteria and fungi. The compound adsorbs onto the lipid portion of the bacterial cell membrane. At low concentrations, triclosan interferes with vital transport mechanisms in bacteria. A concentration of 0.1–0.2% is suitably efficacious with minimal side-effects. Activity is enhanced when the compound is combined with zinc citrate or incorporated into a co-polymer of methoxyethylene and maleic acid. The co-polymer increases the substantivity of triclosan and acts as a reservoir.

ROOT SURFACE INSTRUMENTATION

Non-surgical management (NSM) of periodontal diseases comprises OHI and root surface instrumentation (RSI), the preferred term for what is also known as scaling and root planing (SRP):

- Scaling is the removal of plaque and calculus from the tooth surface.
- RSI is the removal of subgingival plaque and calculus with the aim being to disrupt the subgingival biofilm.

RSI is generally undertaken with various hand instruments and/or ultrasonic scalers. As a result of OHI and RSI, plaque bacteria are reduced and there is resolution of the inflammatory lesion in the periodontium. This leads to shrinkage of the gingival soft tissues (as oedema resolves), increased resistance to probe tip penetration by the tissues at the base of the pocket (as inflammation resolves) and the formation of a long junctional epithelium at the base of the pocket. All these mechanisms contribute to the reduction in probing depths observed after effective NSM, although gingival shrinkage and resolution of inflammation have the most significant effects on pocket reduction.

Clinical research has shown that effective OHI alone can reduce mean probing depths by approximately 0.5 mm, and RSI results in additional reductions of about 1.0–1.5 mm. There is no initial probing depth above which NSM does not confer a benefit to patients. However, RSI performed at sites with minimal or no pocketing is detrimental rather than beneficial. RSI of shallow sites with initial probing depths <3 mm results in loss of attachment to the root surface as a result of mechanical trauma from instrumentation.

Periodontal Instruments

There are a number of instruments required to perform effective RSI.

Periodontal explorers are used to detect subgingival calculus deposits and root surface roughness. A variety of shapes and designs are available; generally, all are very light instruments (to improve tactility) with fine curved tips to reach subgingivally.

Sickle scalers are strong, heavy instruments used to remove supragingival calculus deposits. They have two cutting surfaces that converge in a sharp tip. They should not be used subgingivally as they will traumatise the gingiva. They are inserted under ledges of calculus and used with a pull stroke to remove the calculus from the tooth surface.

Curettes are fine instruments used for subgingival RSI. They are designed to adapt to the root surface and provide good access to deep pockets without causing significant trauma to the soft tissues. Curettes have a spoon-shaped blade with a rounded tip, and there are cutting edges on both sides of the blade. Curettes can be area specific: different curettes are designed to adapt to specific anatomical areas of the dentition and are used to instrument specific root surfaces. Universal curettes have cutting edges that afford access to the root surfaces by altering their position and angulation.

Periodontal hoes are used for removal of ledges of calculus, primarily from broad, flat root surfaces. They are inserted into the pocket, placed against the tooth surface and pulled coronally to remove calculus. They should not be used in furcations as they will score the cemental surface in this anatomically complex region.

Chisels are used to clean the interproximal surfaces of teeth that are too closely positioned to permit access to other scalers, particularly mandibular anterior teeth. They are inserted from the buccal aspect and pushed lingually while maintaining contact against the interproximal surface of the tooth.

Ultrasonic scalers are used for RSI. An electrical generator delivers energy to a handpiece in the form of high-frequency (ultrasonic) vibrations such that the tip vibrates at between 20,000 and 50,000 Hz, depending on the machine. A variety of inserts (tips) are available for instrumentation. Water cooling is essential to dissipate the heat generated by the vibrations; ultrasonic scalers should be operated in a wet field and kept in motion (to prevent heat build-up and also gouging of the tooth surface). The vibrating tip shatters cementum adhering to the tooth surface. Within the water spray mist, tiny vacuums develop that quickly collapse, releasing energy (cavitation). The cavitating water spray also helps to flush calculus debris and plaque from the periodontal pocket. Because of the splatter and aerosol generated by the scaler, proper barrier and respiratory protection infection control measures should be employed. Finally, care should be employed around adhesive and porcelain restorations as these can be damaged or removed by the scaler.

Polishing instruments are rubber cups used with polishing pastes to clean and polish the tooth surface. Rubber cups are used in the slow handpiece and are disposed of after use. Overzealous use of a rubber cup, particularly if combined with a coarse or abrasive paste, can result in abrasion of the tooth surface. Rubber cups are used in preference to bristle brushes as the latter can traumatise the gingival soft tissues and, therefore, should not be used close to the gingival margin.

Techniques

For effective instrumentation, the operator should be comfortably seated, the patient should be supine in the dental chair and there should be good illumination. An assistant should retract the oral soft tissues, where necessary, and maintain a clean operating field through the use of an aspirator. The operator should have a good knowledge of dental anatomy and root morphology, and appropriately selected, sharp instruments should be used. The *modified pen grip* is preferred, in which the instrument is held by the thumb, index finger and middle finger in the same way as a pen is held. The index finger is bent so it can be positioned well above the middle finger on the instrument handle. In this way, a triangle of force is applied to the instrument, and this tripod effect allows for stability and tactility during use. The fourth finger (ring finger) is used as a *finger rest* to stabilise the hand and reduce the likelihood of uncontrolled movements and injury. The finger rest also acts as a fulcrum for working movements of the instrument. Finger rests may be on tooth surfaces in the immediate vicinity of the working area, they may be cross arch (on tooth surfaces in the other side of the same arch), opposite arch or extraoral.

Calculus should be identified prior to RSI. Supragingival calculus can be seen with good lighting and a dry field. The dark colour of subgingival calculus may be visible through thin overlying gingival tissues. An air syringe to retract the gingiva may also reveal subgingival calculus. Interproximal calculus may be visible radiographically. An explorer should be used subgingivally to check for calculus, grooves, furcations and other anatomical structures.

Scaling instruments should be *adapted* to the tooth surface, which means that the cutting edge of the instrument conforms to the anatomy of the root surface. This results in maximal efficiency during scaling and minimal damage to the adjacent tissues. The cutting edge should be *angled* at between 45° and 90° to the root surface: less than 45° and the instrument will not engage the calculus; more than 90° and tissue trauma will be achieved instead. Instruments should be placed apical to the calculus and *pulled* coronally with firm, controlled strokes to remove the calculus. Increasing *lateral pressure* may need to be applied to remove particularly tenacious deposits. Following RSI, debris should be flushed from the pocket with an irrigating solution (e.g. chlorhexidine) in a syringe with a blunt needle.

Historically, dentists aimed to leave root surfaces 'glassy smooth and hard' following RSI (referred to then as root planing). Research has shown that this is not necessary and, indeed, may result in damage to the tooth by removal of cementum. Instead, we now consider that RSI aims to remove plaque and calculus and disrupt the subgingival biofilm as the vehicle to reduce inflammation in the periodontal tissues. The pockets should not be probed sooner than 6–8 weeks after RSI as this may interfere with the healing process. Post-treatment evaluation of the healing response to RSI should be considered together with patient plaque-control capabilities and motivation prior to embarking on further treatments, such as additional RSI, adjunctive antimicrobial usage or periodontal surgery.

SURGICAL TREATMENT

The major limitation of RSI (non-surgical treatment) is that root surfaces cannot be visualised directly, and access for removal of subgingival plaque and calculus may be limited. Periodontal therapies (both surgical and non-surgical) are aimed at the removal of all plaque and calculus, and while this is seldom achieved, improvements in periodontal health are observed nonetheless. Therefore, while total elimination of causative factors is an appropriate goal for periodontists, reduction of plaque and calculus below a certain threshold acceptable to the host may be a more realistic aim. This tips the balance between the host and bacteria in favour of the host, allowing reduction in the signs of inflammation and improvements in clinical parameters.

It is typical, therefore, for patients to receive a course of non-surgical therapy and then to be monitored. For those sites that do not respond favourably to treatment (e.g. because of complicated local anatomy such as grooves or furcation involvements), then a decision may be taken to expose the area surgically for further treatment. The majority of periodontal surgery is undertaken to improve access to the root surface for cleaning, generally via a flap procedure, although there are also several indications for specific surgical procedures. *It is fundamentally important that a high level of oral hygiene is maintained before and after surgery; surgical treatments will fail if plaque is not adequately controlled.*
Other indications for periodontal surgery include:

- crown lengthening to increase clinical crown length
- gingivectomy for the removal of overgrown gingival tissues
- guided tissue regeneration (GTR) to regenerate periodontal supporting structures
- mucogingival surgery for correction of mucogingival and aesthetic defects.

Flap Surgery

Following flap procedures, and the removal of plaque, calculus and chronically inflamed granulation tissue, healing occurs by the formation of a long junctional epithelium. This leads to reduced probing depths, which are easier to maintain in the maintenance phase of periodontal therapy. A new connective tissue attachment may form following flap procedures, although this cannot be predicted with certainty. The long junctional epithelium that forms following periodontal surgery is more susceptible to plaque-induced breakdown than the original connective tissue attachment and, consequently, postoperative plaque control must be of a high standard.

Flap procedures can be classified as involving *replaced flaps* or *apically repositioned flaps*, with or without bone removal (Boxes 1.1–1.3).

Replaced Flap, No Bone Removal

A replaced flap is one that is replaced at (or very close to) its presurgical position and is not apically repositioned. The modified Widman flap is an example of a replaced flap (see Box 1.1).

Indications
- Access to root surface for RSI.
- Elimination of deep pockets.

Box 1.1 Technique for Replaced Flap Procedure (Fig. 1.16).

1. Inverse bevel incision (first incision) (approximately 0.5 mm from the gingival margin) to the level of the alveolar bone.
2. Crevicular incision (second incision) from the base of the pocket to the bone crest.
3. Full-thickness mucoperiosteal flap is raised to expose alveolar bone crest, and the remaining inflamed pocket epithelium and connective tissue are removed with a horizontal incision (third incision).
4. The crest of the alveolar bone is exposed and the root surface is instrumented.
5. The flap is replaced at the original level and sutured. Simple interrupted sutures may be used, although vertical mattress sutures, which position the tissues more coronally, often provide better aesthetics. A surgical pack may be placed if there is continued bleeding but is often not necessary if the flaps are well adapted.

Box 1.2 Technique for Apically Positioned Flap.

The procedure is similar to that for the replaced flap except:
1. The initial incision may be made further from the gingival margin to thin the tissues and allow for better adaptation to the tooth and bone during suturing.
2. Flaps are raised to a greater extent.
3. Flaps are apically repositioned during suturing so that they just cover the bone crest. Trimming of the flaps may be necessary to conform to the shape of the alveolar bone and teeth.
4. Interrupted sutures are placed to hold the tissues in their new position.

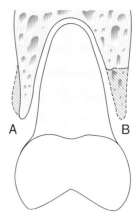

Fig. 1.17 Techniques for bone removal. *(A)* Osteoplasty. *(B)* Ostectomy.

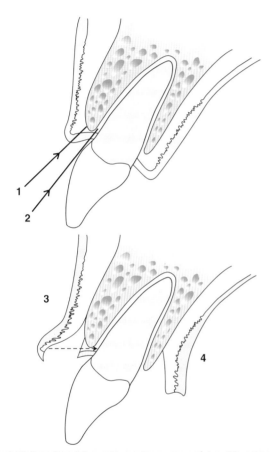

Fig. 1.16 A replaced flap with no bone removal (modified Widman flap). 1 = inverse bevel incision; 2 = crevicular incision; 3 = a full-thickness flap is raised and the remaining inflamed pocket epithelium and connective tissue are removed with a horizontal incision or a sharp curette; 4 = the crest of the alveolar bone is exposed and the root surface is accessible for instrumentation.

Advantages
- Good access to root surface.
- Replacement of flap at presurgical location minimises problems of aesthetics and root hypersensitivity.
- Width of keratinised gingiva is maintained.

Disadvantages
- Deep, infrabony pockets may not be eliminated.
- Long junctional epithelium is formed.

Apically Repositioned Flap, No Bone Removal
The procedure involving an apically repositioned flap is similar to the replaced flap procedure, except that the flap is elevated to a greater distance, exposing more alveolar bone, and is then apically repositioned and sutured just coronal to the alveolar bone crest (see Box 1.2). This procedure is not recommended for anterior teeth, where apical repositioning of the flaps leads to aesthetic problems. However, at posterior sites where aesthetic concerns are not as great, this technique is preferred over the replaced flap as it results in greater pocket reductions.

Indications
- Access to root surface for instrumentation.
- Elimination of deeper pockets, particularly in areas where aesthetics are not important.

Advantage
- Greater probing depth reduction as a result of apical repositioning of the flap.

Disadvantage
- Apical repositioning can create problems of aesthetics and dentine hypersensitivity owing to root exposure.

Apically Repositioned Flap, With Bone Removal
The procedure used for the eradication of deep pockets involves the loss of some alveolar bone and connective tissue attachment (see Box 1.3).

Indications
- Deep, infrabony pockets in areas where aesthetics are not a concern
- Adequate remaining bony support for the tooth once procedure (including bone removal) is completed.

Advantage
- Good reductions in pocket depths.

Disadvantages
- Removal of alveolar bone and connective tissue attachment to the root surface.
- Problems of aesthetics and hypersensitivity as a result of root exposure.

Crown Lengthening
Crown lengthening procedures are essentially apically repositioned flaps with bone removal, usually undertaken to

increase clinical crown height prior to placement of restorations in order to maximise retention and preserve the *supracrestal tissue attachment (biologic width)*. The concept of supracrestal tissue attachment covers the importance of maintaining a distance of approximately 2–2.5 mm between the margins of a restoration and the alveolar bone crest. This space is required for the epithelial and connective tissue components of the soft tissue attachment to the root surface (see Fig. 1.1). If restorations are placed that encroach upon this space, inflammation and attachment loss may occur.

Indications for Crown Lengthening

- Short clinical crowns requiring increased retention for the placement of full coronal restorations (including cases of gross tooth wear requiring full mouth rehabilitation).
- Deep, subgingivally located crown preparation margins, resulting in difficulty finishing margins and taking impressions, and also encroachment on the supracrestal tissue attachment.
- Subgingival caries.
- Root fractures or root resorption in the cervical third of the tooth root.
- Aesthetic improvement of anterior teeth with short clinical crowns and a high lip line.

Gingivectomy

Gingivectomies are primarily used to remove excess gingival tissue in gingival enlargement (e.g. resulting from drug-induced gingival enlargement) (Box 1.4).

Guided Tissue Regeneration

Following periodontal surgery, the newly instrumented root surface is rapidly colonised by gingival epithelial cells that migrate apically to form a long junctional epithelium. This prevents the formation of new connective tissue attachment to the root surface, the ultimate goal of periodontal therapy. GTR aims to manipulate the repopulation of the wound such that pluripotential cells from the periodontal ligament proliferate and migrate into the healing area. These cells have the capability to differentiate into fibroblasts, cementoblasts and osteoblasts and thus can produce new periodontal ligament fibres, cementum and bone to regenerate the lost connective tissue attachment to the root surface.

GTR is achieved by placing barrier membranes over periodontal defects to exclude gingival epithelium and

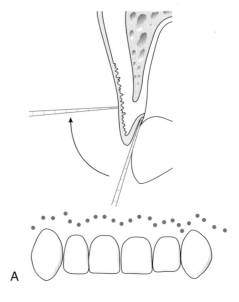

A

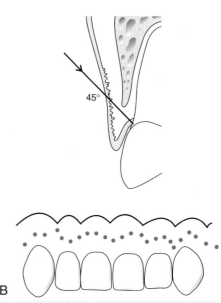

B

Fig. 1.18 Gingivectomy. (A) The depths of the pockets are marked on the gingival surface using pocket-marking tweezers or a pocket probe. (B) A bevelled 45° incision contacts the tooth surface at the base of the pocket.

connective tissues, and to create a space into which proliferating cells from the periodontal ligament and bone can migrate (Fig. 1.19). Key aspects of GTR include exclusion of epithelium, preservation of space under the membrane into which cells can migrate and formation of a stable blood clot under the membrane. Originally, membranes were non-resorbable, but these required removal 4–6 weeks after placement. Resorbable membranes (e.g. polylactic acid or collagen) biodegrade within the tissues over 1–2 months and do not require a second surgical procedure for removal. Membranes can also be reinforced so that the membrane can be 'tented' to create space for the development of a blood clot. Membranes may also be placed over

---

Box 1.4   Technique for Gingivectomy (Fig. 1.18).

1. Pockets are probed, and probing depths are marked on the gingival tissues with a sharp probe (see Fig. 1.18A).
2. A 45° bevelled incision is made apical to the points marking the base of the pockets and directed coronally to the base of the pocket (see Fig. 1.18B).
3. The excised gingival tissues (including the pocket wall) are removed.
4. Remaining granulation tissue is excised and the root surface is instrumented.
5. A surgical pack is placed to protect the healing area. Healing occurs by secondary intention.

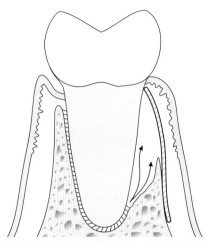

Fig. 1.19 Guided tissue regeneration. A barrier membrane is placed over the bone defect to exclude epithelium and to create a space for blood clot and migration of pluripotential cells of the periodontal ligament (arrows).

implants and in conjunction with bone grafts in an attempt to increase the quantity of available bone.

GTR produces most predictable results in class II furcations and in two- and three-walled osseous defects (Box 1.5). Improvements may be gained in class III furcations, although complete bone fill is rare. Complications include infection, perforation of the flap (sharp corners on the membrane must be trimmed prior to placement), sloughing of the flap and gingival recession (1–2 mm recession may occur following GTR procedures).

Mucogingival Surgery

Surgical procedures for the correction of mucogingival defects are varied and range from simple gingivectomies or crown-lengthening procedures (e.g. to increase the clinical crown length if there is a 'gummy' smile with a high lip line) to complex gingival grafting procedures (Boxes 1.6–1.8). In patients with bone defects, GTR and bone grafting may also be employed to increase the bulk of available alveolar bone. Grafting procedures generally aim to cover exposed roots, to increase the width of keratinised gingiva and to prevent further gingival recession. Grafting procedures include the *free gingival graft*, the *pedicle sliding graft* and the *subepithelial connective tissue graft*. The donor site heals by secondary intention.

Box 1.5   Technique for Guided Tissue Regeneration (Fig. 1.20).

1. A full-thickness mucoperiosteal flap is raised.
2. The root surface is thoroughly instrumented to remove plaque, calculus and granulation tissue.
3. Membrane is selected and trimmed to extend approximately 3 mm beyond the margins of the osseous defect, then it is sutured against the tooth with a sling suture.
4. Flaps are replaced and sutured, ensuring the membrane is fully covered.
5. A periodontal pack is placed if necessary.

Box 1.6   Technique for a Free Gingival Graft (Fig. 1.21).

1. Recipient site where gingival recession has occurred (see Fig. 1.21A) is prepared by raising a split-thickness flap to generate a connective tissue bed to receive the graft (see Fig. 1.21B). The flap (primarily epithelial tissue) is discarded so that only a layer of immobile connective tissue remains.
2. Epithelium and a thin layer of connective tissue are harvested from the donor site, usually the palatal mucosa. A template of sterile aluminium foil may be used to ensure the graft is the right shape and size for the recipient site. The graft is trimmed to fit, and any glandular tissue is removed.
3. The graft is placed, connective tissue side down, onto the recipient site (see Fig. 1.21C). Any clot or debris must be removed from the recipient site to ensure the graft is closely adapted to the underlying connective tissues.
4. The graft is sutured in place, and a periodontal dressing applied.

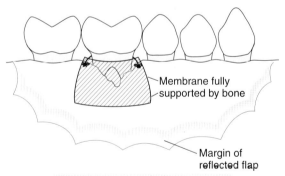

Fig. 1.20 Guided tissue regeneration.

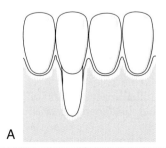
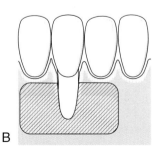
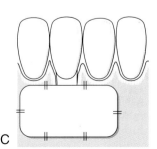

Fig. 1.21 Free gingival graft. (A) Gingival recession. (B) Recipient site prepared by raising a split-thickness flap. (C) Graft from palate placed over recipient site and sutured. Some coverage of the root is achieved but the principal aim is to limit further recession by increasing the width of keratinised tissue.

Box 1.7   Technique for Pedicle Sliding Graft (Fig. 1.22).

1. Pedicle flap is raised by split-thickness dissection from keratinised tissues adjacent to a narrow recession defect (see Fig. 1.22A). A split-thickness flap is preferred because it results in more rapid healing of the donor site.
2. Gingival margins around the exposed root are excised (see Fig. 1.22A).
3. The flap is repositioned laterally to cover the root and sutured, and a periodontal dressing is placed (see Fig. 1.22B).

Box 1.8   Technique for a Subepithelial Connective Tissue Graft (Fig. 1.23).

This procedure to deal with a recession defect (see Fig. 1.23A) is similar to the free gingival graft procedure, except for the following:
1. A split-thickness flap is raised at the recipient site to beyond the mucogingival junction (see Fig. 1.23B).
2. A wedge of connective tissue and overlying epithelium is harvested from the palate (see Fig. 1.23C).
3. The graft is placed with the strip of epithelium located at the cementoenamel junction and sutured (see Fig. 1.23D).
4. The flap is repositioned coronally to cover the graft and sutured.
This technique, which requires a split-thickness graft, has the advantage that the graft receives a blood supply from two sources: the overlying flap, and the underlying connective tissues and periosteum.

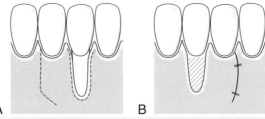

Fig. 1.22 Pedicle sliding graft. (A) Gingival margin around the exposed root is excised and a split-thickness flap raised. (B) The flap is rotated laterally to cover the defect. The donor site heals by secondary intention.

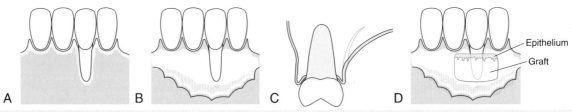

Fig. 1.23 Subepithelial connective tissue graft. (A) Recession defect. (B) A split-thickness flap is elevated. (C) A 'wedge' of epithelium and connective tissue is dissected from the palate. (D) The graft is sutured over the defect with the band of epithelium at the cementoenamel junction and the flap is then sutured over the graft.

Self-Assessment: Questions

MULTIPLE CHOICE QUESTIONS (TRUE/FALSE)

1. Dental calculus:
   a. Is a causative agent in periodontitis
   b. Forms on the coronal aspects of teeth only
   c. Is plaque that has become mineralised with ions from gingival crevicular fluid
   d. Contains predominantly crystals of hydroxyapatite when mature
   e. Does not contain bacteria
2. *Porphyromonas gingivalis*:
   a. Is one of the first bacterial species to colonise a newly cleaned tooth surface
   b. Has the ability to invade gingival soft tissues
   c. Is generally encapsulated
   d. Is a causative organism for molar-incisor pattern periodontitis
   e. Is an obligate aerobe
3. Concerning the following organisms associated with periodontal diseases:
   a. *P. gingivalis* and *A. actinomycetemcomitans* are frequently isolated from healthy sites
   b. Streptococci and *Actinomyces* spp. are early colonising organisms
   c. *F. nucleatum* is an anaerobic motile rod implicated in periodontitis
   d. *A. actinomycetemcomitans* is effectively removed from periodontally involved sites by root surface instrumentation (RSI)
   e. *A. actinomycetemcomitans* can be eradicated by the use of systemic tetracycline
4. The established inflammatory lesion of gingivitis:
   a. Is recognisable histologically within 2–4 days of plaque growth
   b. Represents the transition between gingivitis and periodontitis

c. Is dominated by a T lymphocyte infiltrate

d. Is associated clinically with increased flow of gingival crevicular fluid (GCF)

e. Can be diagnosed clinically by the presence of gingival erythema and oedema

5. Polymorphonuclear leukocytes (neutrophils):
    a. Are not found in the gingival sulcus
    b. Secrete matrix metalloproteinase (MMP) type 1
    c. Contribute to the destruction of the periodontal tissues during periodontitis
    d. Represent the first line of cellular defences against periodontal pathogens
    e. Are almost always found in the gingival tissues

6. Guided tissue regeneration (GTR):
    a. Is essential for class I furcation defects
    b. Is dependent on the formation of a stable blood clot for best results
    c. Typically results in probing depth reductions, attachment level gains and decreased gingival recession
    d. Requires the use of a non-resorbable membrane (e.g. ePTFE) for best results
    e. Results in osseointegration

7. Periodontal flap surgery:
    a. Is indicated when non-surgical treatment is contra-indicated owing to poor plaque control
    b. Results in the formation of a long junctional epithelium
    c. Is the surgical treatment of choice for drug-induced gingival overgrowth
    d. Frequently results in compromised aesthetics through gingival recession
    e. Usually results in loss of the keratinised gingiva

8. Regarding alveolar bone destruction in periodontitis:
    a. Vertical bony defects have a better prognosis than horizontal defects following non-surgical treatment
    b. Fenestrations and dehiscences predispose sites to periodontal breakdown
    c. Three-walled vertical defects are well suited for treatment by guided tissue regeneration
    d. Radiographs provide an accurate representation of sites undergoing active bone loss
    e. Osteoclasts are stimulated to resorb bone by inter-leukin-1β

9. Regarding periodontal surgery:
    a. The gingivectomy incision should commence at the level of the base of the pocket
    b. One major goal of guided tissue regeneration (GTR) is to exclude epithelial cells from the healing area
    c. Split-thickness flaps are raised when repositioning flaps apically
    d. Plaque control is less critical than when considering non-surgical treatment
    e. Gingivectomy wounds heal by granulation

10. A traumatic occlusal force acting on a tooth with a healthy periodontium will likely cause:
    a. Gingivitis
    b. Periodontal disease
    c. Radiographic widening of the periodontal membrane space
    d. Increased tooth mobility
    e. Gingival recession

11. Vertical, infrabony defects are frequently seen on radiographs:
    a. In patients with molar-incisor pattern periodontitis
    b. Adjacent to a tooth which has 'tipped' into an extraction space
    c. Adjacent to an overhanging restoration
    d. On teeth that serve as abutments to partial dentures
    e. On teeth that serve as abutments for bridge retainers

12. In periodontal health:
    a. The width of keratinised gingiva is the same through the mouth
    b. The alveolar bone crest is at the same level as the cementoenamel junction
    c. Gingival crevicular fluid (GCF) is absent
    d. Teeth show no mobility
    e. There are no periodontal pockets

13. The aim of root surface instrumentation (RSI) is to:
    a. Remove calculus deposits and disrupt the subgingival biofilm
    b. Remove the entire cementum layer to expose dentine
    c. Remove the ulcerated epithelial pocket wall
    d. Facilitate healing by formation of a long junctional epithelium
    e. Obtain a new connective tissue attachment to the root surface

14. Chlorhexidine gluconate:
    a. Is a phenolic compound
    b. Demonstrates substantivity
    c. Is bactericidal only against streptococci
    d. Is available in the United Kingdom as mouthrinses of 0.2%, 0.12% and 0.06% concentrations.
    e. Only stains teeth in patients who smoke

15. The Basic Periodontal Examination (BPE):
    a. Should be undertaken using a Hu-Friedy periodontal probe
    b. Was designed as a screening tool to assess treatment need
    c. Records only the maximum scores in each quadrant
    d. Does not identify furcation involvement
    e. Does not identify mobile teeth

16. Clinical measurements of probing depths are likely to be influenced by:
    a. Subgingival calculus
    b. Probing force
    c. Dimensions of the probe
    d. Inflammatory infiltrate at the base of the pocket
    e. Angulation of the probe

17. Drugs that are known to cause gingival overgrowth include:
    a. Ciclosporin
    b. Nifedipine
    c. Insulin
    d. Metronidazole
    e. Tetracycline

18. Molar-incisor pattern periodontitis:
    a. Is highly prevalent in adolescents
    b. Can affect any teeth in the permanent dentition
    c. Is typically characterised by *A. actinomycetemcomitans* infection

d. Commonly runs in families

e. Is associated with neutrophil defects

19. Necrotising gingivitis (NG):
    a. Is a viral infection
    b. Is characterised by vesicles that break down to form yellow–grey ulcers with a red 'halo' of inflammation
    c. Is a painful condition
    d. Is likely to recur in the absence of long-term maintenance
    e. Should always be treated using metronidazole as the first line of treatment

20. Advantages of locally delivered antimicrobials for treatment of periodontal disease include:
    a. Prolonged duration of action of the antimicrobial
    b. High local concentrations of the antimicrobial are achieved
    c. Patients themselves are able to insert the antimicrobial at the appropriate site
    d. The need for patient compliance is eliminated
    e. Incidence of adverse reactions is reduced

21. Powered toothbrushes:
    a. Are more effective in removing plaque than manual toothbrushes
    b. Have brushheads that are designed specifically for patients with fixed orthodontic appliances
    c. Have a 'novelty effect' associated with their use
    d. Are generally cheaper than manual toothbrushes
    e. Should be used with the Bass toothbrushing technique

22. Mandibular first molars with grade I furcation involvement:
    a. Demonstrate horizontal mobility of >1.0 mm
    b. Are almost certainly non-vital
    c. Have horizontal attachment loss of <1/3 the width of the tooth
    d. Should be managed using a tunnel preparation
    e. May be managed using guided tissue regeneration (GTR)

23. Features associated with periodontal disease that may be identified on intraoral periapical radiographs are:
    a. Pattern of alveolar bone loss
    b. Extent of alveolar bone loss
    c. Overhanging restorations of interproximal tooth surfaces
    d. Subgingival calculus
    e. Furcation involvement

24. A periodontal abscess:
    a. Is almost certainly associated with a non-vital tooth
    b. Should be managed initially using systemic antimicrobials
    c. Often tracks through the alveolar bone, resulting in a buccal sinus opening
    d. Is usually painful when the associated tooth is percussed
    e. Should be managed initially using locally delivered antimicrobials

25. According to the random burst model of periodontal disease progression:
    a. Bursts of disease activity are random with respect to previous episodes of destruction
    b. Multiple sites break down within a finite time period
    c. Some sites remain free of disease throughout the life of the patient
    d. Sites of previous disease may remain quiescent indefinitely
    e. Disease activity is present only at sites that bleed

EXTENDED MATCHING ITEMS QUESTIONS

Theme: Periodontal diagnosis

1. The previous classification of periodontal diseases and conditions was published in the *Annals of Periodontology* in 1999. The following is a list of some of these diseases and conditions. For each of the case scenarios (a–e), select from the list (1–15) the single most appropriate diagnosis for the signs and symptoms given.

   Each diagnosis may be used once, more than once or not at all:
   1. Generalised chronic periodontitis.
   2. Periodontal abscess.
   3. Primary endodontic lesion with secondary periodontal involvement.
   4. Plaque-induced gingivitis.
   5. Primary herpetic gingivostomatitis.
   6. Localised mucogingival defect.
   7. Localised aggressive periodontitis.
   8. Generalised aggressive periodontitis.
   9. Chronic periodontitis associated with diabetes.
   10. Necrotising ulcerative gingivitis.
   11 Necrotising ulcerative periodontitis.
   12. Drug-induced gingival enlargement.
   13. Periodontitis associated with cyclic neutropenia.
   14. Gingival trauma.
   15. Pregnancy-associated gingivitis.
      a. A 54-year-old female smokes 20 cigarettes a day. Her main complaint is bleeding gums and of a gap appearing recently between her two upper front teeth.
      b. An 18-year-old student smokes 10 cigarettes a day. Her main complaint is very sore gums at the front of the mouth and bad breath. This has been a problem before but has responded to antibiotics given by her doctor.
      c. A 28-year-old lecturer from Nigeria complains of tooth sensitivity and an inability to eat due to having many loose teeth. Medical history is uneventful and the patient does not smoke.
      d. A 25-year-old nursery teacher complains of extremely sore and painful gums, and roof of mouth. The symptoms were first noticed only 2 days previously and are so severe that she has been unable to eat.
      e. A 15-year-old female complains of excruciating pain from the gums all around the mouth. Many aspects of the history are vague but it appears to have been a problem for many months. She has also recently been in hospital for investigation of severe headaches.

2. Using the 2017 classification of periodontal diseases what is the stage and grade of periodontitis for the following cases?
   A. Generalised periodontitis Stage 1 Grade A
   B. Generalised periodontitis Stage 1 Grade B
   C. Generalised periodontitis Stage 1 Grade C
   D. Generalised periodontitis Stage 2 Grade A
   E. Generalised periodontitis Stage 2 Grade B
   F. Generalised periodontitis Stage 2 Grade C
   G. Generalised periodontitis Stage 3 Grade A
   H. Generalised periodontitis Stage 3 Grade B
   I. Generalised periodontitis Stage 3 Grade C
   J. Generalised periodontitis Stage 4 Grade A
   K. Generalised periodontitis Stage 4 Grade B
   L. Generalised periodontitis Stage 4 Grade C
       1. 50-year-old patient with 50% horizontal bone loss affecting all remaining teeth. (H)
       2. 40-year-old patient with 20% horizontal bone loss affecting all remaining teeth. (D)
       3. 25-year-old patient with 50% horizontal bone loss affecting all remaining teeth. (I)
       4. 75-year-old patient with 25% horizontal bone loss affecting all remaining teeth. (D)
       5. 30-year-old patient with 10% horizontal bone loss affecting all remaining teeth. (A)

SINGLE BEST ANSWER QUESTIONS

1. When applying the Akerly Classification of traumatic incisor relationships, a Class 2 relationship is best described as:
   A. Lower incisors impinge upon the palatal mucosa of the mandible
   B. Lower incisors impinge upon the palatal mucosa of the maxilla
   C. Lower incisors occlude on the palatal gingival margins of the mandibular teeth
   D. Lower incisors occlude on the palatal gingival margins of the maxillary teeth
   E. Lower incisors sheer the palatal gingival tissues from the maxillary teeth
2. You have recently completed a course of non-surgical periodontal treatment under local anaesthetic for a patient diagnosed with generalised periodontitis Stage 3, Grade B with smoking as an identified risk factor. From the following list choose the best statement that describes interventions appropriate for a follow-up visit arranged 2 weeks later.
   A. Plaque control check, smoking cessation advice, root surface re-instrumentation
   B. Smoking cessation advice, bleeding on probing score, root surface re-instrumentation
   C. Soft tissue check, plaque control check, probing pocket depths
   D. Soft tissue check, plaque control check, smoking cessation advice
   E. Soft tissue check, probing pocket depths, bleeding on probing score
3. When considering furcation lesions on a maxillary first molar choose the statement that best describes the expected clinical anatomy to gain access to the trifurcation:
   A. It is distobuccal and distopalatal
   B. It is mesiobuccal and mesiopalatal
   C. It is mid-buccal and distopalatal
   D. It is mid-buccal and mesiopalatal
   E. It is mid-buccal and mid-palatal

CASE HISTORY QUESTION

A 25-year-old healthy female presents to your surgery complaining of gum recession adjacent to one of her mandibular lower incisors. Apparently, this has developed during the previous 3 months and she is very worried that the tooth might have to be extracted.
The tooth is free of symptoms.

1. Describe how you would assess the problem clinically.
2. How would you advise the patient?
3. Discuss your management of the case.

PICTURE QUESTIONS

Picture 1

Study the two radiographs (Fig. 1.24) which are of the same patient at (A) 19 years and (B) 34 years of age.

1. What is the most likely periodontal diagnosis at 34 years of age?
2. What does the initial phase of treatment involve?
3. The patient has a sister who is aged 29 years. What advice might you offer?

Picture 2

Study the position of the probe in the pocket (Fig. 1.25).

1. What type of probe is this?
2. What is the 'score' for the pocket?
3. What does the 'score' infer regarding the extent of attachment loss?

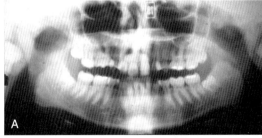
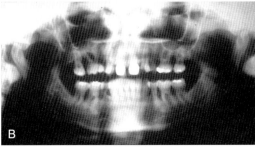

Fig. 1.24 Radiographs of a patient at (A) 19 years and (B) 34 years of age.

Picture 3

This 23-year-old patient (Fig. 1.26) complains of extremely painful gums and a foul taste, both of recent onset.

1. What is the most likely diagnosis for this characteristic presentation?
2. Identify possible risk factors for this condition.
3. Outline your management strategy.

Picture 4

Fig. 1.27 is an intraoral radiograph taken for a 20-year-old female who was complaining of an acute, aching pain from her lower left molar teeth.

1. What is the most likely cause of the pain?
2. Identify the radiographic findings on this film.
3. What is the differential diagnosis for the appearance of the bone defect on the distal aspect of the first molar?

Picture 5

This 20-year-old female complains of severe pain from the ulcers on her gums, mainly in the upper jaw (Fig. 1.28). The history of their onset is extremely vague.

1. Apart from the gingival and mucosal ulceration, what other significant periodontal feature(s) can be identified from the photograph?
2. Consider your differential diagnosis for these ulcers.

SHORT NOTE QUESTIONS

Write short notes on:

1. *Aggregatibacter actinomycetemcomitans*
2. long junctional epithelium
3. random burst model of periodontal disease progression
4. tooth mobility
5. collagenases.

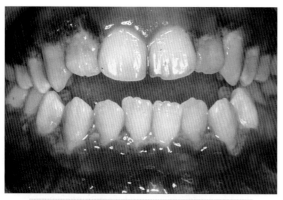

Fig. 1.25 Probe within a pocket.

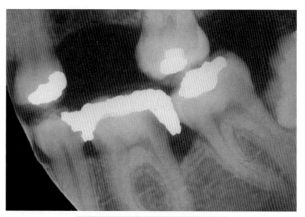

Fig. 1.27 Intraoral radiograph.

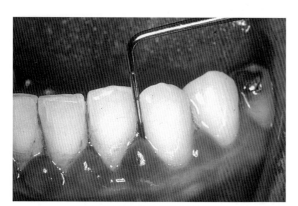

Fig. 1.26 Mouth of a patient with painful gums.

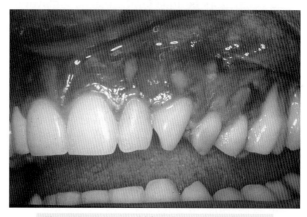

Fig. 1.28 A 20-year-old female with painful ulcers.

Self-Assessment: Answers

MULTIPLE CHOICE ANSWERS

1. a. False. Dental plaque is the key aetiological factor in periodontitis (although calculus is always covered by a layer of unmineralised plaque).
   b. False. Calculus forms both supra- and subgingivally.
   c. False. Plaque is mineralised by calcium and phosphate ions from saliva.
   d. True. Mature calculus contains predominantly crystals of hydroxyapatite and tricalcium phosphate.
   e. False. Calculus contains (non-viable) plaque bacteria that have become mineralised.

2. a. False. *P. gingivalis* is an example of a late colonising species, typically found in mature subgingival plaque.
 b. True. *P. gingivalis* invades and also replicates within gingival epithelial cells.
 c. True. Most strains of *P. gingivalis* are encapsulated, which inhibits phagocytosis of the organism.
 d. False. *A. actinomycetemcomitans* is the organism most strongly implicated in molar-incisor pattern periodontitis.
 e. False. *P. gingivalis* is an anaerobic non-motile rod.
3. a. False. These organisms are associated with periodontally diseased sites.
 b. True. These Gram-positive species are among the first to colonise a newly cleaned tooth surface.
 c. True. *F. nucleatum* is associated with periodontitis.
 d. False. *A. actinomycetemcomitans* invades the gingival soft tissues and, therefore, is not totally eradicated by RSI. Adjunctive antimicrobial therapy or surgery may be indicated.
 e. False. Most strains of *A. actinomycetemcomitans* have developed resistance to tetracyclines.
4. a. False. The established lesion is apparent after 2–3 weeks of undisturbed plaque growth.
 b. False. The established lesion is confined to the gingival tissues.
 c. False. Plasma cells are the predominant inflammatory cell type in the established lesion.
 d. True. Increased vascular permeability, vasodilatation and an increasingly permeable junctional epithelium all lead to increased GCF flow.
 e. False. It is not possible to evaluate the histological status of the tissues from clinical appearance alone, and the diagnosis of gingivitis is made solely using clinical parameters. Furthermore, there are no clear boundaries between the histological changes occurring during the development of gingivitis.
5. a. False. Neutrophils cross the junctional epithelium in response to chemotactic stimuli from subgingival plaque bacteria.
 b. False. The main collagenase produced by neutrophils is MMP-8. MMP-1 is produced by fibroblasts.
 c. True. Lysosomal enzymes, granule contents and products of the respiratory burst can all be spilled into the surrounding tissues from neutrophils, leading to tissue damage.
 d. True. Neutrophils are involved in the initial acute response to plaque, cross the junctional epithelium and form a 'leukocyte wall' between plaque bacteria and the underlying tissues.
 e. True. Neutrophils can be identified histologically even in clinically healthy gingival tissues. They are present to combat bacteria present in the gingival sulcus, even in the absence of clinically diagnosed gingivitis.
6. a. False. GTR is primarily indicated in class II furcation defects. RSI (with or without flap elevation) is the treatment of choice for class I furcations.
 b. True. The space under the membrane must be filled with clot, which acts like a scaffold for the migration of colonising cells from the periodontal ligament.
 c. False. Although probing depths reduce and gains in attachment are seen, there is usually an increase in recession of 1–2 mm following GTR.

 d. False. Many resorbable membranes produce results equivalent to those seen when using a non-resorbable membrane.
 e. False. Osseointegration refers to the intimate contact observed between alveolar bone and the titanium surface of implants.
7. a. False. Plaque control is of paramount importance before and after surgery, and surgery will fail if oral hygiene is not of the highest standard.
 b. True. The long junctional epithelium that forms is more at risk of subsequent plaque-induced breakdown; plaque control must, therefore, be of the highest standard.
 c. False. Gingivectomy is the preferred surgical treatment option for hyperplastic gingiva.
 d. True. Recession, leading to poor aesthetics and also dentine hypersensitivity, is common after flap procedures, particularly when flaps are apically repositioned.
 e. False. The width of keratinised gingiva can be maintained in flap procedures.
8. a. False. Vertical bony defects are harder to treat and maintain; therefore, the prognosis is worse.
 b. False. Providing oral hygiene is good, sites with dehiscences or fenestrations are not more at risk of periodontitis.
 c. True. Three-walled defects are easier to isolate from the epithelium with a membrane than one- and two-walled defects, and the prospects for bone infill are, therefore, enhanced.
 d. False. Radiographs provide a historical representation of which sites have already lost bone and do not provide reliable information regarding active bone resorption.
 e. True. Interleukin-1β is a major stimulator of osteoclastic bone resorption.
9. a. False. The gingivectomy incision should start apical to the base of the pocket and be angled at 45° towards the base of the pocket.
 b. True. The prevention of downgrowth of epithelial cells to form a long junctional epithelium is the main aim of GTR.
 c. False. Full-thickness flaps are raised when apically repositioning.
 d. False. Plaque control is of paramount importance in promoting healing following both surgical and non-surgical periodontal treatment.
 e. True. Gingivectomy wounds heal by secondary intention – there is no primary closure.
10. a. False. Occlusal forces do not initiate an inflammatory response.
 b. False. Forces may exacerbate an existing lesion but will not cause periodontal disease.
 c. True. An adaptive response of the periodontal membrane.
 d. True. The mobility results from the widened membrane space.
 e. False. Recession represents attachment loss which is not precipitated by occlusal trauma alone.
11. a. True. They are typically associated with first permanent molars.
 b. True. The cementoenamel junction to bone crest dimension tends to remain constant. An angular alveolar bone crest is usually evident.

c. True. Local bone loss associated with plaque accumulation, which results from an inability to clean beneath the 'ledge'.

d. False. Occurs, only occasionally, if those abutments are subject to jiggling forces and there is preexisting periodontitis.

e. False. Occurs, only very occasionally, if the occlusal scheme has not been planned and overloading/jiggling of the abutment occurs in the presence of preexisting periodontitis.

12. a. False. The width of keratinised gingiva can show considerable variation throughout the mouth.

b. False. Bone crest is usually at least 1 mm below the cementoenamel junction.

c. False. There is always a flow of GCF, even in health.

d. False. Tooth mobility in periodontal health is minimal but detectable by the naked eye.

e. True. A pocket is defined as a pathologically deepened crevice, which excludes their presence in the healthy state.

13. a. True. Although it is difficult to assess when all the calculus has been removed.

b. False. This may occasionally occur but should not be the aim of treatment.

c. False. Epithelium is inevitably damaged during instrumentation but its removal is not an aim.

d. True. A long junctional epithelium may form as part of the healing response.

e. False. Epithelium downgrowth will preclude new connective tissue attachment.

14. a. False. Chlorhexidine is a bisbiguanide antimicrobial.

b. True. Retention in the oral cavity is one of the most important properties of this agent.

c. False. Chlorhexidine is a broad-spectrum antimicrobial.

d. True.

e. False. Chlorhexidine stains teeth independently of whether the patient smokes.

15. a. False. The examination should be undertaken using the specifically designed WHO (CPITN) probe.

b. True. The screening examination should be supplemented by a detailed periodontal investigation in cases where scores of 4 are recorded.

c. False. Trick. The record is the maximum score in each sextant.

d. False. The asterisk (*) denotes furcation involvement.

e. True. The BPE has no facility to record the mobility of teeth.

16. a. True. Calculus acts as a physical barrier to probing.

b. True. A number of 'pressure-sensitive' probes are available to control the degree of pressure (force) used when probing pockets.

c. True. Many designs of probe exist with variation in length, thickness and dimension of probe tip. To minimise variation in probing depth, measurements in one patient at different visits should be made using the same type of probe.

d. True. The inflammatory infiltrate will facilitate penetration of the probe through both epithelial and connective tissues at the base of the pocket.

e. True. The probe should be maintained, as far as possible, parallel with the vertical root length. The probe tip should then approximate the base of the pocket. Probing depth can be overestimated when the probe is placed at an angle to the vertical root length.

17. a. True. Ciclosporin is a potent immunosuppressant used in the field of organ transplantation.

b. True. Nifedipine is a calcium-channel blocker used for the management of hypertension and angina.

c. False. However, remember that both type 1 and type 2 diabetics appear to be at increased risk for periodontal disease.

d. False. This drug is indicated for the treatment of some periodontal conditions.

e. False. This drug is indicated for the treatment of some periodontal conditions.

18. a. False. Prevalence is <1%.

b. False. There is a localised first molar and incisor presentation with no more than two other teeth affected (if more teeth than this are affected, the diagnosis is generalised rapidly progressing periodontitis).

c. True. Microbial analysis typically reveals elevated levels of this organism.

d. True. Studies show that molar-incisor pattern periodontitis is a heritable trait.

e. True. Patients with molar-incisor pattern periodontitis may have abnormalities of neutrophil chemotaxis and phagocytosis.

19. a. False. Traditionally, the condition has been associated with a fusobacterial–spirochaetal complex, although aspects of the disease are characteristic of viral involvement (e.g. the relatively narrow age range affected and the tendency to recur). As yet, however, no specific virus has been identified as causal.

b. False. These signs are characteristic of acute herpetic gingivostomatitis. Vesicle formation does not occur in NG.

c. True. NG is one of the few periodontal conditions that is associated with acute pain.

d. True. If predisposing factors are not removed, the disease is very likely to recur.

e. False. Metronidazole is indicated in severe, acutely painful disease and when there is involvement of regional lymph nodes. In less severe disease, RSI under local anaesthesia and hygiene phase therapy are of primary importance and antimicrobial therapy is not indicated.

20. a. True. The antimicrobials are released slowly as the vehicle matrix biodegrades/breaks down.

b. True. Placement is site specific so the entire dose of the antimicrobial is targeted to the site where it is required.

c. False. All products have to be placed by the clinician.

d. True. As the product is placed by the clinician, there is no need for patient compliance. Furthermore, the majority of products now available in the United Kingdom have a biodegradable matrix so the products do not have to be removed at a follow-up visit.

e. True. The incidence of adverse reactions will be reduced by avoiding the systemic route of drug administration.

21. a. True. The vast majority of clinical trials have shown powered toothbrushes to be as, if not more, effective for removing plaque than conventional manual brushes. Most of these observations are short term and may well be the result of a 'novelty effect' of using a new brush rather than as a consequence of better mechanical cleaning per se.

b. True. Some powered units have brushheads that are designed specifically for cleaning fixed appliances.

c. True. See (a).

d. False. Powered brushes are more expensive.

e. False. Instructions for use of powered brushes are provided by the manufacturers. Generally, the brushes should be guided around the dental arches with the knowledge that the movement of the brushhead itself is generated by the powered unit.

22. a. False. This is a possibility but the classification of furcation involvement is not linked with tooth mobility.

b. False. A periodontal–endodontic lesion might be present, but the classification does not imply vitality or non-vitality of a tooth.

c. True. The horizontal attachment loss refers to the progression of the disease at the furcation site. Do not forget that pocketing/vertical loss of attachment will also have occurred but is not identified in the grading of furcation involvement.

d. False. A grade I lesion will, by definition, have considerable remaining intra-radicular bone and attachment. This must be preserved, so tunnelling is certainly contraindicated.

e. True. Most class I lesions should be managed conservatively with oral hygiene and RSI. Studies have shown, however, that these defects can be managed predictably and successfully using GTR.

23. a. True.
b. True.
c. True.
d. True.
e. True.

All of these features may be seen on radiographs. The important word in this answer is *may*. Overhanging restorations, calculus and furcation involvement (particularly class I) can sometimes only be detected clinically while not being apparent on radiographs.

24. a. False. The tooth may be non-vital if there is a combined endodontic–periodontal lesion. If the infection is primarily of periodontal origin, the tooth will very likely still be vital.

b. False. Local instrumentation of the site should be the primary treatment. Periodontal abscesses usually drain through the pocket opening, thus reducing the need for systemic antimicrobials.

c. False. A sinus opening on the attached gingiva is usually associated with a periapical infection that tracks along the path of least resistance from the apex of the tooth.

d. True. A periodontal abscess is one of the relatively few periodontal conditions that is painful.

e. False. Drainage and local debridement are the first lines of treatment. The purulent exudate and localised bleeding are likely to restrict the efficacy of local antimicrobial therapy.

25. a. True.
b. False. This is consistent with the asynchronous multiple burst theory/model.
c. True.
d. True.
e. False. This is not a criterion for the random burst model, nor is it a true statement in itself.

EXTENDED MATCHING ITEMS ANSWERS

1.
   a. 1
   b. 10
   c. 8
   d. 5
   e. 14

2.
   1. H
   2. D
   3. I
   4. D
   5. A

SINGLE BEST ANSWER QUESTIONS ANSWERS

1. C
2. D
3. D

CASE HISTORY ANSWERS

1. Record the extent of the gingival recession by measuring the vertical distance from the cementoenamel junction to the free gingival margin. Study models or an intraoral photograph are useful permanent records to which reference can be made at a later date to establish whether the lesion is progressing. Note whether the gingival soft tissues adjacent to the recession are inflamed and whether there are plaque and calculus deposits on the exposed root surface. Record the mobility of the tooth (if any). Identify any factors that might predispose to the gingival recession. For example, an incisor that is displaced labially from the arch may have only very thin or completely absent labial alveolar support. A very prominent midline or labial frenal attachment may restrict access for toothbrushing. It is also important to measure the width of attached/keratinised gingiva adjacent to the affected tooth. When this tissue is compromised, the ability of the soft tissues to resist masticatory and toothbrushing forces is reduced and the depth of the labial sulcus is also affected. The width of keratinised tissue can be identified more clearly by using an iodine solution, which preferentially stains keratinised tissue

bright orange and non-keratinised oral mucosa a deeper purple colour.

2. For gingival recession, a history of the presenting complaint is not always accurate. It is possible that the recession has occurred over a very short period of time. In many cases, however, the lesion may have been present for many months (if not years) before the patient first noticed it. In the absence of tooth mobility, the patient should be reassured that the prognosis for the tooth remains good provided that any plaque-induced inflammation is resolved and stability of the lesion can be achieved. It is also worth mentioning to the patient that gingival recession that affects mandibular incisor teeth is often covered by the lower lip. When patients become aware of this, they do not usually consider the appearance of the recession to be a major problem.

3. In the first instance, the lesion should be managed conservatively. Any causative factors, such as an injudicious toothbrushing technique, should be corrected. Oral hygiene instruction should be given and localised toothbrushing using a single tufted, interspace brush might be indicated when access for a conventional toothbrush is compromised. Deposits of plaque and calculus should be removed from the root surface, although excessive root instrumentation should be avoided to reduce the chance of exposing dentine and the root surface becoming sensitive to hot and cold. Topical desensitising agents, such as a fluoride varnish, should be applied frequently to reduce both the likelihood of sensitivity and the development of root caries in the longer term. Surgical widening of the keratinised gingiva might be indicated over the long term if the patient is unable to practise good oral hygiene procedures because of local mucogingival morphology and reduced sulcus depth. Progression of the recession despite the removal of causative factors and establishment of good plaque control might also be an indication for a surgical procedure to increase the width of keratinised tissue.

PICTURE ANSWERS

Picture 1

1. Generalised rapid rate periodontitis.
2. Initially conventional cause-related treatment is instigated: instruction in toothbrushing and use of adjunctive aids for interproximal and subgingival cleaning, RSI, prophylaxis. Ultimately, treatments such as surgery and the adjunctive use of antimicrobials might be indicated, but conventional treatment is first in line.
3. Periodontal screening and radiographic examination. There is evidence that certain subjects are at high risk of developing rapid rate periodontitis and this risk may be under genetic control. Siblings should be screened and affected individuals with children warned that early signs may develop from around puberty onwards.

Picture 2

1. World Health Organization (WHO) or BPE probe. The black band extends from 3.5 to 5.5 mm from the tip.
2. Part of the band remains visible above the gingival margin giving a score of 3.

3. Nothing at all. The score of 3 tells you that the pocket is greater than 3.5 mm but less than 5.5 mm. This could be a false pocket or a true attachment loss. Both situations require treatment and, therefore, the BPE score gives you an indication of treatment need.

Picture 3

1. The clinical appearance of 'punched-out', yellow–grey ulcers of the interdental and marginal gingiva is characteristic of necrotising gingivitis (NG).
2. Risk factors are:
   - poor oral hygiene
   - pre-existing chronic gingivitis
   - smoking
   - malnutrition
   - stress.

A persistent NG is associated with immunocompromised patients and the possibility of HIV infection must be considered in such cases.

3. Management involves:
   - reduce cigarette consumption
   - oral hygiene advice
   - RSI, ultrasonic scaling (under local anaesthesia)
   - oxygenating mouthrinse (e.g. hydrogen peroxide) to irrigate and cleanse the necrotic tissues and superficial debris
   - if general symptoms (regional lymphadenopathy) are present, treatment with systemic metronidazole (200 mg, three times a day) for 3 days
   - long-term follow-up must include regular visits to reinforce oral hygiene measures and so reduce the likelihood of recurrence.

Picture 4

1. Recurrent caries beneath the distal aspect of the MOD restoration in 36.
2. Findings include:
   - recurrent caries 36
   - missing 26
   - overhanging restoration MOD 36
   - mesio-angular impaction 38.
3. Angular bone defects may be associated with overhanging restorations, when difficult access for cleaning leads to stagnation and an environment in which predominantly Gram-negative anaerobic pathogens will flourish. Such defects are also found on the mesial surfaces of teeth that have tipped into an adjacent edentulous space and on periodontally involved teeth that have been subject to excessive occlusal loading or jiggling forces. In this case, the most obvious causal factor appears to be the overhanging restoration. The patient suffers from molar-incisor pattern periodontitis and identical vertical bone defects were found on the contralateral first molars, neither of which were restored. There is also another clue to this diagnosis, in that 26 has already been lost.

Picture 5

1. The gingival recession adjacent to the maxillary molars is very severe for a 20-year-old patient.
2. Gingival ulceration may occur in a number of conditions: necrotising gingivitis; herpetic gingivostomatitis;

mucocutaneous diseases such as erosive lichen planus, benign mucous membrane pemphigoid and pemphigus vulgaris; and squamous cell carcinoma affecting the gingiva. Recurrent aphthae tend to appear on the more labile oral mucosa rather than on the immobile gingival tissue. In this case, the lesions were self-inflicted, with the diagnosis being factitious gingivitis. Eventually, lesions appeared in contralateral quadrants, on the palate, the lips and extraorally on the face. The lesions did not respond to simple treatment measures including protective dressing and at no time did the patient admit to knowing the cause of the lesions. Eventually, the patient was referred for a psychiatric opinion.

SHORT NOTE ANSWERS

1. *A. actinomycetemcomitans* is a Gram-negative capnophilic rod that is strongly linked to molar-incisor pattern periodontitis. *A. actinomycetemcomitans* has been isolated with molar-incisor pattern rapid rate periodontitis and appears to be associated particularly with progressing periodontal lesions. It is a virulent organism and produces collagenase, leukotoxin, endotoxin, proteases and toxins. These factors are important in the evasion of host defence mechanisms and the destruction of periodontal tissues, including connective tissues and bone. Transmission between family members is common and may constitute a source of reinfection following therapy. *A. actinomycetemcomitans* has the ability to invade gingival soft tissues and replicate within epithelial cells. This means that the organism is difficult to eradicate by RSI alone. Adjunctive antimicrobial therapy (amoxicillin 250 mg > metronidazole 400 mg, three times a day, for 7–14 days) prescribed to coincide with RSI typically results in good improvements clinically. Surgical treatment may be required to allow for improved access to the root surface and excision of infected soft tissues.

2. Following efficacious periodontal therapy, the newly cleaned root surface is rapidly colonised by the downgrowth of gingival epithelial cells to form a long junctional epithelium (JE). Attachment of the long JE to the tooth surface occurs via hemidesmosomes. Rapid downgrowth of the gingival epithelial cells prevents colonisation of the tooth surface by cells migrating from the gingival connective tissues, which would otherwise result in root resorption or ankylosis. In this way, the integrity of the epithelial barrier is maintained, preventing ingress of bacteria into the tissues. Pluripotential cells from the periodontal ligament are also prevented from colonising the root surface, and there is no opportunity for the generation of new connective tissue attachment to the root. Providing a high standard of oral hygiene, the long JE is maintained and probing depths are reduced compared with pre-treatment measurements. The long JE is susceptible to plaque-induced breakdown and, if plaque accumulates, apical migration of the JE will occur, resulting in increased probing depths.

3. Early studies that investigated patterns of progression of periodontitis concluded that there is linear, progressive loss of attachment (LOA) over time, although the rate of progression may vary according to the population studied. This suggests that, once initiated, periodontal disease progresses relentlessly throughout life. The use of more sophisticated probes and statistical models for assessing disease progression revealed that: (1) rates of LOA in some individuals can be too slow/fast to fit a linear model; (2) many sites do not change over long periods (which is inconsistent with the linear progression model) and (3) destruction at a site may arrest and progress no further. Therefore, the random burst model was suggested in which certain sites do not exhibit periodontal destruction at all and other sites exhibit bursts of destruction that may last for an undefined period of time. Those latter sites subsequently may become quiescent or may exhibit one or more bursts of disease activity in the future. The bursts are random with regard to time and previous LOA.

4. Tooth mobility may be either physiological or pathological. Physiological mobility allows slight movement of the tooth within the socket to accommodate masticatory forces without injury to the tooth or its supporting structures. Pathological mobility is increased or increasing mobility as a result of connective tissue attachment loss. Pathological mobility is dependent on the quantity of remaining bony support, inflammation in the periodontal ligament and the magnitude of any occlusal or jiggling displacing forces that may be acting on the tooth. Tooth mobility is measured by displacing the tooth with a rigid dental instrument and a moderate force and is classified according to horizontal (class I <1 mm, class II 1–2 mm, class III >2 mm) and vertical (class III) mobility.

5. Collagenases are enzymes that degrade collagen. Collagen degradation requires special enzymes because its cross-linked molecules resist most proteinases. The enzymes that degrade collagen (and also other matrix molecules) comprise a family of enzymes called matrix metalloproteinases (MMPs). All have a zinc ion at the active site and are synthesised and secreted as inactive precursors. Conversion to the active form occurs outside the cell and requires activation by proteinases, such as plasmin and trypsin, or reactive oxygen species. Production of MMPs is regulated by growth factors and cytokines, such as interleukin-1 (increases MMP synthesis) and transforming growth factor-β (decreases MMP synthesis). Inhibitors of MMPs exist in the serum (α2-macroglobulin) and in the tissues (tissue inhibitors of metalloproteinases (TIMPs)). MMPs are produced by fibroblasts (MMP-1), keratinocytes, macrophages and neutrophils (MMP-8).

References

Caton J, et al. A new classification scheme for periodontal and peri-implant diseases and conditions – Introduction and key changes from the 1999 classification. *J Clin Periodontol.* 2018;45(Suppl 20):S1–S8.

Health and Social Care Information Centre. *Adult Dental Health Survey 2009.* UK: NHS Government Statistical Service; 2011.

Herrera D, et al. Acute periodontal lesions (periodontal abscesses and necrotising periodontal diseases) and endo-periodontal lesions. *J Periodontol.* 2018;89(Suppl 1):S85–S102.

Meyle J, Chapple I. Molecular aspects of the pathogenesis of periodontitis. *Periodontol 2000.* 2015;69:7–17.

2 *Endodontics*

Overview

Pulp and periradicular disease is common and can result in discomfort, pain and potentially premature tooth loss for patients. The understanding of endodontic disease and the way in which it can be managed is progressing rapidly. Although there has been a dramatic evolution in the technology available to make complex treatment easier, the field is beginning to move towards more biologically based principles to diagnose and treat endodontic diseases.

Our understanding of pulpal disease is increasing exponentially and while managing the injured pulp was always thought to be unpredictable, such dogma is being challenged. This revised chapter includes a new section on vital pulp therapies as modern biologically based treatments are shown to be far more predictable than first thought. Pulpal and periradicular disease is principally caused by an infection which is bacterial in origin. The aim of treatment therefore is to protect pulp tissue from infection or eliminate these bacteria from within the complex anatomy of root canal systems if it becomes infected and then seal the canal space to prevent re-entry.

This chapter provides an overview of pulpal and periradicular disease and the methods used to examine the patient and formulate a diagnosis. A section is included on managing the injured vital pulp, followed by a review of both traditional and some of the more recent treatment developments that have proved useful in day-to-day practice in managing the necrotic pulp. The restoration of endodontically treated teeth is discussed before managing failed root canal treatment with non-surgical and surgical approaches.

2.1 Pulpal and Periradicular Pathology

LEARNING OBJECTIVES

You should:
- be able to recognise conditions that may affect the dental pulp and periradicular tissues caused by endodontic disease

- understand the basic pathobiology of pulpal and periradicular disease.

Pulpal and periradicular diseases are inflammatory pathological conditions which result from irritation of these tissues, generally by an infective source or, less commonly so, mechanical or chemical sources.

INFECTIVE SOURCE - BACTERIA

Bacteria, usually from dental caries, are the main sources of injury to the pulpal and periradicular tissues. These enter either directly or through dentine tubules. The link between bacteria and pulpal and periradicular disease is well established as periradicular pathology does not develop in the absence of bacteria. Modes of entry for bacteria – other than caries – include periodontal disease (dentine tubules, furcal canals and lateral canals), erosion, attrition and abrasion (dentinal tubules), cracked teeth, trauma with or without pulpal exposure, developmental anomalies and anachoresis (the passage of micro-organisms into the root canal system from the bloodstream).

MECHANICAL IRRITANTS

Examples of mechanical irritation include trauma, operative procedures including iatrogenic perforations, excessive orthodontic forces, subgingival scaling and over instrumentation during root canal treatment.

CHEMICAL IRRITANTS

Pulpal irritation may result from bacterial toxins or some restorative materials/conditioning agents. Periradicular irritation may occur from irrigating solutions, phenol-based intracanal medicaments or extrusion of root canal filling materials.

PULP DISEASE

The dentine-pulp complex (Fig. 2.1) is a unique mineralised connective tissue that is composed of two integrated

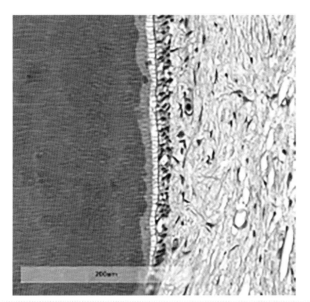

Fig. 2.1 Haematoxylin and eosin staining of the dentine-pulp complex.

constituents: the pulp – an underlying gelatinous soft connective tissue which has a rich vasculature and is well innervated, and the dentine – an outer casing of mineralised tissue.

It is under threat from three main sources: carious attack, trauma and iatrogenic damage. The response of the pulp depends on the severity of the insult and may result in a transient (reversible) inflammatory response or an irreversible one, which may eventually proceed to pulp necrosis. The classical terms of reversible and irreversible still remain useful but are under review as our understanding of the disease improves and our clinical procedures are refined. Current diagnostic terms for pulpal disease are:

Normal pulp: The pulp is symptomless and responds normally to a stimulus.

Reversible pulpitis: Pain or discomfort initiated by a stimulus such as cold or sweet which resolves shortly after the stimulus is removed. The pain and discomfort on occasions may be difficult to localise. On examination suspect teeth are not tender to percussion (unless involved with occlusal trauma) and have a normal radiographic appearance.

Irreversible pulpitis: More intense pain that can be spontaneous or radiating which is long lasting and lingers after removal of stimulus. It can be exacerbated or worsened by lying down.

Pulp necrosis: The pulp is dead and the patient is usually unresponsive to pulp testing.

Other diagnoses related to pulp pathology are:

Hyperplastic pulpitis: Hyperplastic pulpitis, also known as a pulp polyp, occurs as a result of proliferation of chronically inflamed young pulp tissue when exposed to the oral cavity.

Pulp calcification: This results in eventual occlusion of the pulp chamber by either physiological secondary dentine or tertiary dentine which is laid down in response to environmental stimuli as reactionary or reparative dentine. Reactionary dentine is a response to a mild noxious stimulus whereas reparative dentine is deposited directly beneath the path of injured dentinal tubules as a response to strong noxious stimuli. Treatment is dependent upon the pulpal symptoms.

Internal resorption: Occasionally, pulpal inflammation may cause changes that result in dentinoclastic activity. Such changes result in resorption of dentine; clinically, a pink spot may be seen in the later stages if the lesion is coronal. Radiographic examination reveals a punched-out outline that is seen to be continuous with the rest of the pulp cavity. Root canal therapy will result in the arrest of the resorptive process; however, if destruction is very advanced, extraction may be required (Fig. 2.2).

Making an accurate diagnosis of pulp status can be challenging. The information gained from an accurate patient history is supplemented with a good clinical/radiographic examination and pulp testing. It is important not to draw conclusions on one positive or negative finding. All information gathered from the examination, history and special tests should be assimilated and judged in context with one another (Section 2.2 and Conservative Dentistry chapter).

PERIRADICULAR DISEASE

Periradicular periodontitis (also known as apical periodontitis) is an inflammatory disease of the tissues surrounding the root of the tooth which is most frequently caused by an infection inside the root canal system. A complex polymicrobial biofilm can become established within the root canal system once the pulp becomes necrotic and the tooth loses its defence system. Endodontic biofilm is mainly made up of Gram-negative bacteria; however Gram-positive bacteria can also exist. These organisms release virulence factors such as lipopolysaccharides (LPS) and lipoteichoic acid (LTA) inducing a host response which leads to complex interactions resulting in inflammation, resorption of mineralised tissues surrounding the root and potential clinical symptomology.

The terms periradicular periodontitis and more commonly used apical periodontitis can be used interchangeably. Although a semantic point the term periradicular will be used here as it more accurately encompasses pathology that results from endodontic causes that not only exist at

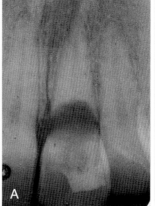
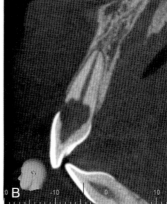

Fig. 2.2 Internal resorption of upper left central. (A) Intraoral periapical and (B) sagittal plane of cone beam computerised tomography scan.

the apex of the root but on any surface of the root. Current diagnostic terms for periradicular disease are as follows:

Normal periradicular tissues: Asymptomatic tooth which responds normally on vitality testing is not sensitive to percussion or palpation testing and radiographically has continuous lamina dura and normal periodontal ligament space.

Asymptomatic periradicular periodontitis: Asymptomatic tooth that does not elucidate any positive clinical signs of disease following examination apart from radiographic evidence of periradicular inflammation that is of endodontic origin.

Symptomatic periradicular periodontitis: Inflammation of the periradicular tissue produces clinical symptoms involving a painful response to biting and/or percussion or palpation. Radiographic appearance can be varied, ranging from minimal widening of the periodontal ligament space to a large area of destruction of periapical tissues.

Chronic periradicular abscess: An inflammatory reaction to pulpal infection and necrosis characterised by gradual onset, little or no discomfort and an intermittent discharge of pus through a sinus tract or periodontal pocket. Radiographically, there are frequent signs of osseous destruction such as a radiolucency.

Acute periradicular abscess: Inflammatory response to micro-organisms or their irritants that have leached out into the periradicular tissues. Symptoms vary from moderate discomfort or swelling to systemic involvement, such as raised temperature and malaise. Teeth involved are usually tender to both palpation and percussion.

In cases where infection is severe or where the immune system is compromised, infection may cause systemic sepsis. There are a number of clinical signs that are deemed high risk for sepsis, including altered mental state, rapid breathing and heart rate, failure to pass urine, low systolic blood pressure, a non-blanching rash or cyanosis of the skin. Interestingly in these cases, there is often a low temperature <36 degrees Celsius; caution should always be taken when dealing with patients who are immunocompromised.

Condensing osteitis: Represents a diffuse increase in trabecular bone in response to irritation. Radiographically, a concentric radio-opaque area is seen around the offending root.

Although lesions noted on radiographs are usually of endodontic origin, this is not always the case. Other causes may be normal anatomic structures, benign or malignant lesions. For example, certain normal anatomic structures may mimic radiolucencies (e.g. maxillary sinus, mental foramen and nasopalatine foramen). In these situations, the associated teeth will respond normally to pulp sensitivity tests, and a radiograph taken from a different angle will reveal that the lesion is not so closely related to the root. Benign lesions that may mimic endodontic pathology include cementoma, fibrous dysplasia, ossifying fibroma, primordial cyst, lateral periodontal cyst, dentigerous cyst, traumatic bone cyst, central giant cell granuloma, central haemangioma, odontogenic keratocyst and ameloblastoma. In some such situations, the lamina dura will be intact around the teeth and final diagnosis relies on histopathological analysis following appropriate biopsy. Malignant lesions to be aware of include squamous cell carcinoma, osteosarcoma, chondrosarcoma and multiple myeloma. These lesions are usually associated with rapid hard tissue destruction.

2.2 Patient Assessment

LEARNING OBJECTIVES

You should:
- be able to follow a structured approach to history taking and conducting a thorough clinical examination
- understand the relevance of special tests
- appreciate the importance of patient-specific treatment planning.

The most common cause of orofacial pain is caused by pulpal or periradicular disease and making an accurate diagnosis for such conditions can be challenging. Successful endodontic diagnosis requires a systematic approach to gathering information through a thorough history and clinical examination followed by the use of appropriate diagnostic aids in order to determine the correct treatment strategy for the patient. Do not draw conclusions on one positive or negative finding. All information gathered from the examination, history and special tests should be assimilated and judged in context with one another.

Diagnosis of pulpal and periradicular disease can be complicated because of the potential for convergence of nerves within the trigeminal ganglion. Pain originating from other tissues such as the periodontium, paranasal sinuses, temporomandibular joints, muscles of mastication, ears, nose, eyes and blood vessels may also be affected by lesions that can mimic pain of endodontic origin. In some cases, the nature of the pain is not coincident with patient's symptoms or the symptoms have not changed as a result of previous treatment, in which case there should always be a suspicion of a non-odontogenic or neuropathic element to this pain.

PATIENT HISTORY

Should be considered as four components: presenting compliant, medical history, dental history and pain history.

- *Presenting complaint*
  The aim of this stage is to record the patient's symptoms or problems, preferably in their own words.
- *Pain history*
  It is important to take the time to listen to your patient, ask broad open questions to start with, then follow-up with more direct questions once the story forms. It can be useful to follow a consistent pattern in questioning and a mnemonic such as SOCRATES below is useful.
  Site – Where is the pain?
  Onset – When did the pain start, and was it sudden or gradual?
  Character – What is the pain like? An ache? Stabbing?
  Radiation – Does the pain radiate anywhere?
  Associations – Any other signs or symptoms associated with the pain?
  Time course – Does the pain follow any pattern?

Exacerbating/relieving factors – Does anything change the pain?

Severity – How bad is the pain?

■ *Medical history*

A detailed medical history should be taken for each new patient or be updated for previously registered patients, dated and signed. Treatment planning can be affected by the patient's medical status. For example, a patient who is at higher risk of osteonecrosis of the jaw due to previous radiotherapy or taking bisphosphonate drugs.

■ *Dental history*

The purpose of the dental history is to summarise current and past dental treatment. Such information may provide clues as to the source of the patient's complaints. It is also an opportunity to establish the patient's attitude towards dental health and treatment that may affect treatment decisions/planning.

On occasions, it is possible to form a provisional diagnosis based purely on the history prior to carrying out any clinical examination. A wise clinician has to be careful not to form opinions that are too fixed at this stage as it can prejudice the objectivity of a clear unbiased clinical examination.

CLINICAL EXAMINATION

Extraoral Examination

As soon as a clinician first sees their patient, they are making a subconscious assessment of their general appearance and wellbeing. An assessment is made of any swelling, facial asymmetry, redness or extraoral sinuses. Lymph nodes are palpated for enlargement and/or tenderness. Clinicians should always be cautious with patients who do have a swelling as the extent and severity of a developing infection/cellulitis is one of the few dental problems that can cause death. A systemic infection should be considered if the patient has general malaise or a raised body temperature. If the patient has dysphagia, any compromise of airway or there is a risk that the swelling is spreading to the orbit, then the patient should be managed immediately by an inpatient team and given appropriate intravenous antibiotics.

To ensure non-odontogenic causes of pain are not overlooked, muscles of mastication and temporomandibular joints are also palpated for tenderness and a note made of the degree of mouth opening. Readers are directed to the diagnostic criteria for temporomandibular disorders (DC-TMD) for further information in this area. Whilst carrying out the extraoral examination, it is important to note the extent of tooth display on maximum smiling.

Intraoral Examination

The oral mucosa and gingival tissues are examined for discoloration, inflammatory change and sinus tract formation. A basic periodontal examination is performed to screen for periodontal disease and the amount of attachment around suspect teeth. Teeth are examined for caries, large restorations, crowns, discoloration, fracture, attrition, abrasion, erosion and restorability. In order to make the restoration of the tooth predictable, there should be at least 2 mm of circumferential supra-gingival tooth structure and not less than 30% of the original coronal tooth structure remaining.

SPECIAL TESTS

All special tests have their limitations and require care in the way they are performed and interpreted. The objective is to find the tooth that is causing discomfort. In general, healthy (control) teeth are tested first.

■ Percussion

Percussion refers to gently tapping or pressing the occlusal or lateral surface of a tooth. A painful response indicates periradicular inflammation. The region over the apices of teeth may also be palpated. Tenderness may be an indication of inflammation, although care should be taken in interpretation when apices are close to the surface.

■ Mobility

A mirror handle is placed on either side of the tooth and a note made of the degree of movement: up to 1 mm scores 1, over 1 mm scores 2 and vertically mobile teeth score 3.

■ Occlusal analysis

It is important to examine suspect teeth for interferences on the retruded arc of closure, intercuspal position and lateral excursions. Interferences in any of these positions could result in occlusal trauma and initiate a symptomatic periapical periodontitis although it may be transient.

■ Pulp testing

Pulp tests determine the response to stimuli and indicate if the pulp has become necrotic or is inflamed. It is usual to try to mimic the stimulus that initiates the pain. Pulp testing may help to distinguish between an infection of periodontal or endodontic origin when a periodontal–endodontic communication is present. Thermal tests are usually the most useful as they give an indication not only as to whether the pulp is alive but also how healthy it is.

Numerous different methods exist in order to determine the viability of the pulp. Most commonly used thermal and electric tests are available in general dental practice. In the first instance, when selecting a thermal test, the practitioner should try and replicate the exacerbating factor the patient identifies with most commonly, be that hot or cold.

■ *Cold test*

Ethyl chloride (−5°C) has been used for many years but non-polluting hydrochlorofluorocarbons (HCFCs) refrigerant spray such as tetrafluoroethane (TFE) at approximately −26°C or propane/butane mix at −50°C are now considered more effective. Cold tests are effective for testing vital and non-vital teeth and generally should be used as a first line test.

■ *Hot test*

Hot gutta-percha or hot water after the application of dental dam may be used to mimic hot stimuli.

■ *Electric pulp test*

Electric instruments can provide an indication as to whether or not there is vital nerve tissue in the tooth; they do not give an indication of different stages of degeneration. Electric pulp tests are accurate when testing vital teeth but poor when testing non-vital teeth.

- *Test cavity*
  Occasionally, as a last resort, an access cavity is cut into dentine without local anaesthesia as an additional way of pulp testing.
- Sinus tract exploration
  Where a sinus tract is present, it may be possible to insert a small gutta-percha point. A radiograph is then taken to see which root the tract/point leads to.
- Transillumination
  Transillumination with a fibre-optic light can be useful in the diagnosis of cracks in teeth.
- Periodontal probing
  Detailed periodontal probing around suspect teeth may reveal a sulcus within normal limits. However, on occasions, deeper pocketing will be noted. A narrow defect may be an indication of a root fracture or an endodontic lesion draining through the gingival crevice. Broader-based lesions are usually an indication of disease of periodontal origin.
- Selective anaesthesia
  Selective anaesthesia can be useful in cases of referred pain to distinguish whether the source of pain is mandibular or maxillary in origin. It is less useful for distinguishing pain from adjacent teeth, as the anaesthetic solution may diffuse laterally.
- Directed cusp loading test
  A plastic bite stick (e.g. tooth sleuth) which allows directed loads to specific cusp tips can be used to aid diagnosis of cracked tooth syndrome (CTS). With CTS it is typical, but not always, for the pain to occur on release of biting pressure.
- Radiographs
  Radiographs should be taken with a paralleling technique using film holders and an associated beam-aiming device. Digital radiography is superseding traditional film radiographs and has the advantage of using software which can enlarge and manipulate the image easily to improve interpretation. If traditional films are used they should be viewed using an appropriate viewer with magnification. Radiographs may provide much important information to help to confirm a diagnosis, but they should not be used alone. Radiographic findings may include the loss of lamina dura (laterally or apically) or a frank periradicular radiolucency indicative of pulp necrosis. Radiographs may show pulp chamber or root canal calcification, which can explain reduced responses to pulp testing, and emphasises the need for considering the results of more than one test. More rarely, radiographs may reveal tooth/root resorptive defects.

Checklist for Radiographic Assessment

All the following can be assessed:

- periodontal bone support
- caries
- crown shape and size
- proximity of restorations to pulp chamber
- quality of restorations, including coronal seal
- the size of the pulp chamber ± calcifications
- crown root ratio
- the number of roots
- root anatomy
- canal anatomy
- canal calcification
- root end proximity to important structures
- presence of lesions of endodontic origin periradicularly or furcally
- root fractures
- extra root canals
- resorptive defects
- quality and effectiveness of previous treatment
- root filling materials used
- iatrogenic complications
- presence of pins/posts.

Following conventional radiography there may be indications for three-dimensional (3D) imaging techniques to be utilised to improve diagnostic yield (Fig. 2.3), inform prognosis to aid treatment planning and provide information to plan execution of treatment. Indications for cone-beam computer tomography include the following:

- Assessment and/or management of root resorption
- Determine anatomically complex root canal systems prior to endodontic management (e.g. dens invaginatus)
- Presurgical assessment prior to complex periradicular surgery (e.g. proximity to sensitive anatomical structures such as the maxillary antrum or inferior dental nerve)
- Detection of radiographic signs of pathology or dentoalveolar trauma when plain film imaging is inconclusive and the diagnosis is unclear
- Non-surgical retreatment of cases where prognosis and treatment strategy is not clear from two-dimensional imagining
- Identification of the spatial location of extensively obliterated canals.

DIAGNOSIS

Following this systematic approach to history taking and the application of appropriate special tests, it will usually be possible to make a diagnosis of the pulpal or periradicular problems. Such diagnoses are covered in Section 2.1. After taking a thorough history and performing appropriate special tests, the clinician may be unsure as to whether the pain is of odontogenic origin. Endodontic treatment is invasive and should not be performed on an ad hoc or 'hit and miss' basis. In cases of difficult diagnosis, a referral to an orofacial pain clinic, a neurosurgeon or an ear, nose and throat specialist may be considered.

CASE SELECTION AND TREATMENT

Once a diagnosis has been reached, an endodontic treatment plan needs to be formulated. The difficulty of an endodontic case can be modified by a number of factors at a patient and diagnostic level. Some of these, such as the medical history and emergency presentations, have been

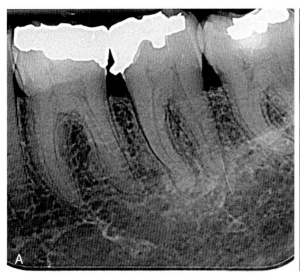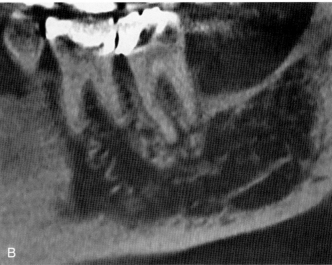

Fig. 2.3 (A) Intraoral periapical showing sound periradicular health of left mandibular second molar and (B) sagittal plane cone beam computerised tomography image of same tooth showing bone loss around apex of mesial and distal roots.

already discussed. However, limitation of opening, the position of the tooth in the arch and the ease of which routine radiography can be taken should not be underestimated. At a tooth level, the following may complicate treatment: presence of large restorations or crowns, significant root curvature, unusual canal anatomy, presence of pulp stones, calcifications, pathological resorption and previous root canal treatment.

The fact that an endodontic procedure is feasible is not sufficient justification for performing it. Endodontic treatment must be considered as part of an overall treatment plan in such a way that it represents the patient's best interests and wishes. Case selection is key to a successful outcome and not all cases will be manageable let alone successful. The past dental history will have provided information as to the patient's attitude towards treatment. Good endodontic treatment takes time, requiring a commitment from both clinician and patient.

On occasions it may be necessary to perform endodontic treatment on teeth which would normally be considered unrestorable due to the patient's medical history. There are an increasing number of patients with a history of radiotherapy or prescription of bisphosphonate drugs which puts them at a high risk of osteonecrosis of the jaw if a tooth was extracted. In these cases extra efforts may be warranted to save the tooth and re-establish healthy periradicular tissues even if the crown of the tooth cannot be restored predictably.

Treatment Planning

Sequencing of treatment involves the management of pulpal or periodontal pain as a priority, and the extraction of unsavable teeth. Teeth with large carious lesions should be stabilised with pre-endodontic cores and a preventive regimen instituted to halt any further progress of periodontal disease or caries. Endodontic and restorative procedures can then be performed in a more stable environment and more predictable results can be obtained.

2.3 Vital Pulp Therapy

LEARNING OBJECTIVES

You should:
- be able to recognise conditions that may affect the dental pulp
- understand the relationship between pulpal diagnosis and appropriate treatment.

The principles of minimally invasive treatment approaches are becoming more established as the importance of conserving dental tissue once the integrity of a tooth is broken is becoming more fully appreciated. Preserving a vital pulp is fundamental to such strategies and has numerous benefits:

- Preservation of the tooth's defence system.
- Preservation of full proprioceptive function of the tooth.
- Root canal treatment is technically demanding and not always predictable.
- Permits normal growth of the tooth and dento-alveolar complex during development.
- Avoids root filled teeth that are weakened are more prone to fracture.

The vitality of the dental pulp can be challenged in many ways, including carious tissue loss, non-carious tooth surface loss, trauma and iatrogenic damage, leading to reversible or irreversible changes. The extent of injury to the pulp is very difficult to determine and clinicians rely on weak empirical evidence, since there is a poor correlation between clinical signs and symptoms and the true histological state of the pulp; however, this standpoint is being questioned. In 1922, not long after the pioneering thesis of Herman (1920) which demonstrated the regenerative capacity of the dental pulp, the exposed pulp was described as a 'doomed organ' (Rebel). Unfortunately, that dogma still blights our approach and anecdotally appears to be followed by some undergraduate teaching programmes even though our understanding of the reparative mechanisms of the dentine–pulp complex is now so much greater. Following pulpal injury, the vitality of the pulp can be maintained therapeutically in one of three ways: indirect pulp cap, direct pulp cap and pulp amputation/pulpotomy.

STRATEGIES FOR VITAL PULP TREATMENT (VPT)

Clinicians carrying out an operative procedure on a vital tooth should be mindful that the heat generated by dental handpieces, the potential damage by over dehydrating dentine and the use of caustic agents in tooth restoration can result in unnecessary iatrogenic pulp damage. Frequently prevention is better than cure and therefore care/attention should be taken when removing tooth tissue/selecting materials to prevent injury to the pulp. Damage to the pulp will not just occur when the surrounding dentine is breached and thus VPTs should not just be considered as procedures to manage the injured pulp but also thought of as a treatment step to prevent pulpal disease. The range of VPTs can be considered as follows with the aim of producing a positive biological response so the pulp can protect itself:

Indirect pulp capping: Application of a material onto a thin layer of dentine which is close to the pulp.
Direct pulp capping: Application of a material directly onto the pulp.
Partial pulpotomy: Removal of a small portion of superficial coronal pulp tissue followed by application of a material directly onto the pulp.
Full pulpotomy: Complete removal of the coronal pulp to the root canal orifice level followed by application of a material directly onto the remaining pulp.
Pulpectomy: Total removal of the pulp from the root canal system followed by root canal treatment where there is no potential seen of producing a positive biological response so the pulp can protect itself.

The following guidelines cover all indications and treatment procedures to treat the vulnerable pulp irrespective of whether dentine is lost due to caries, trauma or previous iatrogenic intervention. In the case of treating caries, a strong evidence base shows that when managing deep carious lesions, a selective caries removal approach should be adopted (one-stage or two-stage stepwise technique) in order to decrease the risk of pulpal exposure.

Numerous different materials have been used in VPTs. The aim of using these materials is to protect the pulp and maintain its normal function. In order to do this the primary properties of such materials are:

- antibacterial
- create a bacterial tight seal and prevention of microleakage
- promote tertiary dentinogenesis and controlled hard tissue barrier formation
- biocompatible – prevention of 'over' irritation and avoidance of induction of a severe inflammatory response
- radio-opaque
- resistant to forces of displacement of any subsequent material placed over them.

It is established that calcium silicate cements (CSCs) such as mineral trioxide aggregate (MTA) induce a more predictable and better pulpal response compared to calcium hydroxide; however, calcium hydroxide still produces good results and is widely available to all practitioners. CSCs are yet to establish themselves as a mainstream material used by all general dental practitioners and although CSCs are the material of choice for VPTs, calcium hydroxide is still considered acceptable.

It is important to note that bismuth oxide containing CSCs should not be used on anterior teeth or on teeth where aesthetics is important. Although these materials have excellent biological characteristics, there is clear evidence that such materials can discolour teeth and should be avoided in these situations. CSCs that do not contain bismuth oxide such as biodentine have not yet shown cause for concern with respect to discolouration; however, users should still be cautious as such materials have not been used for long enough to clearly demonstrate that they will not cause any form of discolouration.

INDIRECT PULP CAPPING

It could be argued that any therapeutic process for the benefit of pulp survival that is adopted during a restoration of a tooth with an unexposed pulp is an indirect pulp cap. Classically, this procedure is carried out when dentine is lost due to caries, trauma or a previous iatrogenic intervention and a cavity exists which is close to the pulp but dentine still remains over the pulp tissue.

Procedure Outline (Fig. 2.4)

The tooth should be isolated with dental dam and the cavity preparation completed as appropriate. The cavity should be disinfected using cotton pellets soaked (removing gross excess) ideally with sodium hypochlorite (0.5–5%). The deepest part of the cavity, closest to the pulp, should be covered ideally with a CSC or calcium hydroxide. If calcium hydroxide is used it should be sealed with glass ionomer cement (GIC) or a resin glass ionomer cement (RMGIC). The tooth is then definitively restored with the appropriate restorative material.

DIRECT PULP CAPPING

This procedure is carried out if dentine is lost due to caries, trauma or a previous iatrogenic intervention and a cavity

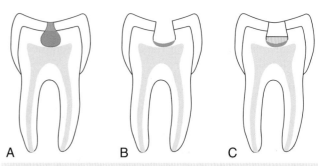

Fig. 2.4 Indirect pulp capping. (A) Deep carious lesion extending close to the pulp. (B) Cavity preparation adopting a selective caries removal approach to minimise the risk of pulp exposure, (C) Calcium silicate cement overlying caries with definitive restoration.

exists where the soft tissue of the pulp is exposed (≤2 mm) and in most cases is bleeding. When carrying out this treatment strategy, if symptoms exist they should be relatively mild and not considered to be indicative of irreversible pulpitis.

Procedure Outline (Fig. 2.5)

As soon as a pulp exposure is realised, it is crucial that the tooth is isolated immediately with dental dam. Once the cavity preparation has been completed, it and the exposed pulp should be disinfected using cotton pellets soaked (removing gross excess) ideally with sodium hypochlorite (0.5–5%). Once bleeding is controlled, the exposed pulp should be covered ideally with a CSC but calcium hydroxide is still suitable if an appropriate CSC is not available. If calcium hydroxide is used it should be sealed with GIC or a RMGIC. The tooth can then be definitively restored.

PARTIAL PULPOTOMY

This treatment strategy is used when dentine is lost due to caries, trauma or previous iatrogenic intervention and a cavity exists where the soft tissue of the pulp is exposed and bleeding and in most cases ≥2 mm. The exposed pulp appears to be inflamed/contaminated or it is not possible to get haemostasis due to the inflammation.

Procedure Outline (Fig. 2.6)

The tooth should be isolated with dental dam. Superficial coronal pulp tissue is removed with a high-speed

handpiece and bleeding controlled using cotton pellets soaked (removing gross excess) ideally with sodium hypochlorite (0.5–5%). If bleeding is not controlled within 8–10 minutes further pulp tissue should be removed. A CSC is placed onto the remaining pulp tissue; however, calcium hydroxide is still suitable if an appropriate CSC is not available. If calcium hydroxide is used it should be sealed with GIC or a RMGIC. The tooth can then be definitively restored.

FULL PULPOTOMY

A full pulpotomy is carried out when there is gross loss of dentine due to caries, trauma or previous iatrogenic intervention and a cavity exists where a large portion of the soft tissue of the pulp is exposed and bleeding. The exposed pulp appears to be inflamed/contaminated or it is not possible to get haemostasis at a superficial level.

Procedure Outline (Fig. 2.7)

The tooth should be isolated with dental dam. The coronal pulp tissue is completely removed to canal orifice level with high speed handpiece and bleeding controlled using cotton pellets soaked (removing gross excess) ideally with sodium hypochlorite (0.5–5%). If bleeding is not controlled within 8–10 minutes further pulp tissue should be removed until haemostasis is achieved or it is determined that a pulpectomy should be carried out. A CSC is placed onto the remaining pulp tissue; however, calcium hydroxide is still suitable if an appropriate CSC is not available.

PULPECTOMY

For completeness this procedure is considered here as it is a form of vital pulp treatment. In treating cases, where it is determined that the pulp is non-viable as it appears to be severely inflamed/contaminated/not possible to get haemostasis or appears necrotic a pulpectomy may be indicated. In such cases it has been shown that success rates are higher when the pulpectomy and root canal treatment is completed in one visit and the clinician should adopt a cautious approach with length control as it is better to be short of the apical constriction. The treatment procedure is outlined in detail in Sections 2.4, 2.5 and 2.6.

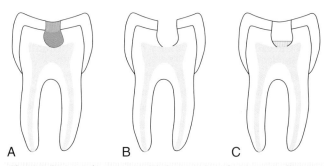

Fig. 2.5 Direct pulp capping. (A) Deep carious lesion extending to the pulp. (B) Carious exposure of pulp following cavity preparation. (C) Calcium silicate cement directly interfacing with pulp and definitive restoration has been completed.

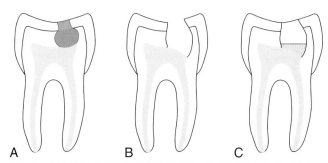

Fig. 2.6 Partial pulpotomy. (A) Deep carious lesion extending to the pulp. (B) Superficial pulp tissue which is inflamed is removed. (C) Calcium silicate cement directly interfacing with pulp and definitive restoration has been completed.

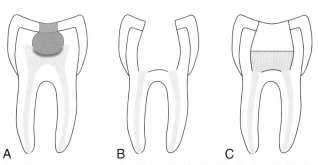

Fig. 2.7 Full pulpotomy. (A) Deep carious lesion extending to the pulp. (B) The whole of the coronal portion of the pulp is removed. (C) Calcium silicate cement directly interfacing with pulp stumps at the canal orifice and definitive restoration has been completed.

FOLLOW-UP AND OUTCOMES FOR VPT

Following VPT, teeth should be carefully monitored by history and clinical examination at 6 months and a periapical radiograph at one year. If symptoms persist or there is uncertainty regarding healing, the tooth should continue to be assessed at regular intervals and a further intervention should be carried out if indicated. Cold and electric pulp testing should be carried out to monitor pulpal response, noting that teeth with full pulpotomy will be unresponsive.

VPT carried out well using aseptic techniques can produce predictable results with a high success rate. Direct pulp capping with either a CSC or calcium hydroxide at one year shows success rates of nearly 90% with partial and full pulpotomy demonstrating 98% and 99% success rates respectively at the same time point.

2.4 Root Canal Morphology

LEARNING OBJECTIVES

You should:
* understand the complexity of root canal morphology
* appreciate the importance of adequate access in root canal therapy.

An understanding of the expected root canal anatomy before embarking on root canal treatment is essential. Intra-oral preoperative radiographs will provide useful information as to the overall anatomy. Shifts in horizontal or vertical angulation of periapical radiography can also help visualise what the likely root canal anatomy will be. In reality, root canal anatomy has significant variability from tooth to tooth and from person to person. In cases where clinical and plain film examination reveals complex anatomy, there may be an indication for a limited field cone beam computerised tomography scan (CBCT) which will provide more information on the morphology. Studies of cleared extracted teeth have shown that all roots enclose at least one root canal system, which frequently consists of a network of branches that often interconnect. Furthermore, developmental anomalies may also impact on the ability to deliver uncomplicated root canal treatment; these include dens invaginatus where folds in enamel and dentine often allow the passage of bacteria into the invagination and communication with the pulp. Similarly, childhood trauma may well have stunted root development leaving teeth with incomplete root development, and if this were to have happened in early childhood, root dilacerations (sharp bends or curves) may further complicate the anatomy seen.

Roots often have communications with the periodontal ligament along their length either in the furcation (furcal canals) or laterally (lateral canals). In addition, the root canal may frequently terminate not at a single point but with an array of accessory canals forming an apical delta. These furcal, lateral and apical communications have been termed 'portals of exit' from the root canal system. Furcal, lateral and accessory canals are created during tooth formation either when there is a break in the sheath of Hertwig or the sheath itself grows around an existing periodontal blood vessel. On occasion, such canals can be as large as the apical

constriction. These may harbour bacteria in niches which are difficult or impossible to instrument, further emphasising the importance of adequate chemical disinfection of the canal system throughout treatment.

The pulp chamber and root canal orifices may be reduced in size as a result of the age-related deposition of secondary, or reactionary and reparative tertiary dentine. Identification of these issues preoperatively will help inform access cavity depth and the need for caution where pulp chamber volume has been decreased. If pulp irritation is severe with extensive destruction of pulpal cells, then further inflammatory changes involving the rest of the pulp will take place and could lead to pulp necrosis. Such pulpal degeneration starts coronally and progresses apically. Necrotic pulpal breakdown products may leach out of the root canal system to form lesions of endodontic origin around the various portals of exit. Sometimes changes may be visible as widening of the periodontal membrane space lateral to the root before they are apparent apically.

IMPORTANT GENERAL CONSIDERATIONS OF PULPAL ANATOMY

Pulp Chamber Anatomy

This alters with age, irritants, attrition, caries, abrasion and periodontal disease. Generally, the pulp chamber is located in the centre of the tooth at the CEJ level, and the outline shape of the root canals apical to this will reflect the external root morphology throughout the length of the root (Fig. 2.8). The walls of the pulp chamber are lighter in colour than the darker floor.

Root Canal Orifices

With the exception of maxillary molars, the root canal orifices lie equidistant from the mesio-distal midline of the tooth where the walls of the pulp chamber meet the floor. Developmental fusion lines on the floor of the pulp chamber will also help to guide identification of root canal orifices.

Root Anatomy

Over 90% of roots are curved but this may not be immediately obvious from plain film radiography as the curvature may be in a bucco-lingual direction. Canals with curvature beyond 45° are extremely challenging to navigate. The only roots that rarely contain two canals are maxillary anteriors, maxillary premolars with two roots and the distobuccal and palatal roots of maxillary molars. All other (note this includes all mandibular) roots may contain two canals.

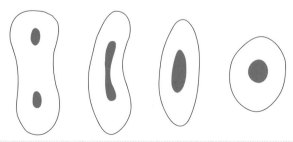

Fig. 2.8 Cross-sections of root canal anatomy showing the relationship between pulpal and radicular shape.

Apical Anatomy Changes With Age

The apical constriction is variable and usually cannot be detected by tactile sense, as dentine laid down in the coronal third of root canals will frequently cause files to bind coronally before they reach the apical third of the root canal.

ACCESS

Access to the root canal system involves both coronal access to the pulp chamber and radicular access to the root canals.

Coronal Access

The coronal access preparation in root canal therapy serves several important functions to:

- provide an unimpeded path to the root canal system
- eliminate the pulp chamber roof in its entirety
- be large enough to allow light in and enable inspection of the pulp chamber floor for root canal orifices or fractures
- have divergent walls to support a temporary dressing between visits
- provide a straight-line path to each canal orifice.

Examination of the tooth will provide guidance as to the position, size and angulation of the access cavity as many teeth are tilted in one or more planes relative to the arch and adjacent teeth. The ideal access cavity will achieve the above objectives but will preserve as much sound coronal and radicular tissue as possible. Occasionally, however, it may be necessary to enlarge and deflect access to enhance the preparation of roots that are especially curved in their coronal thirds. In these situations, access preparation is dynamic, developing as instrumentation progresses.

Radicular Access

The principle of straight-line radicular access cannot be overemphasised as it allows instruments to flow down the cavity line angles into the apical third of the root canal system without interruption and provides maximum tactile feedback while instrumenting the most delicate apical portion of the root canal. Adequate straight-line access reduces the angle of curvature in the coronal third of the root canal where it exits from the floor of the pulp chamber and thus reduces the overall canal curvature. Further advantages are discussed later.

Access to the root canal system is aided by examination of:

- coronal anatomy
- tooth position and angulation
- external root morphology
- the preoperative radiograph (preferably more than one taken at different angles).

Examination of the radiograph affords information on:

- the size of the pulp chamber ± calcifications
- the distance of the chamber from the occlusal surface (overlay the access bur to determine the maximum safe depth)
- the angle of exit of root canals from the floor of the pulp chamber; this provides an indication of the amount of coronal third root canal modification required to obtain straight-line access
- the number of roots, degree of root curvature and canal patency.

ENDODONTIC ACCESS OPENINGS, LENGTHS AND CONFIGURATIONS

Incisor and Canine Teeth

The access cavities for maxillary central and lateral incisors are similar and broadly triangular in shape taking into account the mesial and distal pulp horns. Straight-line access may require extension of the access cavity to include the palatal aspect of the incisal edge (Fig. 2.9). Average lengths for maxillary central incisors are 23.5 mm and they typically have a single root canal; maxillary lateral incisors average 22 mm in length and often have distal curvature to their single root canal.

Access cavities for maxillary and mandibular canines are almost identical and more ovoid in shape (see Fig. 2.9). Upper canine root length averages at 26.5 mm with a single root canal and 23.5 mm for lower canines; around 15% of lower canines have two root canals.

Access for mandibular central and lateral incisors is triangular in shape, and a second canal may be present in 40% which often merge again towards the apex. Identification of the second canal may require extension of the access cavity towards the incisal edge and under the cingulum (see Fig. 2.9). Average lengths of mandibular central and lateral incisors are 21 mm.

Premolar Teeth

Premolar teeth have more variability in their anatomy and canal configurations. The maxillary first premolar in most individuals contains two canals and the access cavity is extended more buccolingually than in single-rooted premolars. Approximately 5% may have a third root/canal placed buccally. In such situations, the access will be triangular in outline with the base towards the buccal side (Fig. 2.10). Maxillary first premolars average 21 mm in length.

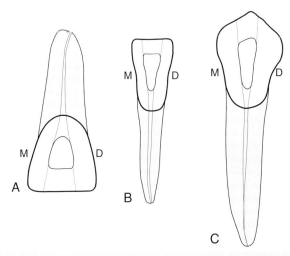

Fig. 2.9 Access cavity outline for anterior teeth. (A) Upper incisor. (B) Lower incisor. (C) Canine teeth. *M*, Mesial; *D*, distal.

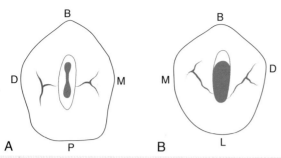

Fig. 2.10 Access cavity outline for (A) upper and (B) lower premolar teeth. *M*, Mesial; *D*, distal; *P*, palatal; *B*, buccal.

The maxillary second premolar (average length 21.5 mm), the mandibular first premolar (average length 21.5 mm) and second premolars (average length 22.5 mm) usually have one centrally located root canal but again there may be variations present. If the canal appears to be situated under either the buccal or lingual cusp, look carefully for a second canal under the opposite cusp. The access opening is a narrow oval shape. The maxillary second premolar access is centred over the central groove. Access for mandibular premolars should be made just buccal to the central groove (see Fig. 2.10).

Maxillary Molars

The maxillary molar access is generally triangular in shape with the base to the buccal and the apex to the palatal, taking care not to overextend the access cavity beyond the transverse oblique ridge. Usually, one palatal and two buccal canals are identified. However, two canals may be present in the mesiobuccal root in 90% of cases with approximately half ending in two foramina (Fig. 2.11). Maxillary upper molars average 21 mm in length.

Mandibular Molars

The mandibular molar access should start broadly triangular in shape and with the base towards the mesial and apex towards the midpoint of the occlusal. Mandibular molars usually have two roots (mesial and distal) with two canals in the mesial root and one in the distal root (see Fig. 2.11). If necessary, the access cavity can be extended into more of a trapezoid in shape if two distal canals equidistant from the midline are identified (33% cases).

Access: Prior Considerations

A number of steps should be taken to prepare for access (Box 2.1).

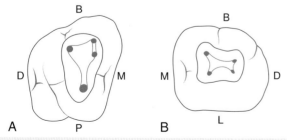

Fig. 2.11 Access cavity outline for (A) upper and (B) lower molar teeth. *M*, Mesial; *D*, distal; *P*, palatal; *B*, buccal.

Box 2.1 Access: Prior Considerations.

- Removal and replace all defective and temporary restorations where possible.
- Ensure that all caries has been removed prior to entering the pulp chamber.
- Assess the restorability of the tooth.
- Extract unrestorable teeth.
- Restorable but broken-down teeth should be repaired with composite or amalgam; some may require an orthodontic band to aid dental dam isolation and reduce the likelihood of fracture between visits.
- Examine radiographs carefully to assess the complexity of treatment, e.g. identify if the root canal anatomy is visible throughout the length of the canal, any variations including curvature, pulp chamber calcifications and existing filling materials.
- If the tooth has a full-coverage crown, be aware that the pulp chamber anatomy may not be orientated to the crown.

Dental Dam

The dental dam is essential for root canal treatment and affords the following advantages:

- asepsis – prevention of saliva contamination
- improved visibility
- soft tissue protection
- confinement of excess irrigant
- reduced liability in the medicolegal sense.

On occasions, particularly where the coronal anatomy has been altered or replaced with large restorations, it may be deemed appropriate to initiate access prior to the placement of dental dam as this allows better appreciation of external root contour and tooth position. The dam should be placed as soon as the pulp chamber is identified for the aforementioned reasons.

Access Technique

Box 2.2 describes the technique used to achieve access.

2.5 Root Canal Preparation – Cleaning and Shaping of the Root Canal System

LEARNING OBJECTIVES

You should:
- understand the technical procedures involved in combating root canal infection
- appreciate some of the problems that may be encountered in root canal preparation
- appreciate some of the technological advancements that have made root canal preparation more predictable.

Herbert Schilder's seminal paper entitled 'Cleaning and Shaping the Root Canal' has been adopted as the ideological approach to managing the infected root canal system. In this, it refers to cleaning and shaping 'as the removal of all organic substrate from the root canal system and the development of a purposeful form within each canal for the

Box 2.2   Access: Technique for Entering a Pulp Chamber.

1. Outline the standard access cavity shape using a water-cooled bur (see Figs 2.9–2.11). The authors' preference is for a tapered diamond bur with around 8 mm of cutting diamonds over the length. Progress is then made pulpally, constantly being spatially aware of the depth of the bur and its orientation, stopping and checking where necessary. A round-ended bur is preferred as flat-ended ones tend to gouge the access cavity walls. The expected depth of the pulp chamber can be compared to the preoperative radiograph; if the cavity depth is at the full depth of the cutting diamonds, then the access may be misaligned or the chamber sclerosed. It is useful to remember that dentine is yellow/brown in colour, and the floor of the pulp chamber is grey.
2. If the canal(s) cannot be readily located, stop and check radiographically.
3. Once the pulp chamber has been identified, it is deroofed and smoothed using a safe, non-end cutting bur such as an endo-z bur; it may be necessary to use a Gates–Glidden bur to remove small overhanging areas of the pulp chamber roof especially in smaller teeth where use of a bur in air rotor would be overly destructive.
4. The pulp chamber space should now be thoroughly irrigated with sodium hypochlorite solution and canal orifices identified using a straight probe or DG16 endodontic explorer. Magnification and lighting are particularly useful in helping to identify small root canal openings and to refine access.
5. Further refinement of the access may now be performed to enable straight-line access to the canals. In addition, troughing may be performed using a long-neck or goose-neck bur; alternatively the careful use of high powered cutting piezoelectric ultrasonic inserts will remove dentine overlying canal orifices, especially in the MB2 region of upper molar teeth.

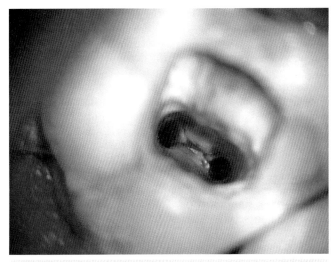

Fig. 2.12 A multirooted tooth with a connecting isthmus between two of the canals, this space may be anatomically complex with various interconnections throughout its length. It is a potential reservoir of tenacious infected biofilm.

reception of a dense and permanent root canal filling'. He established the broad objectives that are still relevant today when carrying out root canal treatment and can be considered separately as the biological and technical objectives of root canal preparation.

BIOLOGICAL OBJECTIVES OF CLEANING AND SHAPING THE ROOT CANAL SYSTEM

Pulp death and subsequent necrosis renders the root canal space undefended and provides an ideal environment which has an abundant nutrient source to support microbial proliferation. To use a military analogy, this chamber acts as a barrack to harbour micro-organisms in which they have the opportunity to develop pathogenicity and induce inflammatory disease of the periradicular tissues. Primary endodontic infections are caused by oral bacteria which are usually opportunistic pathogens. Once the root canal space is infected, endodontic microbiota exist in a fluid phase or, as dense bacterial aggregates/coaggregates adhered to the root canal walls forming multi-layered communities that resemble a biofilm (Fig. 2.12). The root canal space is a complex environment – it is not as simple as round canals passing through the centre of the roots. The anatomy is unique to every tooth and there may be accessory canals, fins, isthumi, branches and other aberrant forms. It is not

possible to mechanically prepare the whole of the root canal system and therefore the operator is reliant on other methods of cleaning this space. The biological objectives suggested by Schilder have therefore evolved but the underlying philosophy remains the same which is to:

- disinfect as much of the root canal system as possible
- remove any potential nutrient source to prevent recolonisation of micro-organisms in the root canal system
- prevent recontamination of the root canal system.

MECHANICAL OBJECTIVES OF CLEANING AND SHAPING THE ROOT CANAL SYSTEM

Cleaning and shaping are processes that are not independent of one another. Mechanically altering the shape of the root canal system facilitates cleaning in two ways: (1) direct removal of bacteria and nutrient sources from the root canal system; and (2) enables active agents that are involved in the disinfection process to penetrate deeper into the root canal system. Schilder proposed design objectives in order to shape the canal so that cleaning could be facilitated but also to produce a shape that would aid obturation to produce an optimal seal. These objectives are summarised as:

- Taper – A continuously tapered preparation should be produced.
- Canal axis – The position of the canal axis should be maintained in the centre of the root.
- Foramen – The original position of the foramen should be maintained and it should not be enlarged.

A continuously tapering preparation is required to deliver and exchange chemically active fluids to the canal terminus in order to remove and destroy bacteria that are driving the inflammatory process in periradicular disease. Sufficient space needs to be created to enable solutions to be carried to the apical part of the canal. It has been suggested that canals should be prepared to larger diameters to achieve this; however, larger canal preparation may lead to destruction of the delicate anatomy of the apical foramen compromising the ability to seal the canal. There is clearly a greater risk of perforation with such an approach and it can also lead to weakening of the dentine thus compromising the long-term survival of the tooth.

In summary, the aim of root canal preparation is to debride the pulp space, rendering it as bacteria free as possible, producing a shape amenable to irrigation and obturation. This apparently straightforward task is clinically challenging through the complex anatomy of root canal systems.

INSTRUMENT MANIPULATION

The two most commonly used motions applied to endodontic instruments (files) are watch winding and balanced force.

Watch winding refers to the gentle side-to-side rotation of a file (30° each way). This motion is useful for all stages of canal preparation, especially initial negotiation and finishing the apical third.

Balanced forces involves rotating a file 60° clockwise to 'set the flutes' and then rotating it 120° anticlockwise while maintaining apical pressure sufficient to resist coronal movement of the file. Balanced forces are an efficient cutting motion and have been shown to maintain a central canal position even around moderate curvatures while allowing a larger size to be prepared apically (compared with other hand instrumentation techniques).

Coronal interferences influence the forces a file will exert within a canal. This is of particular importance in curved canals where files may prepare more dentine along the furcal (danger zone) as opposed to the outer canal wall. It is important to be aware of this, to limit the size of enlargement in curved canals and direct files away from the furcal wall to avoid a strip perforation (Fig. 2.13).

IRRIGATION

Advances in preparation techniques may plateau in the near future, and in order to improve treatment outcome, there will be more reliance on improving methods of irrigation with enhanced biological activity. A philosophy of minimally invasive endodontics is developing, in which access cavities are limited in size in order to preserve as much tooth tissue as possible, to prevent weakening the tooth. Whilst preservation of tooth structure is of course

important, this should never be done at the expense of hindering canal location, access or increase the risk of problems during preparation. There is currently little evidence for the benefit of these very limited size occlusal access cavities when the marginal ridges that provide much of a tooth's flexural strength remain intact. Such an ideology will rely even more heavily on irrigation or more advanced methods of disinfection of the root canal. Our basic demands for irrigating solutions are outlined in Table 2.1; however, in the future, more efficacious irrigants will be required to fulfil a minimally invasive philosophy and an appetite for treatment modalities which are more biologically driven to improve healing.

Irrigating solutions are usually delivered using a syringe with a 27- or 28-gauge side-venting needle. Care should be taken to ensure that the needle tip remains free in the canal and does not bind; if this were to happen there is a risk that the canal becomes an extension of the irrigating needle with the risk of extrusion of irrigating solution into periapical tissues. The role of the irrigant is to remove debris and provide lubrication for instruments. Specifically, an irrigant such as sodium hypochlorite will dissolve organic remnants and, most importantly, also has an antibacterial action. It may be used in a range of concentrations (0.5–5.25%), with 2.5% being popular. It is important that the irrigant is changed frequently; ideally irrigation should be performed between each file, at least every two to three files being the minimum. If removal of the smear layer is desired, then an irrigation solution containing ethylenediamine tetra-acetic acid (EDTA) should be used. There is no clinical consensus to the removal of the smear layer although there is opinion that it may have a positive effect on the outcome of retreatment cases.

Enhancing Irrigant Efficacy

Numerous suggestions have been made to enhance the efficacy of irrigation solutions. For example, by intensifying the energy supplied to the irrigant by mechanical means, heat or ultrasound. It is worth noting that whichever technique is adopted, irrigant use carries a risk of complications, especially with the use of NaOCl; controlled safe practice is therefore essential. Conventionally, irrigant is delivered via a syringe in a passive manner or with simple agitation. The latter is achieved by moving the needle up and down whilst dispensing the irrigant. Other simple methods of manual agitation include using a gutta-percha cone with an 'in and out' pumping action – this has been shown to significantly improve debris removal compared to no agitation.

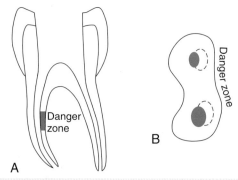

Fig. 2.13 The danger zone where care needs to be taken in order to avoid strip perforation. (A) Lateral view and (B) cross-sectional view.

Table 2.1 Summary of Desired Properties From an Irrigant Solution Used in Endodontics.

Biological	▪ High bactericidal efficacy against micro-organisms in biofilms and their planktonic state
	▪ Inactivate endotoxin
	▪ Nontoxic and hypoallergenic to vital tissues
Mechanical	▪ Flush out debris
	▪ Lubricate the canal
Chemical	▪ Dissolve organic tissue
	▪ Dissolve inorganic tissue and remove smear layer

Other methods may improve the hydrodynamic action of the solution through using additional devices or pieces of equipment. Sonic agitation operating at a lower frequency (1–6 kHz) produces smaller shear stresses than the similarly principled ultrasonic agitation (25–30 kHz). The endo activator (Dentsply Sirona, Switzerland) is a device which is operated in the sonic frequency range. It is an untethered handpiece with a smooth polymer disposable tip that is inserted and activated in a saturated canal. It has been reported to clean debris from lateral canals, remove the smear layer and dislodge clumps of simulated biofilm within the curved canals of molar teeth. Ultrasonic devices can enhance the energy in the irrigation solution through transmission from an oscillating file or smooth wire which induces acoustic microstreaming and cavitation within the solution. Such a technique is known as passive ultrasonic irrigation (PUI). It is suggested that ultrasonic systems remove more dentine debris than sonic ones. A further technique suggested to improve irrigant efficacy follows the principle of developing apical negative pressure to ostensibly drag irrigant into the apical portion of the canal. One such system is known as the EndoVac system (Kerr, USA). Irrigant solution is dragged into the canal by a macro- or micro-cannula which is positioned in the apical part of the canal and connected to a conventional dental suction system. This results in a high volume of irrigant flow/replenishment and reduced risk of extrusion of irrigant solution.

CANAL PREPARATION

Several methods of canal preparation exist; however most contemporary techniques follow this basic sequential framework:

- canal exploration
- pre-enlargement (when necessary)
- straight-line radicular access
- length determination and apical patency
- apical third preparation.

Canal Exploration

Root canals are infinitely variable in their shapes and sizes. Larger canals allow easy placement of instruments and irrigating solutions whereas smaller ones require pre-enlargement coronally prior to the canal exploration. Preliminary assessment of the canal can be made with the smallest and most flexible instruments. It is unlikely that the operator will be able to determine the working length initially as files may be binding coronally.

Pre-enlargement and Straight-Line Radicular Access

Pre-enlargement may be achieved by watchwinding file, small flexible stainless steel hand file sizes 10–20 in series, gradually opening up narrow canal orifices to a size sufficient to take a mechanical bur (e.g. Gates–Glidden) or motor-driven endodontic file to gain radicular access. The pre-enlargement can then be developed further to produce straight-line radicular access taking care to work the bur away from furcal regions of roots. A file should stand upright in the tooth and pass undeflected deep into the canal once this has been achieved.

Radicular access is the process of pre-enlargement of the coronal part of the canal to facilitate a pathway to the characteristically and more anatomically complex apical third of the canal. Typically, in multirooted teeth this means removing dentine to eliminate any curvature in the coronal part of the canal so that subsequent files entering the apical region have straight-line access and an unimpeded pathway. Once the initial opening of the canal has been created with small stainless steel hand files, coronal curvature can be removed with instruments such as traditional Gates–Glidden burs, X-gates (Dentsply Sirona, Switzerland), Protaper Sx (Dentsply Sirona, Switzerland) or Endoflare (Micro-Mega, France) (Fig. 2.14) if required. This crown-down approach allows for bulk removal of infected material early in the preparation. This will also reduce stress on subsequent instruments used deeper in the canal and facilitate better irrigant exchange.

Advantages of pre-enlargement and establishment of straight-line access are as follows:

- It creates sufficient space to introduce files and irrigating needles/solutions deeper in the canal.
- The bacterial count in the more coronal aspects of the canal is reduced.
- A reservoir of irrigant is created that files pass through as they move apically.
- The increased space allows files to fit passively in the canal, making inoculation of infected material into the periapical tissues less likely.
- Pressure on the coronal flutes of the file is decreased thereby increasing tactile sense and control when using files in the apical third.
- Precurved files remain curved, can be easily inserted and freely pass down the canal.
- A greater volume of irrigant is present enhancing pulp digestion.
- The bulk of pulpal and related irritants are removed reducing debris accumulation apically.
- Working length is more accurate because there is a more direct path to the canal terminus.
- Larger files may be used for the working length radiograph.

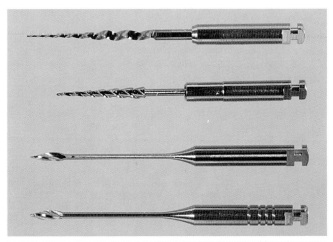

Fig. 2.14 Burs designed for improving straight-line radicular access. Top to bottom: ProTaper Sx (Dentsply Sirona), End of lare (Micromega), X-Gates, Gates Glidden No. 4 (Various).

It is important to ensure that the apical region of the canal is not blocked with dentine debris or pulp tissue when using a crown-down technique. For this reason, it is important that small files ± chelating agents are used to prevent blockage and ensure canal patency. Although apical preparation develops throughout canal enlargement, it is not completed until the end of the procedure when greater control is possible over the files in this most delicate region of the root canal.

Length Determination and Apical Patency

To best meet the biological objectives of cleaning and shaping the root canal system, the operator should attempt to prepare and obturate the whole canal. In terms of determining root canal length, clinically, the aim is to identify the apical constriction. This is the narrowest point of the root canal towards its terminus. Apical to this, the canal space widens to form the apical foramen and beyond is the periodontal ligament (in the absence of disease).

The length of a root canal can be determined in many ways, including radiographic methods, tactile discrimination, paper-point method and with the use of an electronic apex locator (EAL). It is now widely accepted by most operators that the EAL is a mandatory tool in the armamentarium of the dentist. Amongst manufacturers of these electronic devices there is not always consistency about which anatomical point the EAL will identify. It is however recognised by users that the most reliable reference point, regardless of the device, is the zero reading. With modern apex locators considered so reliable, a huge step forward has been made compared with relying on the preoperative radiograph to determine the length. In reality, this previous method was no more than a crude estimation of the length of the canal with the position of the apical foramen in relation to the radiographic apex varying enormously (0–3 mm) (Fig. 2.15). It is essential that care is taken over identification of the correct canal length with the aim to identify the apical constriction that is the narrowest point of the root canal.

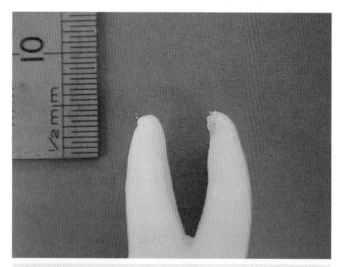

Fig. 2.15 Extracted tooth with patent files illustrating location of the foramen in relation to the tip of the root and therefore what would be the radiographic apex.

The working length can change during the preparation of curved canals. It is therefore important to recognise length determination as a process and not a single stage and therefore should be checked a few times during preparation to accommodate the likely change following removal of coronal interferences. The EAL lends itself well to this approach.

APICAL PATENCY

The concept of apical patency is considered controversial but is becoming increasingly accepted. A patency file is a small flexible instrument (08, 10) that will move passively through the terminus of a root canal without binding or enlarging the apical constriction. The aim is to prevent apical blockage which will, in turn, reduce the incidence of ledge formation and transportation of the root canal. The use of a patency file also helps remove vital or necrotic pulpal remnants from the end of the canal. To use a patency technique, therefore, infers an intention to clean to the full canal length. Care should be taken not to use larger instruments as patency files as these can damage the delicate periapical region and unnecessarily enlarge or transport the anatomical apex.

APICAL PREPARATION

Once straight-line access, glide pathway, patency and the working length of the canal have been established, the remaining part of the root canal preparation is more straightforward. There are countless methods of preparing the remainder of the root canal with the use of stainless steel hand files, ultrasonic instruments and hand/motor-driven NiTi (nickel titanium) instruments. Most recent developments in this area have focused on motor-driven NiTi instruments.

Apical Preparation With Conventional Instruments

Although the use of NiTi instruments is rapidly increasing, most root canals are still prepared today with conventional hand stainless steel files. Such techniques should never be discounted as they still have their place so that clinicians can develop skills to negotiate a complex canal and prepare a glide pathway. In larger, straight canals, the apical preparation is accomplished by preparing the apical portion using a slight rotational action of the file to an appropriate size after straight-line access has been confirmed.

Apical Preparation With NiTi Instruments

Since Nitinol was proposed as a material for the manufacture of root canal instruments in 1988 due to its increased flexibility compared to stainless steel, there has been considerable evolution of instrument design using NiTi alloys over the last three decades. The original NiTi files were based on a design with fixed tapered instruments and passive cutting radial lands file flutes. In order to improve ease of use, safety and efficiency, development from this point has concentrated on the following features of design: cutting flutes, variable tapers, the material, the motion and the cross-section. Cutting flutes were introduced to improve efficiency and variable tapers to limit the cutting portion of the file to a specific point within the canal. More recently, advancement has taken place with NiTi metallurgy, motion and novel cross-sectional designs.

Several novel thermomechanical processing and manufacturing technologies have been developed to optimise the microstructure of NiTi alloys to improve flexibility and fatigue resistance of endodontic instruments. NiTi files such as Reciproc and later Reciproc Blue (VDW, Germany), Twisted Files (SybronEndo, USA), WaveOne (Dentsply Sirona, Switzerland) and ProTaper Next (Dentsply Sirona, Switzerland) have been produced utilising these techniques. To some extent the precise details of the thermomechanical processing remain unknown due to the commercial sensitivity surrounding these products; it is clear however that these modifications have improved flexural fatigue resistance compared to files of similar design made from conventional NiTi alloy. Dentsply Sirona recently introduced what is described as a 'Gold Wire' NiTi alloy used in ProTaper Gold and WaveOne Gold (Dentsply Sirona Endodontics, Switzerland) which has reduced shape memory at room temperature compared to conventional NiTi alloys. This means it is possible to lightly precurve the instrument off the central axis without permanent deformation (Fig. 2.16). This instrument does feel different to most NiTi files when manipulated in the hand. It feels rubbery compared to the feel of flexing other NiTi instruments which bounce back immediately to their original shape when slightly bent. This feature has a technical advantage as the instrument can be precurved slightly in order to aid its placement into difficult-to-reach canals.

The use of NiTi instruments in a continuous rotating motion has been widely adopted by many practitioners. More recently, reciprocating motions have been developed as a new technique to prepare the root canal. This concept is not completely new as engine-driven files directed in an axial and rotational reciprocation motion have been used before, such as the Cursor Filing Contra-Angle in 1928 (W & H, Austria), the Racer in 1958 (W & H, Austria) and Giromatic in 1964 (Micro-Mega, France). These engine-driven reciprocating files never make a complete 360° rotation during the movement sequence. In newer systems, there is an unequal clockwise (CW) and counter-clockwise (CCW) movement. To date, there are two instrument systems which utilise such a motion which are manufactured by Dentsply International, namely, Reciproc (VDW,

Germany) and WaveOne (Dentsply Sirona, Switzerland). The principle behind these systems is that there is a rapid repetitive process of engagement and disengagement of the file with the canal wall through the precise CW and CCW movement as it effectively rotates through 360°. This reduces load on the file and allows it to follow the canal more easily. The files are designed in such a way that in most cases and following establishment of the glide path only one reciprocating file is required to prepare the canal.

Other recent developments in file design include an off-centred cross-section which is used in the following instrument systems: Revo-S (Micro-Mega, France), ProTaper Next and WaveOne Gold (Dentsply Sirona, Switzerland). The principle of this design is to minimise the engagement between the file and the dentine of the canal wall (Fig. 2.17), therefore decreasing the load on the file. Such a cross-section also allows space for debris to accumulate between the flutes of the file and it is driven in a coronal direction. It is anticipated that such a design would enhance cleaning of the root canal system due to efficient debris removal. The off-centred cross-sectional design also allows greater flexibility in the file. This is achieved as this file design creates a larger envelope of motion and will cut a larger preparation compared to a file with a conventional cross-sectional design. Therefore, a greater tapered preparation can be created with a file that has a smaller centred mass which will mean the file is more flexible.

Rotary Nickel–Titanium Instrumentation Technique

ProTaper Universal (Dentsply Sirona, Switzerland) is described here as an example of a rotary NiTi technique as it is a commonly used technique worldwide. It has an innovative instrument design which has a variable taper along its length, no radial lands and cuts very effectively. There are three progressively tapered Shaper files and five Finisher files with tip sizes of 20, 25, 30, 40, 50 and tapers in the apical three millimetres of 7%, 8%, 9% and 6%. The ProTaper Universal Shaper files should be taken to initial resistance and then brushed laterally, away from furcal areas. Each ProTaper Shaper creates its own crown-down shaping in view of the progressive taper (similar to the Eiffel Tower in profile). Finishers are taken sequentially short of the Shapers, not brushed, and removed immediately as soon as they have reached their length. ProTaper Universal files are also available for use by hand.

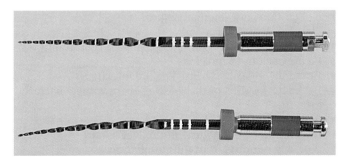

Fig. 2.16 WaveOne Gold primary (25, 0.07) instruments photographed at room temperature. (Top) Instrument is untouched following removal from packaging. (Bottom) Instrument is precurved off central axis without permanent deformation due to reduced shape memory compared to conventional NiTi instruments.

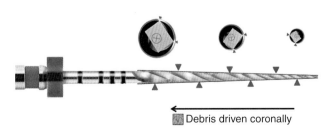

Debris driven coronally

Fig. 2.17 ProTaper Next file design with rectangle off-set cross-section along its length which results in only two points of engagement (*red arrows*). In principle this creates space for debris to be driven coronally when in motion.

Techniques for the use of rotary NiTi instruments are evolving continuously as greater understanding is gained of how best to use them safely. Pre-enlargement, coronal flaring and a crown-down approach are now recognised as being important considerations in getting best results and limiting instrument failure. Each rotary instrument may be dipped in a lubricant prior to use, with their use being preceded by irrigation and passage of a small hand instrument. This will move irrigating solutions deeper into the canal system and maintain canal patency. Apical preparation should be completed at the end.

NiTi has good shape memory so it is difficult to see when files are fatigued. Canal curvature and calcification seem to influence fatigue more than time of use. All files should be inspected following passage into the canal. The sensible operator should have a low threshold for discarding any damaged instruments or instruments that have been used past severe curvature rather than risk breakage. It is important to appreciate that these instruments are for canal enlargement, not canal negotiation.

It is especially important that a quality speed-reduction handpiece with high torque is used with NiTi instruments to allow appropriate defined speeds to be used. Instruments must be used with a light touch, similar to that which would be used with a narrow lead propelling pencil. Introduction into the canal should be gradual, using an in and out motion no more than 1 mm at a time. The instrument should be continuously introduced and removed, never being held at the same point in the canal.

The rotary NiTi instrumentation technique is a major development in canal preparation; however, it is important to be cautious in certain situations:

- Calcified canals (ideally it should be possible to establish a glide path and place at least a loose size 15/0.02 taper file to length prior to using rotary files in the apical third). Alternatively, rotary NiTi Pathfiles (tip sizes 0.13, 0.16, 0.19) or ProGlider files (tip size 0.16) may be used to create a glide path following the use of a 10 file in calcified or severely curved canals.
- Canals having sharp curvature in the apical region.
- Two canals that join into one smaller canal at a sharp angle.
- Large canals that suddenly narrow.

One Visit Root Canal Treatment

Root canal therapy may be performed in one visit if there is adequate time for both instrumentation and more importantly disinfection; the ability to dry the canals is important. Root canal treatment should not be rushed with a potentially compromised outcome just so that treatments can be performed in one visit. An advantage of doing a procedure in two visits is that an intracanal dressing of calcium hydroxide can be placed. This compound has a high pH and will further help to reduce the bacterial flora. Care needs to be taken to ensure that a sound coronal seal of 3–4 mm of temporary dressing material is present to prevent recontamination of the canal between visits. It is also usual to place a small pledget of cotton wool prior to placing the temporary dressing in order to prevent its inadvertent dropping into the canal between visits, or during subsequent removal.

2.6 Root Canal Obturation

LEARNING OBJECTIVES

You should:
- understand the reasons for obturating root canals
- appreciate that there are many different ways of achieving satisfactory canal obturation.

The aim of obturation is to establish a fluid tight barrier to protect the periradicular tissues from micro-organisms that reside in the oral cavity. The concept of a perfect airtight or hermetic seal is sadly unachievable; however, every attempt should be made to get as close as possible to that goal. Providing a well obturated system serves three main functions:

1. Prevent coronal leakage of micro-organisms or potential nutrients to support their growth into the dead space of the root canal system.
2. Prevent periapical or periodontal fluids percolating into the root canals feeding micro-organisms.
3. Entomb any residual micro-organisms that have survived the debridement and disinfection stages of treatment in order to prevent their proliferation and pathogenicity.

REQUIREMENTS BEFORE ROOT CANAL FILLING

The tooth must be asymptomatic, chemomechanical preparation completed and the root canal dry before a root filling is inserted. Any serous exudate from the periapical tissues indicates the presence of inflammation. If there is persistent seepage, calcium hydroxide may be used as a root canal dressing until the next visit. It is advisable to recheck the canal length in situations of persistent seepage as this may frequently result from overinstrumentation and damage to the periapical tissues.

Materials most commonly used for obturation are a combination of semisolid cores combined with a sealing cement. There are some newer two-part semisolid core and cement systems which are system dependent. To manage a wide and open apex, calcium silicate cements offer the best material properties for this clinical situation and are the material of choice.

Ideal properties of a root filling material are as follows:

- Be easily introduced into the root canal.
- Not irritate periradicular tissues.
- Not shrink after insertion.
- Seal the root canal laterally, apically and coronally.
- Be impervious to moisture.
- Be sterile or easily sterilised before insertion.
- Be bacteriostatic or at least not encourage bacterial growth.
- Be radio-opaque.
- Not stain tooth structure or gingival tissues.
- Be easily removed from the canal as necessary.

Now that we are entering a biological age, an additional demand would be to actively induce regeneration of the periradicular tissues rather than just creating a positive environment for them to heal.

TYPES OF ROOT FILLING MATERIALS

Solid and semisolid materials include gutta-percha and the C-point system (formally known as Smart Point – a hydrophilic obturation cone that swells laterally around its central axis and used with a sealer as a single cone technique). Previously silver points and resin-based systems such as Resilon/Real Seal have been considered under this categorisation; however, they are not recommended.
Sealers and cements include Tubliseal, AH Plus, pulp canal sealer, Roths sealer, AH 26 and calcium silicate sealers (CSSs).
Medicated pastes include N2, Endomethosone, Spad, Kri and are not recommended as they may contain paraformaldehyde, which is cytotoxic. Such materials are now considered historic.

Gutta-percha used in conjunction with a sealer is without doubt the most commonly used root canal filling material due to its consistent long-term success and because it can be removed.

GUTTA-PERCHA FILLING TECHNIQUES

Each of the techniques (except where indicated) will produce acceptable clinical results if used correctly. Proponents exist for the different techniques, although personal preference usually determines the final choice:

- Single cone.
- Lateral condensation.
- Thermomechanical compaction.
- Warm vertical condensation.
- Carrier-based techniques.

Single Cone

The single cone technique is not conventionally recommended as it does not provide a good barrier apically, laterally and coronally as little or no effort is made to deform the cone to occupy as much of the volume of the root canal space as possible. With this technique a sealer is introduced into the canal followed by a single well-fitting obturation cone. Due to the space around the single cone there is considerable reliance on the sealer and as many sealers are only designed to be a film thickness there is considerable weakness with such an approach.

This approach is now being reviewed as CSSs have been developed. These materials are capable of existing in a thicker form, may provide an excellent seal (based on the properties of the material they have evolved from – MTA) and show excellent biocompatibility. Although CSSs show great promise, there is little clinical research published to provide support for their use at this stage.

Lateral Condensation of Gutta-Percha

The objective is to fill the canal with gutta-percha points (cones) by condensing them laterally against the sides of the canal walls (Fig. 2.18). The technique requires a tapered canal preparation ending in an apical stop at the working length (Box 2.3).

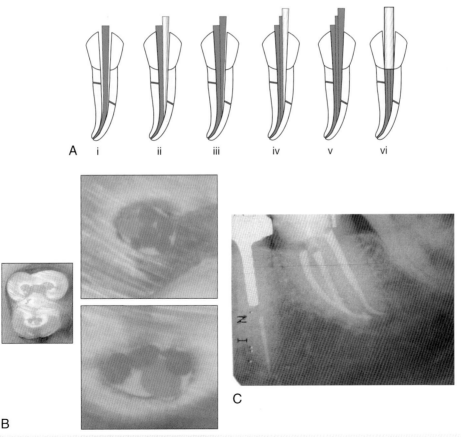

Fig. 2.18 Lateral condensation of gutta-percha. (A) Filling the canal with gutta-percha which is condensed laterally against the walls of the canal (i)–(vi). (B) Cross-section of mandibular molar showing multiple gutta-percha cones surrounded by sealer. (C) Postoperative radiograph of lower molar obturated using cold lateral condensation.

Box 2.3   Technique for Lateral Condensation of Gutta-Percha.

1. A spreader is selected that reaches to within 1 mm of the working length and the length marked with a rubber stopper.
2. A master point is selected that allows a friction fit in the apical portion of the root canal (see Fig. 2.18 Ai). When this is marked it is called 'tug back' (like pulling a dart out of a dart board). This may be difficult to achieve with small-size gutta-percha points; therefore, it is usual to accept a friction fit in narrow canals. A point one size larger than the master apical file is usually selected. If it is not possible to place the point to working length, select a point that passes to full length and trim 0.5 mm off the end using a scalpel (this has the effect of making the point slightly larger). Retry the point and adjust as necessary.
3. Mark the length of the point by nipping it with tweezers at the reference point and take a check radiograph with the cone in place.
4. Sealer placement. The sealer is mixed according to the manufacturer's instructions and introduced into the canal using a small sterile file rotated anticlockwise (omit this stage if there is a danger of sealer passing through the apical foramen, e.g. open apex). The master cone is then coated with sealer on the apical one-third and is introduced into the root canal slowly to aid coating of the canal walls and reduce the likelihood of sealer passing into the periapical tissues.

5. Once the master cone is seated, place a spreader between it and the canal wall using firm pressure in an apical direction (see Fig. 2.18 Aii) (lateral pressure may bend or break the spreader or fracture the root). This pressure, maintained for 20 seconds, will condense the gutta-percha apically and laterally leaving a space into which an accessory point is placed.
6. An accessory cone the same size or one size smaller than the spreader is used. Rotate the spreader slightly, remove it and immediately place the accessory cone. Repeat the procedure until the root canal is filled (see Fig. 2.18 Aiii–v). The finger spreader condenses each cone into position. The final cone is not condensed as this would leave a spreader tract and contribute to leakage.
7. Cut off the gutta-percha, 1 mm below the cementoenamel junction or gingival level (whichever is the more apical), using a hot instrument and vertically condense the gutta-percha (see Fig. 2.18 Avi). This is important as remaining root-filling material may stain the tooth.
8. If two or more canals are obturated with gutta-percha, undertake one at a time unless they meet in the apical third.
9. Seal the access cavity, remove the dental dam and take a postoperative radiograph.

There are two main types of spreading instrument for condensing gutta-percha: long-handled spreaders and finger spreaders. The main advantage of a finger spreader is that it is not possible to exert the high lateral pressure that might occur with long-handled spreaders. The chance of a root fracture is reduced and it is therefore a suitable instrument for beginners.

A modification to the cold lateral condensation technique is to perform it warm as this will soften the gutta-percha and make it easier to condense, possibly resulting in a denser root filling. The spreader may be heated by placing it in a hot bead steriliser before insertion into the canal. Alternatively, the friction of ultrasonic vibration may be used to introduce heat into the root filling.

Thermomechanical Compaction

In this thermomechanical technique, a compactor that resembles an inverted file is placed in a slow-speed handpiece and used to help to plasticise and condense the gutta-percha. Care must be taken to use this instrument only in the straight part of the canal in order to avoid gouging of the walls. The frictional heat from the compactor plasticises the gutta-percha and the blades drive the softened material into the root canal under pressure.

Lateral Condensation and Thermocompaction of Gutta-Percha

A modification of the thermomechanical technique has been described as an adjunct to lateral condensation. Gutta-percha is first laterally condensed in the apical half of the canal, then a compactor is used to plasticise and condense the gutta-percha in the straight coronal half of the canal. The laterally condensed material in the apical half of the canal effectively prevents any apical extrusion and the softened gutta-percha is thus forced against the dentine walls.

Warm Vertical Condensation

Thermal conductivity through gutta-percha occurs over a range of 2–3 mm and it only needs to be raised 3–8 degrees Celsius above body temperature (40–45 degrees Celsius) for it to become sufficiently mouldable. The requirements for vertical condensation of warm gutta-percha include a tapered preparation, accurate cone fit apically, suitable sealer, a heat source and a range of prefitted pluggers. Briefly, the technique of vertical condensation involves applying heat to the gutta-percha, condensing it down the root canal from coronal to apical (the downpack) and then filling the remaining space (the backfill). The downpack procedure results in apical corkage, filling of lateral and accessory canals and an empty canal space coronally. Backfilling of the canal is achieved by using thermoplasticised gutta-percha delivered in increments and condensed (see Box 2.4).

The technique uses a device heat carrier that has interchangeable soft steel pluggers of varying tapers, commonly 0.06, 0.08, 0.10 and 0.12. The pluggers are thermostatically controlled, can be heated to pre-set temperatures and maintain their temperature while condensing the gutta-percha within the root canal system. The appropriate plugger is selected to match the taper of the master cone, activated and used to condense the gutta-percha to just short of its binding point (4–5 mm from the terminus of the root canal). The heat is then reactivated, the plugger drops to the binding point and is removed together with excess gutta-percha, providing an apical plug of gutta-percha. In this technique, the downpack consists of a continuous rather than several interrupted waves of condensation. Backfilling is normally completed using increments of thermoplasticised gutta-percha delivered using a dispensing gun. There are now several other systems available which include the B&L Alpha and Beta (B&L Biotech, USA), Elements IC, (KaVo Kerr, USA) and Gutta-Smart (Dentsply Sirona, Switzerland) systems available for vertical condensation.

The philosophy behind vertical condensation has not changed over three decades. The procedure aims to seal the terminus of the canal with an accurate cone fit and to obturate the coronal end once the surplus gutta-percha has

Box 2.4   Technique for Warm Vertical Condensation of Gutta-Percha.

Phase 1 – The Downpack (Fig. 2.19 A)

1. Try the proposed master cone in a wet canal (i). Fit the master cone (either non-standardised cones or system matching cones) at the working length (WL) in the canal and ensure good 'tug-back' is felt. The cone should be tried into a wet canal and the opportunity to agitate the irrigant should be taken; this is done by pumping the cone in and out of the canal so as to increase the movement of the irrigant for more effective cleaning.
2. Select a heat carrier that binds in the prepared canal at about 4–7 mm from the WL and mark with a silicone stop (ii).
3. Dry the canal with paper points. Coat the master cone lightly with sealer and apply to the walls of the canal. Seat the master cone precisely but firmly.
4. The heat source is best used at a temperature of approx. 200°C.
5. Cut of the coronal part of the gutta percha (GP) at the orifice level and condense vertically whilst the GP is soft (iii and iv).
6. Take the heat source and activate it while driving the heated plugger smoothly through the GP over a maximum of 3 seconds to 4–7 mm from the WL. Switch off the heat (v).
7. Maintain firm apical pressure for a 10-second sustained push to take up any shrinkage that might occur upon cooling of the apical mass of GP (vi).
8. While still maintaining apical pressure reactivate the heat carrier and twist to separate the GP and then quickly withdraw the

heat carrier. This should remove the surplus coronal portion of GP.
9. After removal, use a hand plugger to pack the apical portion of GP lifting any excess GP off the walls of the canal and packing it on to the apical mass (vii).

Phase 2 – The Backfill (see Fig. 2.19 B)

1. Lightly recoat the walls of the unfilled canal space with sealer if required.
2. Introduce the needle tip of the GP gun device until it contacts the apical GP. Hold in place for a few seconds to reheat the GP in the canal.
3. Squeeze the trigger until the gun starts to back out of the canal. Maintain light resistance while letting the needle drive coronally, still keeping it embedded in the mass (ii).
4. Deposit 2–3 mm of gutta-percha, withdraw the needle and immediately apply apical pressure with a hand plugger. Vertically condense until the GP has cooled (iii).
5. Repeat until increments until orifice level is reached, withdraw the needle and immediately apply apical pressure with a hand plugger. Vertically condense until the GP has cooled (iv). This will compensate for cooling contraction.

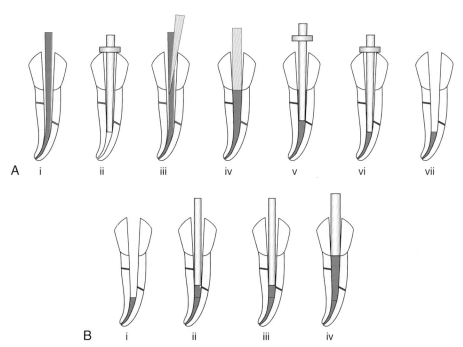

Fig. 2.19 Warm vertical condensation obturation technique. (A) Downpack and (B) backfill.

been removed. The downpack then forces sealer and gutta-percha along the lines of least resistance (Fig. 2.20). Significant changes have been made in armamentarium, simplifying the technique and making it more operator friendly. Vertical condensation is, however, a taxing technique which, together with the expense of the initial purchase of the equipment, probably explains the greater popularity of lateral condensation.

Carrier-Based Systems

Carrier-based techniques consist of a carrier coated in gutta percha (GP). The carriers historically have been made from stainless steel and titanium (Thermafil (Dentsply Sirona, Switzerland)), then plastic (Thermafil (Dentsply Sirona, Switzerland)) and more currently a cross-linked GP (Gutta Core (Dentsply Sirona, Switzerland)) (Fig. 2.21).

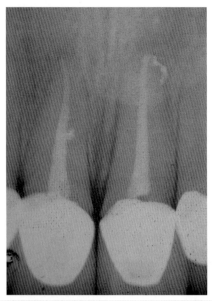

Fig. 2.20 Postoperative periapical radiograph showing excess sealer extruded from upper left maxillary central incisor.

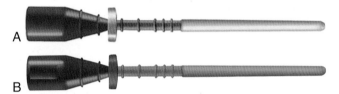

Fig. 2.21 (A) Thermafil carrier with plastic core surrounded with gutta-percha. (B) Gutta core with cross-linked gutta-percha.

This cross-linked GP gets over the problem of difficulties in post space placement and retreatment; however, it is very new to the market. With all of these systems, there is a verifier to check which size carrier to use. The carrier is then heated in the oven for that system for a specified time, the canal coated in sealer and the carrier pushed to the working length. The handle from the carrier is then removed and the GP condensed vertically. There are matching carriers for systems such as Protaper, Reciproc, Waveone, etc. Although this technique is quick, length control and postoperative pain can sometimes be a problem.

MANAGEMENT OF THE WIDE AND OPEN APEX

Calcium silicates cements are currently the materials of choice as an apical filling in immature or 'blunderbuss' apices. These materials have evolved from MTA and are used for obturating the root canal system when the material interface with the periradicular tissues is larger than normal. They provide an excellent seal and biocompatibility. Most calcium silicate cements are presented in a powder and liquid form that are mixed to the required consistency although some pre-mixed versions are gaining popularity. A number of specialised instruments have been developed for placement of these materials such as the MAP system (Produits Dentaires, Switzerland) which enables precise placement of the material to the desired site for both orthograde and retrograde indications. When placing the material to obturate a wide root canal (≥0.7 mm) the CSC should be expelled from the device carefully at the length and should not be packed like other conventional materials; it should be delicately manipulated into place with a plugger or a large flat-ended paper point. The latter has the advantage of absorbing any excess moisture. The periradicular tissues will have a spongy consistency and there will be no resistance form with which to pack against, so care must be taken. Ideally 6-mm apical fill should be placed; however, one must respect the future restorative needs of the tooth and the length of the pulp chamber that remains to gain retention (Fig. 2.22).

CORONAL SEAL

It is important after completing canal obturation that a definitive coronal seal is provided immediately. This does not mean a definitive restoration as this may not be able to be provided immediately; however, a definitive seal can be. Therefore, an appropriate material should be selected to seal the canal orifice even if the definitive restoration is not to be provided until later. This can be achieved by placing a resin composite or glass ionomer material over the floor of the pulp chamber and canal orifices together with a glass ionomer, resin composite or amalgam core.

OVERFILLS

A small amount of sealer may be seen apically on a radiograph after obturation, especially when using warm gutta-percha techniques. Sealer may also be seen opposite large accessory or lateral canals (see Fig. 2.20). It is, therefore, important that a relatively inert sealer material is used. Proponents of vertical condensation argue the distinction between overfilling and vertical overextension of underfilled canal systems, that is, filling materials may be overextended or extruded beyond a canal system that has not been sealed internally. Underfilling of a canal system could also indicate that it has not been debrided satisfactorily. In such situations, necrotic pulp tissue, bacteria and their by-products would be expected to then lead to failure. Overfilling infers that the whole canal system is obturated but excess material has been placed beyond the confines of the root canal and represents a quite different situation. The aim of vertical condensation is not to produce extrusion of filling material; nevertheless, this can occur and histological studies have shown that these overfills do produce an inflammatory response even though patients may not report discomfort.

2.7 Restoration of Endodontically Treated Teeth

LEARNING OBJECTIVES

You should:
- outline why root-filled teeth require careful restorative consideration
- describe a safe technique for direct and indirect post placement
- outline the key features of posts in relation to root canal-treated teeth.

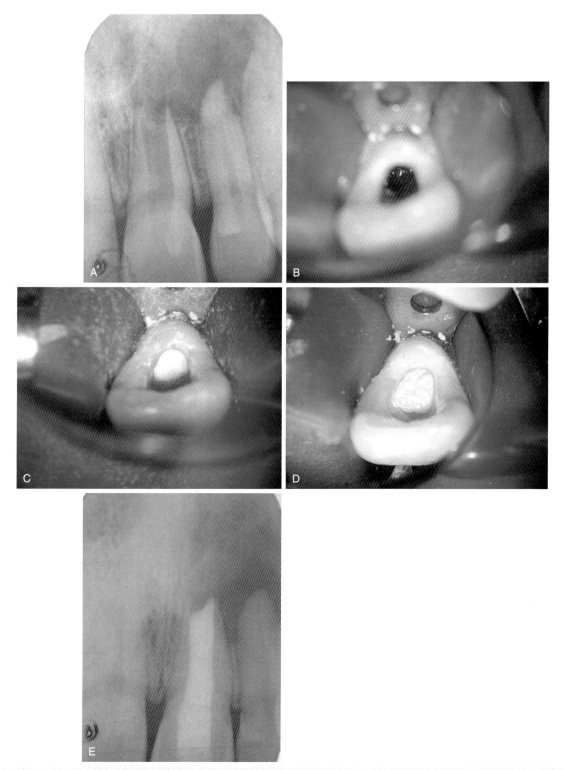

Fig. 2.22 Obturation of upper left central incisor with wide open apex. (A) Preoperative periapical radiograph. Mid op photograph showing (B) apical tissue through wide open apex, (C) mineral trioxide aggregate apical fill, (D) gutta-percha back fill. (E) Post-op periapical radiograph.

Root canal treatment is performed on teeth with varying amounts of remaining tooth structure, the loss of tooth tissue, removal of additional dentine during instrumentation and the use of some irrigants and dressings can leave root filled teeth in a very vulnerable position. The remaining tooth structure should be replaced and reinforced with careful consideration given to whether additional tooth is sacrificed and an extra-coronal restoration provided so as to protect the tooth in the longer term.

The aim is to restore the tooth with a restoration that is both biologically and mechanically sound. Consideration should be given at the very start of a root canal procedure as to what the final restoration may be and therefore it is good practice to assess the restorability of a tooth before embarking upon root canal treatment.

If all or nearly all of the coronal tooth substance has been lost, then predictable long-term restoration may be problematic. Anterior teeth are subject to shearing forces in dynamic occlusion whereas posterior teeth are subjected to more compressive loading. It is important to consider these forces when choosing both the restoration type and whether or not there is a need to help support the restoration with the placement of an inter-radicular post. Posts themselves will not strengthen teeth but will provide support to a coronal restoration.

The ideal time to restore a root canal-treated tooth (at least with a sealing core) is immediately following completion of the root canal obturation as mentioned earlier. The operator has a clear understanding of the anatomy of the tooth and the field is already isolated with dental dam; this way the canal(s) can be sealed immediately to prevent microbial ingress. A slightly wider operating area may therefore need to be isolated when undertaking root canal treatment so that there is access to the contact areas of the adjacent teeth to facilitate matrix placement. Attention to detail is important and access cavities should be free of gutta-percha and sealer prior to restoration, with the use of ultrasonics and particle abrasion being particularly effective.

Anterior teeth with either a single access cavity or minimal interproximal restorations may be restored with direct composite restorations alone. In premolar and molar teeth, where there are intact marginal ridges, and an occlusal access cavity, teeth may be restored directly with an adhesive resin composite restoration or amalgam.

Where there has been loss of significant tooth structure it is sensible to place a post which will help to support the restoration either as the definitive restoration or as a core for a crown. The tooth loses much of its strength when one or both marginal ridges have been lost. Root canal-treated premolar teeth with loss of marginal ridges are particularly vulnerable to crown and/or root fracture and therefore should have a post placed to support the overlying core.

In molar teeth, it is often possible to avoid the need for a post as 2–3 mm of gutta-percha may be removed from the entrances to canals, and restorative materials of either composite or amalgam may then be placed into these to aid retention.

A vast array of different post types are available. It is essential to retain as much sound tooth structure as possible as this helps in reducing leverage forces in the root and potential fracture.

Post choice is therefore influenced by the amount of remaining coronal dentine, root morphology and internal canal anatomy. Post length should approximate to about two-thirds of the root length, ideally with an equal amount of post below and above the alveolar crest. Care should be taken to leave an adequate amount of root canal filling material apically and ideally 4–5 mm of gutta-percha should remain at root end. Should there be a curve in the anatomy of the root, any preparation should stop short of the curve. Post length ultimately is affected by the length of the available root, the anticipated occlusal forces and the level of periodontal bone support. Conflicting opinion exists as to post taper. Tapered posts are most sympathetic to root anatomy; however, there is considerable evidence that parallel posts are more retentive. It is advised that all cases are assessed individually giving due consideration to the root morphology and canal anatomy.

Posts may be pre-fabricated or custom made from cast metal. The most commonly used pre-fabricated posts are either made from metal (e.g. titanium, stainless steel) or glass fibre embedded in resin; these are referred to as fibre posts. Space must be created in the root canal to accommodate a post; the safest way to do this is to remove gutta-percha with a Gates–Glidden bur or heated instrument followed by the proprietary sequence of end-cutting twist drills that correspond to the size and shape of post being used. The post diameter ideally should not exceed the diameter of the optimally shaped and cleaned canal. A wider post does not mean more retention, with post length being the more important factor. It is important that the post channel follows the direction of the main root canal. Failure to achieve this may result in root perforation.

Coronally there should be a minimum of 2 mm of supragingival tooth tissue remaining so that when a crown is cemented, the encircling of both dentine and core with the crown provides a reinforcing 'ferrule effect'. The manufacturer's protocols for placement, cementation and subsequent core build up should be adhered to. Once the core is in place, the tooth may then be prepared for an indirect restoration.

Preparation of the root canal for a cast post is very similar to that for fibre posts; coronally the preparation margin for a crown should also be outlined, and any weak fragments of dentine should be reduced in height. Most proprietary cast post kits (e.g. Parapost X, Coltene/Whaledent, Switzerland) contain a plastic impression post and a stainless steel temporary post. The dental dam will need to be removed and gingival retraction required prior to a silicone impression being taken with the impression post in situ. The tooth is then temporised using a stainless steel temporary post along with either a preformed or chairside made provisional crown. Alternatively, a barrier is placed in the canal and a sealing non–tooth-coloured restoration is placed in the root canal entrance, over which an immediate partial denture can be inserted. Once manufactured by the dental technician, the cast post can be cemented in place and the crown preparation refined as necessary ensuring adequate reduction for the chosen crown type. Custom made cast posts are particularly useful for oval shaped canals.

A summary of some of the key aspects of restoration of endodontically treated teeth is provided in Fig. 2.23.

2.8 Root Canal Retreatment

LEARNING OBJECTIVES

You should:
- appreciate the reasons why root fillings might fail
- understand how to tackle a range of retreatment problems.

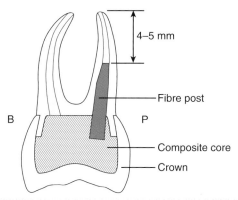

Fig. 2.23 Restoration of a multirooted tooth with a fibre post and composite core following root canal treatment. An apical 4–5 mm of gutta-percha remain and a fibre post bonded into the canal, the other canal remains filled with gutta-percha and is cut back to the canal entrance. The head of the post is then encased in composite providing support to the core. An indirect restoration (in this case a crown) is then placed to provide cuspal coverage.

Success rates for root canal treatments are generally very good, but it is acknowledged that some cases fail. Follow-up after a root canal procedure is therefore important; ideally this should be performed after 1 year (unless symptoms present prior to this) and would include clinical and radiographic examination. Guidelines suggest the absence of symptoms and a radiographic lesion that reduces in size or resolves completely does not justify further radiographic follow-up. A lesion that stays the same should continue to be monitored for an additional year and subsequently, as it may take up to 4 years for some lesions to completely resolve radiographically. Where symptoms dictate or there is clear radiographic evidence that a lesion has increased in size then a timely retreatment (or extraction if this is the patient's choice) is indicated. Failure of the primary root canal treatment and persistent pain may be as a result of a range of different factors including:

Intraradicular causes of failure are:
- failure to identify anatomy at primary treatment (e.g. missed MB2 canal of upper molar or lingual canal of lower incisor)
- failure to adequately disinfect the instrumented root canal system (e.g. bacteria left in accessory canals)
- loss of coronal seal and re-contamination of the previously treated canal space.

Extraradicular causes of failure are:
- persistent periradicular biofilm
- iatrogenic damage
- radicular cysts
- vertical root fractures
- incorrect initial diagnosis (e.g. neuropathic pain, TMD, sinusitis, etc.).

Diagnosis remains critical to implementing the correct treatment, in particular, differentiating pain of odontogenic origin from pain of non-odontogenic origin. Most 'toothache' is of course infective and odontogenic in origin with clear clinical and radiographic signs of disease (e.g. a discharging sinus or radiographic evidence of periradicular

bone loss); however, it is worth noting that pain arising from what appears to be the teeth can manifest from any structures with trigeminal nerve innervation. Therefore, it is worth considering the site and source of the pain to differentiate a case that has a chance of being successfully managed with a retreatment procedure from one that requires an entirely different and in some cases medical management strategy. These include pain resulting from temporomandibular joints and muscles of mastication, headache and vascular disorders along with referred pain and persistent neuropathic pain. Where there is uncertainty or where primary treatment has been conducted optimally with persistent symptoms then referral for a further specialist opinion may be necessary. Whilst extensive initial treatment may have been successful for a number of years, restorations or coronal seals are lost due to marginal breakdown, leading to reinfection of previously disinfected canal spaces. Careful assessment of the preoperative radiograph should be made with regard to whether or not a post has been used, what type it is, the type of root filling material (paste, gutta-percha, silver point) and potential problems such as curves, perforations or ledges.

A further dilemma exists where there is a plan for advanced restorative work (crowns and bridges) on previously root canal-treated teeth about whether or not the teeth should be endodontically retreated prior to undertaking treatment. A decision should be reached based upon the radiographic findings and clinical symptoms. If there have been symptoms or if obvious improvements can be made to the quality of the root canal filling then this seems like a sensible step to take; however, the decision is much more difficult if there is a very small apical radiolucency, yet no symptoms for 20 years. The authors would generally err on the side of caution and retreat conventionally if there is extensive restorative work planned.

If the diagnosis is odontogenic (rather than neuropathic) then careful consideration should be given as to the complexity of the retreatment procedure and the skill of the operator to conduct this. There is an increased expectation that teeth can be retained at all costs, but this is not always sensible; teeth undergoing re-root canal treatment will already have been subjected to significant amounts of restorative dentistry where critical peri-cervical and coronal tooth structure has been lost. Therefore, consideration should be given at the treatment planning phase as to the long-term prognosis for the tooth and the predictability of providing a long-term restoration following re-root canal procedures. There may well be some unknowns and it may be necessary to consent the patient to an initial assessment of restorability following removal of all restorations prior to committing to a retreatment procedure only to identify later that the outcome is compromised.

Failure, depending on its aetiology, may be treated in one of three ways: root canal retreatment, endodontic microsurgery or extraction. Extraction is usually indicated for root fractures in single-rooted teeth or in cases of gross caries where the tooth is non-restorable. On occasions, it may be possible to resect a fractured root in multirooted teeth or to perform crown lengthening when gross caries is present in order to build up a pre-endodontic core making isolation and future restoration possible. Root canal retreatment is usually the first line treatment option where there are clear and obvious deficiencies in the previous root canal retreatment.

RETREATMENT PROCEDURES

The aim of root canal retreatment is to eliminate microorganisms that have either survived previous treatment or have re-entered the root canal system. The feasibility of root canal retreatment depends on the operator's ability to gain access to and undertake further disinfection of the root canal system.

In a retreatment procedure, access is usually complicated by the presence of coronal restorations, retentive devices in the root canals and root canal filling materials. This can be particularly challenging where the anatomy of the restored crown may be different to the underlying root morphology. The use of magnification with enhanced illumination is especially useful in retreatment procedures. Loupes and a headlamp will provide good visibility of the pulp chamber floor and canal orifices; better still an operating microscope will allow treatment under optimum conditions often allowing direct visualisation of the middle and apical thirds of the root canal.

ACCESS FOR RETREATMENT

The quality of the coronal restoration must be considered when gaining access. If there are no clinical or radiographic signs of marginal leakage and the coronal restoration is generally satisfactory, it may be retained and access made through it. Where there is a post and core present, it is sensible to remove all restorations. Care needs to be taken in bur angulation as the original coronal anatomical form may have been lost, core removal is often made even more challenging where there are deep tooth-coloured restorations or restorations that derive retention from inside the canals, as the distinction between dentine and restoration is difficult to see.

Evidence of leakage coronally around the restoration margins usually indicates that it should be removed prior to performing root canal retreatment. Where there is any uncertainty about the integrity of pre-existing restorations, these should be removed and a pre-endodontic build up or provisional crown placed before embarking on retreatment procedures. This may involve sectioning and removal of crowns or bridges, with careful consideration given as to the method of temporisation.

It is usual to encounter a core under an indirect restoration (crown or onlay) in root canal retreatment. These are made from either amalgam or composite with additional retention being derived from the root canal either with a dowel of material into the canal entrances or a post. Integrated cast post and cores may also be present; examination of the preoperative radiograph will inform the likely challenges faced in removal of these restorations. Removal of the bulk of a composite or amalgam is no different to managing a failed restoration, but careful consideration should be given to working near the canal entrances or pulpal floor. Magnification is extremely useful in being as conservative as possible in the removal of core materials and preservation of dentine in the peri-cervical area, particularly if high-speed diamond or tungsten carbide burs are used. Powerful piezoelectric ultrasound is very helpful when removing the final

layers of restorative material overlying a pulpal floor or into the canal entrances where energy can be directed in a controlled way to the tip of the instrument at reduced risk of iatrogenic perforation. Tooth-coloured restorations can prove to be challenging to remove; regular drying of the cavity floor will usually allow differentiation between dentine and composite along with steady and careful removal. In addition, the texture of the restorative material is rougher than the dentine and this can be detected using an endodontic explorer. Once the restorations have been removed, the tooth and access cavity should be thoroughly inspected considering the following:

- assessment of restorability
- ensuring that all caries has been removed
- inspection for cracks and perforations
- access for identifying untreated anatomy.

REMOVAL OF POST AND CORES

Post and cores may comprise all-in-one castings that have been cemented in place or preformed metal, glass fibre or ceramic posts that are cemented in place and a direct core built up around them. When removing a post, the core should be first dissected in order to expose the individual post or posts; note that in multirooted teeth there may be more than one post supporting an overlying core. In some situations, it may not be necessary to remove all the posts, only those in the roots being retreated. Retrieval of a traditionally cemented post is a very predictable treatment procedure but those that are cemented with rigid resin-based cements can prove more challenging. Removal of a well-fitting post carries with it the risk of rendering the tooth unrestorable. Careful judgment is needed at the treatment planning stage as to whether retreatment conventionally, while accepting this risk, is more predictable than a surgical approach. Removal of a post should certainly not be attempted if the force to remove it could result in root fracture or the removal of dentine necessary would result in iatrogenic perforation.

Removing Cast and Metal Posts

Ultrasonic vibration from an appropriate handpiece with water coolant may be used initially to try to break the cement seal. The vibrations should be directed in a coronal direction, which necessitates the cutting of a notch on the side of the cast core. If a specialised tip is not available, then a standard piezoelectric ultrasonic scaler may be used. Care must be taken to control the heat that is generated from ultrasonic vibration; the instrument and tooth must be water or ice cooled at regular intervals to allow heat to dissipate. If this is not done effectively then there is a risk that the periodontal ligament and alveolar bone will become overheated, resulting in localised necrosis. In extreme cases, this may result in exfoliation of the tooth. It is important to use ultrasound with control, as high power will also risk propagating microcracks in the root. If ultrasonic vibration is unsuccessful, it is necessary to use a device to pull out the post and core or dedicated trepan kits such as the Masserann to cut around the periphery to break the cement lute. In this system, a suitably sized trepan is directed along the side of the post in the space created by the ultrasonic tips or burs. A smaller trepan may then be used to grip and remove the fractured portion (additional ultrasonic vibration applied to the trepan may be useful at this point); inevitably some additional dentine is removed. If the post is of the screw-in type, then it may be unscrewed after the use of ultrasonics to weaken the cement seal, either by placing a groove in its end or grasping it with a tight-fitting trepan. In exceptional cases, fractured posts may be drilled out using an end-cutting bur; this procedure is rarely necessary in view of the recent developments in ultrasonic tip design.

Removal of Glass-Fibre Posts

Water-cooled diamond burs should be used to remove the core and expose the head of the post; dedicated long end-cutting fibre post removal burs can then be used to cut down the length of the glass fibres which are embedded in resin. Care must be taken to regularly check and confirm that the bur remains centred on the fibre post as progress is made, reducing the risk of inadvertent lateral perforation.

REMOVAL OF ROOT CANAL OBTURATION MATERIALS

Those most frequently used obturation materials include gutta-percha, sealers and pastes and occasionally older obturation materials such as silver points. The same principles apply to root canal retreatment as primary treatments, with straight-line access being key. In retreatment, access to the middle and apical third of the root is usually restricted by the presence of materials used to obturate the canal.

Removal of Gutta-Percha

Poorly condensed gutta-percha root fillings may be removed by rotating one or braiding together two small Hedstrom files around or between the root canal filling points, pulling and removing them intact. If this is unsuccessful, then removal of the root canal filling should be considered in stages, removing first the coronal, followed by the middle and apical thirds. Gates–Glidden drills may be used coronally and only in the straight part of the canal; these are available in a range of sizes and have a safe cutting tip that reduces the risk of perforation providing too large a size is not used. They should be used at a speed of 1000–1500 rpm taking care not to force the instrument to avoid potential damage to the canal walls.

In the middle and apical thirds of the canal, rotary or reciprocatory NiTi instruments may be used. Some are dedicated retreatment files, e.g. ProTaper Universal retreatment series (Dentsply Sirona, Switzerland), MTwo (VDW, Germany) Retreatment Files, whereas others may be used for canal shaping but have a particularly useful geometry for retreatment as debris is drawn coronally such as Reciproc (VDW, Germany).

It is not always possible to remove gutta-percha by mechanical means alone and a solvent may be needed to soften the material to aid removal. Care should be taken not simply to force hand or rotary instruments as there is a risk of canal transportation, perforation or instrument fracture. Traditionally, chloroform liquid has been the most effective solvent for dissolving gutta-percha. When introduced into the canal it forms a 'soup-like' mixture of chloropercha that can then be removed easily using paper points. The solution can be replenished from an irrigating syringe into the canal along with further agitation, instrumentation and removal of debris until the canal is clear of gutta-percha with progress in a crown-down manner re-establishing patency. Chloroform remains excellent for this purpose but is now less widely available and needs careful storage. Eucalyptus oil has become a widely used alternative. It is important to avoid switching irrigant back to sodium hypochlorite midway through with partial gutta-percha removal. The result of this is reprecipitation of the gutta-percha out of solution which is then difficult to remove.

Removal of Pastes

Soft pastes can usually be easily penetrated using short, sharp hand files and copious irrigation. The use of an ultrasonics with accompanying irrigation can also be helpful in these situations, especially for removing remnants of paste from root canal walls that may remain despite careful hand instrumentation. Rotary NiTi instruments may also be used. Hard pastes can be particularly difficult to remove and usually need to be removed with a small long-neck bur or chipped out using ultrasonics. These procedures can only be used in the straight part of the canal. Magnification with enhanced lighting is invaluable as the risk of going off-line and perforation is high. Irrigation with EDTA and sodium hypochlorite should be employed, together with frequent drying to improve visibility, especially deep within the canal.

Removal of Silver Points

The seal of silver point root canal fillings is rarely as good as their radiographic appearance would suggest, and in many cases the seal relies on the cement used. If this washes out, then corrosion occurs leading to failure of the root canal filling. The approach to removal depends on whether the point extends out of the canal and is visible within the pulp chamber. In such situations, many silver points can be removed easily by grasping with micro-needle holders, Steglitz forceps or pin pliers and pulling gently. If the points cannot be removed easily, then ultrasonic vibrations can be applied to the forceps holding the point. If the silver point has been cut off at the canal orifice, then it is usually not possible to directly grip it. In such situations, an ultrasonic tip may be used to cut a trough around the point; care needs to be taken not to touch the point as the silver is much softer than the steel used for the manufacture of the ultrasonic tip and the point will fracture in small pieces. A Masserann extractor can be used to grip the point and remove it once a trough around the point has been created. Sometimes, it may be necessary to work an ultrasonic file down the side of a point placed deep in a root canal or bypass the silver point using k-files.

Removal of Fractured Instruments

The fracture of root canal instruments is a procedural hazard in root canal therapy. The problem may be kept to a minimum by:

- developing a stress-free glide path with small flexible stainless steel instruments
- inspecting used instruments and discarding any with visible damage
- not forcing hand or rotary instruments
- using instruments in correct sequence.

The removal of fractured instruments is often very challenging; generally speaking the more coronal the fractured portion lies the greater the likelihood of its removal. Instruments that have been fractured around curvatures are particularly challenging. Magnification is essential and will help to remove superficially fractured instruments, once working past the canal entrance in the middle and apical third then an operating microscope is essential. The first part of instrument removal is to identify the fractured portion; in some cases, it may be possible to pass an instrument alongside the fractured one, particularly if it is a small fragment. This becomes more challenging apically as the diameter of the canal narrows and the canal generally becomes more circular in cross-section with limited room to pass an instrument alongside.

Removal of a fractured instrument may be performed using a thin ultrasonic tip that is used either directly around the tip of the fractured fragment to create space to engage the head of it and allow its withdrawal or to vibrate the instrument loose (Fig. 2.24). It may also be possible to pass a cylindrical tube over the instrument head which engages the fractured element, e.g. IRS or using the Cancellier approach with either self-cured composite resin or cyanoacrylate glue.

The presence of a fractured instrument may not necessarily lead to an adverse outcome for a tooth, particularly if the instrument fracture has occurred following a period of disinfection. However, if the fracture occurs early on then it may not have been possible to adequately disinfect the canal system. Either way, if retrieval is unlikely or carries high risk of iatrogenic damage, then the remainder of instrumentation and disinfection should be completed, and the canal(s) obturated to the level of the fractured instrument. The tooth should then be monitored for signs of periapical disease.

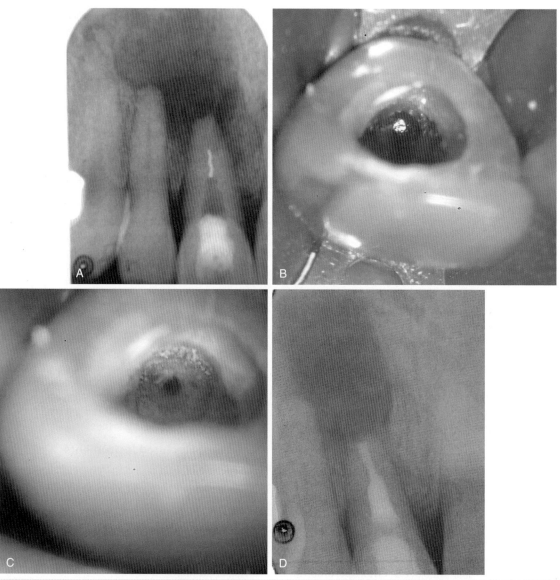

Fig. 2.24 Removal of fractured instrument with ultrasonics. (A) Preoperative periapical radiograph. Mid op photograph showing (B) fractured file at mid root level and (C) file removed. (D) Post-op periapical radiograph.

Success Rate of Root Canal Retreatment

The success of root canal retreatment is good (94–98%) when it is being undertaken to achieve a technical improvement in potential failures. When periradicular pathology is present, the complete healing rate is lower (62–78%). Retreatment itself can bring its own problems: perforation, fractured instruments and compromised cleaning and obturation of the canal system. It is important that patients are informed of such factors prior to embarking on this procedure.

2.9 Surgical Endodontics

LEARNING OBJECTIVES

You should:
• understand the indications for surgical intervention
• have an appreciation of what is involved in surgical endodontics.

The main indication for periradicular surgery is when an endodontic treatment is failing or it is not possible to treat the root canal system by conventional means. Such situations include large posts, sclerosed canals and broken instruments. It must be remembered that the main cause of failure in endodontics is inadequate debridement and bacterial contamination of the root canal system, hence the importance of root canal retreatment whenever possible. A further important indication for periradicular surgery is obtaining tissue for a biopsy.

Conventional orthograde root canal treatment is not always successful and in some cases, e.g. significant canal sclerosis, simply not possible. As a first line treatment, orthograde primary or retreatment is generally preferred to apical surgery, even if it is considered that surgery may be necessary at a later stage. The rationale for this being that periradicular lesions are driven by bacterial contamination of the root canal system and orthograde approaches will enable greater decontamination and reduction of the bacterial load even if the canal can be sealed apically during surgery. Conventional retreatment of a tooth may involve the removal/destruction of expensive crown and bridgework which will ultimately require replacement. Similarly, in cases where crowns are retained with large, well-fitting posts, conventional removal of the post may risk iatrogenic damage and may result in the removal of precious dentine. In such situations, a patient may opt for a surgical as opposed to orthograde approach.

The indications for endodontic surgery are as follows:

■ Failed orthograde primary or retreatment
■ Retrieval of fractured instruments or extruded obturation material
■ Biopsy of suspected pathology, e.g. radicular cyst
■ Repair of iatrogenic damage, e.g. perforation
■ Repair of external inflammatory root resorption
■ Management of periradicular infection where primary treatment is not feasible (e.g. canal sclerosis)
■ Direct inspection and investigation of suspected fractures not visible on radiographic imaging.

SURGICAL ASSESSMENT

Case selection is very important and consideration should be given as to the likelihood of success. Where there is limited chance of success, alternative options should be considered, e.g. extraction and replacement with bridge, denture or implant-retained prosthesis.

It is important that a thorough assessment is made prior to embarking on surgery. History is very important and questioning should be directed to establish the likely underlying aetiology of the patient's presenting complaint. General factors include:

■ medical history
■ the patient's suitability for surgery with local anaesthetic and need for adjunctive conscious sedation
■ a thorough clinical examination noting the gingival biotype, lip line and smile line if surgery considered in the aesthetic zone
■ access to the surgical site including likely proximity to any significant anatomical structures
■ radiographic examination
■ long-term prognosis of the tooth.

Local factors include the strategic importance of the tooth and root end proximity to anatomical structures such as the maxillary sinus, mental foramen or inferior dental canal. These can be evaluated initially from plain film periapical radiographs, possibly utilising parallax techniques. 3D CBCT imaging is generally used for more complex cases (Fig. 2.25) providing valuable diagnostic and prognostic information on the extent of the pathology, anatomical variations such as uninstrumented canals, root fractures, iatrogenic damage, root curvature, and proximity of adjacent anatomical structures, including vasculature. The use of 3D imaging is changing the understanding of persistent disease and directly influencing the treatment planned.

Clinical evaluation should also include a periodontal examination noting any loss of attachment, or areas where there are deep periodontal probing depths. Teeth with periodontal attachment loss may not always be ideal candidates for endodontic surgery; removal of root length apically coupled with historical bone loss coronally may leave a tooth with very little bone support and in a very compromised position. Isolated deep periodontal probing depths may indicate a root fracture or endodontic periodontal lesion (see Periodontology chapter for diagnosis and management).

Apical lesions are by far the most common; however, lateral pathology may indicate the presence of lateral canals, perforations, root fractures or cystic lesions. Access interproximally and palatally/lingually is usually much more challenging and carries the risk of damaging adjacent teeth. It is important also to not make assumptions about the likely cause of any persistent pathology; adjacent teeth should therefore be routinely examined and pulp testing undertaken where appropriate.

CONSENT

It is good clinical practice to obtain written consent from patients prior to endodontic surgery. This process should clearly outline what the procedure will involve and it should be explained and written in language that is easily

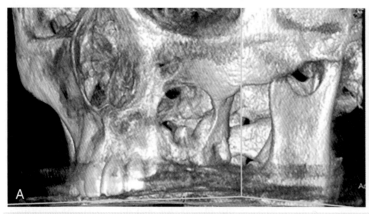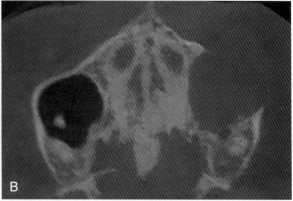

Fig. 2.25 (A) A 3D reconstruction of a cone beam computerised tomography scan of the maxilla: a large radicular cyst centred around the UL5 has eroded the maxilla; there is also mild buccal expansion present of the soft tissues as indicated on the axial view (B). Surgical enucleation and histopathological analysis is important to identify the underlying pathology.

understandable to the patient. Ideally this should include the intended benefits (removal of source of infection/retention of the tooth) and risks that are important and pertinent to that particular patient. For example, those risks normally associated with and expected during any surgical procedure including pain, swelling, bruising and bleeding, but also perhaps what might happen if the tooth is deemed clinically unrestorable at the time of surgery. For those patients with high smile lines, thin gingival biotypes and where there is gingival pigmentation, there may be a risk of gingival recession (depending upon the flap design) or scarring which is equally important. For most, endodontic surgery is a minor surgical procedure and can be successfully managed with local anaesthesia alone; for patients with heightened anxiety, conscious sedation may also be appropriate.

PROCEDURE

Once appropriate assessment has been made, the procedure can be planned. This includes:

- local anaesthesia
- flap design, elevation and retraction
- bone removal
- identification of root end
- periradicular curettage
- root resection
- root end preparation and filling
- haemostasis
- debridement and closure.

Site Preparation and Local Anaesthesia

Prior to surgery, bacterial load of the surgical site should be reduced with a preoperative chlorhexidine or hydrogen peroxide mouthwash for a minute prior to administration of local anaesthetic. Anaesthesia is required for patient comfort and to enhance visibility for the operator by controlled haemostasis. Regional anaesthesia is administered as appropriate, followed by multiple local infiltrations around the apex of the tooth. Lidocaine (2%) with 1:80,000 epinephrine is preferred to in view of its superior vasoconstrictive action. Ten minutes should be allowed

from local anaesthetic administration prior to incision to allow dispersal of the solution, as further attempts at improving anaesthesia or haemostasis during the procedure are usually only met with limited success.

Flap Design, Elevation and Retraction

Flap design should offer access to the full extent of the surgical site; care should be taken in the planning and execution stages to try and minimise the scarring, particularly in the aesthetic zone (Fig. 2.26). For this reason the three mucoperiosteal flap designs most commonly used for root end surgery are:

- papilla base (papillae spared in flap)
- full thickness (papillae included in flap)
- Ochsenbein-Luebke (para-marginal incision).

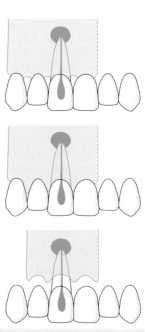

Fig. 2.26 (A) Two-sided papilla-based incision; dotted lines represent additional relieving incision if required, this can be taken further round the arch if necessary or to hide scarring. Note gingival margin crossed at 90° and relieving incisions are vertical. (B) Full thickness incision. (C) Paramarginal incision.

Other flap designs that have been previously indicated include a semilunar incision but the access offered is poor and there is often significant scarring. Relieving incision(s) will reduce the tension on the flap; these should be vertical so as to maintain maximum blood supply to the flap. Care should be taken to place these in a position where there is unlikely to be significant tension (e.g. away from root eminences and away from a bony defect). Only use what is necessary to gain adequate access and reduce postoperative discomfort to the patient. Incisions should be carried out with a sharp blade (e.g. Swann–Morton 11, 15, 15c, 69 micro blades); this author's preference is for a microblade preserving the incisive papillae and a separate 15c to make the relieving incisions. When crossing the gingival margin, incisions should be made at 90° so that closure results in minimal scarring and gingival recession.

Elevation of the flap should start at the attached gingiva using a periosteal elevator, e.g. Buser type on the vertical relieving incision, then progress laterally (undermining elevation) to prevent damage to the flap margins associated with the cervical areas of the teeth. Once reflected, the flap should be retracted, taking care to place and maintain the retractor on bone so as not to compress, damage or compromise the blood supply of the flap. Such damage may lead to excessive postoperative swelling or discomfort.

Bone Removal

Where there is a large bony defect, loss of the cortical plate may make access to the root tip straightforward. In many instances, a round, sterile, water-cooled surgical bur may need to be used to create a small osteotomy site by removing bone overlying the root. These osteotomy sites can also be created using ultrasonics, e.g. Piezosurgery (Mectron, IT), which are designed to cause less trauma to the bone and soft tissues. Care must be taken when creating the osteotomy site not to damage adjacent tooth roots or other anatomical structures.

Once access to the root end has been achieved, it is necessary to curette any granulation tissue or in some cases cyst lining from the defect. If the lesion is tethered to the underside of the mucoperiosteal flap then this should be carefully dissected away with a sharp blade taking care not to cut through the full thickness of the reflected flap. Where possible such tissue should be sent for histological examination. It is not necessary to remove every last remnant of soft tissue and care should be taken when curetting adjacent to anatomical structures such as the mental foramen, incisive nerve or maxillary sinus.

Root End Resection

The root ends may be resected with high-speed crown/endo-z type burs as long as they are used in a surgical air-driven handpiece where the air is directed away from the bone, e.g. Impact Air 45 (Palisades Dental LLC, USA). Failure to do so may result in a surgical emphysema. Alternatively, the root end may be resected using piezosurgery or using a water-cooled fissure bur. Resections should be carried out using appropriate sterile water or saline coolant. Any of these techniques can be used to cut back or section through the root end. In general, about 3 mm of root should be removed as this will result in removal of accessory canals forming part of the apical delta (Fig. 2.27). The

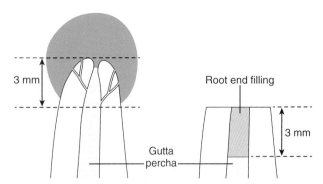

Fig. 2.27 There is frequently branching of the root canal in the apical third; these are areas for biofilm to remain untouched during canal preparation and be source of recurrent infection. Removal and resection of the final 3 mm preserves root length while removing a large proportion of the branching. Any granulomatous or cyst-like material is removed, 3 mm of preparation is carried out with ultrasonics down the long axis of the tooth; the root end filling with a bio-comparable material provides a good apical seal.

resection should also go right through the root but care should be taken to avoid adjacent teeth or other anatomical structures. Ideally the resection should be at 90° to the long axis of the tooth keeping any bevel to a minimum in order to avoid excessive exposure of dentine tubules. In multi-rooted teeth, it may be possible to resect an entire root, particularly where there has been a vertical root fracture maintaining the remaining roots and still providing a stable platform onto which a restoration may be placed.

Haemostasis

It is important that the periradicular surgical site be kept dry whilst the retrograde obturation material is placed both to improve vision and allow appropriate handling of the material. This may necessitate packing the cavity with local anaesthetic impregnated gauze, use of styptic agents, e.g. sterile ferric sulphate or other haemostatic adjuncts, e.g. collagen sponge, Surgicel, bone wax or calcium sulphate. The choice of material depends upon individual preference, but care must be taken to remove all remnants (except some collagen-based products and calcium sulphate, which are resorbable) as, if left, they will act as a foreign body and delay healing.

Root End Preparation

Root end preparations are now almost universally carried out using small contra-angled ultrasonic tips (Fig. 2.28); the removal of softened gutta-percha from the root end preparation allows debridement of the canal space and then compaction of material inside the canal. The preparation can be examined using a miniature retro-mirror. Historically, preparations were performed with small round or inverted cone burs, either in a straight or a miniature handpiece. The benefit of using ultrasonics over conventional handpieces is that preparation can take place down the long axis of the tooth removing gutta-percha and also cleaning any previously uninstrumented parts of the canal. Using traditional techniques, preparations were often orientated lingually/palatally with poor shape and ultimately a poor apical seal; primarily as a result of limited access this

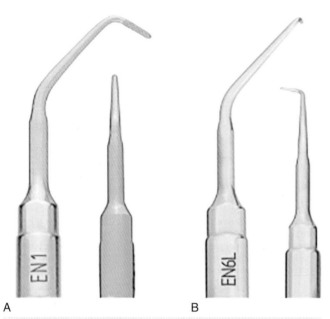

A   B

Fig. 2.28 Examples of fine ultrasonic tips that are used to prepare the resected root end. The cutting tip is diamond coated and is approximately 3 mm in length; the shafts are angled to allow easier access into small osteotomy sites.

occasionally resulted in a palatal perforation. Fine ultrasonic tips must be used at an appropriate power setting in order to minimise the risk of root cracking or tip fracture. Several designs are available, with different angles for easier access to posterior regions of the mouth. In addition, narrow designs are available for running out isthmus areas, which are now considered to be a previously unrecognised reason for failure in multirooted teeth.

Root End Filling Materials

Calcium silicate bioceramic cements such as MTA are considered to be the root end filling material of choice. MTA has excellent biocompatibility, is notably alkaline on setting with excellent osteoinductive properties, it seals well and is sufficiently radio-opaque to be visible radiographically. Historic approaches used amalgam as the retrograde filling material and may still be seen radiographically on a number of cases; failures with amalgam were seen as a result of its much poorer sealing ability, corrosion and aesthetic problems of staining and tattooing of the soft tissues.

Other materials that have proven success include super ethoxybenzoic acid (EBA) and intermediate restorative material (IRM). Due to the moisture control needed, glass ionomer cements and composite resins are more challenging to use; therefore calcium silicate materials are used as the first line option. Care needs to be taken when placing the retro filling that the root end and prepared cavity are adequately isolated and dry. Materials should be mixed according to the manufacturer's instructions, and care taken to avoid excess material out with the retro cavity. There are newer premixed calcium silicates in putty form that are becoming increasingly popular due to their handling characteristics. Micro-apical placement (MAP) systems are available akin to a small amalgam carrier and are very helpful in placing many of these materials into a prepared cavity; once placed the material should then be compacted coronally. Ideally, a radiograph should be taken prior to suturing to ensure that the retro preparation and filling are adequate (Fig. 2.29).

Debridement and Closure

The surgical area should be thoroughly debrided and then rinsed with sterile water or saline, and the flap should then be compressed for about 3 minutes prior to suturing. In general, small, size 5/0 interrupted non-resorbable monofilament sutures will prove adequate for most situations. Suture removal should be performed 3–5 days later; in some cases with good primary closure this can be done as soon as 48 hours postsurgery.

It is usual for a patient to have some discomfort and swelling postoperatively. This, however, is normally minimal and can be controlled using analgesics. The area can be kept clean by continuing the chlorhexidine mouthwash until suture removal allows improved toothbrush access.

Corrective Surgery

Corrective surgery may be required to seal a perforation or resect a root. The position of the perforation is of paramount importance in determining whether it is surgically accessible; parallax radiographs will help to determine the site. Perforations in the apical third of the root may be handled by removal of the apex and sealing the canal with a retro grade filling. Ideally, perforations resulting from post crowns should have the offending post removed and a new one placed within the root canal. Surgical correction then resembles the placement of a retro grade filling in the side of the root. If the post is not removed, it must be cut back sufficiently to allow an adequate margin for finishing the retro filling. Many perforations are now managed by internal perforation repair with MTA, precluding the need for surgery.

Surgical root resection may be indicated on multirooted teeth that have not responded to treatment or have a

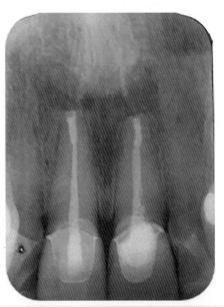

Fig. 2.29 Shows retrograde obturations of UR1, UL1 with MTA putty to around 3 mm in length. There has been good bony healing up to the root end restorations (image taken at 1-year follow-up).

hopeless periodontal prognosis. Other reasons for root resection include extensive resorption and root fracture in a multirooted tooth.

Extraction With Subsequent Replantation

Atraumatic extraction with intentional replantation is a recognised technique that can offer good success rates in cases where there is an experienced operator. The procedure involves extracting the tooth as atraumatically as possible for example using a periotome or extractor device, the root is handled carefully and root resection or repair carried out swiftly before replanting the tooth. The tooth will require splinting in the same way as for a traumatic injury. This procedure may be indicated when a conventional orthograde or surgical approach is not possible or advisable.

Self-Assessment: Questions

MULTIPLE CHOICE QUESTIONS (TRUE/FALSE)

1. The following are important factors in restoring an endodontically treated tooth:
   a. Preserving as much coronal tooth substance as possible
   b. Creating a ferrule effect
   c. Removing all coronal dentine
   d. Providing a wide post
   e. Producing a long post without compromising apical seal
2. Efficiency of irrigation is affected by:
   a. Depth of needle penetration
   b. Coronal pre-enlargement
   c. Frequency of use
   d. Volume and type of irrigant
   e. Temperature of irrigant
3. Major causes of failure in root canal therapy are:
   a. Placing small instruments through the foramen
   b. Presence of bacteria remaining within the root canal
   c. Presence of small amounts of filling material in the periradicular tissues
   d. Presence of necrotic material within the canal system
   e. Loss of coronal seal and reinfection of a cleaned canal system
4. Rotary nickel–titanium instruments:
   a. Require a patent canal prior to use
   b. Are used for canal negotiation
   c. Can be used round any curvatures
   d. Are used for canal enlargement
   e. Should be used with a light touch
5. The following are features of irreversible pulpitis:
   a. Response lasts for minutes to hours
   b. Pain may develop spontaneously
   c. Heat may be more significant in the later stages
   d. Pain does not linger after stimulus
   e. All of the above
6. An ideal access cavity should:
   a. Provide unimpeded access to the root canal system
   b. Have convergent walls
   c. Be only large enough to allow files in to canals
   d. Provide straight-line access to each canal orifice
   e. Eliminate the pulp chamber roof in its entirety
7. Coronal pre-enlargement:
   a. Is always necessary
   b. Blocks the canal
   c. Reduces the bacterial count coronally
   d. Decreases the effect of irrigation
   e. Enhances apical tactile feedback
8. Periradicular surgery is indicated:
   a. For all endodontic failures
   b. When it is not possible to treat the root canal system by conventional means
   c. To clean the root canal system
   d. To obtain tissue for a biopsy
   e. As an investigative procedure
9. Ultrasonic root end preparation:
   a. Is an improvement over steel burs
   b. May cause root cracking
   c. Should be used dry
   d. Enables preparation up the long axis of the root
   e. Needs more space for access
10. The following are features of reversible pulpitis:
    a. Pain lingers after application of stimulus
    b. Pain is difficult to localise
    c. Tooth is tender to percussion
    d. Pain does not linger after stimulus is removed
    e. Normal appearance on a radiograph
11. A patency file:
    a. Should be small and flexible
    b. Is used to deliberately enlarge the foramen
    c. Helps to eliminate apical blockage
    d. Should be used vigorously
    e. Is a generally accepted technique
12. Root canal filling materials should:
    a. Be easy to insert into the canal
    b. Absorb moisture
    c. Expand on setting
    d. Be difficult to remove
    e. Not stain the tooth
13. The following are accepted obturation techniques:
    a. Silver points
    b. Laterally condensed gutta-percha
    c. Continuous wave
    d. Carrier devices
    e. Single point gutta-percha
14. Fractured instruments may be avoided by:
    a. Not precurving them
    b. Not sterilising them
    c. Jumping between different sizes of instruments
    d. Discarding damaged instruments
    e. Not forcing instruments
15. Root canal blockage:
    a. May be caused by dentine chips
    b. May lead to perforation
    c. May be reduced by use of a lubricant
    d. Is increased if the coronal two-thirds is prepared first
    e. Is avoidable

SINGLE BEST ANSWER QUESTIONS

1. A 23-year-old patient attends having fallen over whilst drunk the night before, there was no loss of consciousness or soft tissue trauma. Your examination reveals a complex crown root fracture of the upper left central incisor tooth and less extensive fractures. Which radiographs should be your first line images?
   A. Full maxilla CBCT
   B. Periapical UL1
   C. Parallax views of all upper anteriors
   D. Vertical bitewing
   E. Limited field CBCT

2. A 35-year-old patient attends with mesio-occlusal caries affecting an upper first molar; during your caries removal there is a small pulpal exposure (<2 mm); you clear the periphery and isolate the tooth. Following disinfection with sodium hypochlorite, the most appropriate treatment is:
   A. An indirect pulp cap with calcium hydroxide
   B. A direct pulp cap with a calcium silicate cement
   C. A partial pulpotomy with calcium hydroxide
   D. A coronal pulpotomy with calcium silicate
   E. A pulpectomy and root canal treatment

3. A 34-year-old patient complains of pain from a lower left molar tooth; the onset of pain is following hot or cold drinks and lingers for a few minutes; the pain is poorly localised. There is no need for analgesics. A periapical radiograph suggests secondary caries beneath a large restoration and the periodontal membrane space appears normal. The most likely diagnosis is:
   A. Asymptomatic irreversible pulpitis with normal apical tissues
   B. Irreversible pulpitis with normal apical tissues
   C. Normal pulp with symptomatic apical periodontitis
   D. Reversible pulpitis with normal apical tissues
   E. Reversible pulpitis with symptomatic apical periodontitis

4. A 45-year-old patient complains of pain on biting from an upper first premolar; there are no other symptoms. History reveals that a large MOD amalgam restoration was placed recently; the tooth is TTP but only on the palatal cusp; it responds normally to pulp testing. There are no radiographic findings other than the deep MOD restoration. The most likely diagnosis is:
   A. Cracked tooth
   B. Pulp necrosis, symptomatic apical periodontitis
   C. Pulp necrosis, acute apical abscess
   D. Irreversible pulpitis, asymptomatic apical periodontitis
   E. Reversible pulpitis, normal apical tissues

5. A 56-year-old patient attends complaining of pain from a lower molar tooth; clinical examination reveals deep probing depths around the distal root with associated suppuration. The tooth is TTP but not mobile and nonresponsive to pulp testing. A periapical radiograph reveals a deep restoration, there is 'J' shaped radiolucency that extends distally from the periapex of the distal root and a smaller apical radiolucency around the mesial roots. BPE codes reveal some increased periodontal probing depths elsewhere in the mouth. What is the most likely diagnosis?
   A. A true combined periodontal–endodontic lesion
   B. Localised periodontitis, Stage 4, Grade C
   C. Normal pulp, periodontal abscess
   D. Pulp necrosis, symptomatic apical periodontitis
   E. Pulp necrosis, chronic apical abscess

6. A 30-year-old patient complains of a 'lump on the gum' adjacent to an upper premolar. The swelling has been present 'on and off' for almost a year and gentle pressure leads to discharge of pus from the gingival margin. The patient is periodontally healthy but there is an isolated area of deep probing (10 mm) in a single site where the discharge is coming from. Radiographically bone levels are good but there is a periapical radiolucency. What is the most likely diagnosis?
   A. Localised periodontitis, Stage 4, Grade C
   B. Pulp necrosis, acute apical abscess
   C. Pulp necrosis, chronic apical abscess
   D. Pulp necrosis, condensing osteitis
   E. Symptomatic irreversible pulpitis, symptomatic apical periodontitis

7. A 25-year-old patient attends for obturation of an upper incisor; you have previously performed initial access, extirpation and canal shaping and cleaning at the last visit. The patient reported pain for 3 days following the last visit which has improved but the tooth is still tender to bite on. In addition to the previously initiated therapy, what is the most likely periapical diagnosis?
   A. Acute apical abscess
   B. Normal apical tissues
   C. Chronic apical abscess
   D. Symptomatic apical periodontitis
   E. Asymptomatic apical periodontitis

PICTURE QUESTIONS

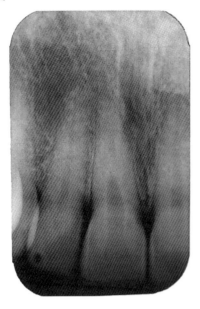

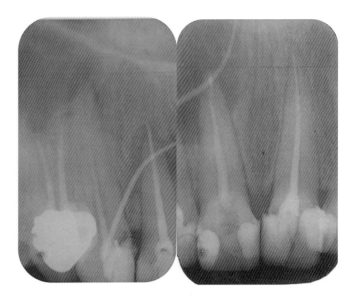

1. This 25-year-old patient attends with a discoloured upper right central incisor; the patient sustained previous facial injuries after being hit by a horse when they were a child. You are considering elective root canal treatment and non-vital bleaching. The tooth has not previously been accessed. Describe the radiographic appearance of the tooth.

3. This 32-year-old patient presents with pain from a discharging buccal sinus adjacent between the upper right canine and upper right lateral incisor teeth. The GP point inserted travels from the sinus tract opening to the upper right central incisor. The UR4, UR3, UR2, UR1, UL1 all appear to be heavily restored and have existing root canal treatments with pathology noted around UR3, UR2, UR1. Describe the treatment planning approach for these teeth.

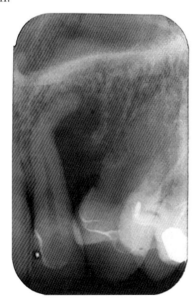

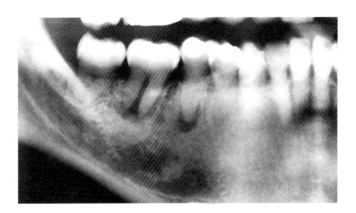

2. This 23-year-old patient has a history of an impacted canine that has been removed from the palate. The lateral incisor has an all ceramic crown to camouflage the peg shaped tooth; the tooth has subsequently become non-vital. Describe why this tooth may be challenging to carry out root canal treatment on and what interoperative techniques can be used to overcome these challenges.

4. This 50-year-old female patient attends complaining of multiple dental abscesses; they have two children each of whom is under the care of a paediatric dentist for similar problems affecting the primary dentition. The patient is fit and well and has no other medical problems. The teeth clinically appear relatively sound and moderately restored, the crowns are bulbous and the root canals in many of the teeth appear indistinct or obliterated. What is the most likely cause and what treatment may be offered?

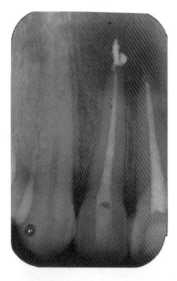

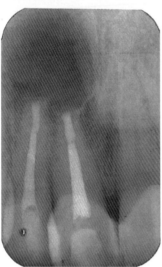

the most likely causes of this persistent swelling, the stages involved in carrying out an apicectomy and the follow-up regime for this patient.

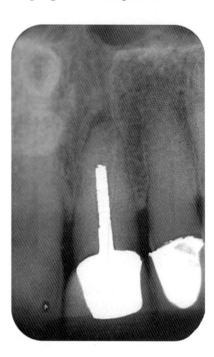

6. A 60-year-old patient attends with pain above an upper left central incisor tooth. Clinically the margins appear intact and despite historical Stage 2 grade B periodontal disease it is currently stable. Radiographic view shows a mesiodens, a post-crowned tooth with no obvious root canal treatment beyond the post. Describe the treatment strategies available to this patient.

5. A 42-year-old patient attends with persistent swelling overlying the apices of their upper right central and lateral incisor teeth. These teeth have been root canal treated on a number of occasions without improvement in symptoms. An apicectomy has been carried out and the image shown is immediately postoperative. Outline

SHORT NOTES QUESTIONS

Write short notes on:
1. reactionary and reparative dentine
2. pulp sensitivity tests
3. cracked tooth syndrome
4. balanced forces
5. the accuracy of electronic apex locators

Self-Assessment: Answers

MULTIPLE CHOICE ANSWERS

1. a. True. It is essential that sound coronal tooth tissue is retained as this enables the tooth to be restored as strongly as possible. See (b, e).
   b. True. Retention of coronal dentine allows a collar to be placed around the remaining tooth structure. This ferrule effect strengthens the remaining tooth structure.
   c. False. Removing coronal dentine unnecessarily weakens the tooth, makes it more difficult to create a ferrule and produces a shorter post. See (e).
   d. False. Wide posts weaken roots.

   e. True. A long post is more retentive than a short one. Leaving coronal dentine enables a longer post to be provided. It is essential however that the apical seal is not disturbed. After post preparation, 3–5 mm of root filling should remain.
2. a. True. It is important to get deep needle penetration; this can only be achieved if the canal is large enough. Irrigant solution does not travel much further apically than the needle tip.
   b. True. Early radicular access increases the space available for needle penetration and irrigant exchange.

c. True. It is important to refresh irrigating solutions frequently as this removes debris and ensures an active solution.

d. True. A larger volume of irrigant has an increased flushing effect. Sodium hypochlorite has been shown to be more effective than water or local anaesthetic as it will kill bacteria and dissolve pulp remnants.

e. True. Increasing the temperature of irrigating solutions increases their reactivity and makes them more efficient.

3. a. False. Small instruments placed through the foramen do not increase the likelihood of failure. It is important, however, not to overenlarge the foramen or cause damage to the periradicular tissues by using large instruments in such a manner.

b. True. Successful endodontics involves removing as many bacteria as possible from the root canal system. The more bacteria that remain, the greater the likelihood of failure.

c. False. Small amounts of filling material outside the root cause localised inflammation, which may be detectable histologically; it is not, however, a major contributing factor to failure and does not usually cause clinical symptoms.

d. True. Any necrotic tissue remaining within the canal acts as a continuing irritant.

e. True. Loss of coronal seal allows reinfection of the root canal system and is a major cause of failure.

4. a. True. Rotary nickel–titanium instruments require a patent canal as they should be used for canal enlargement, not negotiation.

b. False. Using rotary nickel–titanium instruments to negotiate canals increases the risk of fracture.

c. False. Rotary nickel–titanium instruments may be used around gradual curvatures; however, sharp curves and recurvatures put extra stress on the instruments and can lead to fracture.

d. True. See (a).

e. True. If too much force is used in an attempt to drive a rotary nickel–titanium file down a canal, there is an increased risk of binding and file fracture.

5. a. True. Pain from irreversible pulpitis is long lasting and may be severe.

b. True. Pain may develop spontaneously, while lying down or wake the patient at night.

c. True. Heat frequently becomes a more significant feature in the later stages when in fact cold may act as a relieving factor.

d. False. Pain usually lingers after the stimulus is removed.

e. False. See above.

6. a. True. It is important that the access is large enough to allow canal identification and easy placement of instruments.

b. False. The walls should be divergent to enable good visualisation and support of a temporary dressing.

c. False. The access should be large enough to allow unimpeded access of files into canals. This may mean offsetting it to enable straight-line coronal access.

d. True. The file handle should stand upright in the canal when straight-line access has been achieved.

e. True. This allows canal orifices to be identified. Commonly the roof of the pulp chamber is not completely removed over the orifice of the second mesio-buccal canal in upper molars.

7. a. False. Pre-enlargement is not necessary in medium to large root canals.

b. False. Debris is produced during pre-enlargement; however, correct use of irrigation and a small file to disturb the dentine chips will prevent blockage.

c. True. Pre-enlargement removes dentine coronally that is infected with bacteria.

d. False. Pre-enlargement improves irrigation because there is improved access for the needle.

e. True. Pre-enlargement removes coronal dentine, which may restrict the passage of a file deeper into the root canal.

8. a. False. Root canal retreatment is the preferred option in the majority of cases.

b. True. It may not be possible to treat the root canal by conventional means if a very large post is present, the root canal is blocked by a fractured root canal instrument or the apical third anatomy has been destroyed by overinstrumentation.

c. False. Periradicular surgery aims to remove the apical 3 mm and clean a further 3 mm of canal system but is no substitute for conventional cleaning and shaping procedures.

d. True. The collection of biopsy material at the time of surgery is an important part of the procedure.

e. True. Surgery offers the opportunity to look for root fractures or perforations.

9. a. True. The introduction of ultrasonic techniques has been a major advancement in endodontic surgery.

b. True. Care needs to be taken to use ultrasonic vibration at the lowest effective power. If it is used at too high a power, for long periods or in thin roots, then fracture may occur.

c. False. Ultrasonic vibration produces heat. Water spray cools the tip as well as removing debris.

d. True. One of the major problems of instrumentation with steel burs was that it was not possible to get the retro-preparation in the long access of the root.

e. False. Ultrasonic tips are much smaller than conventional burs and handpieces; therefore, less space is required.

10. a. False. Pain from reversible pulpitis is short lasting.

b. True. The pulp does not contain proprioceptive receptors; consequently pain is difficult to localise until the inflammation involves the periodontium.

c. False. See (b).

d. True. See (a).

e. True. The inflammation is contained within the tooth; therefore, there are no changes to be seen in the periodontium.

11. a. True. Small flexible files help to prevent blockage without overenlarging the foramen.

b. False. The purpose of a patency file is to clear the foramen, not enlarge it.

c. True. This is the main purpose of the patency file.

d. False. A patency file should be used with a gentle touch to avoid overenlargement of the foramen.

e. True. Maintaining patency is important to ensure that there is adequate exchange of irrigant and disinfectant around the apical terminus.

12. a. True. Ease of handling is an important property.
   b. False. Root canal filling materials should not absorb moisture as this could lead to expansion or contamination.
   c. False. Expansion on setting could predispose to root fracture.
   d. False. It is important to be able to remove root filling materials easily for ease of retreatment and post space preparation.
   e. True. This is important, as staining of tooth structure leads to an unaesthetic appearance for the patient.

13. a. False. Silver points do not seal the canal laterally or coronally and may cause staining.
   b. True. Lateral condensation is a well-recognised technique as it seals the root canal laterally and coronally.
   c. True. Continuous wave is a simplified version of vertical condensation of gutta-percha and has the potential to seal lateral canals as well as the main canal system.
   d. True. Such devices have been shown to provide an adequate canal seal. Popular examples include Thermafil and 3D GP.
   e. False. A poorly fitting single gutta-percha cone will not seal the root canal laterally or coronally.

14. a. False. A correctly curved instrument should not have any sharp bends in it; these would increase stress in the instrument. Therefore, it will not predispose the file to fracture.
   b. False. Sterilising instruments is an essential part of root canal therapy; it does not weaken them. However, root canal instruments should not be re-used.
   c. False. Jumping between different sizes of instrument is not recommended; they should be used in an ordered sequence.
   d. True. A good quality-control programme is an essential part of endodontic therapy.
   e. True. Root canal instruments should never be forced as they can break.

15. a. True. Irrigation and recapitulation with a small file will help to reduce blockage as a result of dentine chips.
   b. True. Attempts to get past a root canal blockage may result in the file going offline and perforating the root.
   c. True. Lubrication helps to keep debris in solution and emulsifies pulp tissue in vital cases.
   d. False. Coronal two-thirds enlargement improves irrigation and, therefore, helps reduce the incidence of canal blockage.
   e. True. Canal blockage is avoidable if sufficient care is taken in canal preparation.

SINGLE BEST ANSWER QUESTION ANSWERS

1. Answer C. Parallax views are particularly helpful. A single PA would not provide any information about the involvement of adjacent teeth and may not capture a root fracture. A limited field CBCT may be indicated but only after initial plain film radiography and if diagnosis or management would be affected.
2. C
3. B
4. A
5. A
6. C
7. D

PICTURE QUESTIONS ANSWERS

1. There has been pulp chamber obliteration in the mid third of the root most likely as a result of dental trauma, the dentine deposition is likely to be irregular in nature and it is often possible to bypass the apparent blockage. The canal appears wide coronally (consistent with the age of trauma) and patent beyond the blockage and amenable to root canal treatment.
2. The coronal access may be difficult through an all ceramic crown; the morphology of the crown may be different to the underlying anatomy. The canal has significant curvature in its apical third and there is a higher risk of canal transportation, ledging and instrument fracture. Careful straight-line access is required, ideally with good light magnification. Initial glide path should be developed with precurved flexible stainless steel instruments or NiTi glide path files to reduce the risk of transportation. Superflexible heat-treated NiTi rotary or reciprocatory instruments will allow canal preparation at reduced risk of procedural error
3. Initially the patient's pain should be relived, the UR1 should have the existing RCT removed as a priority, disinfected with sodium hypochlorite and then dressed with a non-setting calcium hydroxide. Then, teeth planned for re-RCT should have any existing restorations removed, caries removed and each assessed for restorability. Working composite cores are helpful. Gutta-percha can be removed with hand or rotary instruments with or without the use of solvent. Re-RCT can be carried out prior to placement of cores ± fibre posts prior to preparation for new crowns. The status of the remaining upper anteriors on the left side should also be considered.
4. This patient has dentinogenesis imperfecta (without osteogenesis imperfecta), as do their children. Further investigation in the form of a CBCT scan is indicated as to whether or not the teeth with chronic apical abscesses are amenable to either orthograde or retrograde endodontics. A larger volume scan could be justified as there is strong likelihood of multiple dental abscesses in other areas of the mouth. If not possible then this can be used to plan for replacement with dental implants.
5. This is most likely a periapical granuloma or infected odontogenic cyst. Stages for apicectomy – consent, local anaesthetic, raising of mucoperiosteal flap, osteotomy site, curettage of the lesion, root end resection, root end filling, irrigation, compression of flap, sutures, post-op advice (bleeding, diet, analgesics, emergency contact information) and specimen sent for histopathology. Review should be for suture removal, and at 1 year.

6. The challenge here is removal of what is a very long post; this would involve sectioning the crown and either trying to vibrate using ultrasonics, pull out the post or alternatively trephine around it with a Masserann kit. Orthograde root canal treatment could then be carried out followed by post-crown restoration. Surgery is an option but would potentially leave the tooth in a weakened state. Removal of the ideal 3 mm of root end would leave little space for a root end filling and would leave the tooth with a limited amount of bone support. Extraction and RBB or implant are also possible treatment options.

SHORT NOTES ANSWERS

1. Reactionary and reparative dentine are both types of tertiary dentine, as distinct from physiological secondary dentine. Reactionary dentine is a response to a mild noxious stimulus; reparative dentine is deposited directly beneath the path of the injured dentinal tubules as a response to strong noxious stimuli.
2. Pulp sensitivity tests can be divided into thermal and electrical. Their purpose is to identify the offending tooth, although it is usual to start with a tooth expected to respond within normal limits in order to establish a baseline. Thermal tests are usually the most useful as they give an indication as to whether the pulp is alive and how healthy it is. Cold tests include EndoIce or ethyl chloride spray on a cotton pledget, ice or dry ice; hot tests include hot gutta-percha or hot water. Electric pulp tests are less useful as, although they provide an indication as to whether there is vital nerve tissue in the tooth, they do not give an indication of different levels of degeneration.
3. Cracked tooth syndrome is an increasingly common clinical problem and can be very difficult to diagnose in its early stages. Pain is usually short lasting but can be very sharp, especially on release of the biting pressure. A plastic bite stick (tooth sleuth) may be used over individual cusps in an effort to find the offending one. Lower second molars and upper premolars are frequently affected. Extensively cracked teeth require extraction; if the crack is less severe, then extracoronal restoration may prevent further progression.
4. Balanced forces is a method of instrument rotation introduced by Roane in 1985. The initial technique involved rotating the instrument 90° clockwise to set the flutes and then rotating 180° anticlockwise while maintaining apical pressure to cut dentine. It is efficient and has been shown to maintain a central canal position even around moderate curvatures. It is usual nowadays to use a slightly less aggressive technique, which involves a 60° clockwise rotation and 120° anticlockwise rotation with the apical pressure being just sufficient to prevent the instrument backing out of the canal.
5. Electronic apex locators are used to help to determine canal length. They are accurate about 85% of the time; however, canal length should be confirmed with a radiograph. Problems can occur with the accuracy of electronic apex locators if the canal is very wet and there is fluid in the pulp chamber. These may lead to short circuiting with files in other canals or to metallic restorations. Further problems may be encountered if the file size does not closely resemble the width of the root canal.

Reference

Roane et al. The 'Balanced Force' Concept of Instrumentation of Curved Canals. *J Endod.* 1985;11:203–211.

3 Conservative Dentistry

Overview

This chapter reviews current methods for the restoration and replacement of teeth using direct and indirect restorations. These contemporary techniques have evolved more or less simultaneously with developments in dental materials. The selection, properties, advantages and disadvantages of various materials are discussed.

3.1 Examination, Diagnosis and Treatment Planning

LEARNING OBJECTIVES

You should:
- describe the relevant anatomy of enamel and dentine
- assess the risk factors for the progression of dental caries
- outline the strategies for caries risk assessment and management
- describe the principles of cavity preparation and finalisation
- be familiar with the principles of resin bonding and adhesive dentistry.

Examination of patients with a view to carrying out conservative procedures should follow the general principles for dental examination and history taking; treatment should address the underlying aetiology of the pathological process (Table 3.1).

RELEVANT ANATOMY

Enamel

Enamel has a rigid and highly crystalline structure, which confers a hard outer coating to teeth. It has translucent and opalescent properties important to the appearance of a tooth. It is largely made up of crystals of hydroxyapatite (95–98% by mass) which makes enamel prone to acid demineralisation, from both caries and erosion. It is also brittle and liable to cracking, especially when unsupported by dentine, which provides both resilience and toughness. The inorganic component comprises 86–95% hydroxyapatite by volume. The organic component comprises 1–2%, while water contributes 4–12%. Enamel prisms are the main structural units and are generally orientated at 90° to the external surface of the tooth.

Dentine

Dentine comprises 45–50% inorganic hydroxyapatite crystals, with 30% organic matrix and 25% water by volume. It is vital, moist, flexible and permeable and its colour varies with its value tending to increase with age. Dentine is slowly deposited throughout a patient's lifetime; this is referred to as secondary dentine. Tertiary reactionary dentine, which is deposited much more quickly, has a more irregular structure. It is deposited in response to chronic low-grade trauma such as attrition, erosion, abrasion, progressive caries and tooth preparation.

Dentine consists of:

- *intertubular dentine*: the primary structural component, comprising hydroxyapatite embedded in a collagen matrix
- *peritubular dentine*: which provides a collagen-free hypermineralised tubular wall
- *dentinal tubules*: filled with odontoblastic processes, which form the interface between the dentine and the pulp.

No specific nerve endings lie within the tubules; therefore dentine sensitivity and its pathological derivative, hypersensitivity, have been hypothesised to arise from fluid movement within the tubules. This is called the hydrodynamic theory of dentinal sensitivity and explains how certain stimuli, such as thermal changes and those creating osmotic gradients, can result in painful sensations. Persistent sensitivity can lead to peripheral nerve sensitisation and, as a result, relatively low-grade stimuli can elicit an exaggerated painful response.

3.2 Caries

In order to understand the management of dental caries, we must begin by understanding how the caries process is initiated and progressed (Fig. 3.1). Caries is a disease of the

Table 3.1 Principles of Dental Examination and History Taking.

PATIENT DESCRIPTION OF COMPLAINT	
Complaint	E.g. pain (see Chapter 2) teeth wearing away, appearance, can't eat etc.
History of presenting complaint	E.g. 6-month history of intermittent sensitivity, recently getting more frequent and lasting longer
Systematic enquiry of symptoms	
Site	Where in oral cavity?
Onset	Sudden/gradual onset currently improving/worsening
Character	Sharp, dull, aching types of pain
Radiation	Referral to other oro-facial structures
Duration	Short, lingering, spontaneous
Exacerbating and relieving factors	Pain with hot/cold/sweet/pain on biting. Analgesics effective?
Severity	Numerical or visual analogue scales can be helpful
Dental history	Frequency of attendance, previous experience, concerns and expectations about dental treatment
Medical history	Full systematic enquiry, noting relevant factors to planned examination, investigations and provision of treatment
Social history	Smoking, alcohol consumption, occupation, oral habits
CLINICAL EXAMINATION	
Extraoral	Facial asymmetry, swellings, nodes, temporomandibular joints, muscles of mastication, skin lesions
Intraoral	Soft tissues: lesions, lumps, asymmetry, dryness, swellings, sinuses
	Periodontium: gingival appearance, plaque/calculus deposits, periodontal probing depths, recession, mobility, fremitus, drifting
DENTAL HARD TISSUES	
Caries assessment	Clinical diagnosis following visual, tactile, radiographic examination. Caries: cavitated, non-cavitated; TSL,
Existing restorations	NCCLs, hypoplasia, stain. Restorations: marginal breakdown, fractures, secondary caries, fractures, cracks,
Tooth surface loss	wear of teeth or restorations. Relationship to periodontium, deficient margins, positive/negative ledges, food trapping (contact points)
Periodontal and endodontic Considerations	See relevant chapters
Aesthetic and prosthodontic considerations	Aesthetics, occlusion, edentulous areas: potential abutment angulation, opposing teeth positions
Diagnostic tests	Pulp vitality, percussion, pain on pressure/release of pressure, radiographs, CBCT see Chapter 2
Adjunctive assessments	Study models, articulation, photographs, diagnostic wax-ups, occlusal analysis, digital smile design

CBCT, Cone Beam Computerised Tomography; *NCCL*, non-carious cervical lesion; *TSL*, tooth surface loss.

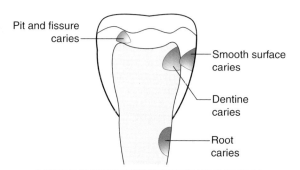

Fig. 3.1 Development and progression of caries.

mineralised hard dental tissues that is caused by the action of micro-organisms present in plaque biofilm (e.g. *mutans streptococci* and *Lactobacillus* spp.) on dietary carbohydrates. Though specific bacteria are associated with caries, the overall nature of the biofilm is important, with the 'ecological plaque hypothesis' currently the favoured model of initiation and progression. This in turn produces an acidic environment in which demineralisation occurs and the early stages of breakdown begin. Caries is not a continuous process. Saliva and fluoride are protective, promoting remineralisation, alongside providing other beneficial effects. Caries progresses, however, if a cariogenic biofilm is frequently exposed to sugars, and dissolution progresses at a faster rate than remineralisation. This net loss of structure is the process of caries. Dentine caries shows a demineralised (caries affected) zone deep to the bacterially infected zone (caries infected), and this is important in the operative management of the disease (see later).

PRINCIPLES OF MANAGEMENT

In spite of greater awareness of prevention and public health measures, dental caries remains prevalent within the population. Identifying a patient's risk for dental caries forms an essential part of providing patient-centred management. Historically caries was treated by complete excision of the lesion with a further extension of the prepared cavity to allow placement of a mechanically retained restoration. Contemporary caries management places risk management, preservation of tooth structure and preservation of pulp vitality at its core, with the aim of preventing new carious lesions from becoming established and halting the progress of existing pathology. This change in philosophy and move in emphasis, from a surgical approach to a conservative approach, enables non-operative treatment of early lesions and a more conservative operative approach to advanced lesions. There remains a place for operative treatment of caries but this now takes into account the tooth's propensity for repair, as well as developments in techniques for preserving pulpal vitality.

CURRENT SYSTEMS OF ASSESSMENT AND MANAGEMENT

The International Caries Classification and Management System (ICCMS) takes this philosophy and outlines how caries can be risk assessed allowing implementation of a personalised plan of care for a patient. Further information on ICCMS can be obtained at https://iccms-web.com.

RISK ASSESSMENT

The first phase is to determine caries risk, which may vary throughout a patient's lifetime. Risks can be classified as clinical, medical, social and behavioural. They are in turn used to determine a risk status for a patient; this can be low, moderate or high. The first stage in management of dental caries is to address any modifiable risk factors. Clinical risks are those that can be assessed by directly examining the patient and include recent past caries experience, the presence of active caries and inadequate oral hygiene, including visible stagnation of plaque biofilm. It is also possible to identify clinically whether or not the patient has oral dryness (xerostomia). Xerostomia may be present for a variety of reasons, including medical conditions, such as Sjogren's syndrome or previous damage to salivary glands from head and neck radiotherapy, or as a result of certain medications, e.g. tricyclic antidepressants, antihistamines, antimuscarinics or recreational drugs. Social, medical and behavioural risks include diet, social status, compliance with hygiene practices, dental attendance patterns and other special educational needs or physical disabilities. Obvious milestones in a patient's life, e.g. reliance on caregivers to prepare food and drinks, as well as help with oral hygiene practices either early or later in life, or adapting to independent living can all impact on caries risk. The most frequently encountered risk factor is a high intake (both amount and frequency) of free sugars in meals, snacks or drinks. The timing of sugar consumption in relation to meals and bedtime is also important and should be ascertained. High sugar consumption is a common risk factor for obesity, diabetes and cardiovascular disease, and the patient should be made aware of the potential impact on their general, as well as their oral, health.

A patient may be unaware of the impact of certain foods on their oral health. For example, there is a perception that smoothies and fruit juices are healthy, which in moderation they can be, but patients are often unaware of the large amounts of sugars they contain. If consumed frequently, or over a prolonged period of time, free sugars will have a significant impact on caries risk. This is often coupled with the impact of socio-economic status and so called 'health literacy'. Patients either may not be able to eat healthily for financial reasons, or understand that there is a benefit to making healthy lifestyle and diet choices for both oral and general health.

It is also important to establish whether or not the patient is already modifying the disease risk in any way. This could include toothbrushing twice per day using a fluoride containing toothpaste (ideally 1450 ppm or greater), and engagement with preventive care, for example effective toothbrushing, or regular professional application of topical fluoride. Living in an area of water fluoridation will also modulate risk, for example.

CLINICAL ASSESSMENT

The next stage of the caries management process is in detection and diagnosis of caries. Visual and radiographic examination of teeth (wherever this is practical depending upon the setting) is essential for understanding the extent, sometimes referred to as the 'stage' and activity of the lesion. Observation of each tooth (free from plaque and in dry and wet conditions) with good lighting, magnification and where available, transillumination, will all aid accurate diagnosis. Clinical assessment should take into account whether the tooth surface has:

- no visible changes of the enamel surface (sound)
- initial visible changes in enamel, for example opacities or brown discolouration but with an intact enamel surface and no shadowing (initial caries)
- a white or brown spot lesion with early enamel surface breakdown or visible shadowing of the underlying dentine (moderate caries)
- a distinct cavity with visible or detectable breakdown with dentine visible (extensive caries).

Caries may be obvious clinically, but often, in posterior teeth where there are substantial restorations that obscure direct visualisation or prevent transillumination, caries can be more difficult to detect. Non-cavitated posterior interproximal caries is often difficult to detect and therefore radiographic examination should be undertaken to help aid diagnosis. Radiographs should be undertaken on a risk basis and should be justified and optimised. Bitewing radiographs are particularly useful for posterior teeth, but no radiograph should be relied on entirely and must be used in conjunction with the clinical picture. In fact, caries visible on radiographs may underestimate the clinical extent of the lesion. For those at low risk, bitewing radiographs should be taken at 2-yearly intervals, for those at moderate risk, annually and for high risk patients every 6 months. If caries risk changes over time then radiographic examination (and examination recall) intervals should change accordingly.

Radiographs may reveal relative radiolucencies indicating potential caries. These areas must be compared to the appearance of intact enamel and dentine. If a carious lesion can be detected radiographically, the extent of progression should be documented in the clinical record. The extent of the lesion will have a direct influence on how it is later managed. Initial caries may be visible in enamel and the outer third of dentine (distance measured from the amelo-dentinal junction (ADJ) to pulp); moderate caries will be visible within the middle third of dentine and extensive lesions will reach the inner third of dentine or even extend into the pulp. Initial caries may not be cavitated, whilst moderate and extensive caries are almost always cavitated clinically.

It is sometimes difficult to determine whether or not a carious lesion is active or inactive. Sharp probing of suspected lesions should be avoided due to a risk of inadvertently cavitating an early lesion. Some idea of texture can be helpful in determining activity and can be obtained by gently running a World Health Organisation probe over the suspected area. Extensive active caries extending into dentine will feel soft or leathery whereas inactive lesions will feel shiny or hard on similar application of pressure. Active enamel lesions are likely to be rougher than inactive lesions and there are also sometimes visual differences between the two. Inactive enamel lesions are likely to be covered with less plaque, having a shinier brown/black appearance rather than a duller whiter/yellow/opaque colour of an active lesion.

The clinical and radiographic findings coupled with identification of risk factors for dental caries will allow the clinician to determine caries risk and from this, formulate a tailored management plan with a focus on prevention and minimally invasive operative treatments, whilst planning an appropriate recall and radiographic interval to be vigilant for new disease.

RISK MANAGEMENT

Preventive (non-excisional) methods to address caries and caries risk look to reduce demineralisation and increase remineralisation, and can be categorised as public health measures, behavioural measures or clinical measures, although clinical advice can lead to behavioural changes, and behavioural changes (or lack of change) can lead to the need for further clinical measures. It is therefore important to appraise and monitor these factors on a regular basis. Initial management should look to address any modifiable risk factors and utilise remineralisation strategies (Box 3.1) Patients should be encouraged to take ownership of their

---

Box 3.1 Preventative, Non-Excisional Caries Management in Adults.

Public Health Measure Examples:

Fluoridated water (public health measure).
Addressing sugar consumption through taxation etc.

Homecare examples.

Reduction of amount and frequency of fermentable carbohydrate intake (through dietary counselling).
Optimised plaque control (advice should be tailored, using appropriate interproximal aids (mechanical ± chemical)).
Prescription of fluoride toothpastes:
  low risk 0.32% NaF (1400 ppm F⁻)
  medium risk 0.619% NaF (2800 ppm F⁻)
  high risk 1.1% NaF (5000 ppm F⁻)
Fluoride mouth rinses ranging from 0.05% to 2% NaF for daily/weekly use.
Use of saliva substitutes/salivary stimulation for xerostomia.
Casein phosphopeptide — amorphous calcium phosphate application
Calcium based snacks, e.g. cheese or xylitol chewing gum after sugar intakes

Clinical Examples:

Professionally applied fluoride 2.26% NaF (22 600 ppmF⁻) NaF varnish.
Fluoride gels, e.g. 0.4% stannous fluoride.
Placement of fissure sealants in vulnerable pits and fissures.
Caries infiltration strategies.

---

dental disease and it is the role of the practitioner to motivate and support them to do so.

Initial Management

When structuring a personalised plan of care, it may be necessary to have an initial phase of care that manages any acute symptoms, and/or where there is frank cavitation, simply occludes the cavity, covering sensitive dentine and making the tooth comfortably cleansable, following which there is an intensive phase of prevention. This will allow a practitioner to determine the patient's response to any initial preventive advice before embarking on a potentially extensive restorative treatment plan. If disease is not controlled, and restorative treatment undertaken, then the patient is likely to rapidly experience recurrent caries around new restorations. Preventative care for a patient is likely to evolve over time and require regular encouragement and reinforcement.

ROOT CARIES

Caries is not limited to the coronal aspect of a tooth and can occur on the root surfaces of teeth where there are areas of exposed dentine and cementum. Exposed areas of dentine are more prone to caries than enamel due to the higher (less acidic) critical pH of demineralisation of dentine (pH 6–6.5 compared with pH 5.5 for enamel). Therefore, the prevalence of root caries increases with age as a consequence of older adults retaining more of their teeth for longer which may have been subjected to periodontal bone loss and recession. The surfaces that are most susceptible are those that are prone to plaque accumulation and stagnation, which may be greater in interproximal sites, around fixed and removable prostheses and may not be removed effectively. Older adults are more likely to be medically compromised and as a result may have poorer manual dexterity. Treatment for root caries therefore will likely focus on prevention and minimally invasive treatment approaches.

NON-OPERATIVE MANAGEMENT

Initial carious lesions may be reversed by addressing the risk factors as outlined above, often in combination with adjunctive strategies such as topical fluoride application or possibly resin sealants in an attempt to inactivate or arrest the caries.

OPERATIVE MANAGEMENT

When a tooth has cavitated and is uncleansable, it is highly likely that the lesion is active and operative intervention is required. This should be carried out in a conservative manner, attempting to rationally preserve as much of the natural tooth tissue as possible whilst maintaining pulp vitality. Restorations should ideally restore the shape of the tooth to cleansable, pain-free function, protecting the pulp-dentine complex, whilst taking into account the patient's aesthetic requirements. Where there is extensive caries, a decision will need to be made about the long-term prognosis of a tooth, and in some cases this may result in its removal.

Operative intervention usually necessitates removal of infected or damaged enamel and dentine and preparation of a cavity that will help to both support and retain the restorative material. Caries removal should begin by removing sufficient enamel to adequately access the infected dentine below. Once any unsupported enamel has been removed, caries management should begin peripherally at the ADJ. Caries at the ADJ should be cleared to firm dentine before moving to the internal aspects of the cavity. Excavation of caries should take place with a combination of rotary and hand instruments. Visual and tactile assessments should be carried out throughout the excavation process. All of the carious lesion does not need to be removed, with the endpoint of excavation being a source of contention. The endpoint is generally assessed by the hardness of the dentine. Caries-affected dentine can be left as it can remineralise, though clinically ascertaining the point of the carious process is not predictable. Some caries-infected dentine may be left over the pulp, as it has been shown that sealing in such caries with an appropriate restoration can kill the bacteria present. This may however negatively impact the lifespan of the subsequently placed restoration.

DEEP LESIONS

Where there is concern over pulpal involvement, carious tissue can be left over the pulp in an attempt to avoid pulpal exposure. Exposure may negatively impact survival of the pulp (though again this is a point of contention – see Chapter 2). Leaving carious dentine over the pulp is called a selective or partial excavation technique, and the sealed remaining dentine referred to as an indirect pulp cap. Other strategies involve clearing the periphery, as described, but removing a very minimal amount of central caries. The cavity is then sealed (with GIC for example) prior to a further operative procedure 3–6 months later, when hopefully the lesion has arrested and become firmer, and the pulp has receded, allowing a safer caries excavation by minimising risk to the pulp prior to definitive restoration placement. This is known as the stepwise excavation technique. There is no consensus as to which technique is superior, but the limited evidence currently available favours the selective excavation technique and definitive restoration at the first visit.

Management of the carious lesion is dependent on a pulpal diagnosis, and this impacts on pulpal management. This is explored further in Chapter 2.

CAVITY FINALISATION

Once a decision has been made as to how much carious tissue requires removal, the cavity may subsequently need modification to help retain the chosen restorative material. Non-bonded amalgam restorations are mechanically retained. This means they are reliant on undercuts to resist displacement of the restoration. Provision of undercuts may require additional preparation, sacrificing tooth structure. Adhesively retained restorations are less reliant on these features, so cavity preparation is based primarily on the lesion or existing restorations. They are therefore deemed more conservative, but do rely on a bond between tooth structure and the restorative material (see later).

Margins should be smooth and placed in areas accessible for finishing, cleaning and maintenance where possible, which commonly means not at the contact area either occluso-apically or bucco-lingually. Cavities for composites are commonly C-shaped, open and flared, whereas for mechanically retained amalgam, they are more box-like, closed and upright (Fig. 3.2).

Finalisation of the preparation with airborne particle abrasion is beneficial to clean the cavity and margins, and homogenise the smear layer (see later) prior to adhesive bonding.

Anterior teeth requiring restoration often benefit from the placement of a buccal intra-enamel bevel. This improves bonding through increasing the surface area of enamel engaged, and exposing transversely cut enamel prisms. It also aids with aesthetic blending of the tooth-restoration interface.

Where direct posterior composite materials are used, the question of bevel placement remains controversial, with evidence for and against placement in different locations. It is generally safer not to place bevels in posterior teeth to avoid more sacrifice of tooth structure when replacing the restoration; putting thin, weak sections of material on the occlusal surface which are prone to fracture; and to avoid moving from an enamel margin to a dentine margin, which is more prone to breakdown.

Liners

Liners are no longer recommended in shallow and moderately sized cavities. In deep cavities, it may be beneficial to use a liner such as GIC or calcium silicate cements (e.g. Biodentine or MTA) in association with an indirect pulp cap.

Isolation

Isolation is critical for adhesively bonded restorations, with a well-adapted dental dam being the ideal technique used to achieve this. Adequate relative isolation may be achieved by using cotton wool rolls and saliva ejectors, for example. Isolation is not critical for the placement of amalgam, making amalgam more predictable in difficult situations, such as in patients with limited cooperation or with subgingival cavities.

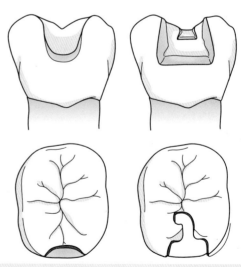

Fig. 3.2 Cavity preparation designs for composite and dental amalgam. Note the more rounded and non-undercut preparation for composite and angular undercut preparation for amalgam. An occlusal "key" is frequently advocated to aid mechanical retention of an amalgam restoration in function.

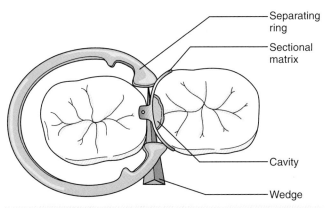

Fig. 3.3 Sectional matrix with separating ring and wedge to ensure stabilisation and tight adaptation of the matrix at the base of cavity, and tooth separation to achieve contact points.

Matrix Use

Matrices can be used to help rebuild teeth where walls have been lost. These come in numerous shapes and sizes, from specific putty matrices (commonly used to help rebuild anterior teeth – see later), to generic metal and clear matrices, which may be contoured or flat, and sectional or circumferential. Sectional matrices, which are commonly contoured, used in conjunction with wooden wedges to seal cavity boxes and provide separation of the teeth, are very useful to achieve contact points both anteriorly and posteriorly with composite, which can be difficult if not impossible to achieve with circumferential bands due to the relatively passive nature of composite placement. This can also be facilitated by the use of separating rings (Fig. 3.3). Given that amalgam is actively packed during placement, contact points can be achieved much more easily with the use of burnished circumferential bands.

3.3 Resin Bonding

Resin bonding agents allow the functional attachment of a restorative material to tooth structure. Enamel is non-living and essentially dry, allowing the formation of predictably strong and long lasting bonds, whereas dentine is living, mutable and wet, making bonding variable, technique sensitive and prone to degradation. Appropriate isolation of a tooth to prevent contamination with oral fluids and debris is critical to optimise the bonding process.

Bonding to both enamel and dentine currently relies on etching them with an acid. This involves dissolution and removal or modification of the mineral component of these substrates.

Acid etching can be achieved by applying an acid and then rinsing it away, which is known as 'total-etching', or by applying an acidic primer which is left on the tooth and not rinsed away. This is known as 'self-etching'.

ENAMEL BONDING

Bonding to enamel is principally micromechanical in nature. It relies on the differential acid etching of enamel.

Different acids are used depending on bonding technique. Total-etch systems employ phosphoric acid, whereas self-etch systems employ weaker acidic primers. Clinical data suggests that etching enamel using phosphoric acid (30–40%) results in reduced staining and marginal breakdown of restorations compared to self-etch systems. It may therefore seem that the use of self-etching systems is inadvisable; however they do offer certain advantages when it comes to bonding to dentine (see later) and the issue of the inferior enamel bond can be overcome. It is therefore advised that when using self-etching techniques, the enamel (only) should initially be etched with phosphoric acid. This is then rinsed and dried prior to application of the self-etching bonding agents which now achieves an optimal enamel bond. This is called 'selective enamel etching'. A gel formulation is advised to aid this process as it allows selective application to the enamel only.

Enamel should be etched for a minimum of 15 seconds. The resultant pitted surface allows a low viscosity resin bonding agent to flow into the pits and form resin tags, which, once polymerised, provide micromechanical retention. The bonding resin is then chemically bonded to a composite resin restorative material, or resin-based luting agent to bond an indirect restoration – see later.

DENTINE BONDING

Bonding to dentine is achieved through the penetration of tags of resin into dentinal tubules, but primarily through demineralisation of dentine. This exposes a collagen lattice structure, allowing resin to infiltrate in and around this exposed collagen which is then polymerised forming a 'composite' functional structure which is called the hybrid layer (Fig. 3.4).

When dentine is instrumented during cavity preparation (except when using some chemo-mechanical techniques), a loosely adherent layer of debris lies over the surface. This is called the smear layer, and it prevents access of the bonding agent to the underlying intact dentine. It therefore must be removed or disrupted to allow the formation of a functionally useful bond.

Total etch systems remove the smear later, whereas self-etch systems disrupt and penetrate it. Removing the smear layer opens up the tubules, meaning dentinal fluid will flow out. Therefore when using the total-etch technique, bonding is taking place in a wet environment, which is why it is also referred to as 'wet bonding'. The smear layer is not

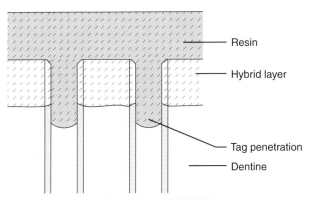

Fig. 3.4 Dentine bonding.

removed in self-etching techniques, so the tubules aren't opened, and hence it is also described as 'dry bonding'.

Dentine is naturally wet; therefore hydrophilic resins, containing adhesives such as 2-hydroxyethyl methacrylate, are required to infiltrate the collagen lattice. This is helped by the use of various solvents. Different solvents require different management to effectively evaporate them, so it seems prudent to highlight the critical importance of following the manufacturer's instructions at this point, as all bonding agents are made up of different constituents, which should be applied and handled in different ways.

Total-etch systems are much more technique sensitive than self-etch systems. When using a total-etch technique, there are risks of over-etching the dentine, and over-drying the dentine, which can have negative effects on the bond formed, potentially leading to poor bond strengths, microleakage and sensitivity. Neither of these risks exist for self-etch systems.

Over-etching can lead to demineralising too deep a zone of dentine. The resin cannot then infiltrate to a sufficiently deep level, resulting in an unreinforced 'gap' between the mineralised dentine and the hybrid zone, which is weak and prone to breakdown.

Freshly cut dentine should therefore not be etched for more than 15 seconds. This is not the case for dentine that has been exposed to the oral environment for a long period, which has responded by laying down more mineral, becoming glassy and dark in appearance. This is termed sclerosed dentine, and is commonly seen in root dentine and tooth surface loss (TSL). In these cases it is advised to roughen the surface and increase the etching time to 30 seconds.

Over-drying the dentine can collapse the exposed collagen lattice compromising the hybrid layer (see Fig. 3.3). So how much should we dry? The dentine should be damp without having pooled water, but it must not be bone dry, as we are wet bonding. Dabbing the cavity with cotton wool appears to remove an optimum amount of water as this achieves the best bond strengths to dentine; however gentle air-drying with a 3-in-1 from around 4–5 cm has been shown to result in acceptable bond strengths.

High bond strengths are important, but not absolutely critical for the reason we intuitively think of: retaining the restoration. A high early bond strength is critical, because resin-based restorative materials shrink when they set (polymerisation contraction) and pull on the bond. The bond must have sufficient strength to resist this polymerisation contraction stress (see later). For this reason and also to prevent displacement of the bonding agent, it is beneficial for the bonding agent to be set prior to applying the restorative material, which is one of the reasons why light-cured bonding agents are preferred, as they can be set quickly on command. Most bonding agents have sufficient strength to resist the contraction stress, based on laboratory studies, but it should be remembered that clinically, we are not bonding in an ideal environment to pristine dentine, we are often bonding to caries affected dentine in far from ideal conditions.

Bond Degradation

There are many mechanisms of bond breakdown over time, including thermocycling and cyclical loading, but fluids getting to the hybrid layer resulting in hydrolytic breakdown is important in this process. This is problematic given that hydrophilic resins are required to infiltrate dentine during the bonding process, but they also allow water to penetrate them. Separating the primer and adhesive into two bottles (total-etch three-step and self-etch two-step systems) allows the initial application of primarily hydrophilic resins in the first 'primer' bottle, and subsequent application of hydrophobic resins (for example, bis-glycidyl methacrylate (GMA)-based resins) in the second 'adhesive' bottle. This results in the formation of a hydrophobic layer which helps to reduce hydrolytic degradation of the hybrid layer over time. In the single bottle systems (total-etch two-step and self-etch one-step systems), all of the resins and monomers are mixed together, which results in less durable dentine bonds. This appears to be more critical clinically when restoration margins are in dentine. Researchers continue to look at increasing the stability of the hybrid layer.

Certain monomers, such as 10-Methacryloyloxydecyl dihydrogen phosphate (10 MDP), can bond chemically to hydroxyapatite, as well as many restorative materials (see later). It appears that they also confer stain resistance to the bonding agent, which is important in preventing premature replacement of restorations, as marginal staining is often mistaken for caries, and is a common reason for patients to request restoration replacement.

3.4 Materials for Direct Restorations

LEARNING OBJECTIVES

You should:
- know the clinical indications and materials for direct restorations
- be able to make an informed choice of the most appropriate material for each clinical situation
- understand the advantages and disadvantages of the materials used to restore teeth.

Classifying a restoration as being direct or indirect refers to the place of fabrication of the restoration, i.e. whether it is made outside of the mouth (usually by a laboratory) – an indirect restoration, or if it is placed entirely within the mouth – a direct restoration. A tooth-borne indirect restoration is therefore cemented or bonded in place, and must have an appropriate path of insertion. It is therefore important that the tooth preparation does not have any undercuts relative to this path of insertion (see later). This is not the case for direct restorations as they are built with an initially soft, workable material, which hardens either chemically or on command, and can therefore engage undercuts.

Classifying a restoration as being intra- or extracoronal refers to the portion of a tooth that is replaced by the restoration. An intracoronal restoration replaces lost structure within the confines of a tooth, which generally means where there are cusps, or the general form of the tooth is remaining. Whenever a surface of a tooth, or cusp(s) are replaced or overlaid, the restoration is said to be extracoronal.

INDICATIONS FOR RESTORATION

- Treatment of caries.
- Replacement/repair of an existing restoration.
- Repair of a fractured tooth.
- Restoration of form/function/aesthetics (e.g. of a congenitally malformed tooth).
- As part of other restorative needs (e.g. core placement prior to crown or in preparation for removable prosthodontics).

DIRECT RESIN COMPOSITE RESTORATIVE MATERIALS

Unset composite materials are made up of a fluid resin matrix and solid filler particles, which are chemically combined by a silane coupling agent. They also incorporate an initiator to commence polymerisation of the resin and this may be mediated chemically, by light activation (using visible light at the cooler, blue end (460–480 nm) of the spectrum, to minimise any pulpal impact), or a combination of both, referred to as dual curing. Chemically cured or dual-cured composites are most often used as luting agents in adhesively retained indirect restorations and posts, whereas light-cured materials are most commonly used as restorative materials (see later).

Composites can also be classified by the size of the filler particles they contain. Hybrid composites have a range of filler particle sizes, whereas microfill composites have only small filler particles. Hybrid composites have a higher percentage of filler by volume, which in turn has an effect on the material properties in both set and unset states. Nanofilled composites are essentially hybrid composites, due to clumping of nanoparticles into nanoclusters. The filler particles are often forms of quartz, silica or glass.

Composites are classified at a basic level by whether they are flowable or not when unset, though this is complicated by the fact that standard viscosity 'paste' composites can be made more flowable by application of heat, and some by application of sonic energy. Yet another classification has been introduced with the development of bulk-fill composites which can be placed in larger increments than conventional light-cured composites, with the aim of reducing placement time.

Increasing the filler content as seen in hybrid composites increases the viscosity of the material, which can impair the adaptation of the material to a cavity; however it reduces polymerisation contraction (see later) and improves the physico-mechanical properties, including strength, rigidity, wear resistance, fracture resistance, reducing the water adsorption and coefficient of thermal expansion of the composite material. Microfills are generally inferior, aside from their ability to be polished and to retain their polish. This makes them ideal for use in low load-bearing situations where aesthetics are important; however in the vast majority of situations, hybrids are more appropriate.

Resin-based materials shrink when they set, which leads to polymerisation contraction stress at the interface between the tooth and the restoration. This can cause cracking or flexure of tooth substance, or gap formation between the tooth and the restoration. These can result in fracture, microleakage, sensitivity and potentially recurrent caries, all of which can result in premature failure of the restored tooth unit.

Increasing the filler content reduces the amount of polymerisation contraction stress. Chemically cured composites set more slowly and develop less stress than light-cured composites, but generally have inferior physico-mechanical properties. They are increasingly being used as bulk-fill composites. Bulk-fill light-cured composites develop less stress at the interface, not through increasing filler content, but by manipulating the chemical properties of the resins used.

Many other factors can also influence the development of interfacial polymerisation contraction stress, including the configuration of the cavity (C factor) and light curing mode for example. Composite placement techniques have therefore developed in an attempt to minimise this damaging stress.

PLACEMENT TECHNIQUES

Placing composite in layers minimises the surface area of composite that is bound to the cavity wall in relation to the unbound surface area. This allows 'flow' within the material, which limits the interfacial contraction stress. This essentially mitigates against the C-factor effect. Layering also respects conventional composite depth of cure. These increments should be no more than 2 mm in thickness and ideally would not connect walls. Light-cured bulk-fill composites can be placed in 4–5 mm increments, and chemically cured, or dual-cured composites have no maximum increment limits.

ADVANTAGES AND DISADVANTAGES OF COMPOSITE RESTORATIONS

Resin composites have been developed in a wide range of shades, tints and opacities, allowing production of aesthetic restorations, capable of matching almost any natural tooth shade and appearance. Colour stability is generally good, but shade will change over time. Extrinsic staining may result with time as a result of surface deterioration, but especially at the tooth restoration interface. Given that composite can be bonded to enamel and dentine, cavity preparation can be initially more conservative of tooth tissue (see Fig. 3.2). Composite in general is sufficiently strong and has improved in wear resistance to allow it to be used in almost any situation. It is however much more technique sensitive than amalgam, taking longer to place and is therefore more costly to the patient. The contraction during setting can lead to many problems as discussed and it can be difficult to achieve contact points without specialised equipment (see Fig. 3.3). There are also higher rates of secondary caries around composite restorations than other materials, with composite appearing to be more supportive of a cariogenic biofilm.

AMALGAM

The continued use of dental amalgam has become a controversial topic in recent years with environmental concerns being raised. It has been phased-down, with restrictions placed on its use in children and pregnant and breastfeeding women in the United Kingdom. There is no firm scientific evidence to indicate an association with any systemic disease other than lichenoid reactions. Some EU countries have banned its use but, at present, no direct restorative material exists that has the same ease of handling, technique insensitivity and cost-effectiveness.

Amalgam is an alloy of mercury with other metals including silver, copper and tin and zinc. High copper alloys are most commonly used which results in elimination of the weak gamma 2 phase, reducing its tendency to corrode.

Advantages

Amalgam has many advantages, such as:

- strength
- technique insensitivity, facilitating its use in subgingival cavities and in patients with limited cooperation
- relative ease of obtaining a contact point
- wear resistance
- reduced microleakage, resulting from slow corrosion
- good survival
- cost-effectiveness.

Disadvantages

The disadvantages of amalgam are:

- poor aesthetics
- may require more extensive cavity preparation due to mechanical retention and weak in thin sections
- lack of inherent bonding to tooth substance, though it can be bonded using adhesives
- potential mercury hazard to operator and associated staff and the environment
- potential galvanic issues
- develops strength slowly, at increased risk of fracture immediately after placement.

GLASS IONOMER CEMENTS

Glass ionomer cements (glass polyalkenoates) set by an acid–base reaction between weak polymeric acids (e.g. polyacrylic acid) and powdered glasses (e.g. fluoroaluminosilicate glass). Once these components are combined either by hand mixing or through encapsulated automated mixing (for convenience and ease of application), they may be adapted to the tooth surface. Following preparation of the cavity, the tooth surface should be prepared by dentine conditioning to remove the smear layer using a polyacrylic acid; this increases surface area and potential for micromechanical retention. Over time, the material matures and will gradually form a strong resilient ionic bond at the interface with the tooth. One advantage of using glass ionomers is that they will release fluoride rapidly over the first 2 weeks following placement; after this the fluoride release is limited and perhaps not clinically significant.

Traditional glass ionomers have been modified to incorporate resins in order to overcome some of the less desirable properties such as its solubility, compressive strength and lengthy setting time; these are referred to as resin-modified glass ionomers (RMGICs). RMGICs can therefore be command set in a similar way to composite resins which allow them to be shaped and adjusted at placement but then continue to undergo further maturation (of the glass ionomer component) over the next 24 hours.

Clinically GIC and RMGIC are useful materials and are predominantly used in the conventional luting of mechanically retained indirect restorations. They may also be used to repair fractured restorations and as medium-term provisional restorations. Whilst some of the RMGICs are advocated for load bearing restoration of posterior teeth, the handling, wear and aesthetic properties of these materials mean that they are generally not favoured in load bearing cavities by these authors.

3.5 Tooth Surface Loss

TSL is the pathological loss of tooth structure that is not attributable to caries or trauma. It is increasing in prevalence and can be a significant problem in patients of all ages. The clinical appearance of the TSL and associated history are important in diagnosing the aetiology, which is important to effectively manage the condition. The main causes are erosion, abrasion and attrition and these often occur in combination. There is limited evidence for one further type of tooth surface loss, abfraction, which has also been reported in the literature.

EROSION

Erosion denotes the non-bacterially derived, chemically mediated pathological loss of tooth tissue. The appearance of primarily erosive TSL is often of cupped lesions in the occlusal aspect of teeth, where progression occurs more rapidly in the less mineralised dentine than in the enamel, and the enamel edges are often ragged and chipped. Smooth surface lesions often have a smooth dished out appearance. The clinical pattern of TSL is often suggestive of the source of the acid which can be either intrinsic or extrinsic:

- Intrinsic acids are gastric acids arising from within the individual, and causes can include gastro-oesophageal reflux disease (GORD), recurrent vomiting in alcoholism and eating disorders. TSL is commonly seen on the palatal surfaces of the maxillary teeth and the occlusal surfaces of posterior teeth, particularly in the mandibular arch.
- Extrinsic acids are acids brought from an external source into the oral cavity, mainly of dietary origin and mainly from carbonated drinks, citrus fruit, fruit juices and acidic foodstuffs (e.g. vinegar/pickles). They can also originate from environmental sources, as seen in certain industries, and in heavily chlorinated swimming pools, for example. Extrinsic TSL is commonly seen on the buccal and occlusal surfaces.

ABRASION

Abrasion is frictional loss of tooth structure from a source other than tooth to tooth, or tooth to restoration contact. Toothbrushing is a commonly cited cause; however it is probably the relative dentine abrasivity (RDA) of the toothpaste which is the more important factor. 'Occupational' aetiologies have been reported for those working in dusty environments with inadequate protection. Abrasion is most commonly seen at the buccal cervical margins of teeth, especially where gingival recession has exposed root surface, and these areas are often known as non-carious cervical lesions (NCCLs) (though these are not solely attributable to abrasion). They often have a multifactorial aetiology, which has been described as biocorrosion in an attempt to allude to this.

ATTRITION

Attrition is loss of tooth structure resulting from tooth to tooth or tooth to restoration contact. Minimal physiological tooth wear occurs throughout life, but aberrant chewing pathways and parafunctional activity such as bruxism can cause abnormal attrition and TSL. The clinical appearance of abnormal attrition presents initially as faceting, which may progress to flattening of occlusal surfaces and incisal edges. More rapid rates of wear may be observed in natural teeth opposing rough ceramic restorations. Cheek ridging along the occlusal line and tongue scalloping may be present.

ABFRACTION

Some lesions cannot easily be explained by erosion, abrasion or attrition. Abfraction is the pathological loss of tooth tissue resulting from biomechanical forces distant from the point of loading and has been posited as a potential cause. It is suggested that cervical flexure and microfractures result in wedge-shaped NCCLs.

MANAGEMENT

TSL management should initially look to address any presenting pain complaint, which could be tooth based, having pulpal or periapical origins, or soft tissue based, where the oral mucosa is traumatised by sharp worn teeth. It is important to understand the patient's concerns if they have any, which may be functional, aesthetic or worry over the progressive loss of tooth structure. Understanding and managing patient expectations is important from the outset. Conservative management should look to address any underlying causes. This may involve education of the patient and provision of:

- dietary counselling
- oral hygiene advice (including use of a low RDA toothpaste, e.g. Sensodyne Pronamel)
- promotion of remineralisation
- protective appliances (splints)
- referral to general medical practitioner if intrinsic acid aetiology suspected.

Thereafter, intervention is governed by the patient's wishes and the extent of damage sustained by the dentition. Simple maintenance and monitoring through the use of intraoral scanning techniques, photographs or serial study models may be the best policy where limited damage has occurred. Various classification systems have been described, but haven't been widely adopted, primarily because the classifications do not effectively guide management.

Restorative intervention requires careful diagnosis and planning, assessing all aspects of the dentition and its prognosis. It commonly involves restoration of multiple teeth in a proven hostile oral environment. These restorations will require maintenance and periodic replacement, which is often termed the restorative burden. The patient must understand these implications particularly when embarking on an extensive rehabilitation.

It is important to assess whether the TSL is localised or generalised, as this will guide the approach to restoration. Teeth that have lost tooth structure exposing appreciable amounts of dentine should ideally be restored if, after conservative managements have been exhausted, symptoms persist, or the TSL is progressive, whilst those that haven't would ideally avoid restoration, to reduce the restorative burden. Sometimes, however, it may be convenient to treat such teeth if they are biomechanically compromised, or they can aesthetically stabilise an occlusion by levelling an occlusal plane.

Commonly, all teeth still contact in intercuspal position (ICP) even though they are worn. Interocclusal space is often lost in both generalised and localised TSL, most commonly through dentoalveolar compensation. Interocclusal space must therefore be gained to allow restoration. This can be achieved in the following ways, which may often be combined:

- Moving the teeth (orthodontics – controlled; Dahl effect – uncontrolled through localised opening of vertical dimension (see later)).
- Lengthening teeth by moving the incisal edge and facial aspect of teeth buccally (caution advised).
- Adjustment of the opposing teeth.
- 'Distalising' the mandible, taking advantage of a horizontal discrepancy between retruded contact position (RCP) and ICP.
- Increasing the occlusal vertical dimension (see later).

Restorative management may involve the following strategies alone or in combination:

- Simple intracoronal restorations to protect exposed dentine.
- Direct or indirect adhesively retained extracoronal restorations.
- Indirect mechanically retained extracoronal restorations.
- Doming of extensively worn teeth and provision of overdentures.

The choices made when managing TSL restoratively are often complex and multifactorial, taking into consideration aesthetics, function and the structural and biological compromise of the teeth. The planning of such cases and restorative options mentioned are explored further in later sections.

3.6 Indirect Restorations

LEARNING OBJECTIVES

You should:
- outline how indirect restorations may be classified according to coverage, material and retention method
- identify the biomechanical principles of treatment planning and tooth preparation for indirect restorations
- describe the methods for transfer of clinical information for accurate indirect restoration manufacture.

Indirect restorations are made outside of the mouth and are generally placed for the following reasons:

- To improve the structural integrity of a compromised tooth.
- To restore form and function.
- For aesthetic reasons.
- To replace missing teeth (bridges), or help facilitate their replacement (design elements to aid retention and/or stability of partial dentures).

Indirect restorations are generally classified in three different ways:

- coverage
- material
- retention method.

The tooth preparation required for an indirect restoration will vary depending on each of these three elements. The decision as to the coverage, the material choice and the retention method should all have been treatment planned prior to picking up a handpiece to perform the preparation.

COVERAGE

Extracoronal

- Full coverage
  - Crown
- Partial coverage
  - ¾ crown
  - Onlay
    - Partial occlusal coverage
    - Full occlusal coverage
  - Veneer/shim

Intracoronal

- Inlay

The classification by coverage has become increasingly blurred, as restorations continue to evolve, with many terms being used for similar restorations. For example, 'onlays' may also be called partial crowns, or overlays. An onlay is essentially any restoration replacing a cusp, but without providing full encircling coverage of the clinical crown as an indirectly made crown would. The term veneer is generally used to refer to a thin extracoronal restoration replacing or overlaying the facial part of a tooth, whereas 'shim' is most commonly used to refer to a thin restoration covering the occluding surface of a tooth. The term shim appears to be falling out of favour, with the term onlay now pretty much covering all partial occlusal coverage eventualities. These different partial coverage designs are driven by a desire to reduce the amount of tooth preparation to hopefully prolong the lifespan of the tooth.

MATERIAL

- All metal
  - Precious (high gold alloys)
  - Non-precious (cobalt chromium alloys)
- All ceramic
  - Etchable (lithium disilicate (Emax); feldspathic)
  - Non-etchable (zirconia)

- Porcelain fused to metal (PFM)
- Composite
- 'Resin-ceramics'

MANUFACTURE

Precious metal restorations are made using casting techniques, with invested wax patterns. Non-precious metals can be made in the same way, but are increasingly being milled through computer-aided design–computer-aided manufacture (CAD–CAM) processes. Gold alloys are softer and less rigid than non-precious metals generally, which means they can be more easily burnished to improve marginal adaptation of a restoration, but will allow more flex which is a concern in longer span PFM bridges. This likely predisposes them to fracture of the veneering porcelain. Achieving a resin bond to non-precious metal is easier to achieve and is stronger than precious metal bonds. Metal restorations are very strong, will not chip or fracture and are less abrasive to the opposing teeth.

Ceramics are often favoured by patients for their aesthetic appearance. However historically, and still today, they have disadvantages in comparison to indirect full metal restorations. They have required increased tooth preparation to allow the restoration to be made in sufficiently thick section to resist fracture of all the ceramic material (though this is changing with newer materials), or to block out the shine through of a metallic coping in a PFM crown. They can chip or break and have a propensity to wear the opposing teeth if not appropriately finished and polished. Polished lithium disilicate and zirconia are very well tolerated by soft tissues, however.

The vast majority of high-strength modern ceramic restorations (lithium disilicate and zirconia-based restorations) are milled, though lithium disilicate can be cast and pressed. Feldspathic porcelains are much weaker than the new higher strength ceramics favoured today, but are still used where aesthetic requirements are high, and these are commonly made on a refractory die.

Both zirconia and lithium disilicates are strong, with zirconia being the stronger material; however its strength varies as the formulation changes. The original zirconias were very opaque and unaesthetic, but also very strong. The newer materials are more translucent and aesthetic, but are generally comparatively weaker. These materials are still stronger than lithium disilicates, which are also very strong, but there is a key difference between these two materials which can impact on how they are used.

Zirconia is a non-etchable ceramic. This means that its surface cannot be easily modified to allow micromechanical bonding to a resin cement. Lithium disilicate (and feldspathic porcelains) on the other hand can be etched (an etchable ceramic) and can therefore be predictably bonded to with resin cements. This affects the method used to retain restorations made of these different materials, and hence the preparation designs (see later).

Zirconias can be chemically bonded using a 10 MDP monomer; however this bond is currently relatively weak. There is abundant research progressing in this area, however. See Table 3.2 for a summary of management of the intaglio (fitting) surfaces of different materials for adhesive bonding.

Table 3.2 Management of Intaglio Surface Prior to Adhesive Bonding.

Material	Preparation of Surface[c]
Etchable ceramics	Hydrofluoric acid (HF), cleaned with phosphoric acid, silane coupling agent
Composite[a]	Particle abrasion[d], silane coupling agent
Non-precious metal[b]	Particle abrasion,[d] 10 MDP
Precious metal	Particle abrasion,[d] sulphide monomers, e.g. VBATDT
Zirconia[b]	Particle abrasion[d], 10 MDP (not to be relied upon for adhesive retention)

[a]Newer resin-ceramic material preparation will depend on the nature of the ceramic particles, i.e. are they etchable or not. If they are, HF etching will be beneficial.

[b]Any surfaces that rely on a chemical bond through the use of 10 MDP (non-precious metals and zirconia) should be cleaned after being tried on without rubber dam, as they will have been contaminated by saliva resulting in reduced bond strengths. The intaglio surface should not be cleaned with phosphoric acid. The phosphate groups in the acid (and saliva) prevent access of the bonding agent to the active binding sites resulting in hugely reduced bond strengths. Cleaning should be performed with particle abrasion, or Ivoclean.

[c]Though so-called 'Universal' bonding agents contain mixtures of most of these active ingredients and can be used, the bond strengths aren't as high as when specific surface preparation agents are used.

[d]Particle abrasion can be carried out with alumina, or with particles leaving a tribochemical coating (e.g. CoJet), which can then be utilised for bonding through the use of a silane bonding agent.

10 MDP, 10-Methacryloyloxydecyl dihydrogen phosphate; *VBATDT*, 6-(4-vinylbenzyl-n-propyl)amino-1,3,5-trizaine-2,4-dithiol

Material developments are occurring at a rapid pace as patients and dentists require ever more aesthetic options with lower biological costs, and this development in materials is driving an evolution in preparation designs for indirect (and direct) restorations.

Layering

PFM crowns have a metal coping which provides a rigid base for the porcelain to be built up in layers over the top and support the rigid, brittle material. The high strength ceramics, zirconia and lithium disilicate, were commonly used as a base coping in a similar way, to rigidly support weaker, but more aesthetic, ceramics which were layered over the top. This is still the most common way of producing an aesthetic restoration at the front of the mouth, but posteriorly, and indeed increasingly anteriorly, these materials are being made monolithically, i.e. without layering the weaker porcelain over the top. This means they are much more resistant to fracture, which in turn means they can be used in thinner section than was advised in the past. The ability to achieve a predictable and high-strength bond between the tooth and the restoration also means that adhesively retained materials can be used in thinner section (see later). This reduces the required tooth preparation thus conserving tooth structure. They are also becoming more and more aesthetic, with graded shade blocks available to mill restorations, and surface characterisation with stains giving the appearance of depth.

Retention of Indirect Restorations

As with direct restorations, indirect restorations can be retained either primarily mechanically or adhesively. We are essentially talking about how well a restoration stays on, and what the characteristics of the preparation are that enable it to stay on under different forces that are encountered in the oral environment. We will therefore define the terms retention and resistance as they refer to restorations.

Retention is defined as obstruction to removal along the path of insertion of a restoration. A direct restoration, as previously discussed, is generally placed in a soft state which then hardens during its setting reaction. It may therefore engage undercut in the tooth preparation in relation to the path of insertion, which therefore provides an excellent retention form. An indirect restoration cannot engage undercut, as it is essentially rigid and made outside of the mouth, so must have a relative path of insertion. The restoration must therefore be retained some other way. It is retained either primarily mechanically, or adhesively.

Resistance is described as the ability of a restoration to withstand lateral or oblique displacement forces, as may be encountered during function or parafunction.

Mechanical Retention

Mechanical retention is primarily dependent on the geometric form of the tooth preparation to provide the retention and resistance to displacement of the restoration.

This is reliant on the preparation height, which would ideally be above 4 mm and to a lesser extent the preparation width (with a narrower preparation offering superior resistance form, all else being equal).

The taper, or the total occlusal convergence of the preparation, is also very important for retention and resistance of a restoration in both bucco-lingual and mesio-distal aspects. This describes an angle measuring the taper of one wall in relation to the opposite wall, and this should ideally be between 10 and 12°. A more parallel-sided preparation would provide superior retention and resistance form, but would not allow adequate extrusion of the lute during the cementation stage, which could result in incomplete seating of the restoration.

The strength of the cement used to retain the restoration is not so important, and the ability of the cement to bond to the tooth or the restoration is also unimportant; therefore conventional (non-resin) cements are primarily used. These include zinc phosphate, RMGICs, GICs and zinc polycarboxylates.

Adhesive Retention

Adhesive retention on the other hand is primarily dependent on the strength of the cement, and the ability of the cement to bond to the tooth and the restoration. This relies on a resin-bonded cement, and the cement provides the retention and resistance to displacement. The geometric form of the preparation is not of primary concern. Given the functional bond between the tooth and the restoration, the restorative material and the tooth work synergistically to improve the strength and rigidity of the restored tooth unit.

Generally, an adhesively retained restoration is more conservative of tooth structure, so, when deciding on the most appropriate preparation design for a compromised tooth, the first decision to make is if an adhesively retained restoration is appropriate. This will depend primarily on the presence of enamel around the periphery of the preparation. Where enamel exists all the way around the preparation, the tooth is generally a good candidate for an adhesively retained restoration. This is because the bond to enamel is strong and predictable in the long term. Whilst the bond to dentine can initially be good, it varies based on the location and quality of the dentine, is technique sensitive and critically will decay rapidly over time and should therefore not be wholly relied upon to retain a restoration. Other tooth specific factors are also thought to be important, such as the height of the preparation, with shorter preparations requiring taller restorations being less favourable, while general patient-related factors may also be of importance, such as aesthetic concerns.

Isolation of the preparation to perform a meticulous adhesive cementation is critical for adhesively retained restorations and this process is highly technique sensitive. The position of the preparation margin in relation to the gingival margin is therefore also critical when considering an adhesively retained restoration. It is advised that dental dam is used for any adhesive procedures. Heavy dental dam will retract the soft tissues to aid cementation, and floss ligatures can aid this process. The adhesive process must involve phosphoric acid etching of the enamel, and a chemically cured, or dual-cured, resin cement is advised to ensure polymerisation when using metallic restorations or where restoration thickness exceeds 2.5 mm. Where tooth coloured restoration thickness is less than 2.5 mm, a light-cured resin can be used.

Where dentine margins are present, as is often the case where deep interproximal carious lesions have been managed, it may often be deemed more appropriate to prescribe a mechanically retained restoration which can be retained using a conventional cement.

Whilst conventional cements aren't as strong as resin cements, and cannot bond as well (if at all), they do have some advantages. They can tolerate moisture and are therefore not particularly technique sensitive, so can be used with less concern when cementing restorations with deep subgingival margins. Clearing excess extruded cement is also much easier, and they are much cheaper than resin cements. The cementation phase is therefore much easier than when using resin cements.

WHY INDIRECT RESTORATIONS?

When we perform an indirect restoration, we are commonly removing more tooth structure. This seems to defy our oft quoted principle of minimal intervention dentistry. It is therefore necessary to consider which parts of the tooth are critical to retain, and which parts, if retained, may compromise the lifespan of the tooth. This requires a consideration of the clinical evidence, and the biomechanical behaviour of the structurally compromised and restored tooth.

Clinical Evidence

Indirect Restorations and Root Filled Teeth

Posterior root filled teeth (premolars and molars) have a better survival when cuspal coverage is provided compared to when it is not; however providing coronal coverage for root filled anterior teeth showed no advantages over intra-coronal restoration where possible.

Why Are Root Filled Teeth Extracted?

Data suggests that around 10% of root filled teeth are extracted for endodontic reasons, 20% for periodontal reasons and 70% due to the root filled tooth being unrestorable through caries and fracture. Stabilising disease processes, as previously discussed, and maximising retention of tooth structure in critical areas to reduce fracture risk would therefore seem to be a sensible approach to prolonging the lifespan of compromised teeth. This will be explored in the following section.

3.7 Biomechanical Considerations

As previously stated, enamel provides a rigid outer layer to a tooth. The underlying dentine is much more flexible but tough, providing resilient support for the enamel. Tooth rigidity is affected as tooth structure is lost, for example through caries. Root filling a posterior tooth with minimal access only has a small effect, whereas as a cavity extends, especially to involve loss of connected marginal ridges, this leads to a marked decrease in the rigidity of the remaining tooth. This loss of rigidity is important, because the remaining thin cusps are subjected to tensional stress under loading, which causes them to flex apart. This in turn can result in cracking or fracture of the cusps, or cyclical fatigue, marginal leakage around a restoration and potentially secondary caries.

Restoring teeth with amalgam has no effect on the rigidity of the restored tooth unit, whereas using adhesively retained composite or bonded amalgam will restore some of the lost rigidity. It has been shown however that under cyclical loading (to mimic functional loading in the mouth) this restored rigidity will be lost reasonably quickly.

By reducing thin cusps and overlaying them, the flexure is hugely reduced, converting tensional loading of the remaining tooth structure to compressive loading at the restoration interface, which stabilises the cusps and is therefore much more favourable for the long-term retention of the tooth.

It is therefore not at all critical to retain thin occlusal portions of tooth, especially where marginal ridges are lost, and their retention could be considered to be actively compromising the structural integrity of a restored tooth unit.

In complete contrast to this situation, it has been shown that maintenance of tooth structure in the cervical region of a tooth is critical to the prognosis of a tooth. This critical tissue, which is commonly referred to as the peri-cervical dentine or quantified as the residual dentine thickness, should be maintained through minimal preparation wherever possible. This should be borne in mind when performing restorative preparations to the external aspect of a tooth, but also when performing endodontic preparations to the internal aspect.

STABILISATION AND MANAGING RISK

Prior to providing a definitive indirect restoration, it is prudent to stabilise any disease processes at the tooth level, and in the mouth as a whole. Treatment planning should be holistic, considering the individual tooth, but also the individual patient, obtaining consent for any treatment prescribed. Expectations should be assessed and managed from the outset and the dentist should realistically appraise their own competence for the prescribed procedures and refer to a more appropriate clinician if appropriate. Patient-centred factors are important in the decision to attempt to retain a tooth, as are considerations of the importance of the tooth in the mouth as a whole.

The restorability of compromised teeth should be assessed, considering whether the remaining tooth structure will be able to retain a core, and then whether that tooth and core can predictably support a definitive restoration. This is usually best ascertained by removing any existing restorations and caries in the tooth. There are no hard and fast rules as to what constitutes a restorable tooth, and it must consider the amount and location of tooth structure remaining (with the peri-cervical location being critical), marginal substrate, presence of cracks in dentine and the subgingival extension of the cavity. It is quite commonly possible to restore a very compromised tooth, but the long-term prognosis of the restored tooth is quite another consideration entirely. We should be looking to predictably restore teeth wherever possible in a financially logical way (i.e. would the money spent restoring the tooth be more effectively invested in another treatment, for example, a dental implant).

The caries status, periodontal status and endodontic status should be stabilised prior to considering expensive definitive indirect restorations. A diagnostic radiograph of the tooth under consideration, including the periapical tissues, should be obtained prior to prescribing an indirect restoration and all teeth without a root filling should be vitality tested, recognising the limitations of these techniques. It is important to assess other factors, such as tooth surface loss and any occlusal factors that may be of importance (see previous and later sections). Though the dentist has a responsibility to provide appropriate management with care and skill, the patient must understand and take responsibility for their role in maintenance of their dentition. Failure to adequately manage these factors may lead to problems which can be difficult, stressful and costly to resolve.

INDIRECT RESTORATIONS AND LOSS OF PULP VITALITY

Teeth prepared for crowns can lose vitality in the short and longer term. This is thought to primarily relate to overheating of the pulp during preparation, and the exposing and opening up of dentinal tubules, through which restorative chemicals and bacteria can access the pulp. Estimates vary as to the incidence of this complication. For example, heavily restored teeth tend to lose vitality more than lightly or unrestored teeth, and the incidence appears to be higher in teeth diagnosed with cracked tooth syndrome. Teeth involved in conventional bridgework (see later) also have a higher incidence of loss of vitality than those prepared for single crowns. The incidence of loss of vitality for bonded ceramic onlay restorations has been estimated to be around 3%, which is another reason to favour these more minimally invasive restorations where possible. It should be remembered however that more heavily broken down teeth with dentine margins often are not indicated for these more minimally invasive restorations, so the true difference between preparations for these different restorations may not be quite as marked in equally compromised teeth.

It is important to have a balanced discussion of the advantages and disadvantages of treatment versus no treatment (or alternatives) with the patient to obtain consent, and this discussion should be documented for medicolegal reasons.

PLANNING AESTHETIC CHANGES

Any aesthetic changes prescribed would ideally be based on a facially generated treatment plan, i.e. making changes based around how the teeth appear in the patient's face, whilst considering any functional occlusal issues (see previous and later). Clinical photographs are a useful adjunct to any form of aesthetic treatment, protecting the dentist from potential medicolegal problems and reminding the patient of their preoperative situation. They are also useful for the dentist and technician team in planning and shade matching the case.

This planning can be converted into a diagnostic 'wax up' performed in a classic analogue way by modification of a stone model of the patient's existing dentition with wax, or with more modern digital methods using optical impressions and appropriate software. This allows the proposed changes to be transferred to the patient's mouth in a reversible way (known as a mock-up, using unbonded composite or conventional or milled provisional crown material), allowing the impact on the patient's teeth, smile (and speech) to be assessed by both patient and dentist, and any modifications required made prior to preparation. The accepted mock-up is also important to define the final prosthodontic plan, so that any tooth preparation requirements can be related to the final restoration and this can be determined prior to picking up a handpiece. This will allow an assessment of the invasiveness of preparation required to achieve the desired aesthetics, and may mean that, for example, veneers are not appropriate. It also means that tooth preparation may not be required at all in some instances where, again, for example, veneers are moving the teeth facially. Communicating an understanding of these requirements and their potential sequelae to the patient is important in obtaining robust consent for the procedure. The same process is also beneficial when using direct composite additions, for example, as is often utilised in managing tooth surface loss, or making changes to the shape of teeth.

OCCLUSAL CONSIDERATIONS

Where a restoration is being provided in a conformative approach (i.e. where the patient's existing ICP, which is also known as the static occlusion, is stable and can be used as the reference treatment position), the use of a face-bow registration is often not required. This is the situation most commonly faced, especially when carrying out single indirect restorations, but also direct restorations. However where this restoration is likely to impact on the dynamic occlusion, i.e. in functional pathways or excursive movements, the use of a face-bow registration and a semi-adjustable articulator is beneficial. The face-bow registration relates the position of the condyles to the maxillary teeth, allowing this information to be approximately replicated on a semi-adjustable articulator, which allows a technician to more accurately build the guidance surfaces of a restoration. When the treatment is being performed conformatively, the mandibular cast is mounted against the maxillary cast in ICP. This can be performed digitally by scanning a portion of the teeth in ICP, or conventionally in an analogue way. When performed in an analogue way, if the casts can be hand articulated, no interocclusal record is required. If they cannot be hand articulated, an appropriate interocclusal record should be taken in ICP.

Similarly, where a change in occlusal vertical dimension is deemed appropriate or being considered (a reorganisational approach), a face-bow mounting on a semi-adjustable articulator is also advised. When taking a reorganisational approach, the teeth can no longer be used as a reference position, and another position must be used. The most commonly used reference in these situations is centric relation (CR) which is a jaw joint position, and it is used because it is reproducible. There are many different techniques used to find this position, including bimanual manipulation, leaf gauges, Lucia jigs and Kois Deprogrammers. An interocclusal record of CR should be taken with the teeth apart. This record relates the mandibular cast to the maxillary cast in CR on the articulator (or virtual digital articulator). This will allow assessment of the most appropriate approach to rehabilitation, which often involves the use of a functional diagnostic wax-up (analogue or digital) as part of the planning procedure. When making functional changes with crown and bridgework, this would ideally be trialled in a more prolonged provisionalisation phase, allowing adjustments to be made to the provisionals which can then be transferred to the design of the definitive restorations. This is much harder to achieve when using indirect adhesively retained restorations. Reorganisational approaches to managing the worn dentition are often planned in a similar way, but are increasingly being performed adhesively, with milled or printed indirect composite (or newer so called resin-ceramics which can be produced very economically), or direct composite restorations, using matrices to accurately transfer the functional wax-up to the mouth. In comparison to ceramic, composite and resin-ceramics are kinder to opposing teeth, easier to repair and more resilient, which may well be advantageous, reducing chipping and fracture in attritively worn dentitions. They are also easier to adjust and may be used as a long-term interim solution to assess aesthetic changes and the stability of functional changes before moving to ceramic restorations if required.

TOOTH PREPARATION

A summary of preparation details for various materials and designs is given in Table 3.3, and common preparations are shown (Figs 3.5–3.9).

Over-preparation can endanger the pulp and weaken a tooth, whereas under-preparation can lead to a thin, weak restoration, which is prone to fracture, or an overbulked restoration which is commonly unaesthetic. This extra bulk can also predispose to biofilm accumulation, putting the patient at risk of caries and periodontal disease, and occlusal issues through introduction of interferences, commonly to the dynamic occlusion.

All internal preparation line angles should be rounded when preparing teeth for all ceramic restorations (veneers, onlays and crowns), as sharp preparation angles lead to sharp internal angles in the fitting surface of ceramic restorations, which can be sites of crack initiation and propagation. This can potentially result in fracture of the restoration. For restorations with metallic fitting surfaces, this is less of an issue, but while it is recognised that sharper preparation transitions will confer benefit to retention and resistance form of mechanically retained restorations, sharp preparation line angles will act as stress concentrators in the tooth, again tending to promote crack initiation and propagation, potentially compromising the lifespan of a tooth.

Measuring Reduction

Teeth should be prepared with respect to the proposed final restoration. Different restorations require different preparations (Table 3.3); therefore we must control the amount of reduction we perform, for the reasons previously discussed. Options to precisely prepare teeth include the following options, and they can be used alone, or in combination.

Depth cuts, respecting the changing planes of a tooth surface. Using depth cuts is dependent on the tooth to be prepared being of ideal form (which is not always the case), but this is not always the case. Depth cuts should ideally be placed with parallel-sided burs or round burs of known dimension. Depth cutting wheel burs are also available.

Reduction guides – for example, a simple putty impression of the tooth to be prepared that is then sectioned bucco-lingually, which can help to visualise the reduction performed. Guides are used in combination with depth cuts. If the tooth is not of ideal form, a digital or analogue wax-up can be performed, and a putty reduction guide made

Table 3.3   Shows Required Tooth/Core Reductions to Accommodate the Chosen Indirect Restoration.

Material/Restoration	Occlusal Reduction (mm)	Margin
Metal crown/onlay	1–1.5	0–0.5 mm knife edge/light chamfer
Porcelain fused to metal crown	2 mm ceramic	1–1.2 mm heavy chamfer(ceramic-buccal) Metal collar same as metal
High strength etchable ceramic (lithium disilicate) crown	1.5–2	0.7–1.2 mm chamfer (monolithic vs layered)
High strength etchable ceramic (lithium disilicate) onlay	1.5–2	Butt joint/0.7 mm flared buccal chamfer
Etchable ceramic (lithium disilicate) veneer	1.5	0–0.4 mm light chamfer
High strength non-etchable ceramic (zirconia)	1–2	0–1 mm knife edge/chamfer (monolithic vs layered)

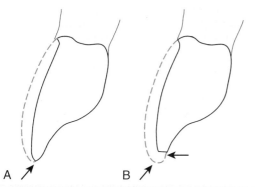

Fig. 3.5 Veneer preparation. Light chamfer. (A) Labial face only and (B) butt joint incorporating incisal edge.

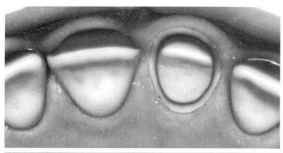

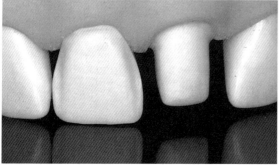

Fig. 3.6 Chamfer preparation, lithium disilicate crown. Occlusal and facial views with adjacent veneer preparation.

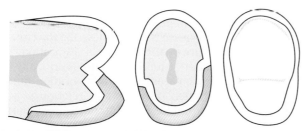

Fig. 3.7 Light chamfer palatal, heavy chamfer buccal. Porcelain fused to metal crown.

from this, or reduction guides can be milled or printed from digital wax-ups.

Provisional crown and bridge material can be placed on a tooth or teeth using a matrix made from a wax-up of an ideal form and then depth cuts can be prepared through this.

Opposing occlusion – this relies on assessing interocclusal clearance in ICP. Flexible bite tabs of known thickness can be used to gauge reduction, as can greenstick or beading wax, which can then be measured using callipers.

Adjacent teeth help to assess the bucco-palatal reduction through assessing the curvature of the arch.

CROWN PREPARATIONS

Crown preparations can be broken down into three aspects: the occlusal reduction, the axial reduction and the marginal configuration (see Figs 3.6–3.8).

Occlusal Reduction

This is the critical part of any indirect restoration as it is the component which resists fracture of the underlying tooth. A slightly increased preparation is recommended for the functional cusp and a functional cusp bevel is also generally advised to accommodate an increased thickness of restorative material, as this cusp will take more functional load. The functional cusps are commonly the buccal cusps of mandibular teeth and the palatal cusps of maxillary teeth except when the teeth are in cross-bite.

Axial Reduction

This is performed to remove hard tissue undercuts which facilitates a path of insertion for the indirect restoration, and to provide retention and resistance form, using the principles already discussed. It is not generally beneficial to the lifespan of the tooth.

Marginal Configuration

This is linked to the axial reduction and generally provides a finishing line which prescribes the position of the restoration margin to the laboratory. The depth and shape advised varies depending on the restorative material prescribed. Common designs include a shoulder, a heavy chamfer, a light chamfer and a knife edge preparation. So called 'vertical' preparations are perhaps a variant of a knife edge, but there doesn't seem to be a currently accepted definition for this preparation, with various factions disagreeing over subtle points of the preparation. Shoulder preparations were often advised for all ceramic and PFM crown margins where porcelain is included; however this design is

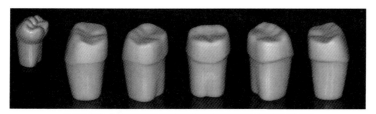

Fig. 3.8 Knife edge preparation. Metal/zirconia crown.

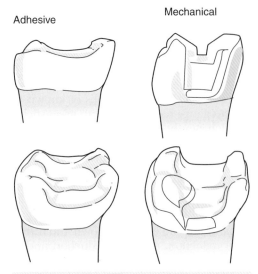

Adhesive   Mechanical

Fig. 3.9 Adhesive vs mechanical onlay preparations.

becoming less favoured as we understand that sharp internal line angles can result in sites of crack propagation in the tooth. Deep chamfers have taken their place; though again, as materials develop, we move to ever more conservative marginal designs which include light chamfers, and knife edge or 'vertical' tooth preparations which preserve the critical peri-cervical dentine. Monolithic zirconia restorations are increasingly being provided for teeth prepared with vertical, or knife edge margins, allowing a tooth coloured restoration to be placed as an alternative to the classic metal crown preparation with a similar, minimally invasive preparation. Such marginal preparation can pose issues in prescribing margin location, and providing cleansable margins; therefore communication with laboratories is critical to design an appropriate restoration. When the preparation is finished deep within the subgingival area it could potentially lead to issues of impingement on the biologic width (the supra-crestal periodontal attachment), with potential inflammatory sequelae. These impacts have yet to be fully elucidated however and periodontal responses may be counterintuitive.

Margin Location

This brings us nicely to a consideration of where we place our restoration margins. We will consider this positioning in relation to the gingival margin, in relation to adjacent teeth and in relation to existing restorations.

In Relation to Gingival Margins

Margin placement can be supragingival, equi-gingival or subgingival. In the anterior dentition, margins are often placed equi-gingivally or slightly subgingivally, just into the gingival sulcus in an attempt to hide the margin. It should be noted that placing a restoration margin subgingivally does not necessarily mean that it will remain hidden in the long term, especially where a patient has a thin biotype and reduced bone support, as recession can occur throughout life. With posterior teeth, or anterior teeth where the patient has a low smile line and will accept a supragingival margin, it is favourable to place margins

supragingivally where possible. There are a number of advantages to this positioning, which are technical and biological in nature. Technically the preparation is easier to perform as it can be more easily seen; the impression is easier to successfully record as the surrounding gingival tissues don't need to be managed. Provisionalisation is simpler in terms of making the restoration and allowing easier removal of excess cement, and the definitive cementation is easier, in terms of isolation and clearance of excess extruded cement. Biologically, the periodontium is more likely to tolerate supragingival margins better than subgingival margins, and the margins will be easier for the patient to clean. As we extend our preparation apically down a tooth, most teeth get narrower, and so the axial reduction has to increase to perform the appropriate marginal preparation. This is destructive in the most critical area of the tooth, the peri-cervical region, while also further endangering a vital pulp.

Sometimes however, where the clinical crown height is limited, as is commonly seen in lower second molars for example, it is prudent to extend the preparation subgingivally to gain sufficient preparation height to provide mechanical retention and resistance form. This is always a trade-off between predictable retention of the restoration and respecting the periodontium. Where the risk to the periodontium is deemed too great, or the margin is already subgingival and preparation height is still limited, retention can be improved through the use of parallel grooves and boxes, or use of resin cements. Self-adhesive resin cements, although not as strong as more conventional resin cements, may be advisable to reduce the potential for contamination. Retraction cord can be useful for isolation during cementation.

Surgical crown lengthening can also provide more preparation height where the clinical crown height is limited, and this often goes hand in hand with gaining supragingival tooth structure to engage with a ferrule (see below). It requires meticulous treatment planning and surgical expertise with careful management of both soft tissue and underlying bone.

It may also be prudent to extend a preparation subgingivally where there is limited sound supragingival tooth structure to engage. Ferrule is used to describe the engagement of tooth structure by the collar of a restoration. The amount of engagement of tooth structure is critically important in resisting displacement of a restoration during function. It is most often referred to in relation to very heavily broken down root filled teeth that require a post to retain a core. It is an important element to consider for all mechanically retained crowns however. Simply engaging the core alone, while potentially satisfying retention and resistance form requirements, puts all of the stress on the interface between the remaining tooth and the core, which will commonly lead to either debonding of the core and crown, or fracture of the root where a post is retaining the core. The minimum requirement for vertical ferrule, to predictably restore a tooth, is often stated as 1.5–2 mm, and while it is accepted that the horizontal dentine dimension is important (we return to the concept of critical peri-cervical dentine or residual dentine width), quantifying a minimum amount has proved elusive. Maintaining as much tooth structure as possible by avoiding destructive marginal preparations in this critical area seems prudent. Rapid orthodontic extrusion, or surgical extrusion, has also been used to gain supragingival tooth structure where it is limited.

In Relation to Adjacent Teeth

Margins for crown preparations should be extended beyond contact points. Adhesively retained restorations, or conventionally retained onlays, do not always require breaking of the contact area, but if this is the case, the margin should be left just coronal to the contact. If the margin is placed at the contact, this puts a margin at one of the most caries susceptible areas of the tooth and prevents the technician from adequately sectioning the working cast. If the margin finishes at the contact point, it should be extended to just clear it in posterior teeth, and in anterior teeth an interproximal strip should be used to separate the contacts sufficiently to allow the cast to be sectioned (see later).

In Relation to Restorations

In light of the previous discussion of ferrule, it is also prudent to place restoration margins on sound tooth structure circumferentially around the preparation. It should be noted that a preparation may go subgingivally in relation to a deep restorative margin, but it does not follow that the whole of the margin then needs to be subgingival. It should be appropriately positioned in different areas of the tooth based on the restorative status, retention form and aesthetic requirements.

ONLAY PREPARATIONS

Onlay preparations aim to provide the beneficial element of a crown preparation – the occlusal reduction, while avoiding the negative elements – axial reduction and marginal placement in the critical peri-cervical region where possible. This means that subsequent failure of the restoration is usually non-catastrophic, i.e. there is a chance to re-restore the tooth, whereas for conventional crown preparations, failure is more likely to be terminal for the tooth in question.

Preparations for onlays pose a unique set of considerations, as onlays can be designed to be adhesively retained, mechanically retained, or both (see Fig. 3.9). Adhesively retained restorations do not require conventional retention and resistance form, as this is provided by the resin-bonded cement. Metals, etchable ceramics and composites can all be adhesively cemented, but all require different surface preparations of the intaglio (fitting surface). These are summarised in Table 3.2.

The preparation should be smooth and flowing, with no sharp internal angles (see Fig. 3.9). The elimination of undercuts, to allow a path of insertion, can be created by tooth preparation, or more conservatively through 'immediate dentine sealing' (placement of a bonding agent over the exposed dentine) and the addition of bonded composite, a process known as 'cavity design optimisation'. These procedures also reduce sensitivity during the provisionalisation stage, and provide a better bond to dentine, than if dentine bonding is performed at the fit appointment. The major drawback is that it can cause the provisional restoration to stick to the preparation, making removal difficult, if precautions aren't taken. Curing the exposed bonding agent and composite under glycerine to reduce the oxygen-inhibited layer can help mitigate against this. Marginal designs advised are slightly gingivally bevelled butt joints in the occlusal aspects of the preparation, to create a so-called 'compression dome' effect, or more open chamfer margin designs buccally to aid an aesthetic blend and seating. Margins are commonly visible with these restorations.

Deep margin elevation is another approach often used with adhesively retained onlays and is performed to provide a preparation form of convenience, raising deep cavity margins just above the gingival margin to allow adhesive cementation of an indirect onlay restoration. It is performed with a matrix to seal the base of a deep cavity, and direct composite is then placed, often in deep box areas. The indirect restoration margin is then placed in the restorative material in this area. This can overcome the issue of isolating deep margins allowing a simple rubber dam placement to meticulously control the environment to bond an indirect restoration. It also makes the impression and the cement clean up easier. This is still currently an experimental technique, with little clinical evidence, despite the concept being initially described over 20 years ago. Anecdotally it has been shown to work excellently when performed meticulously, and when there is still an abundance of enamel available for bonding around the remainder of the periphery of the preparation. Detractors cite the increased number of restorative interfaces involved, all of which are potential failure points for the restoration. With more extensive dentine margins and more heavily broken down teeth, it is currently advised that this technique should be avoided, and a mechanically retained restoration is advised.

To avoid this issue of meticulously isolating deep margins, and the need to raise margins thus creating multiple interfaces, mechanically retained onlays can be used. They rely on gaining retention and resistance form from the internal aspect of a preparation. This involves preparing upright walls and boxes with minimal taper. Again, undercuts can be removed through preparation, or additively. If performed additively, the restorative material used should not be present at the exposed preparation margins. As the retention of the restoration is provided by the internal cavity geometry, an adhesive resin cement is not required, allowing the use of a conventional cement. This confers the benefits already discussed. Materials advised for this type of restoration are primarily metal alloys.

POSTERIOR INDICATIONS FOR INDIRECT RESTORATIONS

Full cuspal coverage (not necessarily a crown) restorations for posterior teeth are generally advised where root canal treatment has been successfully carried out. There are no hard and fast rules to managing compromised posterior teeth with vital pulps. Teeth with dentine cracks, those with thin cusps which are unsupported or minimally supported by dentine and those that have lost much tooth structure (including those with connected marginal ridges), would seem to be good candidates to reduce occlusally and overlay the cusps to reduce the risk of fracture. This can be performed with direct restorations, which offer the advantages of avoiding the need for provisionalisation impressions, further appointments and reducing the up-front cost to the patient. These restorations are often technically difficult to achieve however, with issues being adaptation of matrix bands in deep subgingival cavities, obtaining contact points and optimising occlusal contacts. Indirect materials tend to fare better over time in the oral environment and tend to be stronger and stiffer than direct materials. Indirect restorations are therefore often favoured in these situations.

COMPROMISED ANTERIOR TEETH

Teeth with extensive restorations that have their integrity compromised, including root filled teeth, should be managed with additive techniques where possible. Minimally invasive techniques are available to address aesthetic concerns and commonly can be combined to produce a satisfactory result for the patient. These include vital or non-vital bleaching, remineralisation, resin infiltration, microabrasion and localised composite restorations. These should be considered prior to prescribing indirect restorations. It is often worthwhile exhausting more minimally invasive techniques in an attempt to address a patient's concerns, with a thorough explanation of why this is being done. More invasive techniques can be considered when these concerns haven't or can't be met, but it is prudent to reassess if the patient's expectations are realistic and can predictably be met, whilst also assessing if you are the clinician to meet them.

VENEERS

The porcelain veneer has become a popular aesthetic restoration used primarily to modify the appearance of anterior teeth. This restoration is a thin shell of porcelain that is applied directly to a tooth and is commonly used for teeth that require changes to their colour, shape, spacing or orientation. Orthodontics should be discussed as an alternative approach to correcting issues of spacing and orientation, with a discussion of potential disadvantages and the need for long-term maintenance and upkeep of both approaches. Composite can also be used to make changes to the shape and orientation of teeth and can be placed in combination with minimally invasive approaches described previously, but in comparison to porcelain, it is biomechanically inferior, requires more maintenance over time and can be more technically demanding of the clinician to effectively place. It is often a cheaper alternative however and is commonly performed with no, or more minimal, tooth preparation. Removing failed composite veneers or additions without damaging the underlying tooth can be difficult and time consuming; however special burs are available to aid this process.

Despite often being minimally invasive, the patient must be made aware of any irreversible loss of tooth structure involved in veneer provision. They must also be made aware that periodical replacement will inevitably be required, for example, as a result of fracture, debonding and marginal discolouration of the restoration(s), with an inevitable further loss of tooth structure.

Tooth preparation is commonly required to provide the best cosmetic and functional result with porcelain veneers. Veneer preparations should be kept within enamel where possible, as veneers are adhesively retained and therefore benefit from a more predictable, stable bond, aiding long-term success. Because veneers are adhesively retained, the material used for the veneer must be capable of achieving a strong and predictable resin bond; therefore an etchable ceramic, such as lithium disilicate, or feldspathic porcelain should be used. Reduction of tooth tissue will depend on the prosthetic plan as previously discussed. The thickness of porcelain required will also vary on the underlying shade of the tooth, with a darker tooth requiring an increased thickness to mask the discolouration. Given that enamel thickness at the gingival margin is reduced in comparison to the remainder of the crown of the tooth (when unaffected by tooth surface loss), reduction should be kept to 0.3 mm in this area in an attempt to stay within enamel. This may well be insufficient to mask discolouration however, so planning on a case-by-case basis remains important. No preparation porcelain veneers are possible in certain select situations, but are more suitable for experienced operators, as the resulting restorations can appear bulky and unaesthetic without appropriate planning and care.

Veneer preparations may involve the incisal edge or they may not (see Fig. 3.5). It is quite rare to prepare a veneer that does not involve the incisal edge, but such designs are possible and can be prepared with a window, or feather-edged design. A veneer restoration does not commonly involve changing a patient's static occlusion. It can however impact on the dynamic occlusion when it involves the incisal edge. Preparations for veneers often involve the incisal edge where the length of a tooth is to be altered, and designs described include a butt joint and an incisal wrap.

When considering the design of veneer preparations involving the incisal edge, it is prudent to consider the basic biomechanical behaviour of anterior teeth, specifically the maxillary anterior teeth as these are the teeth most commonly veneered. When teeth with a positive overjet are dynamically loaded, the palatal surface is placed under primarily tensional stress and the buccal surface under compressive stress. Tooth coloured dental materials are generally weak in tension, and strong in compression. It is therefore better to avoid putting a thin section of brittle material into an area of high tensional stress. It is better to rely on the strength conferred by material bulk, and therefore a butt joint (see Fig. 3.5) is biomechanically favourable over an incisal wrap design. Wrapping over the incisal edge is also more destructive of tooth tissue and often leaves a very thin tooth preparation, whereby it is hard to avoid sharp internal line angles within the fitting surface of the veneer. As previously discussed, this results in stress concentration in the internal aspect of the ceramic veneer, which is then prone to crack initiation, propagation and fracture of the restoration. It also limits the path of insertion, meaning it has to be placed down the long access of the tooth, which commonly requires more tooth preparation to avoid relative undercut, in comparison to a butt joint incisal edge design, which permits a range of insertion paths, including from the facial. In the incisal wrap design we see a reluctance to trust modern adhesive technologies, and an obsession with mechanical retention.

Interproximally, care should be taken to hide the margin, commonly by extending the preparation sufficiently into the embrasure spaces, particularly cervically and especially in situations where the natural tooth has darkened.

INDIRECT RESTORATION IMPRESSION TECHNIQUES

Nearly all conventional indirect restoration impression materials are now based on rubber polymers, which means they tend to be somewhat hydrophobic. As a result, it is vital that careful moisture control is achieved prior to impression taking. Optical impression techniques also currently require the teeth to be clean and dry to produce an accurate digital representation.

Indirect restoration preparations often result in margins that are at the gingival crest or just within the gingival sulcus. The gingival tissues should therefore be healthy before recording an impression. The presence of gingivitis and traumatised gingivae increase gingival crevicular fluid flow and the risk of gingival haemorrhage during impression taking, leading to a loss of accuracy of both conventional and optical impressions.

If the preparation margins are all supragingival, there is no need to manipulate the gingival tissues prior to impression taking. If the margins are equi- or subgingival however, the tissues will require management. There are a number of ways to manipulate the gingival tissues to optimise the chance of achieving a workable impression, the most common being the use of gingival retraction cord (GRC). Alternatives described include expansion pastes or use of electrosurgery, lasers or rotary curettage to trough around a preparation. Polytetrafluoroethylene tape twisted into a cord can also be useful when used in a similar manner to GRC. It has the benefit of being easily picked up by optical impression techniques. It should therefore be placed to allow complete visualisation of the preparation margin and left in situ when recording the optical impression. GRCs tend to be either braided or woven cotton, often impregnated with an astringent material. Astringent materials include aluminium sulphate, ferric sulphate and aluminium chloride and help to stop bleeding of the gingival tissues. Single GRC and double GRC techniques have been described, with the authors favouring a double cord technique (Fig. 3.10). This involves the placement of the finest diameter cord available subgingivally where the preparation is subgingival, in an attempt to prevent gingival crevicular fluid contamination of the preparation surface when taking the impression. The entirety of this cord should be tucked into the gingival margin and it is left in place when taking the impression. The cord should be placed carefully with slight pressure towards the last placed part to reduce the tendency for it to pull out of the sulcus again. A second, wider diameter cord is then placed, lying partially in and partially out of the gingival sulcus with the intention of deflecting the free gingival margin laterally. This cord is left to expand the tissues for around 5 minutes and removed immediately prior to impression taking. The aim is to capture an impression of the preparation beyond the preparation margin with a good thickness of impression material.

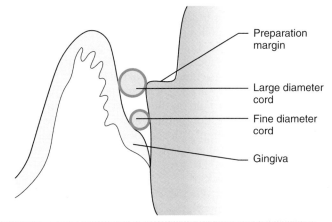

Fig. 3.10 Double retraction cord technique, superficial cord to be removed prior to impression taking.

This makes accurate trimming of the master cast easier for the laboratory technician, reducing the chance of errors in the fabrication of the restoration at the margin. In the single GRC technique, the first fine cord, as described in the double cord technique, is omitted, with just the larger cord placed, which is then removed immediately prior to taking the impression.

Impressions can be taken optically or with an elastomeric material to provide an accurate digital, digitally printed or stone model of the prepared tooth and surrounding tissues for the technician to produce a functionally and cosmetically satisfactory restoration. Occlusal detail of the arch should be adequately recorded and potential contact points with adjacent teeth must be accurately represented.

Conventional materials most commonly used for indirect restoration impressions are:

- polyvinyl siloxane materials (addition cured silicones)
- polyether materials.

These materials are very accurate and dimensionally stable; however polyethers can imbibe water, so shouldn't be stored in water or left in a disinfectant solution for too long, as this can affect their accuracy. Polyethers are also very rigid when set, which means they can be difficult to remove from the mouth or the poured cast. The cast may then fracture. The rigidity is seen as an advantage by some for implant related impressions; however addition silicones are generally seen as the gold standard conventional indirect impression material.

Most materials are supplied in a range of viscosities and setting times and are commonly used in techniques where different viscosities are combined in one impression. Putty and light body wash or medium/heavy and light body wash combination impression techniques are commonly used. Putty materials are quite rigid and can distort flexible plastic impression trays on seating. This can lead to rebound and distortion of the impression when the impression is removed. Putties are therefore better used in a two-stage technique with a spacer. The more rigid, heavier bodied materials support the lighter bodied material, being slightly more dimensionally stable whilst also reducing the problem of material running down a patient's throat, which can be uncomfortable and distressing. Light bodied materials are less viscous and have the ability to flow around a preparation resulting in an accurate, high surface detail representation of the preparation. They are applied using a syringe with a fine tip, to allow injection of the material into the gingival sulcus and around the preparation attempting to avoid inclusion of air pockets. This is best achieved by placing the tip of the applicator against the preparation whilst expressing the material. Any air pockets or fluid on the preparation can result in errors on the impression surface and consequently produce blebs and other irregularities on the cast which can affect the accuracy of the final restoration.

Rigid trays should be used where possible to avoid distortion. Metal rim lock trays are available but are difficult to clean and sterilise. When stock trays are not ideal, custom-made light-cured acrylic special trays should be considered.

Optical impressions offer the advantage of being more patient friendly, but the sensor units can be difficult to manipulate posteriorly and obviously involve a large initial financial outlay. In the longer term, they have the potential to be highly cost-effective.

An accurate impression of the opposing arch should be recorded optically, or conventionally in alginate or elastomeric material, taking care to capture the occlusal surfaces. Direct application of the material onto the occlusal surface of the teeth with a finger can help to avoid air blows, which will then make articulation of the casts accurate (see previous section for consideration of interocclusal records).

PROVISIONALISATION

This can be performed freehand, especially where the preparation has an intracoronal element, such as those for onlays. It can be performed with the use of matrices, formed from an impression of the pre-operative tooth form, or from an intraorally modified tooth (for example with added composite, where the existing tooth is under-contoured in relation to the ideal shape), or from an analogue or digital wax-up of the ideal shape. Provisional restorations can also be made with the use of preformed shells, which can be stock shapes or laboratory manufactured which can then be relined with a suitable material. Commonly now provisional restorations can be rapidly milled or printed following optical impressions with on-site CAD–CAM technology and full digital workflows. They can be made from a variety of materials, such as composite, bis-acryl, polymethylmethacrylate and metals. All have the same aims however, which are to prevent fracture of the tooth, protect any operatively exposed dentine and to stabilise the position of the prepared tooth in relation to both the adjacent teeth and opposing teeth by maintaining pre-existing contacts. Provisional restorations can also have an important role in assessing any proposed functional and aesthetic changes as previously discussed. It is important that it has a good marginal fit, especially when close to the gingival margin, to prevent inflammation of the gingivae. This is important for impression taking, particularly if performed at a subsequent appointment, and at the cementation appointment to minimise bleeding.

Veneers and adhesively retained restorations can be more difficult to provisionalise because of the lack of retention form, though spot etching of enamel can be employed, and undercut between teeth engaged when provisionalisation is for short periods only.

With optical impressions and on site CAD–CAM technology, full digital workflows are now commonplace and it is possible to omit the provisionalisation phase in less complex situations.

CEMENTATION

The cementation process has been previously discussed; however many potential errors can occur between recording an impression of a preparation, and receiving the final restoration from the laboratory. A common issue is a failure of the restoration to seat, which can result from preparation errors such as peripherally lipped margins and impression errors such as blows and drags, both of which can lead to errors on the cast. The operator must therefore critically appraise the preparation and impression and make any necessary adjustments to eliminate these issues. Commonly however, a failure of the restoration to seat is caused by tight interproximal contacts. With analogue manufacture, the cast is typically pinned (to allow relocation of the prepared tooth die between the adjacent teeth) and sectioned through the space between the prepared tooth and the adjacent teeth, so the technician can directly access all aspects of the preparation when making the restoration. This means that there is often a little wiggle room in the cast, and it can result in worn contact points of the adjacent teeth on the master cast, as the restoration is taken on and off the cast during manufacture. This means that often the restoration is made to fit these worn contacts and will therefore be prevented from seating in the mouth. This can be overcome by pouring up a second model of the impression which is not sectioned, and this model is then used for finalisation of the restoration contact points, marking tight areas with fine articulating paper to allow appropriate adjustment. There should be a light smooth contact area that will allow passing of floss with some resistance. In digital manufacture, contact tightness can still be a problem, and it is therefore important to appropriately calibrate the contact tightness in the computer-aided design process.

When cementing a definitive restoration at the patient's existing ICP, the occlusion of adjacent opposing teeth should be checked with shimstock foil without the restoration or provisional restoration in place, noting at least one holding contact between opposing pairs of teeth in the existing dentition. This holding contact should be present after the definitive indirect restoration is cemented. The indirect restoration should be tried in and assessed in both the static and dynamic occlusion checked with thin articulating paper, and with feedback from the patient prior to definitive cementation. Any interferences to finding the existing ICP should be removed and contacts in the dynamic occlusion altered as required. Any adjustments to the occlusal surface of the restoration should be appropriately polished to minimise wear of the opposing teeth.

LABORATORY PRESCRIPTION

Laboratory prescriptions must include sufficient details for the dental technician to produce the required restoration. While this seems obvious, many problems can be prevented by good communication with the laboratory.

SURVIVAL OF INDIRECT RESTORATIONS

The evidence, as ever, is far from conclusive, and materials used when trials start have often been superseded by the time a trial has any meaningful data on longevity. It has become clear that the operator is a critical factor in the survival of restorations, as is the setting in which the restoration is provided. Indirect restorations placed in general practice under publicly funded systems of provision have been shown to have a much reduced survival compared to survival data reported in clinical trials, which are often carried out in secondary, tertiary or specialist environments, with patients at high risk of failure excluded. Survival will depend on multiple other clinical and patient dependent factors, and these should be borne in mind when giving a patient an estimate of survival. Current evidence and opinion suggest it may be reasonable to give an estimate for the average lifespan of an indirect restoration of 5–8 years. It is always appropriate to inform a patient of any caveats, and that the value stated is an average, which means some will survive for a shorter period of time, and others will survive longer. Under promise and over deliver is a sensible approach to take.

For more detail on indirect tooth preparation and procedures, the reader is referred to more comprehensive texts.

3.8 Bridges

LEARNING OBJECTIVES

You should:
- outline the clinical assessment required when considering fixed bridgework to replace missing teeth
- consider different bridge design configurations to optimise retention, occlusal stability and aesthetic outcome.

Where natural teeth are missing, the options for replacing them include removable partial dentures, fixed bridges and dental implants. Not replacing a lost tooth is also an option that should be discussed, as this may be a healthier option for the remaining dentition.

A fixed bridge is a false tooth (the pontic) that is physically attached to an adjacent tooth or teeth (the abutment tooth or teeth) by means of a connector or connectors (the retainer[s]). Fixed bridges can be rigidly attached to teeth on one side of the edentulous saddle (a cantilever design) (Fig. 3.11), or both sides (a fixed–fixed design) (Fig. 3.12).

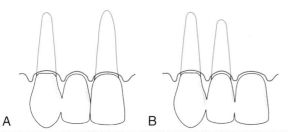

Fig. 3.11 Cantilever design for bridgework. (A) A single abutment (canine) cantilever replacing the lateral incisor (pontic). (B) A double abutment (canine and lateral incisor) cantilever replacing the central incisor (pontic).

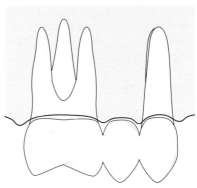

Fig. 3.12 Fixed–fixed bridge design replacing the second premolar (pontic) using the first premolar and first molar as the abutments.

Fixed bridges can be either conventional bridges, based on mechanical retention principles, most often utilising conventional crown style preparations to the abutment tooth or teeth with at least one full coverage retainer, or alternatively, resin-bonded bridges, based on adhesive retention principles which have at least one thin retainer (also known as a wing), that is bonded to an abutment tooth by the use of a resin cement.

CLINICAL ASSESSMENT

For any bridge design, appropriate planning is required as previously discussed for indirect restorations, but also involves additional considerations. These include the position, periodontal and restorative status of the abutment teeth, the length and location of the edentulous span, the nature of the occlusion and functional requirements, and how the bridge will be retained. Any parafunctional activity, and other patient-related risk factors, may also influence design and whether a bridge is appropriate.

Periodontal Health

A stable periodontium is essential prior to provision of bridges. Teeth that have previously experienced periodontal bone loss may be used as bridge abutments provided the disease has been treated and stabilised. There should be sufficient remaining bone support for abutment teeth to contribute satisfactorily to support of the bridge without detriment to themselves or to the function and longevity of the restoration. The suitability of individual teeth will depend on a number of variables, for example, crown to root ratio, furcation involvement, tooth location, as well as patient-related factors. Assessment is therefore required on an individual basis.

Tooth Positions in Relation to the Edentulous Span

Teeth that are opposing and adjacent to the edentulous span are important to assess in relation to their position and angulation. Overeruption of an opposing tooth into an edentulous saddle may mitigate against bridgework for that saddle, unless treatment to address the overeruption is carried out. Similarly, tipped and tilted teeth adjacent to a saddle area will prevent construction of a conventional fixed–fixed bridge, if their long axes are not aligned, as preparation to allow a mutual path of insertion with no relative undercut will be overly destructive of tooth tissue. Orthodontic alignment can be used to overcome this problem, or utilisation of bridges with fixed-moveable joints (Fig. 3.13). Resin-bonded bridges could also be considered.

PREVIOUS RESTORATION

The extent to which an individual tooth has previously been restored will likewise govern its suitability as an abutment for bridgework. The restorative status of a root filled tooth, i.e. the loss of tooth structure, is deemed to be more important than the loss of vitality per se, when considering these teeth for use as bridge abutments. Where a post has been required to retain a core, such teeth should be viewed with much caution as potential bridge abutments.

Unrestored, or minimally restored, teeth should be considered as abutments for adhesively retained resin-bonded bridgework. As ever when assessing suitability for adhesively retained indirect restorations, presence of enamel to bond to is critical. This influences decisions on preparation design.

Fixed–Fixed or Cantilever Design?

Though a cantilever design utilises support from only one side of the saddle area, support may be derived from more than one tooth (see Fig. 3.11). Using two abutments on one side of the saddle is known as double abutting. Whilst this design seems sensible at first glance, it should be used with extreme caution, because, due to the nature of the forces, and differential tooth movements, there is a heightened risk of debond of the distal most retainer from the abutment without loss of retention of the bridge. This can often occur with the patient and dentist unaware that it has happened, which leads to loss of marginal integrity at the debonded site, potentially resulting in rapid carious destruction of the abutment.

A similar issue can arise with a fixed–fixed resin-bonded bridge design (with two wings), where one of the wings debonds, but the other does not and the bridge stays in place. This is one of the major reasons that such designs are not universally advocated; this is especially the case anteriorly due to the nature of the differential force vectors applied to teeth at different points on a curve during function. Their clinical success has also been shown to be lower than

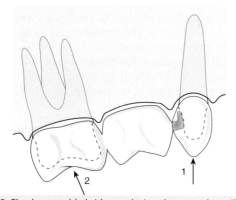

Fig. 3.13 Fixed–moveable bridge replacing the second maxillary premolar has a fixed retainer on the first molar with a moveable dovetail attachment to the distal of the retainer on the first premolar. Arrow 1 indicates path of insertion for the premolar retainer with groove - this is cemented first. Arrow 2 indicates path of insertion for molar retainer with pontic and movable attachment cemented second.

when using cantilever designs. So, if a two-space gap is to be filled with resin-bonded bridgework, it is considered more favourable to use separate cantilevers than a fixed–fixed design. Cantilevered pontics should be limited to a single tooth unit. It is sometimes advised post-orthodontics to use a fixed–fixed design of adhesive bridgework to replace missing teeth, as this also helps to retain the teeth in their new positions. However, given the issues just discussed, it is often better to use a cantilever design and an appropriate other form of orthodontic retention.

Conventional fixed–fixed bridge designs often have favourable survival outcomes and can spread the load over the abutment teeth. They do however come with significant biological costs as previously discussed. This means that the mode of failure is often unfavourable/catastrophic compared with resin-bonded bridgework, which generally have slightly reduced survival outcomes, but more favourable/recoverable modes of failure.

Resin-bonded bridges most commonly fail through debond of the bridge. When a conventional bridge fails, there is a much greater chance that an abutment tooth will be rendered unrestorable. The retrievability of any restoration placed, through consideration of its likely failure mode should therefore be considered.

Pontic Design

Pontic design is important in allowing the patient to maintain satisfactory oral hygiene to prevent recurrent caries or periodontal inflammation, while providing an aesthetic replacement for the missing tooth where appropriate. Designs include (Fig. 3.14):

- sanitary pontics
- bullet-nosed pontics
- ridge-lap pontics
- modified ridge-lap pontics
- ovate pontics.

Of these, a ridge-lap design is undesirable as it does not allow for cleaning between the pontic and the mucosa. Sanitary pontics are primarily historical but bullet-nosed pontics may be preferred posteriorly where aesthetics is less of a concern and cleansibility is more important. A modified ridge-lap design allows cleansibility with improved aesthetics by overlying part of the ridge to mimic emergence of the pontic from the gingival tissues in a similar way to the natural tooth. Ovate pontics are the most aesthetic option, as they do emerge from the soft tissue of the edentulous span. They often require site development however with soft, and sometimes hard tissue grafting and involve more complex techniques.

Material Choices

Resin-bonded bridge retainer wings are most commonly made of non-precious metal due to their high rigidity in thin section and the ability to easily and predictably bond to it. Optimising coverage of the abutment with the retainer is advised to aid retention. A minimum thickness of 0.7 mm of the wing has been advised to reduce flexure and therefore risk of debonding. A disadvantage of using a metal wing is that it can shine through the incisal region of abutment teeth, causing discolouration. Opaque resin cements can be selected to minimise this effect. Zirconia wings are

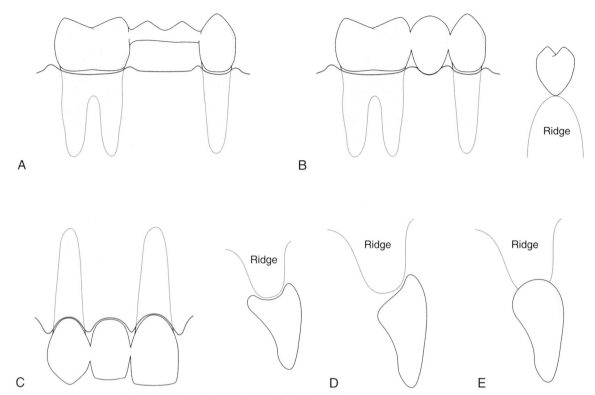

Fig. 3.14 Pontic designs. (A) Sanitary pontic. (B) Bullet-nose pontic. (C) Ridge-lap pontic. (D) Modified ridge-lap pontic. (E) Ovate pontic.

also being used, but, as previously alluded to, the achievable bond strength to zirconia is relatively low (relying solely on a chemical bond using 10 MDP), and therefore preparation for an element of mechanical retention is also often advised. Lithium disilicate wings have been used, but are comparatively weaker than the alternatives, and often require more destructive preparations to achieve a sufficient connector thickness between the retainer and the pontic to avoid fracture.

Conventional bridges are often of PFM design, but are increasingly now being made from zirconia, with or without veneering porcelain. Lithium disilicate bridges are also being used anteriorly where aesthetics are of prime concern, but do require thicker connectors as previously stated as they are relatively weaker than the other materials discussed.

Adhesive Bridgework: To Prepare or Not to Prepare?

Marginal Preparation of Teeth

Marginal finishing lines are often prepared to prescribe the apical extent of the wing to the laboratory. As with veneer preparations, this should be minimised, as the cervical enamel is thin, and remaining within enamel is advised where possible. This margin is increasingly not prepared, as metal wing positioning and thickness can be prescribed through communication with the laboratory and thinned down to a knife edge at the cervical margin thus minimising the impact on biofilm accumulation and access for cleaning. Preparation of a groove just palatal to the contact point adjacent to the pontic site can aid seating and help to hide the transition between the wing and the pontic. It also improves the accessible bonding area between

the wing and the tooth where a tooth has a high bulbous contact point. In posterior teeth, mesial and distal rest seats, or coverage of palatal and lingual cusps may be provided. The path of insertion is also important to consider to provide an aesthetic pontic, as this is only possible if the cervical aspect of the pontic can overlap or engage the soft tissues to give the appearance of emergence from the soft tissues. The path of insertion must therefore have a vertical component to it.

Obtaining Interocclusal Space

Interocclusal space can be obtained through:

- relative axial tooth movement
- tooth preparation.

Preparation of space for the retainer and/or connector of a resin-bonded bridge is a contentious point. It would appear that preparation is not always necessary. The 'Dahl principle' (in a loose sense) has been utilised, whereby no tooth preparation is performed and the restoration is bonded 'high' (in supra-occlusion). This results in a localised contact in occlusion, which will hopefully lead to intrusion of these contacting teeth and extrusion of the non-contacting teeth until harmonious contacts are re-established (relative axial tooth movement). This concept is often used in the management of localised anterior TSL, where commonly at least canine to canine are restored in supra-occlusion with the posterior teeth left out of contact allowing relative axial tooth movement. This commonly occurs with no ill effects; however, on occasion this is not the case. If this option is used to gain space, it is advised to have a stable stop contact to provide axial loading of the contacting teeth. A contact on an incline away from the long axis of the tooth should be avoided if at all possible, which is commonly more difficult to achieve anteriorly. Localised incline contacts can result in unwanted issues, such as positional displacement of the retainer tooth (with pontic), loosening and pain of the retainer tooth, debond or fracture of the restoration and TMD.

Pontics should, wherever possible when providing any bridge, have a holding contact in ICP but immediately disclude in function or excursions. On fitting a bridge, the occlusion should also be checked when contacts have reestablished, as it is impossible to predict the resulting nature of the contact with the pontic. Occlusal adjustment may well be required to achieve immediate disclusion. When using such principles to gain space for a restoration, it has the obvious advantage of no or reduced requirement for tooth preparation; however there is always an element of lack of control and predictability with this approach. Location and clear seating of the restoration in the correct position can also be difficult without preparation, especially in the anterior, but the retainer can be made with location lugs that hook over the incisal edge to overcome this issue. The lugs can subsequently be removed following bonding. In addition, the same principle – relative axial tooth movement – has also been used to provide occlusal coverage to single compromised teeth in the posterior region.

Preparation of Teeth to Provide Interocclusal Space
Tooth tissue can be removed from the abutment tooth or the opposing tooth to provide interocclusal space. This should be performed in a planned manner. When adjusting opposing teeth the potential structural, biological and aesthetic impacts on the teeth should be communicated to the patient prior to preparation. Maintaining the preparation on the abutment tooth within enamel is always advised where possible, to optimise the long-term retention of the restoration. Commonly a combination of preparing both teeth may be deemed appropriate to minimise the impact of each. It is prudent to then prevent loss of any space gained by bonding composite to the opposing tooth to produce a holding contact. This can then be removed at the fit appointment. Preparation should also allow for restorative space in dynamic occlusion. If this is not accommodated, the guidance angle will be steepened and though this will often be tolerated by the patient it is not always. It may impinge on the patient's functional occlusal envelope (providing an incline interference) with potential unwanted sequelae as previously discussed.

Placement of rest seat style preparations on posterior teeth, and cingulum rests on anterior teeth, can also aid the seating of resin-bonded bridges at the cementation appointment.

Self-Assessment: Questions

SINGLE BEST ANSWER QUESTIONS

1. A patient attends reporting short-lived but very intense pain from the upper right quadrant of the mouth when drinking cold or hot drinks. Your clinical examination reveals no clinical or radiographic caries but there appears to be some dentine exposure around the UR5 & UR6 with non-carious cervical lesions adjacent to the gingival margin. Which term best describes the patient's symptoms?
   A. Dentine hypersensitivity
   B. Gingival recession
   C. Irreversible pulpitis
   D. Pulp necrosis
   E. Symptomatic apical periodontitis

2. You have removed extensive caries from a deep two-surface cavity and you are concerned about pulpal proximity. Which of the following materials is the most biocompatible sealing material for an indirect pulp cap?
   A. Dentine bonding agent
   B. Calcium hydroxide
   C. Calcium silicate cement
   D. Glass ionomer cement
   E. Zinc oxide eugenol

3. A medically fit and well patient experiences an area of frequent ulceration and discomfort with spicy foods adjacent to a large, old amalgam restoration. The area has been biopsied, histopathology revealing a distinct T cell inflammatory cell infiltrate below the epithelium. What is the most likely diagnosis for this condition?
   A. Folate deficiency
   B. Lichenoid reaction
   C. Mucous membrane pemphigoid
   D. Pemphigus vulgaris
   E. Squamous cell carcinoma

4. A patient presents with early enamel dental caries affecting a number of smooth surface and posterior interproximal areas. Your initial management is conservative; how frequently should you recall this patient to re-evaluate their caries risk?
   A. 3 months
   B. 6 months
   C. 12 months
   D. 18 months
   E. 24 months

5. A patient presents with multiple carious lesions affecting a number of smooth surface and posterior interproximal areas. Medical history reveals anxiety with a medication of amitriptyline. You determine that the patient is high risk for dental caries. How often can you prescribe fluoride varnish in very high-risk cases such as this?
   A. 3 monthly
   B. 6 monthly
   C. 12 monthly
   D. 18 monthly
   E. 24 monthly

6. What concentration of fluoride toothpaste should be prescribed to a patient with active dental caries who has a history of head and neck radiotherapy?
   A. 1000 ppm
   B. 1350 ppm
   C. 1450 ppm

D. 2800 ppm
E. 5000 ppm

7. One side effect of tricyclic antidepressants is xerostomia; which of the following should you recommend to your patient to improve the comfort of their mouth?
A. Drinking regular cups of coffee
B. Drinking regular sips of water
C. Drinking citrus fruit flavoured drinks
D. Regular use of chewing gum
E. Sucking on pineapple chunks

8. A fully dentate patient attends with worn down surfaces of their anterior teeth. Your examination reveals widespread loss of anatomy with exposure of dentine and in some areas, occluded pulp spaces are visible. You are planning a reorganised approach to restoration of the dentition. What is the most appropriate method of recording the relationship of the maxillary teeth to the position of the mandibular condyles?
A. A diagnostic wax-up
B. A face-bow transfer
C. A wax bite registration
D. A silicone bite registration
E. Lateral check wafers

9. The most appropriate way of determining the activity of a carious lesion is to assess the:
A. Dry tooth with good light, magnification and a blunt ended probe
B. Lesion with a bitewing radiograph
C. Stickiness of the lesion with a sharp explorer
D. Tooth with quantitative laser fluorescence
E. Vitality of the tooth

10. Application of an acid etchant such as 37% phosphoric acid to dentine for 1 minute is likely to result in:
A. Resin not fully penetrating the demineralised dentine and weaker bond strengths
B. Greater bond strengths as a result of a deeper etch into dentine
C. Greater penetration of resin into dentine and a greater bond strength
D. Collapse of the amelodentinal junction at the cavity margin
E. Lower polymerisation contraction when dentine bonding agent is cured

11. An 18-year-old patient attends your surgery within 1 hour of falling off her bicycle with a fractured central incisor. It involves coronal enamel and dentine, and the pulp is visible beneath a thin sliver of dentine. You decide to place a small indirect pulp cap of:
A. Calcium hydroxide
B. Calcium silicate cement
C. Dentine bonding agent
D. Glass ionomer cement
E. Zinc oxide eugenol cement

12. A 64-year-old patient complains of worn upper incisor teeth (they have lost over 50% of the original height). The patient is suffering minimal sensitivity but is keen to reduce the sharp edges of enamel (which is circumferentially present around the affected teeth) and improve upon their appearance. The most appropriate initial cost-effective treatment to address the patient's concerns is to provide:

A. Direct composite build ups
B. Metal-ceramic anterior crowns
C. Overdentures
D. Soft splint
E. Zirconia anterior crowns

13. A 42-year-old patient with a high smile line attends complaining that a number of anterior composite restorations are discoloured and the margins are visible. Your clinical examination reveals that there is a patchwork of restorations from UR3 through to UL3, but with much enamel available to bond to. Otherwise the patient is currently caries free and gingival health is good. You prescribe six upper anterior veneers. What marginal preparation should ideally be prescribed for an etchable lithium disilicate veneer?
A. 0.3-mm light chamfer
B. 0.7-mm shoulder
C. 1-mm knife edge
D. 1.2-mm heavy chamfer
E. 2-mm heavy chamfer

14. A 50-year-old patient has asymptomatic lichenoid lesions on the buccal mucosae adjacent to some large and elderly mesio-occluso-distal restorations in the molar teeth. They have a history of bruxism and previous cuspal fractures restored with pin-retained amalgams in some cases. They are not aesthetically driven and are keen to avoid a crown at present; what is the most appropriate restoration type for this patient?
A. Direct composite
B. Gold onlay
C. Indirect composite
D. Lithium disilicate onlay
E. Replace amalgam under rubber dam

15. You have been removing a large posterior restoration in a young patient, and you notice a pulpal exposure. Which of the following should be used directly onto the pulp to stop the bleeding prior to placement of a direct pulp cap?
A. Calcium hydroxide
B. Triamcinolone acetonide
C. Sodium hypochlorite
D. Epinephrine containing local anaesthetic
E. Clindamycin hydrochloride

MULTIPLE CHOICE QUESTIONS (TRUE/FALSE)

1. The following factors are important in remineralisation and demineralisation of early carious lesions:
a. Plaque composition
b. Frequency of sugar intake
c. Fluoride content of dentifrices
d. Gingival inflammation
e. Salivary flow rate

2. Which of the following may be used in a cavity to be restored with composite?
a. Non-setting calcium hydroxide
b. Dentine-bonding agent
c. Glass ionomer
d. Unmodified zinc oxide eugenol
e. Zinc polycarboxylate

3. The following definitions in occlusion are correct:
a. Group function is the presence of bilateral tooth contacts in lateral excursion

b. Retruded contact position (RCP) is equivalent to relation (CR)
c. Freeway space is a positive interocclusal space arising as the difference between resting face height (RFH) and occlusal face height (OFH)
d. A deflective contact is a tooth contact deviating the mandible from natural path of closure
e. More than 80% of the dentate population will have a centric relation (CR) to CO slide

4. The following are methods of recording the relationship of mandibular teeth to maxillary teeth:
a. Occlusal wax registration
b. Transfer copings
c. Gothic arch tracing
d. Face-bow transfer
e. Diagnostic wax-up

5. Bleaching:
a. Always requires rubber dam isolation
b. Can only be carried out on non-vital teeth
c. A 'walking bleach' uses carbamide peroxide
d. Is always effective in severe tetracycline staining
e. External bleaching is more effective if heat is applied

6. With reference to resin-bonded bridges:
a. A double-winged design is favoured
b. The wing should normally be of a Rochette design
c. The preparation should be ideally only in enamel
d. Cementation should be with a glass ionomer cement
e. May not be aesthetically acceptable due to the metal of the retainer

CASE HISTORY QUESTIONS

Case History 1

A 35-year-old female patient attends complaining of gradual discoloration of an upper right central incisor tooth over the last 2 years. It is presently symptom free, but she is unhappy about its appearance and wishes this to be improved.

1. What questions would you ask in relation to the history?
2. What investigations would you carry out?
3. What treatment options exist?

Case History 2

A 50-year-old male patient attends complaining of intermittent discomfort from a lower molar tooth, mainly on chewing or biting on the tooth in one position. The tooth has been restored a few years previously with a large mesio-occluso-distal (MOD) amalgam. The pain is sharp in nature, related to the one tooth, and each episode lasts only a few minutes at most.

1. What investigations might you carry out?
2. What is the differential diagnosis?
3. How would you treat it?

Case History 3

A 20-year-old female patient attends with a complaint of severe sensitivity of many teeth, especially to thermal stimulus (hot and cold). She looks frail and underweight.

1. What might you expect to see intraorally?
2. What might be its aetiology?
3. How would you deal with the patient?
4. How would you deal with her dentition?

Self-Assessment: Answers

SINGLE BEST ANSWER QUESTIONS ANSWERS

1. A. Dentine hypersensitivity is the most likely cause of the patient's symptoms given the non-carious tooth surface loss.

2. C. Calcium silicate cement is the most biocompatible material that will provide the best indirect pulp cap, examples of which are Biodentine and MTA.

3. B. A contact lichenoid reaction is the most likely diagnosis; this may be confirmed with a biopsy. Histological features are similar to the autoimmune condition oral lichen planus.

4. A. It is recommended that dental recall intervals be based on risk; low-risk individuals may not need to be recalled for 2 years whereas someone with a high risk of dental caries and/or periodontal disease may be recalled as frequently as every 3 months. Three months would be prudent here.

5. A. Fluoride varnish should be applied to those at risk of caries on a 6-monthly basis, in very high-risk cases such as this it can be applied on a 3-monthly basis.

6. E. A patient with a history of head and neck radiotherapy is likely to have some oral dryness and therefore problems with clearance of food and reduced buffering potential. Whilst modern radiotherapy techniques are planned to direct the beam away from at least one of the major salivary glands, there is an inevitable impact that this treatment has. They are therefore at high risk of caries and 5000 ppm fluoride is appropriate.

7. B. Patients should be encouraged to drink regular sips of water, caffeine containing drinks should be avoided, citrus fruit drinks are likely to be both acidic and contain sugars, regular use of chewing gum is acceptable as long as it is specified as sugar-free. Sucking on pineapple/consuming citrus fruits will stimulate saliva but will be both erosive and cariogenic.

8. B. Whilst all of the answers may be used, it is the face-bow transfer which prescribes the relationship requested.

9. A. It is often difficult to assess the activity of a carious lesion, sharp probing should be avoided as an early

lesion that could be managed conservatively could accidently be cavitated, bitewings will only be helpful if there is a comparison taken previously, quantitative laser fluorescence will provide information about demineralisation but not necessarily activity, vitality of the tooth is important but not used to determine caries activity.

10. A. Etching time can be extended if there is clear evidence of sclerotic dentine as a result of tooth wear. There is a risk that over-etching will result in the subsequent resin not fully penetrating the dentine resulting in a bond that is relatively weak and prone to breakdown.

11. B. The most biocompatible indirect pulp capping material is a calcium silicate cement. GIC and calcium hydroxide have also been advocated in these situations, though the use of calcium hydroxide is becoming more contentious with the availability of calcium silicate cements. They are however more expensive and more difficult to use than calcium hydroxide, with longer setting times.

12. A. Composite build ups are often the first line treatment in such cases. Bonded indirect composites are becoming more affordable and may be considered as an alternative to directly placed composites. There may be an indication for further indirect restorations at some point, though there is likely to be further sacrifice of tooth tissue to be able to do so. Overdentures are an option for severe tooth wear but in this instance would likely be inappropriate. A soft splint may be appropriate for the patient once treatment is complete to protect the restorations if the aetiology of the wear was deemed to be attritive.

13. A. 0.3-mm light chamfer.

14. B. Amalgam may be better avoided as the replacement, given the patient's proclivity to lichenoid reactions. An onlay restoration would be a suitable alternative to prevent fracture of the weakened remaining tooth structure. Lithium disilicates or composites may also be suitable alternatives but in this patient, with a history of bruxism, may be more prone to fracture.

15. C. If pulpal bleeding can be arrested through the use of sodium hypochlorite applied on a pledget or similar within 5 minutes and the tooth is appropriately isolated, a direct pulp cap can be placed.

MULTIPLE CHOICE ANSWERS

1. a. True. The thickness and viscosity of plaque, in addition to the types of bacteria incorporated in it, will have an effect on the transfer of ions into and out of a carious lesion.
   b. True. The plaque ecology will be altered by regular consumption of refined sugar allowing the pH level to reduce (Stephan's curve) and increasing demineralisation.
   c. True. Any form of topical fluoride will provide free fluoride ions, which will be incorporated in the remineralisation process.
   d. False. Gingival inflammation, while being an effect of plaque accumulation and toxin production, does not

in itself affect the remineralisation/demineralisation process.
   e. True. Salivary flow rate, if reduced, will reduce the available ions for remineralisation. Saliva generally has an important function in modifying caries development.

2. a. False. Non-setting calcium hydroxide is used as an interim root filling material. It is not suitable for lining a cavity.
   b. True.
   c. True.
   d. False. Unmodified zinc oxide eugenol is too slow setting and may also interfere with setting if composites are used.
   e. True.

3. a. False. Group function is defined as multiple tooth contacts on the working side during lateral excursion but with no non-working side contact.
   b. False. Retruded contact position (RCP) is the first tooth contact on an arc of closure when the condyles are seated in centric relation. Centric relation (CR) is a joint position.
   c. True.
   d. True.
   e. True. Only 20% of the population have coincidence of the most retruded mandibular position with maximum interdigitation of the teeth.

4. a. True.
   b. True.
   c. True. Occlusal wax registrations, transfer copings and the gothic arch tracing devices are all means of recording the intermaxillary relationship.
   d. False. A face-bow only records the relative position of the maxilla to the hinge axis.
   e. False. A diagnostic wax-up is used as a tool to assess changes in occlusion or tooth shape prior to an advanced restorative procedure.

6. a. False. A 'walking bleach', where the active agent is sealed within the tooth, by its nature does not require rubber dam isolation, although dam should be used during placement.
   b. False. Vital and non-vital bleaching can be carried out.
   c. False. The agents commonly used for a 'walking bleach' are usually hydrogen peroxide (30%) and/or sodium perborate (Bocosan). Carbamide peroxide is the active agent in recent vital bleaching agents (e.g. opalescence).
   d. False. Severe tetracycline staining, while it may be improved by bleaching in many cases, does not always improve.
   e. False. Whilst heat speeds up the rate of chemical reaction, the result would be largely a dessication effect and has been implicated in an increased risk of external cervical resorption.

7. a. False. If debonds occur, marginal leakage and caries may go unnoticed.
   b. False. Rochette designs were the original type of resin-bonded bridge. Debonds were more common than with full coverage wings. Rochette designs are useful as immediate bridges which can be more easily removed.

c. True. Preparations into dentine result in a lower bond strength. In some cases, where occlusion is favourable for instance, no preparation may be required.

d. False. Cementation should be with a self- or dual-cure resin cement with silanation of the metal wing.

e. True.

CASE HISTORY ANSWERS

Case History 1

1. You should ask for the:
   - history of trauma: its nature, severity, timing
   - incidence and timing of previous symptoms: sensitivity, pain, gingival swelling/discharge, mobility
   - history of previous treatment: restorations, endodontic treatment
   - patient's views on appearance and on improving appearance.

2. Investigations would include:
   - clinical examination: careful examination in good light, assessment of degree and nature of discolouration (including comparison with shade guide as necessary), quality of existing restorations, periodontal status, mobility, presence of gingival sinus
   - pulp vitality tests: electric, hot (heated gutta-percha), cold (ice, ethyl chloride)
   - radiographs: to identify the morphology of the root canal system and the presence of any apical or other pathology
   - assessing the nature and quality of previous dental treatment (root fillings, restorations).

3. Treatment could include root canal treatment as required, bleaching (internal/external), a veneer or a crown based on the restorative status of the tooth. All relevant options, with their advantages and disadvantages, should be presented to the patient to obtain valid consent.

Case History 2

1. Examination would include:
   - clinical examination: assessment of existing restoration (presence of crack lines, recurrent caries, occlusal contacts), assessment of remaining tooth structure (caries, crack lines – careful use of transillumination often required), careful periodontal probing around the tooth
   - vitality testing: thermal and electric
   - radiographs to identify recurrent caries, deficient restoration, possible fracture (although fractures are rarely identifiable in these circumstances on radiograph)
   - occlusal tests: percussion tests using a Tooth Slooth or FracFinder placed over individual cusps and with patient occluding on the instrument with the opposing tooth; a positive response for a cracked cusp/tooth is for the patient to experience a sharp pain on release of the occlusal pressure, which arises from flexure of the two parts of the tooth.

2. Differential diagnosis includes cracked cusp/tooth syndrome, recurrent caries, symptomatic apical periodontitis, occlusal trauma

3. Treatment will vary with the diagnosis, but from the information given, the most likely cause is cracked tooth syndrome. Treatment should look to remove the restoration, visualise the crack and provide a direct bonded restoration (i.e. composite) involving coverage of the affected cusp or cusps. If there is a deep periodontal probing depth associated with a vertically orientated crack, the prognosis is very poor, and extraction may be the best option.

Case History 3

1. In such cases, extensive erosive tooth wear may be seen affecting almost all natural tooth surfaces and resulting most commonly from frequent vomiting. The tooth surfaces may be eroded through to dentine and, if the condition is severe enough and progressing rapidly, sensitivity will result from thermal stimuli because the rate of wear is more rapid than the ability of the pulp to generate secondary dentine. Cusps will be rounded and the tooth surface will tend to be smooth and glossy. Any restorations previously present in teeth may lie proud of the tooth surface. The patient may be dehydrated and have a dry appearance to the skin and oral tissues. There may also be extensive caries.

2. A patient of this age who appears very underweight may well suffer from an eating disorder such as anorexia or bulimia. If this is the case, sensitivity is required in eliciting a history, as the patient may be reluctant to admit to this. Tooth surface loss can result from intrinsic or extrinsic acids, therefore diet analysis should also be performed, and oral habits around the time of any acidic challenges should be elicited.

3. It is important, where possible, to identify the aetiology of the disease process and symptoms and management targeted towards addressing the underlying problem. If the patient can acknowledge the nature of their problem, liaison with their medical practitioner for further investigation and treatment of the condition is desirable. Failure to do so will make dental treatment more difficult and lead to more rapid failure.

4. Management should look to address the patient's initial complaint – widespread sensitivity, in the short term, and depends on the extent and aetiology of the erosion. Use of desensitising toothpaste and fluoride varnish application may be beneficial. Remineralisation therapy should be prescribed, alongside behavioural management- such as avoiding toothbrushing after vomiting, and perhaps using a fluoride mouthwash for example. Management will likely require involving medical practitioners, if the patient's consent is forthcoming, and looking to manage the underlying aetiology. Adhesive restorations of the affected teeth can then be considered, often at an increased OVD, requiring complex planning.

4 *Prosthodontics*

Overview

As people are living longer and retaining their dentitions into later life, the demands on the prosthodontist have changed to match the increasing needs of a changing population. The discipline of prosthodontics has evolved significantly over the last 15 years from being a discipline heavily weighted to complete denture construction into a specialty concerned with removable, fixed, implant-supported prosthesis and maxillofacial prosthodontics. Prosthodontics is now a specialty which includes a broad clinical skill set, one which is too broad to incorporate into a single chapter. This chapter addresses the clinical stages involved with complete and partial denture construction and highlights other areas of interest to the prosthodontist. Detailed information on material science, preprosthetic surgery and prosthetic laboratory techniques has not been included and indeed this text should be seen as an introduction and summary of the areas covered.

4.1 Complete Dentures

LEARNING OBJECTIVES

You should:
- appreciate the importance of correct patient assessment
- recall and link the key clinical and laboratory stages in complete denture construction
- develop understanding of solving complete denture problems.

PATIENT ASSESSMENT

Assessment of a patient who requires any form of dental treatment should begin at the earliest stage of meeting that patient. On first meeting the patient, there are points that should be subconsciously noted, even before any dialogue occurs: gender, age, physical stature, their appearance and, finally, their present dental status. Initial impressions of a new patient often give a very valuable insight into a patient's potential expectations of the dental care, and one can develop ideas of how to meet their expectations. Nevertheless, it is vitally important not to definitively categorise patients as a result of initial impressions. A patient's appearance and demeanour may be misleading; a detailed history alongside a more structured history is required. Recognising their oral status, dental demands and psychological attitude towards treatment are imperative in the pursuit of a successful outcome. A concise evaluation of the presenting complaint or reason for attendance, and identifying the patient's perspectives of the problem, should be used to enable the clinician to formulate patient-centred solutions. Structured questioning should then be used to clarify concerns and prioritise which aspects of their problem are of greatest importance. A detailed denture wearing history is built up gradually. This may include the following points:

- **When** did you become edentulous?
- **Why** did you lose your teeth?
- Have you worn partial dentures or complete dentures previously?
- Did you have immediate dentures fitted?
- **How many sets** of dentures have you had?
- **How long** did each set of dentures last?
- Did you attend the dentist for any denture maintenance visits?
- **How old** is your present set of dentures?
- Which set of dentures was the most successful in your opinion?
- Do your present dentures cause you any discomfort?
- Do you wear your dentures at night?
- Do you like the appearance of your present dentures?
- Can you eat with your present dentures?
- Are there any foods which you avoid eating and why?

A clear and concise medical history is also required (Table 4.1). In this respect, it is important to appreciate the possible oral manifestations of systemic disorders, as elderly patients often present with complex medical conditions. The role of polypharmacy in developing oral dryness should also be considered.

An extraoral assessment of temporomandibular joint, facial asymmetry, lymph node enlargement, lower face height and soft tissue support are all routine clinical requirements. Following this, the patient should be asked to remove their dentures and an intraoral assessment should be carried out. All soft tissues should be inspected, including the floor of mouth and tonsillar fossa and the health of

Table 4.1 Important Medical Factors for Denture Wearers.

Area	Significant Factors
Physical disabilities	Disability (mental or physical), arthritis
Neuromuscular disorders	Parkinson's disease, epilepsy, stroke
Airway/breathing disorders	Asthma, bronchitis
Skin/mucosal disease	Pemphigus, pemphigoid, lupus erythematosus
Medication	Any medication that may cause dry mouth

the tissues evaluated. Patients may present with oral lesions, either related or unrelated to their dentures. Complete denture wearers attend less frequently than their dentate counterparts; a dentist may therefore detect mucosal conditions which might otherwise go unnoticed.

The ridges should then be palpated and a note made as to the remaining hard tissue support. Once the health of the extraoral and intraoral hard and soft tissues has been examined, a thorough examination of the dentures themselves should be carried out away from the mouth to assess their cleanliness and condition. Each denture in turn should then be placed intraorally to assess:

Retention

Definition: Resistance of a denture to vertical movement away from the tissues.

It is often beneficial to classify retention as being good, adequate or poor; reasons for lack of retention should be listed, such as under- or overextension of the periphery, position of post dam and adaptation of the fitting surface. Paucity of the underlying anatomy and lack of an adequate salivary function should also be noted.

Stability

Definition: The resistance of a denture to displacement by functional forces.

A scale of good, adequate or poor should be used and the reasons for lack of stability are listed such as mobility of the ridge, unsupported ridge, extensive resorption or inadequate muscle control, tooth position which encourages displacement either at rest or in function.

Occlusion

Definition: Any contact between the teeth of opposing dental arches.

A classification should be used to describe the incised and buccal occlusal relationship of the dentures, and a general assessment of occlusal contact and support should be made; an assessment of the freeway space (interocclusal clearance) provided by the existing dentures is also important.

It is pertinent to remember that previous dentures may provide useful information on the appropriate jaw relationship, occlusal plane, incisal level and the relationship of teeth to soft tissues (polished surfaces). Any intended alterations to these factors that may be required should have been noted at the treatment-planning stage. Consideration

of what changes and why they are being made should also influence treatment-planning decisions.

A classification system of the type shown in Fig. 4.1 may be of benefit. It is important to recognise that there is considerable variation in the outline, morphology and constitution of any edentulous mouth. A well-formed ridge may be made as challenging as a heavily resorbed ridge due to the nature of the functional sulcus, interarch space, mucosal resilience, adaptive capacity of the patient, quality and quantity of saliva.

Once the assessment has been completed, it is important that a diagnosis and treatment plan should be developed for every patient, which will be dependent upon the presenting complaints together with the findings from the clinical examination. It is not satisfactory for the treatment plan to be simply 'the construction of complete dentures'. The proposed treatment should include any preliminary requirements, treatment of mucosal conditions or preprosthetic surgery, followed by the intended technique of denture construction including any special considerations. It should also clearly indicate the objectives of impression making, impression materials, intended freeway space, balanced occlusion, tooth selection and selection of denture base. Specific references should be given to the indications for copy dentures, functional impressions, neutral zone technique, lingualised occlusion or flat-cusped teeth.

CLINICAL TECHNIQUES

Visit 1: Preliminary Impressions

Preliminary impressions are taken in stock trays using impression compound or another suitable impression material of choice. Impression compound is used in teaching establishments as it often records a slightly overextended first impression which is preferable for tray construction. The additional advantage of impression compound is that it allows the impressions to be modified to correct any errors or deficiencies without the need to take a whole new impression. Alginate may also be used, although its recording of the sulcus is largely dictated by the extent of the chosen stock tray. These stock trays may need modification (reduction or border moulding) to improve their suitability for the patient – in some cases, first using compound then modified to record detail using an alginate wash. There is little point in taking preliminary impressions if the subsequent special tray uses exactly the same technique, without any modification to the requested special tray.

Laboratory Prescription

As the next appointment will be for recording master impressions, it is essential at this and subsequent stages to indicate precisely your technical requirements. The prescription on the laboratory card should be clear and comprehensive. If there is any possibility of confusion, it is most valuable to discuss the patient personally with the technician involved. If a laboratory card is not completed and dated properly, the work may not be available at the next appointment.

Requirements for Trays

UPPER AND LOWER TRAYS. *Custom made special trays* should be prescribed for use with a specified impression material to enable the technician to space the tray accordingly.

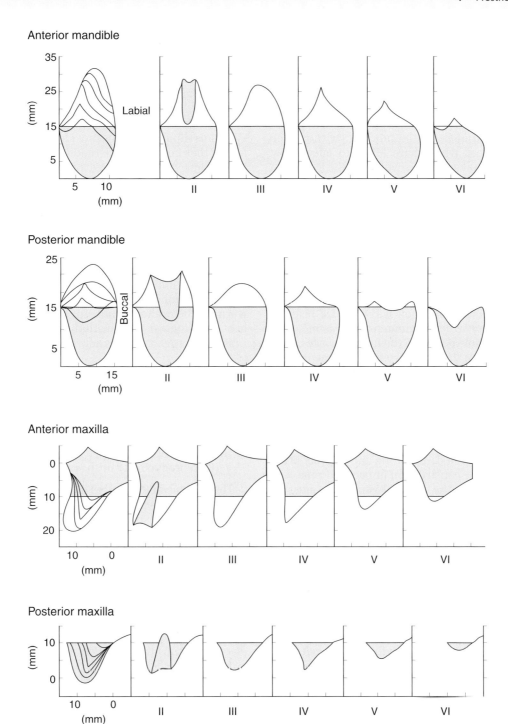

Fig. 4.1 A classification system for edentulous jaws. (Reprinted from Cawood JI, Howell RA. Reconstructive preprosthetic surgery I. Anatomical considerations. *Int J Oral Maxillofac Surg.* 1991;20:75–82 with permission from Elsevier.)

Close-fitting (0.6 mm spacer) light-cured trays for use with zinc oxide/eugenol paste can be requested. If extensive undercuts are present, a spaced tray for alginate or silicone may be required.

BORDERS. The peripheral border of all trays should finish 2 mm short of the depth of the sulcus recorded by the primary impression, when the spacer is in place. This is an estimate of the position of the mucogingival line and will assist the clinician in recording the functional sulcus depth in the master impression.

Visit 2: Master Impressions

The master impression should record detail of the denture-bearing area together with the depth *and* width of the functional sulcus so that the finished denture maintains an effective facial or border seal. In some cases, the tray will require modification to its peripheral border and this should be carried out using a material of sufficient viscosity to be mouldable and self-supporting such as medium body silicone, silicone putty or greenstick compound prior to the impression being recorded.

Greenstick may also be used to create functional post-dam recording. A layer of greenstick is placed along the posterior 2–3 mm of the fitting surface aligning with the vibrating line of the hard soft palate junction. This differentially compresses the tissues in this area. Care is then taken to remove any excess material extending beyond the vibrating line. An advantage of this thermoplastic material is that it can be modified without the need to re-take areas which have failed to adequately capture the functional sulcus, as would be the case with any of the set elastomers. The final impression is taken with the material selected, ideally those with hydrophilic low viscosity properties which will record surface detail. Low viscosity silicones are often used, but alginate may also be effective.

These impressions are not to be considered complete until ribbon wax is placed approximately 2 mm from the periphery of the impression in order to provide a land area and protect the width of the sulcus on the resultant master cast. This placement of ribbon wax is called beading (Fig. 4.2). In the cases where alginate is used, a line must be drawn with indelible pencil on the facial surface of the impression 2 mm from the periphery for the same reason. This area must not be removed!

It is always advisable after pouring the master casts to retain the individual trays until all treatment has been completed.

Laboratory Prescription

Casts should be poured in dental stone and a prescription provided regarding the construction of occlusal rims. The material to be used for the occlusal rim bases must be specified. This may be temporary, but sufficiently stable and robust as to avoid distortion during any of the future clinical and laboratory stages; for this reason wax only bases and occlusal rims are best avoided. A temporary base is discarded before final processing of the denture. Alternatively, permanent acrylic bases offer the advantage of allowing a check of the comfort and retention of the final denture to be assessed at an early stage, as well as optimising the accuracy of recording jaw relations. Where problems are identified and new impressions indicated these are undertaken without involving unnecessary use of additional clinical time. The disadvantages are additional cost and the small possibility of distortion (about 1%) of the permanent base during a second cure when the denture is flasked and packed (Fenlon et al, 2008). This can largely be avoided, however, by use of stone capping during processing.

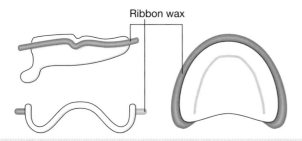

Fig. 4.2 Positioning of red ribbon wax for beading to create a land area on a master model.

Visit 3: Recording Jaw Relations

Before embarking on this stage it is important to refer back to the treatment plan and to verify with the patient that what you are doing meets their requirements.

Clinical Procedure

Wax rims should ideally be provided on heat-cured bases, or failing that an alternative rigid temporary base. If the occlusal rims are constructed on acrylic bases, the fitting surfaces should be examined for sharp edges and excessive undercuts. A permanent heat-cured base offers the opportunity to effectively check and modify the retention and stability of the base, and to determine if a second master impression is required. If the acrylic resin has been extended into bony undercuts, disclosing wax or pressure relief cream may be used to locate any area requiring adjustment. To minimise any distortion of the wax, the use of a rigid base is important, as is ensuring it does not become too warm in the oral environment; removing it regularly and gentle cooling will assist with this.

The upper record rim is adjusted so that:

- lip support is correct
- incisal height is correct
- occlusal plane is correct (parallel to the lower ridge, alar-tragus and interpupillary lines)
- labial and buccal contour is correct (allowing for buccal corridors to be present)
- the centre line is marked and lateral check marks to verify reproducibility of the path of closure.

The presence of dentures in the mouth will modify the rest position of the mandible. Measurements of the resting face height should normally be made with the upper rim in place.

The lower rim should be adjusted to correct the buccolingual contour posteriorly and correct the labial contour anteriorly. The rim should sit in the neutral zone. It should be trimmed to establish even, bilateral contact along the retruded arc of closure (centric relation). In this respect, the patient should be asked to close until the rims first contact. Excessive pressure may cause them to tilt or be displaced into the alveolar mucosa, giving the appearance of even contact when, in fact, it does not exist. In some cases, the patient may be helped to find the retruded arc by asking them to curl the tongue back to contact the posterior border of the upper occlusal rim. An assessment should be made of both resting vertical dimension and occlusal vertical dimension. This may be assessed from facial appearance and confirmed from an estimation made using some kind of measurement from two facial reference points, commonly using a Willis gauge. This should identify an adequate interocclusal clearance or freeway space. In an elderly patient who has been a denture wearer for many years, often providing slightly more freeway space can be beneficial.

When satisfied that the patient is consistently occluding on the retruded arc of closure at the correct vertical dimension of occlusion, make locating marks in the midline and buccally in the canine region. Remove the rims and place them together outside the mouth using the locating marks. The jaw relation is now ready to be recorded: locating indices are cut into the occlusal rims to aid rearticulating once the record blocks are removed from the mouth.

The rims are placed in the mouth and a thin layer of silicone jaw registration material or a similar recording material is applied along the entirety of the lower rim. Stabilise the rims with fingers and encourage the patient to close into retruded jaw relation (check locating marks are coincident) and wait until the material has set. After removing rims from the mouth, check that casts can be placed into the rims without any premature contacts distally, either between the heels of the casts or between the posterior extensions of the denture bases (avoidance of heel clash). Also ensure that the rims can be separated and relocated accurately.

Select teeth that are an appropriate shade and mould for the patient. Reference may be made to previous dentures if the patient was happy with their appearance.

If a functional impression of the posterior extension of the upper denture has not been used, a post dam is cut into the master cast prior to final processing. If the patient has consistently had problems with complete dentures or had a gross skeletal abnormality, it may be worth considering using a face-bow registration of the upper rim to allow for a more reliable location of the cast on the articulator in the laboratory, although there is little evidence to show this is of benefit. Use of permanent bases to optimise stability and retention of the record blocks should also be considered.

Laboratory Prescription
Record the shade, mould and material to be used for the artificial teeth on the laboratory card. Indicate the type of articulator (average movement or semi-adjustable) on which the dentures are to be set up and indicate any aspects of the anterior tooth setup that are to be copied in the trial dentures. Indicate the type of bases required for the trial dentures. All casts should be mounted using a split-cast technique.

Visit 4: Trial Dentures

An examination of the completed setup on the articulator should be carried out before trying in the mouth, and any discrepancies noted. If the trial dentures are not correct on the articulator, this must be evaluated before a decision to proceed to place these trial dentures in the patient's mouth. If some technical or occlusal fault is evident a decision about how to effectively rectify this is required.

In the mouth, carry out a complete assessment of the trial dentures including the following:

- Stability and retention, more difficult to assess when using temporary bases. When using a permanent base this should verify that the retention and stability are consistent with your finding during recoding of jaw relations.
- Peripheral extension.
- Positioning of teeth in relation to neutral zone and shape of polished surfaces.
- Occlusion should be assessed visually (articulating paper is *not* necessary at this stage, but care must be taken to stabilise the bases on their respective supporting tissues). Occlusal interferences may displace denture bases away from the tissues disguising occlusal errors.
- Verify with the patient that the contact feels even and simultaneous.

- Interocclusal clearance to give a satisfactory freeway space. Speech sounds and mouth feel give clues as to the appropriateness of this.
- Appearance including the shade, mould and position of the anterior teeth and the contour of the labial flanges; check that the appearance is natural (a completely even arrangement of teeth usually looks *unnatural*), and modify if necessary.
- Recheck occlusion if the positions of the anterior teeth have been modified as this may result in occlusal interference.

After carrying out any necessary corrections, obtain the patient's comments. *Do not proceed to finish unless the patient is satisfied, especially with the appearance* (record this in the notes).

Anything other than minor localised discrepancies of occlusion and vertical dimension will require a new jaw registration using the trial denture as an occlusal rim. A decision about what has caused the error will determine which teeth will need to be removed and replaced with wax, before once more sealing them together using occlusal registration paste prior to rearticulating the casts and resetting the teeth.

The dentures would then proceed to being reset and tried in again at the next visit. It is important to have an approach which uses the 'try in' stage as an opportunity to confirm that all of the planned treatment objectives have either been achieved or that those which conflict with other objectives have been agreed and discussed with the patient. Any such discussion should highlight that compromises have been agreed between both clinician and patient.

Final Laboratory Prescription
The prescription should state definitely whether dentures can be finished or if a further trial is required. If the jaw relationship has been re-recorded, the casts are remounted on the articulator and a second trial stage is carried out. When the dentures are processed, use of the split-cast technique will minimise occlusal errors during processing.

Porosity
One of the possible faults that can occur in the laboratory is porosity within the acrylic resin or tooth movement during the processing cycle.

Contraction porosity results when insufficient acrylic dough has been placed to create an excess or flash. Alternatively, the application of insufficient pressure during curing can lead to porosity voids dispersed throughout the whole mass of the denture base.

Gaseous porosity results when the temperature of the dough is raised significantly above the boiling point of the monomer (100 degrees Celsius), producing spherical voids in the hottest part of the curing dough. This occurs most commonly in the lingual flanges of a lower denture.

Granular porosity results from evaporation of the monomer during preparation. Proportioning of the powder to liquid ratio is dependent on allowing each powder particle to become wetted by the monomer. The mixture is left to stand until it reaches the right consistency suitable for packing into the gypsum mould. During this standing period, a lid should be placed on the mixing vessel to prevent evaporation of the monomer. Loss of monomer during this stage can produce granular porosity in the set material, which is characterised by a blotchy opaque surface.

Visit 5: Final Dentures

The processed dentures should be checked for any sharp edges, acrylic 'pearls' or excessive undercuts on the fitting surface. Insert each denture separately and check on fit and comfort to the patient. An examination of the occlusion in the mouth can be done either visually or using articulating paper.

Visual assessment is made by observing and by asking the patient if the teeth are meeting with equal pressure on both sides of the mouth when the mouth is closed gently.

Articulating paper is used to confirm these findings and to precisely locate any premature contacts. A heavy mark made by the paper may indicate where the initial contact is being made. Fossa rather than cusp tips should be ground at this stage only. Beware of artefacts, such as those produced by tilting of the dentures. This would produce marks from the articulating paper on both sides of the mouth, whereas initial observations may have indicated that the first occlusal contact is only on one side.

If any occlusal faults are diagnosed, it is liable to be a clinical and not a laboratory error providing that the split-cast technique has been used. Relatively minor occlusal discrepancies may be adjusted at the chair side until:

- the occlusal pressure on both sides of the mouth is the same
- the occlusal *contacts* indicated by articulating paper are primarily on the premolar and first molar teeth; heavy contacts distally or anteriorly should be avoided as these may cause tipping of the dentures
- lateral and protrusive movement is possible without cuspal interference causing displacement of the dentures.

Significant chair-side occlusal adjustments are particularly difficult; where there is any doubt, a check record should be obtained. This often saves time if a large occlusal error is found at the initial insertion stage.

Check Record

A check record is advisable for the correction of occlusal errors that are too large to adjust easily at the chair side. This technique is also more reliable and accurate than major adjustment made at the chair side using articulating paper. Narrowed wax wafers, constructed from one thickness of pink modelling wax, are sealed to the occlusal surfaces of the lower posterior teeth and adjusted so that the patient occludes evenly on the wafers in retruded jaw relation with the teeth separated by a distance less than the freeway space. The teeth should not penetrate through the wax; otherwise tooth contact may cause displacement of the dentures and/or the mandible. This occlusal registration may be refined using registration paste. The dentures are then remounted on an articulator.

The articulator is closed with the incisal pin removed, and the occlusal contacts are checked visually and with articulating paper. Adjustments are carried out until an even occlusion is obtained. The dentures are reinserted and the occlusion checked in the mouth.

EVIDENCE BASE FOR THIS CLINICAL APPROACH TO COMPLETE DENTURE CONSTRUCTION. As with lots of areas of clinical dentistry, there is little evidence to support clinical approaches recommended; however, the following does suggest that master impressions may not be required to provide the same degree of patient satisfaction.

SIMPLE COMPLETE DENTURE TECHNIQUES CAN PROVIDE PATIENT SATISFACTION. When complete dentures are required, are simplified techniques as effective as complex traditional ones for their manufacture? A randomised controlled trial (RCT) was carried out in a hospital environment by Kawai et al (2005). A total of 122 edentulous individuals, aged 45–75 years, were randomly allocated into groups to receive dentures made using either traditional or simplified techniques. Individuals allocated to the traditional arm had a final impression taken in a custom-made tray and a face-bow recording and a semi-adjustable articulator were used, with articulator remount after delivery. Those in the simplified technique group had impressions taken in stock trays and no face-bow recording and a monoplane articulator were used, with no articulator remount after delivery. There were no significant differences between the two groups in patient ratings for overall satisfaction at 3 or 6 months. These results suggest the use of simplified techniques, which are easier to master and which should reduce treatment costs.

CRITICAL REVIEW OF SOME DOGMAS IN PROSTHODONTICS (CARLSSON 2009)

- A scrutiny of the prosthodontic literature indicates that many common clinical procedures lack scientific support. In the era of evidence-based dentistry, ineffective interventions should be eliminated and decisions should be made on best available evidence.
- Studies have demonstrated that dentists' and patients' interpersonal appraisals of each other were most significant factors, accounting for patients' evaluation of treatment outcome.
- Reviews of the literature on this topic have suggested that the creation of a good relationship with the patient seems to be more important than a technically perfect denture construction for achieving patient satisfaction.

ADVICE TO PATIENTS

Instructions in respect of new dentures should be discussed with your patient after the final dentures have been inserted, preferably using a printed leaflet. In particular, the importance of good denture hygiene should be emphasised. If an immersion cleaner is recommended, a hypochlorite type is the most suitable. Any mechanical cleaning should be done with a brush that allows access and has good adaptability to all surfaces of the denture.

If the patient has to leave the new dentures out because of pain or soreness, request that the dentures be worn for 24 hours before the review appointment, in order that the cause of the discomfort may be more readily detected. Under no circumstances should the patient attempt adjustment of the dentures.

Denture Maintenance

Unfortunately, evidence-based guidelines for the care and maintenance of removable complete denture prostheses do not exist. Based on the best available evidence, the following are guidelines for the care and maintenance of dentures (Felton et al 2011):

1. Careful daily removal of the bacterial biofilm present in the oral cavity and on complete dentures is of paramount importance to minimise denture stomatitis and to help contribute to good oral and general health.
2. To reduce levels of biofilm and potentially harmful bacteria and fungi, patients who wear dentures should do the following:
   a. Dentures should be cleaned daily by soaking and brushing with an effective, non-abrasive denture cleanser.
   b. Denture cleansers should ONLY be used to clean dentures outside of the mouth.
   c. Dentures should always be thoroughly rinsed after soaking and brushing with denture-cleansing solutions prior to reinsertion into the oral cavity. Always follow the product usage instructions.
3. Although the evidence is weak, dentures should be cleaned annually by a dentist or dental professional by using ultrasonic cleansers to minimise biofilm accumulation over time.
4. Dentures should never be placed in boiling water.
5. Dentures should not be soaked in sodium hypochlorite bleach, or in products containing sodium hypochlorite, for periods that exceed 10 minutes. Placement of dentures in sodium hypochlorite solutions for periods longer than 10 minutes may damage dentures.
6. Dentures should be stored and immersed in water after cleaning, when not replaced in the oral cavity, to avoid warping.
7. Denture adhesives, when properly used, can improve the retention and stability of dentures and help seal out the accumulation of food particles beneath the dentures, even in well-fitting dentures.
8. In a quality-of-life study, patient ratings showed that denture adhesives may improve the denture wearer's perceptions of retention, stability and quality of life; however, there is insufficient evidence that adhesives improve masticatory function.
9. Evidence regarding the effects of denture adhesives on the oral tissues when used for periods longer than 6 months is lacking. Thus, extended use of denture adhesives should not be considered without periodic assessment of denture quality and health of the supporting tissues by a dentist, prosthodontist or dental professional.
10. Improper use of zinc-containing denture adhesives may have adverse systemic effects. Therefore, as a precautionary measure, zinc-containing denture adhesives should be avoided.
11. Denture adhesives should be used only in sufficient quantities on each denture to provide sufficient added retention and stability to the prostheses.
12. Denture adhesives should be completely removed from the prosthesis and the oral cavity on a daily basis.
13. If increasing amounts of adhesives are required to achieve the same level of denture retention, the patient should see a dentist or dental professional to evaluate the fit and stability of the dentures.
14. While existing studies provide conflicting results, it is not recommended that dentures be worn continuously (24 hours per day) in an effort to reduce or minimise denture stomatitis.
15. Patients who wear dentures should be checked annually by the dentist, prosthodontist or dental professional for maintenance of optimum denture fit and function, for evaluation for oral lesions and bone loss and for assessment of oral health status.

COMMON COMPLAINTS OF THE EDENTULOUS PATIENT

Most prosthetic complaints can be prevented or minimised by adequate diagnosis, treatment planning and treatment plus attention to detail during the construction phase. A pre-prosthetic radiographic investigation can prevent the finding of retained roots, unerupted teeth and bone pathology after the new dentures have been constructed; however, this should not be done as a matter of course. Pretreatment case history and clinical investigation with a detailed assessment of any existing dentures should aid the resolution of such problems as correct face height, tooth position and polished contour. However, problems and complaints will still occur with new dentures. Table 4.2 lists some of the more common complaints, their probable causes and suggested treatment.

RELINES OR REBASES

A reline involves the addition of a material to the fitting surface of a denture base. A rebase involves the removal and replacement of virtually all the denture base, namely the fitting and polished surface of the denture. There are always risks with both relining and rebasing that the resultant denture may be made worse. There are few indications these days for a full rebase as it is often more satisfactory to consider a copy technique of the denture that would have been rebased. This will not necessitate the removal of the denture from the patient.

Advantages of a Reline

- Can be done at the chair side or in the laboratory
- Can be permanent or temporary
- Will improve the retention of an ill-fitting denture
- A resilient lining can be added to a previous denture base

Advantages of a Rebase

- Will not increase the thickness of the palate
- Will remove the majority of the previous denture base if, for example, bleaching has occurred

4.2 Copy/Duplicate Dentures

LEARNING OBJECTIVES

You should:
- understand the indications and advantages of a copy/duplicate denture technique over a more conventional approach to complete denture construction
- appreciate the clinical and technical stages involved in such a technique.

Table 4.2 Common Complaints of Patients With Dentures.

Complaint	Probable Cause	Treatment
Generalised discomfort over the denture-bearing areas	Increased occlusal face height	Occlusal adjustment or, more commonly, remake
	Occlusal interference in lateral and protrusive movements	Balanced articulation with free sliding contact
	Movement of denture bases over basal tissues	Reline/remake using copy technique
	Incorrect anteroposterior relationship of dentures (i.e. non-coincidence of tooth and muscular positions)	Occlusal adjustment
	Increased free monomer	Remake with correct curing cycle
Lack of chewing pressure, 'collapsed face', generalised facial discomfort	Decreased occlusal face height	Use cold-cure acrylic (occlusal pivots) or splint to build up occlusal face height then remake one or both dentures
Angular cheilitis	Lack of facial support (rarely occlusal face height). Maceration of cutaneous tissues by repeated wetting of angular folds This may lead to superinfection with *Staphylococcus aureus*	Build up canine prominence or move anterior teeth forward; use antifungal cream; increase denture hygiene
Pain over crest of ridge (especially lower anterior region)	Irregular bony contour following abnormal healing pattern	X-ray for diagnostic and treatment planning, osteoplastic surgery
Localised pain	Irregular soft tissue following socketed immediate dentures	Relieve/reline. Consider pre-prosthetic surgery
	Irregularities on fitting surface	Adjustment
	Premature contact	Occlusal adjustment
	Buried roots, unerupted teeth, cysts, etc.	X-ray, surgery
	Excess undercut utilised	Partial blocking out of undercut. Localised use of soft lining material
Pain in sulcus		
Ulcer	Overextension	Relieve
Denture-induced hyperplasia	Overextension	Severe relief; may not resolve, then surgery
Localised pain in lower premolar region	Pressure on superficial mental nerve	Relieve denture, surgery: repositioning only to be used in exceptional cases Resilient lining Viability of implant supported denture
Pain on one side	Premature contact, poor articulation	Analyse occlusion (check record) and articulation, then adjust
Pain from cheek and tongue	Teeth not set in neutral zone; especially if no horizontal overlap	Reduce width of teeth and provide horizontal overlap
Denture displaces on opening or in speech	Overextension of border	Reduce border, develop new border and replace in acrylic resin
	Underextension of border	Develop new border and replace in acrylic resin
	Anterior teeth too far forward of ridge	Reposition anterior teeth, F/F will probably have to be remade
Upper denture	Inadequate post dam	Trace and reprocess or cold cure
	Excessively deep post dam	Remove excess and polish post-dam area
	Interference of coronoid process on opening	Reduce thickness of flange
	Bulky flange	Reduce thickness of flange
Lower denture	Incorrect shape of polished surfaces	Recontour
	Excessive thickness of flange in region of modiolus	Reduce
	Posterior teeth outside neutral zone	Reduce width of teeth or remake
	Insufficient room for tongue	Increase/remake
Speech defect	New F/F	Encouragement and perseverance Reduce thickness of denture to provide more tongue space Speech analysis and adjustment
Poor mastication	Worn teeth increase in freeway space	Correct OVD-remake
	Lack of freeway space	Correct OVD-remake
Dry mouth	Systemic factors and medication	Salivary substitute
General inability to accommodate	Adaptive capacity: age, oral dryness, high oral awareness	Meticulous attention to detail and encouragement
	Errors in occlusal vertical dimension	Correct errors in OVD
	Psychological factors	
	Change in denture shape	Consider copy technique

Table 4.2 Common Complaints of Patients With Dentures.—cont'd

Complaint	Probable Cause	Treatment
Nausea	Denture extended onto soft palate	Reduce
	Lack of retention	Correct
	Reduced tongue space	Recontour polished surface
	Inability to accept such a large amount of acrylic	Horseshoe design for upper
'Teeth meet too soon', 'can't open mouth far enough for food'	Increased occlusal face height	Reduce or remake F/F
Appearance	Insufficient attention at try-in	Correct
	Unwillingness of patient to put function before aesthetics	Attempt to reach understanding
Denture stomatitis	Ill-fitting denture	Reline/remake
	Fungal infection	Denture hygiene; antifungal cream
	Increased free monomer	Remake: correct curing cycle
Midline fracture	Ill-fitting dentures	Reline/remake
	Teeth set excessively off the ridge	Remake
	F/– against lower standing teeth	Metal palate/sufficient overjet
	Fatigue	Rebase

OVD, Occlusal vertical dimension.

The process of history taking and examination of the patient and their existing dentures presents valuable information about the patients' previous denture-wearing success. Recognising the limitations of an existing denture whilst noting any successful aspects may inform the choice of a conventional technique of denture construction, which incorporates some of the beneficial features of the existing denture. Patients who have worn dentures satisfactorily over a long period of time and have developed a neuromuscular feedback in relationship to the spatial relationship of the denture to the surrounding tissues may benefit from a copy denture technique. In this respect, however, it is important to realise that the copy denture does not simply replicate the current dentures worn by the patient. It is designed specifically to reproduce the favourable aspects of the current prosthesis such as tooth position and polished surfaces, while improving the adaptation and occlusion. Copy dentures are particularly useful for elderly patients with good denture-wearing experience. There are numerous ways to reproduce beneficial features of existing dentures incorporating both conventional remake and copy techniques. These range from the use of impressions to create models of anterior tooth setup, shape and size of teeth, to using an Alma gauge to measure the incisal height and labial position of anterior teeth to reproduce lip support and aesthetics.

INDICATIONS

There are a number of situations where copy dentures are advisable:

- Correct position of teeth in the neutral zone or correct zone of adaptation and the polished surfaces are satisfactory
- Loss of retention in otherwise favourable dentures requiring replacement
- Wear of the occlusal surfaces

- Replacement of immediate dentures
- Spare set of dentures. This might be a consideration for patients who live in care homes and who have cognitive impairment.

Typical dental history that would suggest an indication for copy dentures:

- Elderly patients presenting with satisfactory complete dentures
- Worn occlusal surfaces, indicating long-term acceptability without significant loss of occlusal vertical dimension and change in the horizontal jaw relationship
- Deterioration of denture base materials
- Patient requests 'spare set' of dentures
- Patients with a history of denture problems make controlled modifications to copy previously most successful dentures.

Clinical Advantages

- No alteration or mutilation of existing dentures
- No period for the patient without their dentures (as compared to a reline or rebase)
- Three clinical stages
- Simple duplication procedure, less time than conventional impressions

Technical Advantages

- No individual trays or record blocks required
- Infrequent rearticulation of teeth for try-in necessary
- Elimination of repolishing after border adjustments
- No thickening of palate in the finished denture, as occurs in some reline procedures

ALGINATE COPY BOX/SILICONE COPY TECHNIQUE

First Clinical Stage

Any modifications are made at the first clinical stage (Box 4.1).

Box 4.1   Technique for Copying Existing Denture.

1. Correct any under- or overextension using greenstick or acrylic border moulding material.
2. Add labial flange (if required) to open face denture using impression compound.
3. Use a wax wafer to provide desired occlusal face height and decide whether increase to be on F/ alone or /F alone or shared between the two.
4. Choose shade.
5. Copy denture utilising alginate and copy boxes (Fig. 4.3).
6. Send copy boxes to laboratory with prescription.

Laboratory Stage

Wax-acrylic replicas are poured by adding wax into the mould to 1 mm past the gingival margins of the teeth and allowed to set. The base of the wax is then scored and self-cured acrylic is poured into the closed mould through previously cut sprue holes and allowed to polymerise. A stone duplicate is cast into the mould once the wax and acrylic copy has been removed. This stone mould can be used for comparison of the copy try-in. The denture templates are then removed from the moulds and articulated using the wax wafer provided. The wax teeth are then removed and replaced by acrylic denture teeth of appropriate shade and mould. This will provide trial dentures for the second clinical stage. Grooves are cut in the palate and filled in with wax (Fig. 4.4) to allow removal of the palate at a later stage.

Second Clinical Stage

At the second clinical stage, the trial dentures are assessed by the clinician and the patient and any errors in occlusion or tooth position are corrected, necessitating a retry. When the trial dentures are satisfactory, they should be prepared for impression taking. This involves removing any undercuts, reduction of the peripheral border and modification using greenstick or a border-moulding self-cured acrylic resin. The polished surfaces of the replica are coated with yellow petroleum jelly. Wash impressions are recorded using zinc oxide/eugenol or low-viscosity elastomer (if hard tissue undercuts are present in the mouth) using the closed-mouth technique. Occlusal relationships should be maintained. The position, width and depth of the required post dam are determined.

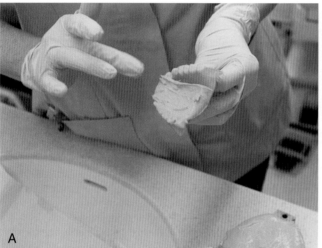

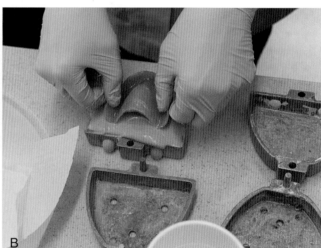

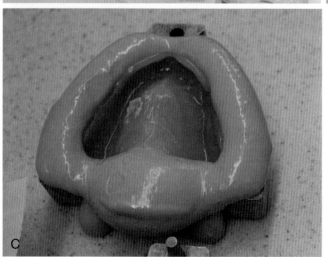

Fig. 4.3 Denture copied by insertion in a copy box. (A) Coating the polished surface with alginate to avoid air inclusion. (B) Seating the denture to be copied, aligning it with the sprue holes and ensuring slow seating to exclude air. (C) Excess alginate extruded above the level of the flange periphery should be trimmed back.

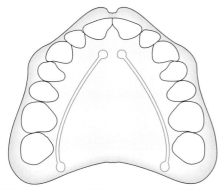

Fig. 4.4 Grooves cut in the palate to allow its removal later.

Final Laboratory Stage

The functional borders are preserved and stone casts are poured. The acrylic palate is removed and an even-thickness palate is waxed up.

Third Clinical Stage

The new dentures are checked for fit, extension and occlusion. A subsequent review is arranged.

COMMON PROBLEMS

The dentist may have several problems:

- Unfamiliarity with technique leading to failure to use closed-mouth technique with light and even occlusal contact
- Attempting a copy denture technique in a patient for whom it is clearly not indicated
- Copy flasks; some flasks are costly, but if they are used frequently and repeatedly the cost is minimal
- Forgetting to take the shade
- Finding a laboratory that is comfortable with the technique, fees additional to conventional complete denture construction charged by the laboratory
- Inadequate information on the prescription.

Similarly, certain problems are encountered by technicians:

- Duplicating the dentures; many laboratories duplicate the denture completely in wax or self-cured acrylic. Wax will distort especially at the stage of closed-mouth impressions
- Articulating the copy
- Setting up, copying the previous arrangement
- Waxing up
- Finishing, removing the palate and replacing a wax palate
- Grinding of denture teeth to fit acrylic base
- Registration problems
- Fees in comparison to the laboratory fee and the time taken to provide treatment.

There is no published evidence base available comparing conventional techniques to this approach to suggest that a copy/duplicate denture technique is superior.

4.3 Immediate Replacement Dentures

LEARNING OBJECTIVES

You should:
- understand the concept of immediate replacement dentures
- comprehend the clinical stages involved in immediate denture construction.

An immediate denture is defined as a denture that is made prior to the extraction of the natural teeth and which is inserted into the mouth immediately after the extraction of those teeth. It may involve total or partial replacement. Generally it is unacceptable to patients that they should be rendered edentulous without replacement of teeth for functional and aesthetic reasons. As overall dental health has generally improved, the total removal of teeth followed by the provision of complete dentures has become less common. It is now more usual to provide simple immediate additions to existing dentures or to provide an immediate partial denture which then transitions gradual tooth loss with future additions. A transitional denture may therefore be considered one which is designed as a partial denture, to which teeth of doubtful prognosis might be added, as they fail; the ultimate prognosis is for complete tooth loss within that arch.

Over the last 10 years we have seen a shift in the delivery of removable immediate dentures to immediate loaded implant-retained prostheses, in situations where good primary stability of implants has been achieved. These are generally a fixed alternative to the traditional removable immediate denture. However, whilst this represents a treatment option which may be beyond the affordability of many patients, it nevertheless offers significant advantages in terms of psychosocial adaptation, quality of life, bone preservation and functionality. Treatment planning for tooth loss, final restoration, long-term maintenance and optimisation of implant placement requires specialised clinical skills beyond the scope of this chapter.

ADVANTAGES OF IMMEDIATE DENTURES

There are several advantages for the patient:

- Maintenance of the soft tissue contour of the face:
  - dentures will support the soft tissues around the face in their correct position once teeth are lost and thereby prevent collapse of facial tissues
- Maintenance of mental and physical wellbeing:
  - the patient is not seen to be edentulous; this is important for business, domestic and social purposes
  - aesthetics are maintained by placing the artificial teeth in a position similar to natural teeth or improved by changing the position.
- The advantage of a more seamless adaptation to dentures is aided by:
  - maintenance of tooth position
  - maintenance of muscle balance

- prevention of the formation of abnormal mandibular movements
- aiding chewing and mastication.

■ Patients are likely to adapt to immediate dentures rather than waiting several months until healing and postextraction resorption is complete. Subsequently a copy denture technique may then be utilised to reproduce successful design features and maintain some continuity, where desirable, to the patients' original dentition.

There are also advantages for the dentist:

■ The use of existing dentition to reproduce occlusal relationship: teeth may act as occlusal stops, which will provide the intercuspal position and the correct occlusal vertical dimension.
■ Aesthetic consideration: shape and size of the teeth are known, which will assist selection (this may prove to be a problem rather than an advantage if teeth have drifted owing to periodontal disease).
■ Haemorrhage control.

DISADVANTAGES OF IMMEDIATE DENTURES

Immediate dentures do have a number of disadvantages:

■ Good cooperation is required, with the need for several follow-up appointments. Aftercare may require many visits including relines/rebases/new dentures.
■ As alveolar bone resorption occurs rapidly, there is loss of tissue adaptation and retention.
■ Increased cost: the provision of relines and further denture provision makes the treatment costly.
■ A trial denture stage is not always possible: this is a big disadvantage as it is not possible to show the patient what the teeth will eventually look like.
■ Gross irregularities of teeth make processing difficult (e.g. class II division 2, bulbous tuberosities/tori).
■ Surgical challenges may present difficulties Special care for infective endocarditis/diabetes/coronary heart disease/risk of medication related osteonecrosis of the jaws.

Types of Immediate Denture

Immediate dentures can be flanged or socket fit.

Flanged dentures:
- are retentive
- are easier to reline and rebase
- may be difficult to place where there is an undercut – use of partial flange.

Socket-fit dentures:
- are contraindicated in mandible
- the necks of the teeth sit into extraction sockets and are aesthetically good initially
- are prone to loss of aesthetics as resorption progresses
- are difficult to reline/rebase or to add flange
- have poorer retention
- are technically easier to provide, though unless strongly indicated are suboptimal.

Diagnosis

The decision to render a patient edentulous should not be undertaken lightly, and a clear understandable discussion about the risks and benefits of treatment and alternatives should be entered into. A record of the patients' decisions to accede to being rendered edentulous should be noted. The difficulties involved with immediate denture provision must be explained to patients. The patient needs:

■ clear explanation of the technique
■ visits to be planned
■ the staging of planned extractions
■ appropriate cooperation.

The health of the oral and facial tissues must be assessed:

■ Soft tissues: basic periodontal evaluation, probing depths give an indication of the initial collapse/retraction of soft tissues; pre-extraction scaling and polishing
■ Hard tissues: edentulous areas, charting of teeth, use of appropriate justified radiographic images.

Treatment Planning

For a one-tooth immediate denture when no denture is present:

1. Preliminary and/or master impressions, usually in alginate. Impression of opposing arch and suitable interocclusal record
2. Select shape and shade of tooth
3. Extraction of tooth/teeth and delivery of dentures.

For a one-tooth addition to an existing denture:

1. Impression of mouth with denture in situ. Impression of opposing arch and suitable interocclusal record
2. Addition of denture tooth/teeth as soon as possible
3. Extraction of tooth/teeth and delivery of denture.

For multiple-teeth immediate denture, one of the three options is possible:

1. Extract all the teeth at one time and insert immediate dentures.
   or:
2. Extract posterior teeth prior to making immediate dentures to replace anterior teeth.
   or:
3. Post-immediate dentures – difficulties can arise because of ongoing resorption of ridges during denture construction.

Clinical Stages

The clinical stages are the following:

1. Preliminary impressions in alginate with or without impression compound
2. Master impressions in alginate
3. Occlusal record rims for existing edentulous areas
4. Trial stage
5. Delivery of dentures and extraction of teeth
6. Review appointments.

Laboratory Stage

Trimming of casts occurs between try-in and before processing of dentures. The cast should ideally be prepared by the dental surgeon as they alone have seen the patient and undertaken the clinical examination. The cast is marked with a pencil to show the gingival margin, the long axis of the teeth and the length of the teeth. The teeth are removed from the cast. The stone is removed to a depth that is predetermined by the probing depth around the teeth and information from any radiographs. In a flanged denture, the stone is trimmed to simulate the ridge following tooth extraction.

Surgery

In extreme cases, surgery (septal alveolotomy and labial alveolectomy; very rare nowadays) of the ridges is undertaken at the same time as tooth extraction. This may be indicated if there is a large particularly labial undercut or if marked repositioning of the teeth is to be undertaken. It is undesirable to remove the cortical plate of bone as it accelerates bone resorption.

Review Appointments

It is important to review a patient with an immediate denture at regular intervals especially in the first few weeks and months. The initial days are primarily concerned with the postoperative care of the healing tooth sockets, while the later reviews are directed at the management of the resorption. Advice on ensuring that the denture is not removed for the first 24 hours will help limit any inflammatory changes. These changes may become a problem where the denture is left out of the mouth for any length of time and reinsertion then becomes either painful or intolerable. A 24-hour review is therefore essential to make appropriate adjustments.

A timeline of reviews is suggested as follows:

At 24 hours: a general check is made of the overall comfort of the dentures and to ensure no major ulceration has occurred and that the clot is still in situ.

At 1 week: a more detailed check and adjustment of dentures can be made.

At 1 month: the socket has healed and a chair-side temporary reline may be required.

At 3–6 months: the management of loss of fit of the dentures owing to bone resorption is undertaken; this may involve relines and/or rebases, which are undertaken at either the chair side or with the aid of the production laboratory.

At 12 months: a replacement denture is made using the copy denture technique.

There is no evidence base available to suggest that an immediate denture technique is of any clinical benefit although clearly this is an area that has gained much attention recently in the implant field.

4.4 Overdentures

LEARNING OBJECTIVES

You should:
- understand the advantages of overdentures over more conventional dentures
- acknowledge the different overdenture preparations that can be prepared and the advantages and disadvantages of each.

An overdenture is a prosthesis that gains additional support by covering one or more teeth, prepared roots or implants beneath its impression surface. Dental implants have created a new category of overdentures, namely the implant-retained or implant-supported overdenture. This section focuses on tooth-supported overdentures but analogies can be drawn for implant-retained or implant-supported overdentures.

The need for meticulous planning is necessary when undertaking the use of precision attachments in tooth-borne overdentures, their use increases complexity as well as both financial and biological cost.

INDICATIONS

- Converting a partially dentate individual to complete dentures
- Elderly patient with a few remaining teeth and a mucosal-borne partial denture
- Severe attrition/erosion/abrasion
- Cleft plate and surgical defects
- Hypodontia
- Potentially difficult complete denture requirements

CONTRAINDICATIONS

- Poor oral hygiene
- Rampant uncontrolled caries in the remaining dentition
- Uncontrolled periodontal disease
- Inadequate interarch space

ADVANTAGES OF OVERDENTURES

- Maintenance of alveolar bone
- Proprioceptive feedback
- Assistance in control of masticatory force; a patient with an overdenture is able to exert higher forces during mastication with more precision
- Recognising size and texture of objects
- Position of mandible during function
- Minimal load thresholds
- Reduction of psychological trauma

The ideal overdenture scenario would be the retention of four root-filled teeth in the lower arch, the canines and the first molars. This situation, however, is highly improbable as the first molars are commonly among the first teeth to be lost and, therefore, are unlikely to be one of the four remaining teeth. The canines are important teeth as they have long roots and are highly proprioceptive but also command an important position in the line of the arch.

ABUTMENT

Abutment selection depends upon: (Ettinger (2004))

- periodontal status
- number and location in arch
- canines and molars where possible
- conservation status
- need for root canal therapy
- presence of bony undercuts
- extra retention from teeth
- economics.

PERIODONTAL DISEASE

With respect to periodontal disease in patients wearing overdentures, it has been shown that:

- 35% show a significant loss of attachment within the first 3 years
- only 50% of dentures are plaque free, and the majority of patients wear their dentures at night
- disease is related to both poor denture and poor oral hygiene.

Caries prevalence within 5 years of placement in studies of overdenture abutments varies from 13% to 35%. The use of topical fluoride is indicated for these patients, which may be delivered as fluoride varnish at maintenance and recall visits. The daily use of a high fluoride toothpaste is the most cost-effective form of delivery.

Preparation of Coronal Root Surface

Table 4.3 describes various preparations of the coronal root surface for overdenture placement.

The presence of overdenture abutments allows the loads from occlusal forces to be dissipated over a larger area as the support of the periodontal ligament is brought into function. This along with the increase in tactile discrimination and the maintenance of alveolar bone levels make the benefits of this technique invaluable in dealing with certain clinical denture problems.

The use of implant-retained or implant-supported lower overdentures particularly in the mandible is becoming more widespread. An atrophic mandible can be prosthetically very difficult to manage; planning to maintain residual alveolar ridge using dental implants or retained roots confers significant benefit, enhanced retention and improved stability, for a patient who would otherwise have to cope with the limitations of a conventional complete denture.

Evidence Base for This Clinical Approach to Overdenture Denture Construction (Crum and Rooney 1978)

- Patients with complete maxillary dentures and mandibular overdentures showed a mean vertical reduction of 1.8 mm for the anterior part of the maxilla and 0.6 mm for the anterior part of the mandible over a period of 5 years postextraction compared to vertical bone loss on the maxilla of 1.7 mm, while the mandible showed 5.2 mm of bone resorption in conventional patients over the same 5-year period.

- The findings were taken at yearly intervals and showed that the greatest portion of the loss of alveolar bone (approximately 50%) occurred during the first year after extractions.
- This work has been replicated numerous times since in patients with implant-retained or implant-supported overdentures.

The McGill Consensus Statement on Overdentures (Feine et al 2002)

The evidence currently available suggests that the restoration of the edentulous mandible with a conventional denture is no longer the most appropriate first-choice prosthodontic treatment. There is now overwhelming evidence that a two-implant overdenture should become the first choice of treatment for the edentulous mandible.

Mandibular Two Implant-Supported Overdentures as the First Choice Standard of Care for Edentulous Patients – The York Consensus Statement (Thomason et al 2009)

With the advent of dental implants there is now more than one available treatment for edentulous patients. Current evidence suggests that the restoration of the edentulous mandible with a conventional denture is a much poorer alternative than the use of an implant-supported prosthesis. There is now a large body of evidence that supports the proposal that a two–implant-supported mandibular overdenture should be the minimum offered to edentulous patients as a first choice of treatment.

4.5 Removable Partial Dentures

LEARNING OBJECTIVES

You should:
- understand the basic concepts of partial denture construction
- appreciate the importance of design for the prevention of further dental disease
- be able to classify and describe a partial denture using terminology that will be understood by colleagues.

Treatment planning for partial dentures should follow an assessment of the oral health of the patient. Partial dentures carry significant risk in terms of increasing risk for both caries and periodontal disease. The provision of a partial denture should consider the benefits as well as the risks, and all

---

Table 4.3 Preparation of the Coronal Root Surface for Overdenture Placement.

Preparation	Advantages	Disadvantages
Flat facing	Plenty of occlusal clearance; no lateral forces applied; easy to place attachments	Risk of gingival overgrowth; difficult to keep clean; no real additional stability
Dome-shaped facing	Favourable crown:root ratio; efficient plaque control; sufficient occlusal clearance	RCT normally required; may provide less retention and stability than thimble shape
Thimble-shaped facing	Provides maximum retention and stability; RCT may not be required; patient is aware that a tooth still remains	May be insufficient occlusal clearance; unfavourable crown: root ratio; minimal room for attachment placement; protection of tooth surface may be required

RCT, Randomised controlled trial.

alternatives should be discussed with the patient. The need for ongoing maintenance and the responsibilities of the patient in order to maintain and enhance their oral health should be explored. Each partial denture should be designed specifically for each patient, taking into account the capacity of the patient. Consider what appropriate professional support would be required to maintain their oral health encumbered by a partial denture, more importantly the risks and benefits to a patient (of a partial denture) where their capacity to maintain their dentition is impaired, even with appropriate professional support. Fixed alternatives and implants may be of greater benefit, as indeed may accepting the status quo and not providing a partial denture. Not all missing teeth should be or indeed need to be replaced. Stabilisation of existing disease should be undertaken before embarking upon prosthetic treatment, unless incurring a delay would be detrimental to the wellbeing of the patient, where a provisional or interim denture is advisable to restore aesthetics and function. Preliminary impressions are taken for the planning and design of the partial denture. The resulting models will require mounting on an articulator prior to design. There might be significant advantage in undertaking these during the stabilisation of disease as the design of the denture may influence treatment planning, for example, rest seats incorporated into class II restorations, full veneer crowns contoured to provide undercut areas for retention or tooth extraction as a result of overeruption.

Partial denture design intends to:

- preserve what remains
- restore what is missing
- prevent future disease.

When making a partial denture, the following questions need to be addressed:

- Is the prosthesis necessary?
- Is the patient healthy?
- Is the patient suitable for the prosthesis?
- How large a space is to be restored?
- By what structures is the prosthesis to be supported?
- How is the prosthesis to be made?

PARTIAL DENTURE CLASSIFICATION

A simple and effective classification is one that describes partial dentures in terms of the nature of the support utilised by the partial denture:

- Teeth – the only true tooth-borne removable prosthesis is a telescopic bridge
- Mucosa
- Teeth and mucosa.

Further information can be gained by a classification of the partially edentulous arches which relates the edentulous spaces to the remaining teeth (Fig. 4.5; Kennedy 1928).

The following points should be noted when using this classification:

- The most posterior edentulous area determines the class.
- Additional edentulous areas are called modifications.
- The size of the modification is not important.
- If a third molar is missing and not to be replaced, it is not considered in the classification.

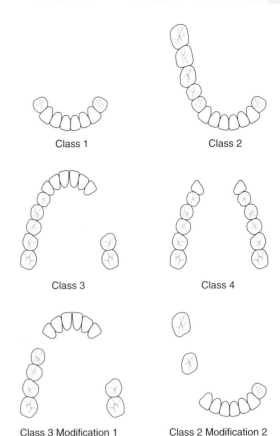

Fig. 4.5 Classification of the partially edentulous arches. Class 1, bilateral free-end saddles; class 2, unilateral free-end saddle; class 3, unilateral bounded saddle; class 4, single-bounded saddle anterior to abutment teeth. Class 3 modification 1 shows an additional bounded saddle; Class 2 modification 2. A unilateral free end saddle with two additional bounded

PRELIMINARY IMPRESSIONS

This preliminary impression will be used to produce a preliminary model which in turn is used to fabricate a special tray, record blocks for the recording of a preliminary registration and then to be surveyed in the process of designing the final partial denture. For this reason these preliminary impressions need to be evaluated with each of these clinical stages in mind. The clinician should be discerning in what constitutes an adequate impression fit for each of these purposes and to avoid the temptation of thinking, 'I can compensate when using the special tray'. A special tray compromised in quality by the standard of the preliminary impression will produce a final impression which is then likely to be compromised. One of the greatest challenges in recording a preliminary impression for a partial denture is ensuring that the stock tray is able to record both the dental hard tissues and the alveolar hard and soft tissues. There is often significant vertical difference between occlusal and incisal levels and the vestibular and buccal sulcus depths. It may very well be desirable to modify the stock tray with impression compound or silicone putty to support alginate. This should ensure recording of all the features required to support and retain the final partial denture.

LABORATORY PRESCRIPTION

The prescription on the laboratory card must be clear and comprehensive. If there is any possibility of confusion, it is essential to discuss the case personally with the technician involved. If preliminary record blocks are required they should be stable and rigid enough to support a wax rim without danger of distortion either by occlusal loading or the effects of prolonged exposure to the oral environment. Special tray design should be compatible with the impression material and technique to be deployed for the working impression. If the laboratory card is not completed and dated, work may not be available for the next appointment.

DESIGN

The design of a partial denture should always be determined before the master impressions are recorded. In this respect, the preliminary casts should be mounted on an articulator and surveyed prior to producing the desired design. In some cases where there are sufficient teeth, casts can be placed in occlusion by hand prior to mounting. In other situations, it will be necessary to construct occlusal rims to register the jaw relationship of the patient. A provisional design should then be produced and, at this stage, a decision should be made on the need for possible tooth preparation or modification.

This may indicate that the following may be necessary:

- Rest seat preparation to provide sufficient space and horizontal surface for any support component.
- Modification of tooth contour preparation to lower survey lines or the addition of light-cured composite resin to create adequate retentive undercuts for clasp arms.
- Altering the path of insertion to enhance retention along the path of natural displacement.
- Preparation of guide planes designed to facilitate paths of insertion or eliminate dead spaces at the abutment-saddle interface.

The proposed design should then be transferred to the laboratory prescription and study cast, which should be retained for reference until the trial stage has been completed. The design prescription must be clear and comprehensive. The design will describe:

- saddles
- support
- retention
- bracing and reciprocation
- connector
- path of insertion.

Second Clinical Visit

Normally, the second visit will be devoted to recording the jaw relationship of the patient prior to mounting casts on the articulator and developing a design. However, the second visit may be for master impressions where the occlusion is sufficiently clear for the casts to be mounted and a design determined.

Recording Jaw Relationships

For the purpose of jaw relationships and their registration, partially dentate patients can be divided into two categories:

1. Patients without an occlusal stop to indicate the correct intercuspal position or vertical dimension of occlusion
2. Patients with occlusal contact in the intercuspal position.

If an occlusal stop is present in the mouth, it may be that the associated intercuspal position is acceptable. If there is horizontal deviation of the mandible after the initial occlusal contact, it may be necessary to correct the deflective occlusal contact by tooth modification. If there is no stable contact or loss of occlusal vertical dimension (OVD), the appropriate OVD will have to be determined by adjusting occlusal rims in relation to the rest vertical dimension (RVD). The OVD is determined by establishing the RVD and modifying the occlusal rims until the OVD is some 2–4 mm short of the RVD, this distance indicating the amount of interocclusal clearance. The horizontal jaw relationship recorded should be the retruded position. Box 4.2 outlines the procedure.

Occlusal Contact in Intercuspal Position

If there is occlusal contact, the rims should be adapted until the natural occlusal contact is observed (Box 4.3). These may be checked visually, by asking the patient if there is even contact, using articulating paper and shimstock. Shimstock is valuable when determining contacts in cases with deep overbites and long labial palatal contacts which cannot otherwise be easily seen.

Box 4.2 Technique to Establish Jaw Relationships in Patients With an Occlusal Stop.

1. Occlusal rims should be supported by a temporary base made to resist both thermal and mechanical distortion. Care should be taken to ensure wax does not fracture or delaminate.
2. In the mouth, the fit and extension of the rim should be modified if necessary to produce acceptable stability.
3. Occlusal contacts should be recognised with the natural teeth in occlusion.
4. The upper occlusal rim should be adjusted so that the occlusal plane is appropriate in relation to the remaining upper natural teeth.
5. If when the patient closes the occlusion shows a premature contact between a tooth and the opposing occlusal rim, the offending part of the rim should be adjusted until the occlusal stop is re-established. If there is an anterior saddle, the rim must indicate the correct incisal level and degree of lip support. Removal of wax from the palatal aspect of this rim might be necessary in order to allow closure of the mandible into the tooth position while retaining the incisal level.
6. The lower rim should then be adjusted until the occlusal stop has again been established.
7. Wax should be removed or added from the buccal and lingual surfaces of the rims align with the natural teeth.
8. The lower rim should be modified so that there is a small gap (about 1 mm) between the occlusal surface of the rim and the opposing teeth or rim when the natural teeth are in contact.
9. The intercuspal or retruded contact position should be recorded using an occlusal registration material such as Bite Registration Paste. This should be thin and only record the cusp tips and incisal tips.
10. The casts should be placed in occlusion using the occlusal rims and checked to determine that the tooth relationship on the casts is the same as that in the mouth. Excessive thickness of particularly elastomeric registration pastes will lead to the wax rims springing apart.
11. Check if there is a premature contact between the heels of a cast and the opposing block or cast, this should be eliminated.

Box 4.3 Technique to Establish Jaw Relationships in Patients Without Occlusal Contact.

1. The maxillary and mandibular rims are trimmed to conform to selected reference points for the remaining natural dentition.
2. The lower rim should be adjusted until there is an even occlusion along the retruded arc of closure at the chosen occlusal vertical dimension. Allowing adequate freeway space between the record blocks at rest.
3. Locating notches should be cut in both rims, a thin and even application of registration paste applied to the occlusal surface of the lower rim, and the patient guided into their path of retruded closure.

Laboratory Prescription

The prescription will cover a number of points. If the next stage is the try-in of a metal framework, the design should be drawn on the laboratory card and full instructions given, including the path of insertion decided by the clinician. Shade, material and mould of artificial teeth should be chosen if the next stage is try-in. It is advisable to undertake framework try-in separately to the tooth setup try-in.

MASTER IMPRESSIONS

Master impressions are obtained at the second or third clinical visit. A suitable impression material is selected based on accuracy and, particularly if the impressions are not being cast promptly, dimensional stability.

Stops may be placed on the fitting surface of the individual trays before correcting peripheral extension. These will aid in ensuring an adequate thickness of the impression material. When free-end saddle areas are present, border moulding should be undertaken:

- The study casts should be retained as a guide for the technician.
- If the metal denture is restoring lower free-end saddles, consider the need for the altered cast technique (see later): if the technique is to be employed, request the addition of acrylic trays to the framework in the saddle areas.

The impression is recorded as described in Box 4.4.

Laboratory Prescription

The laboratory prescription should indicate that casts are to be poured in hardened dental stone. Bearing in mind that the occlusion has already been determined naturally or by

occlusal rims prior to establishing a design, the subsequent stage should be either trial dentures or the production of a metal casting. In the former situation, a shade and mould of teeth must be selected.

The Metal Framework

1. The framework must conform to the original design.
2. The framework must fit the cast. If the fit is unsatisfactory on the cast, it will also be unsatisfactory in the mouth.
3. The casting should be free from porosity or other imperfections.

Note: if any of the above points are not met, the casting should be returned to the laboratory.

The position of the retentive and bracing arms should be checked relative to the survey lines:

1. All components that are designed to be clear of the gingival margin area should be checked to ensure that the clearance is adequate.
2. In the mouth, these aspects should be checked again, remembering that the likelihood of some instability in free-end saddle designs may be caused by spacing beneath the mesh retention.
3. The occlusion is examined to ensure that there are no premature contacts; this should be done by visual examination, from comments by the patient and with the use of articulating paper or disclosing wax. Any premature contact must be removed at this stage.

If the metal framework is satisfactory, request the setting of the teeth on the framework after choosing an appropriate shade and mould of tooth.

Altered Cast Technique

The altered cast technique is an impression method designed to compensate for the differential support provided by the abutment teeth and the mucosa of the edentulous part of the alveolar ridge to a lower partial Kennedy I or II denture base (Box 4.5).

In many cases there is no indication for the use of this technique; indeed it is more often used to correct faults created by a suboptimal master impression.

THE TRIAL DENTURE

The trial denture is the last stage at which modifications can be made before the wax is replaced by acrylic. A careful

Box 4.4 Recording the Impression.

1. The tray is dried and a thin layer of adhesive is applied to the whole of the inner surfaces of the tray and to an area extending 3 mm beyond the periphery of the tray. The adhesive is allowed to dry before loading the tray.
2. A low-viscosity alginate is used to record the impression. In some cases, it may be beneficial to use silicone-based or rubber-based materials.
3. If the impression is satisfactory, a cast should be poured in improved hardened dental stone as soon as possible.
4. All individual trays should be retained until treatment is completed.

Box 4.5 The Altered Cast Technique.

1. The cobalt–chromium (CoCr) casting is tried in the mouth to ensure it adapts correctly.
2. A 0.6-mm fitting tray is added to the free-end saddle of the CoCr framework and border moulded using an appropriate material.
3. The recording of an impression uses zinc oxide/eugenol, with pressure only applied to the rest seat areas of the framework. No direct pressure is applied to the edentulous saddle area.
4. The original master cast is sectioned, removing the posterior part of the model that had recorded the free-end edentulous ridge area.
5. The framework is seated back on the sectioned model and a new posterior section cast into the tray area.

routine must be followed to prevent any mistakes continuing through to the finished dentures. The dentures should be examined first on the mounted casts for:

1. fit of dentures on the casts
2. occlusion
3. position of artificial teeth with regard to adjacent natural ones
4. the arrangement of anterior teeth
5. extension and contouring of wax flanges.

The trial dentures are then examined in the mouth for:

1. fit of the dentures
2. occlusion and OVD
3. contouring of wax flanges with regard to peripheral extension, shaping of polished surface, coverage of gingival margins
4. appearance: modify positions of teeth and incisal edges of anterior teeth to achieve a pleasing result that is acceptable to the patient
5. patient's comments on appearance: as seen in the mirror and ensure that they are satisfied.

If, at this stage, the occlusion is incorrect, modifications must be carried out before continuing with the next stages. Consideration how best to correct this may range from minor chair-side adjustment of the acrylic teeth either within the wax, to re-recording the occlusion and rearticulating the casts, in which case it will be necessary to have a retry to check that any changes are satisfactory.

Laboratory Prescription

Carefully list and describe any modifications you wish the technician to carry out before finishing the dentures. Modifications at this stage should always be minor unless a retry is to be undertaken.

To avoid problems on insertion of the final denture:

1. Undercuts should be blocked out in wax on master cast, in respect of vertical path of insertion.
2. The master cast should be duplicated.
3. Denture should be processed on duplicate cast.
4. The processed denture should be fitted back onto the master cast.

FINAL DENTURE INSERTION

The denture should be checked to see that there are no sharp edges or acrylic 'pearls' on the fitting surface of the saddle areas. Insert the denture into the mouth. Occasionally, the denture cannot be seated because acrylic has been processed into an undercut area on the cast; this results from inadequate blocking out of the undercuts. If the area of acrylic to be removed is not immediately apparent, use pressure relief cream. Always remove the acrylic by approaching with the bur from the fitting surface. The contact between the denture and the tooth in the non-undercut area should not need adjustment.

In the mouth, check:

1. fit of components
2. retention and stability
3. aesthetics
4. occlusion.

Occlusal contact is checked by asking for the patient's comments, by visual inspection and by the use of articulating paper. Articulating paper should be inserted bilaterally.

Occlusal adjustment should be continued until both the patient's comments and visual inspection confirm that even contact has been achieved in intercuspal position. Attention should be given to occlusal contacts in lateral and protrusive positions. In many patients, the dentures will be adjusted so that they conform to the occlusal guidance provided by the remaining natural teeth.

Advice to the Patient

The patient must be shown and taught the correct way to handle the denture for insertion and removal and vulnerable components must be pointed out. A printed sheet of instructions should be provided for the patient. This will mention, in particular, aspects such as cleaning/eating/wearing at night/pain/need for regular recall, including recall with the hygienist.

It is important to discuss these points verbally with the patient first of all. The purpose of such a sheet is simply to act as an aide-mémoire. Finally you should ensure that the patient knows whom to contact in the event of problems arising with the denture.

The responsibility for the prosthetic care of the patient does not end with the insertion of a denture.

Review Appointment

The patient should be asked for comments on the first week of wearing the dentures. A history must be taken of any complaint. Subsequent examination must be directed to diagnosing the cause of the complaint before making any adjustments. Whether or not there are any problems reported by the patient, the denture-bearing tissues must be examined and the occlusion must be checked. At times, a patient may claim to be perfectly comfortable even though extensive ulceration is present.

Any inflammation of the denture-bearing tissues that is not related to the peripheral area is most likely from occlusal causes. Therefore, a careful inspection must be made of occlusal contact in tooth position and excursive movements, and the necessary adjustments made. The impression surface of the denture should only be adjusted where there is clear evidence of excessive pressure. Should attention of the impression surface be required, a disclosing material such as pressure indicator paste should be used.

A check must be made on the patient's oral and denture hygiene. This can be done with the use of a disclosing solution. Steps to reinforce plaque control must be taken.

Evidence-Based Approach to the Provision of Partial Dentures (Graham et al 2006)

1. Existing research suggests that 30–50% of patients who are prescribed a removable partial denture (RPD) never or only occasionally wear the prosthesis.
2. This study has identified key factors that influence professional provision and patient use of RPDs.

3. For patients, wearing an RPD is not simply a matter of aesthetics, but of avoiding the social stigma associated with tooth loss.

Why Do Dentists Struggle With Removable Partial Denture Design? An Assessment of Financial and Educational Issues (Lynch and Allen 2006)

1. Financial factors did not have as significant an effect on the quality of prescription and fabrication of cobalt–chromium removable partial dentures (CCRPDs) as compared to educational factors.
2. Serious deficiencies in the teaching of CCRPDs during vocational training were identified, and these deficiencies lead to deskilling of newly qualified dentists.

Critical Review of Some Dogmas in Prosthodontics (Carlsson 2009)

1. Kayser, in 1981, published his opinions on the shortened dental arch (SDA). His message was that there is sufficient adaptive capacity in subjects with SDA when at least four occlusal units are left. Kayser's and his successor's research groups have conducted a series of clinical cross-sectional and longitudinal studies on SDA.
2. The World Health Organization guidelines published in 1992 provided strong support by suggesting that the SDA concept was a possible clinical alternative in situations when economy and service resources are limited.

Self-Assessment: Questions

MULTIPLE CHOICE QUESTIONS (TRUE/FALSE)

1. Complete denture assessment should include:
   a. A history of tooth loss
   b. A denture history
   c. A medical history
   d. A social history
   e. A summary of the patient's expectations
2. Impression compound contains:
   a. Stearic acid
   b. Borax
   c. Talc
   d. Paraffin wax
   e. Copper
3. An immediate denture is advisable for:
   a. A single tooth replacement in the anterior region of the mouth
   b. A patient who will require the surgical removal of the broken down tooth
   c. A patient who is at risk of tooth movement if a replacement unit is not placed soon after extraction
   d. A patient losing an upper second molar tooth
   e. A case where haemorrhage control may be required
4. A partial denture clasp made of cast cobalt–chromium:
   a. Should not be used as an occlusally approaching clasp arm on a premolar
   b. Is more flexible than a wrought gold clasp of similar length
   c. Engages 0.5 mm undercut
   d. Is a potential food trap
   e. Can be circumferential, occlusally approaching or gingivally approaching in design
5. The altered cast technique is used to:
   a. Account for the differential compression between hard and soft tissues
   b. Remount flasked dentures to perfect the occlusion
   c. Destroy unwanted models
   d. Construct a master cast that is altered by partial replacement with a cast of an additional impression
   e. Modify a cast to allow for rest seat preparation intraorally
6. The indications for the 'copy denture' technique include:
   a. Recurrent fracture of a previous upper denture base
   b. A spare set of satisfactory dentures
   c. An elderly patient who has worn a satisfactory set of dentures for many years
   d. Incorrect positioning of the anterior teeth
   e. Replacement of immediate dentures
7. The choice of denture teeth:
   a. Is dependent on the age of the patient
   b. Is dependent on the patient's complexion
   c. Should be determined by the patient
   d. Should conform to the patient's facial contour
   e. Is related to the upper lip length
8. The neutral zone technique:
   a. Can be used in the maxilla
   b. Should have the upper denture in place while it is being recorded
   c. Is used to record the zone of minimal conflict
   d. Helps to determine the pre-extraction position of the natural dentition
   e. Requires the use of laboratory stents to locate the teeth
9. Elastic impression materials include:
   a. Plaster
   b. Alginate
   c. Zinc oxide/eugenol
   d. Agar
   e. Silicone
10. At the jaw registration stage in complete dentures:
   a. The freeway space of the dentures should be determined
   b. The horizontal relationship of the jaws is recorded
   c. The tooth shade is chosen
   d. The tooth mould is selected
   e. Heat-cured base plates may provide increased stability
11. Surveying for partial denture construction:
   a. Is only carried out on the preliminary model
   b. Is always carried out at 90° to the occlusal plane
   c. Should use an analysing rod prior to deciding the angle of survey

d. Determines naturally occurring guideplanes
e. Is not necessary in acrylic partial denture construction

12. Various techniques used in the management of the free-end saddle situation include:
    a. Split-cast technique
    b. RPI (rest, plate, I bar) design
    c. Altered cast technique
    d. Balance of forces
    e. Flexible connectors

EXTENDED MATCHING ITEMS QUESTIONS

Theme: Partial dentures
For each of the statements (a–e), select from the list below (1–10) the single most appropriate component or function of component of partial dentures that matches the statement. Each diagnosis may be used once, more than once or not at all:

1. Saddles
2. Support
3. Occlusal rests
4. Retention
5. Bracing
6. Stability
7. Reciprocation
8. Connector
9. Indirect retention
10. Clasps.

    a. The resistance to vertical force directed towards the mucosa.
    b. The resistance to horizontal forces provided by rigid components of the denture.
    c. Function, anatomical constraints, hygiene, rigidity and patient acceptability all influence the choice of what?
    d. This resists pivotal movement of a denture through the hinge axis of the clasp tips.
    e. The principle of horizontal resistance to tooth movement that may occur during clasp engagement.

CASE HISTORY QUESTIONS

Case History 1

A 60-year-old male presents complaining of a loose upper denture. He has been edentulous for over 20 years and has had two sets of complete dentures in this time. On examination, his palate presents as seen in Fig. 4.6.

1. What questions in the history of this patient are important in this problem?
2. What are the priorities in the management of this patient?
3. What are the differential diagnoses?

Case History 2

A 50-year-old lady presents with an unretentive upper denture and a lower denture that causes recurrent ulceration (Fig. 4.7).

1. What are the likely causes for the symptoms that this patient presents with?

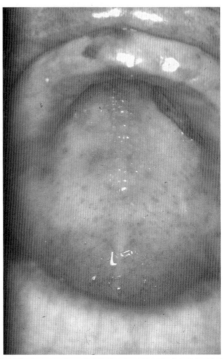

Fig. 4.6 60-year-old male with loose upper denture.

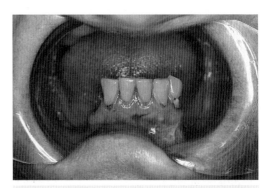

Fig. 4.7 Ulcerated lower arch of a 50-year-old female.

2. How could you resolve the problem of the unretentive upper denture?
3. What treatment would be suggested to resolve the problems of her lower arch?

SHORT NOTE QUESTIONS

Write short notes on:

1. disinfection of impression materials
2. special trays
3. heat-cured base plates
4. the important features in complete denture construction that contribute to the retention of a denture, naming three anatomical features that may affect the retention of complete dentures
5. an Every denture design
6. gingival stripping caused by partial dentures
7. spoon dentures

8. the properties that a clasp should exhibit and list three commonly utilised materials used to construct denture clasps
9. denture stomatitis
10. angular cheilitis
11. denture hygiene.

ESSAY QUESTION

List the basic principles of removable partial denture design and describe their importance in relation to the maintenance of oral health.

Self-Assessment: Answers

MULTIPLE CHOICE ANSWERS

1. a. True. A history of tooth loss will provide an approximate timescale for the resorptive processes of that individual patient.
   b. True. A denture history will give some indication as to the tolerance of the patient to a prosthesis.
   c. True. A medical history may provide information regarding current medication that could result in a dry mouth and, therefore, affect the possible retention of a prosthesis. Several other factors in a medical history may also affect complete denture construction.
   d. True. A history of smoking and/or drinking will increase the prevalence of oral malignancy and may necessitate more frequent reviews to monitor the oral mucosa.
   e. True. It is important to assess the patient's expectations as these can often be unrealistic and may affect the patient's acceptance of a prosthesis.
2. a. True. Because stearic acid improves flow properties of material.
   b. False. Borax is used as a retarder in gypsum products.
   c. True. Talc increases the viscosity of the material, reducing its thermal contraction.
   d. True. Determines the softening temperature.
   e. False. Copper is metallic and is not an impression compound.
3. a. True. An immediate denture can provide an aesthetic replacement of an anterior tooth.
   b. False. An immediate denture would not be indicated as the bone contour of the area after surgical intervention is uncertain.
   c. True. An immediate denture can be used as a space maintainer.
   d. False. It is rarely necessary unless an addition to an existing partial denture can be carried out to replace a posterior unit in this manner.
   e. True. Although this point is often one of debate, it is generally accepted that an immediate denture can assist in haemorrhage control if constructed carefully.
4. a. True. A cast cobalt–chromium clasp of this length will not be flexible enough to engage an undercut.
   b. False. A gold clasp is more flexible.
   c. False. Engages a 0.25 mm undercut.
   d. True. Partial dentures themselves could be considered as food traps but the clasp component particularly causes a problem.
   e. True. These are the three traditional designs of clasp arm.

5. a. True. This is the concept of the altered cast technique.
   b. False. That is the split-cast technique.
   c. False. This is not the purpose of the technique.
   d. True. This is how an altered cast is carried out.
   e. False. This is not the purpose of the technique.
6. a. False. The reason for the recurrent fracture of the denture base would need to be addressed prior to remaking the denture.
   b. True. This is a method of duplicating dentures.
   c. True. If a patient has become accustomed to the polished surfaces of an existing denture then it is often advantageous to copy this.
   d. False. There would be no advantage of a copy technique if the tooth position had to be changed.
   e. True. This would mean that the original tooth position was copied.
7. a. True. The age of the patient will dictate tooth colour and length.
   b. True. This will determine tooth colour.
   c. False. Often patients will choose tooth colour to be too white; therefore, their approval should be sought after the dentist's selection.
   d. True. This will help to determine the tooth mould.
   e. True. The length of the upper incisors will be partly determined by the upper lip length.
8. a. False. The neutral zone can only be used in the mandible.
   b. True. Upper lip support is essential to record the neutral zone.
   c. True. The neutral zone is often called the zone of minimal conflict.
   d. True. The technique helps to determine the likely position of the original dentition.
   e. True. This is how the technician positions the teeth from the neutral zone impression.
9. a. False. Plaster is a non-elastic impression material.
   b. True. Alginate is an elastic impression material.
   c. False. Zinc oxide/eugenol is a non-elastic impression material.
   d. True. Agar is an elastic impression material.
   e. True. Silicone is an elastic impression material.
10. a. True. The occlusal face height of the denture should be recorded at the jaw registration stage.
    b. True. The relationship of the mandible to the maxilla in the retruded contact position is recorded.
    c. True. The technician needs this information for the try-in stage.
    d. True. The technician needs this information for the try-in stage.

e. True. The use of heat-cured bases does provide a more stable record rim for the registration stage.

11. a. False. The master model has to be surveyed also.
    b. False. Although this is often the first choice of survey, it is often the case that the path of insertion should follow a different path.
    c. True. The use of an analysing rod helps to assess the path of insertion prior to the initial survey.
    d. True. The use of naturally occurring guideplanes will aid greatly in the retention of a denture.
    e. False. Undercut areas must be blocked out prior to processing an acrylic partial denture.

12. a. False. This technique is used to remount casts after processing.
    b. True. The use of a mesial rest, distal plate and I bar design is commonly applied in this situation.
    c. True. The altered cast can be used to address this clinical situation.
    d. True. This design concept has been used in the free-end saddle situation.
    e. True. The use of stress-breaking or flexible connectors can be used in this clinical situation.

EXTENDED MATCHING ITEMS ANSWERS

a. 2
b. 5
c. 8
d. 9
e. 7

CASE HISTORY ANSWERS

Case History 1

1. History taken would reveal:
   - social history: this patient was a heavy smoker who smoked around 60 cigarettes a day. He was also a heavy drinker.
   - dental history: the patient had experienced surgery to his front teeth prior to their extraction 10 years ago. The lesion in his palate was first noticed 6 months ago and has progressively got larger since then resulting in his denture no longer fitting.
   - medical history: this may have some relevance to the problem but did not in this case.

2. Resulting from this patient's presentation and history, it is unlikely that the lesion in the palate is a simple traumatic ulcer and, therefore, an urgent referral to an oral maxillofacial surgeon or an incisional biopsy must be carried out. The suggestion that the denture should be left out for a week and the situation reviewed given the history and presentation of the lesion would be ill-advised.

3. Differential diagnosis. The main palatal lesion was an adenoid cystic carcinoma, but it could have been a squamous cell carcinoma, a pleomorphic adenoma or a mucoepidermoid carcinoma. The histological appearance would have confirmed the diagnosis. The lesion on the ridge was an amalgam tattoo.

Case History 2

1. The upper denture problem is likely to be related to a flabby ridge that has developed as a result of the retention of the lower natural dentition. This often results in the patient having a problem of support or stability of the denture, although there can also be a problem of retention. The recurrent oral ulceration of the lower ridge is likely to be a result of an unretentive and unstable lower denture caused by the lack of denture-bearing area and also the height discrepancy between the occlusal plane and the residual ridge.

2. The management of an unsupported or flabby ridge is by use of a selective compression impression technique or the use of a mucostatic impression technique. A brief summary of these two techniques should be included.

3. The problem of the lower arch is complex; however, the extraction of the remaining lower dentition may just transfer the problem from that of a partial denture problem to one of a complete lower denture problem. This particular case was managed by root filling the lower canines and using stud attachments to retain an acrylic partial lower denture. This solved the presenting complaints because the stud retainers stopped the movement of the lower denture, thus eliminating the traumatic ulceration.

SHORT NOTE ANSWERS

1. Answer should include a summary of the guidelines on the disinfection of dental impressions (Control of Substances Hazardous to Health Regulations 1999). An impression should be rinsed under running water on removal from the mouth to remove any saliva, blood or debris. The impression should then be disinfected. Possible disinfectant solutions should be listed and the duration of soak stated (e.g. sodium hypochlorite 10 000 ppm for 5 minutes minimum). The effects of such disinfectants on the stability of the impression material should also be commented on.

2. Special trays are constructed of a variety of materials including shellac, acrylics and light-cured composite materials. The use of adhesives can be complemented by the addition of perforations within the tray design. Trays should be extended ideally to 2 mm short of the functional sulcus depth. The spacing of a tray is dependent on the impression material being used and varies from 3 mm spacing for impression plaster to 0.5 mm for zinc oxide/eugenol.

3. Heat-cured base plates can be used at the jaw registration stage of complete denture construction. They provide increased stability to the denture for use at this stage and give a good guide to the likely retention and stability of the completed denture. They potentially can have disadvantages in that if there is minimal interarch space then premature contact of the base plates between the maxillary tuberosity region of the upper plate and the retromolar pad region of the lower can occur. The processing of the final denture can potentially cause distortion of the base plate if it is not carried out carefully.

4. Features that contribute to retention include:
   - peripheral (border) seal
   - area of impression surface
   - accuracy of fit
   - adhesion between the saliva, denture and oral mucosa
   - cohesion within saliva film
   - orientation of the denture-bearing structures: the shape of the palate, for example, will influence the retention, a flatter palate providing better retention but less stability
   - correct positioning of the denture base in relation to displacing forces, namely soft tissue forces of the lips, cheeks and tongue
   - anatomical features: for example, maxillary and mandibular tori, frenal attachments, muscle attachments, genial tubercles, hard/soft palate junction, maxillary tuberosity.

5. An Every denture conforms to a specific design to ensure gingival health. It is restricted to use in the upper arch. The denture design requires the presence of bounded saddles. The design should incorporate the following features: point contact between natural teeth and artificial teeth, wide embrasures, uncovered gingivae, distal stabilisers and a 'free occlusion'. The general principles of partial denture design should be followed.

6. An acrylic or cobalt–chromium connector of a denture can cover the gingival margins of teeth. If insufficient support for the partial denture exists, then gingival stripping can occur of the dentition under load. This can be avoided by providing adequate tooth support for the denture, using dental connectors that do not cover the gingival margins of teeth and by the maintenance of good oral hygiene.

7. Spoon dentures are simple acrylic dentures made to replace one or more anterior maxillary teeth. They derive their support from the ridge and palate. They are used commonly as they are cheap, easy to construct and modify. However, such a denture is weak and non-rigid and it is commonly unretentive and poses a possible airway risk.

8. Properties should include the following:
   - Strength. Should be strong enough in thin cross-section to withstand oral forces. Adding molybdenum in small amounts to cobalt–chromium alloy increases its strength; however, the addition of nickel decreases its strength while increasing its ductility.
   - Ductility. In cobalt–chromium, the grains tend to be large and, therefore, there are only two to three grains across the thickness of a clasp. This reduces its ductility and it is easily broken or distorted.
   - Malleability. A malleable material can be worked into thinner sections; this property is of importance in wrought clasps.
   - Proportional limit. The limit beyond which a clasp will permanently deform or fracture.
   - Torsional elasticity. The rigid position of a clasp arm should be above the survey line. The torsional elasticity of the metal in the more rigid upright part provides flexibility to the horizontal arm and a more effective distribution of stress throughout the structure.
   - Modulus of elasticity (resilience). The higher the modulus, the shallower the undercuts that can be engaged.
   - Appearance. A tooth-coloured clasp may be more aesthetically pleasing but may not provide other optimal properties. Often gold alloys are more aesthetically acceptable intraorally than 'silver'-coloured alloys.
     Three commonly used materials could be chosen from cast cobalt–chromium, wrought stainless steel, cast gold, wrought gold, tooth-coloured resin clasps.

9. Denture stomatitis is a multifactorial condition. The aetiological factors include poor denture hygiene, trauma, *Candida albicans* infection, endocrine imbalance, iron deficiency anaemia, reduced salivary flow, folate deficiency and diabetes mellitus. The clinical picture is normally a diffuse erythematous area associated with denture support. Treatment includes the establishment and control of the relevant aetiological factors.

10. Angular cheilitis is usually as a result of an infection with *C. albicans*, *Staphylococcus aureus* and/or *Streptococci*. It is commonly related to denture stomatitis, but other causes include iron deficiency, hypovitaminoses, malabsorption conditions, HIV infection and other immune defects. Investigations can include blood pictures, smears for fungal hyphae and bacteriological cultures. The treatment should involve the resolution of any systemic predisposing factors where possible and the use of topical antifungals and antibacterial agents.

11. Denture hygiene should involve a regimen of brush, soak, brush. The adherence of plaque to both acrylic and cobalt–chromium requires that hygiene measures are carried out at least twice daily. The initial brushing will remove any food debris and then the use of a proprietary soaking solution will loosen and remove stains, plaque and calculus deposits. The final brushing stage will remove any residual debris. It is essential that a brush or cleanser that is not too abrasive is used as otherwise this will scratch the acrylic and potentially provide a rougher surface for plaque attachment.

ESSAY ANSWER

This essay plan is to be seen as a template to the structure of the essay. The content is not exhaustive but gives an example in each area of the content that could be included.

Introduction

All removable prostheses will by their nature attract or retain more plaque in the mouth than if an appliance were not present. However, various features of design can influence this, as well as factors of patient motivation and instruction on cleaning techniques and materials. The maintenance of oral health is also not purely dependent on oral hygiene but also relies on the design of the prosthesis, which should aim to preserve what remains and prevent future disease.

Important Features to Discuss

Saddles. Number of saddles and the need to replace all missing units to prevent overeruption or drifting has important implications.

Support. The choice between tooth support or mucosal support of the denture will influence the load distribution to the oral structures and could, therefore, affect the health of the oral tissues.

Retention. All forms of clasps will cause plaque retention; therefore, the correct number and positioning of clasps is essential to maintain oral health.

Bracing/reciprocation. The prevention of movement of a denture base during function will aid in the protection of the dental tissues.

Connector. If a connector is designed to cover as little gingival margins as possible, this will minimise gingival damage and limit plaque and debris accumulation.

Indirect retention. The provision of indirect retention will help to prevent rotational forces being applied to abutment teeth and will, therefore, be important in the maintenance of oral health.

References

Carlsson GE. Critical review of some dogmas in prosthodontics. *J Prosthodont Res.* 2009;53(1):3–10.

Crum RJ, Rooney GE Jr. Alveolar bone loss in overdentures: a 5-year study. *J Prosthet Dent.* 1978;40(6):610–613.

Ettinger RL, Fang Q. Abutment tooth loss in patients with overdentures. *J Am Dent Assoc.* 2004;135(6):739–46.

Feine JS, Carlsson GE, Awad MA, et al. The McGill consensus statement on overdentures. Montreal, Quebec, Canada. *Int J Prosthodont.* 2002; 15:413–414.

Fenlon MR, Sherriff M. An investigation of factors influencing patients' satisfaction with new complete dentures using structural equation modelling. *J Dent.* 2008;36:427–34.

Felton D, Cooper L, Duqum I, et al. Evidence-based guidelines for the care and maintenance of complete dentures: a publication of the American College of Prosthodontists. *J Am Dent Assoc.* 2011;142:1S–20S.

Graham R, Mihaylov S, Jepson N, et al. Determining 'need' for a removable partial denture: a qualitative study of factors that influence dentist provision and patient use. *Br Dent J.* 2006;200:155–158.

Kawai Y, Murakami H, Shariati B, et al. Do traditional techniques produce better conventional complete dentures than simplified techniques? *J Dent.* 2005;33:659–668.

Kennedy E. *Partial Denture Construction.* Brooklyn, NY: Dental Items of Interest Publishing Co; 1928.

Lynch CD, Allen PF. Why do dentists struggle with removable partial denture design? An assessment of financial and educational issues. *Br Dent J.* 2006;200:277–281.

Thomason JM, Feine J, Exley C. Mandibular two implant-supported overdentures as the first choice standard of care for edentulous patients – the York Consensus Statement. *Br Dent J.* 2009;207:185–186.

5 *Restorative Management of Dental Implants*

Overview

Assisting patients to attain a healthy, functional and aesthetic dentition is one of the primary goals of any dental practitioner. Unfortunately, there are many reasons why this goal might not be achieved, and there is then a requirement for intervention to repair or replace what is damaged or lost over time. Osseointegrated dental implants have been developed over the last fifty years and, in addition to removable dentures, bridges and tooth transplants, provide a further option for replacing missing teeth. This chapter provides an intentionally basic overview of implant dentistry.

After an introduction to basic terminology, the chapter is organised to follow a patient's pathway through presurgical planning, implant placement, provisional and then definitive restoration, followed by the maintenance phase of management. The use of dental implants for both fixed and removable restorations is described.

In the United Kingdom, the knowledge and skills to provide implant restorations is regarded as an area that requires clinicians to undertake additional training following basic qualification as a dentist.

5.1 Basic Implant Terminology and Componentry

LEARNING OBJECTIVES

You should:
- be familiar with the basic elements that go to make up typical implant-borne restorations
- understand the basic difference between primary implant stability and osseointegration.

A basic understanding of implant treatment requires knowledge of the component parts that go to make up implant-borne restorations. Implant dentistry is a rapidly changing area of clinical practice with ever-evolving products and techniques. It is not the intention here to provide a detailed review of implant dentistry of individual implant brands, but rather to provide an understanding of the underlying principles of implant dentistry from a generic perspective.

A basic implant-borne restoration may be considered as comprising three distinct elements: one that interfaces with the hard tissues; an element which interfaces with the soft tissues and an element that interfaces with the oral environment. These different structural elements may take the form of either one, two or three separate components. Fig. 5.1 shows the three separate components diagrammatically and how they are associated with one another in a typical single crown implant restoration. The component that is osseointegrated with bone is usually referred to as the implant itself. The implant in Fig. 5.1 would be expected to have bone up to the region of the implant–abutment interface. The abutment is the component that is connected to the implant by a holding screw known as the abutment screw. It traverses the overlying soft tissue to provide a connection between the implant in bone and the overlying restoration: it is the *transmucosal* part. The final component of the system is the restoration or superstructure that gains support and retention from the implant through the abutment. Although this is a basic overview of a generic implant system, it may be applied to many products whether they comprise separate implant, abutment and restoration, or whether, for example, the implant and abutment are one physical unit.

IMPLANTS

Osseointegrated implants are available in a vast array of sizes, shapes, surface morphologies and implant–abutment interface-linking configurations. In all cases, the primary aim of the implant is to integrate rapidly and reliably with the bone in order to provide long-term stability and retention for the overlying restoration. The tightness in bone upon insertion of an implant is partly responsible for what is referred to as *primary stability*. Good *primary stability* assists in achieving osseointegration at the outset and is influenced by implant thread design and whether, for example, an implant is tapered or parallel sided in overall shape. *Primary stability* is also influenced by what is termed bone quality (related to cortical and cancellous bone density) and the shape of the site in bone (the osteotomy)

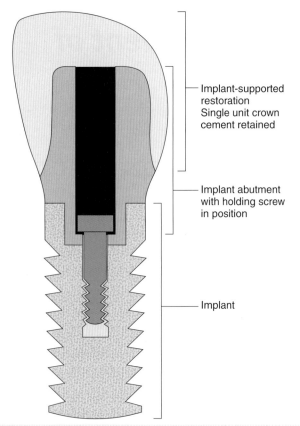

Implant-supported
restoration
Single unit crown
cement retained

Implant abutment
with holding screw
in position

Implant

Fig. 5.1 Diagram to show the basic elements of an implant restoration.

where the implant is to be inserted. The long-term function of the implant is dependent upon establishment of biological osseointegration, or *secondary stability*. Many factors influence the establishment of osseointegration, but fundamental to the process are the presence of a biocompatible implant material (usually titanium dioxide which forms naturally on the surface of titanium), a healthy infection-free bony recipient site, avoidance of heat generation during osteotomy preparation and implant insertion and good *primary stability*. Successful osseointegration results in direct connection of living bone onto the surface of the implant and is indicated by a completely non-mobile implant that gives a high-pitched/bright note when percussed. Failure of an implant to osseointegrate or loss of *secondary stability* is apparent when an implant is mobile, in which case it may eventually exfoliate.

ABUTMENTS

An abutment links the implant to the restoration in the mouth. It provides support and retention for the overlying restoration through either a fixed physical link (e.g. a permanently cemented or screw-retained single crown) or a breakable physical link (e.g. a magnetically retained implant-assisted overdenture). Somewhere along the surface of the abutment or at the coronal end of the implant, a circumferential soft tissue (mucosal) seal is established consisting of epithelial and connective tissue elements.

IMPLANT RESTORATIONS

Implant-supported restorations serve to replace the tissues which have been lost, and it is convenient to consider these as either replacing teeth or replacing a combination of teeth *and* supporting tissues. A further way to classify restorations is according to whether they are fixed, so that they cannot be removed by the patient (e.g. cemented or screw-retained implant crowns or bridges), or removable restorations that are designed so that the patient can disengage them (e.g. partial or complete dentures that are connected to abutments by means of retentive anchors of various sorts: implant-assisted overdentures).

5.2 Planning Implant Restorations

LEARNING OBJECTIVES

You should:
- be familiar with the indications and contraindications of using dental implants
- be aware of the stages involved in planning for dental implant restorations.

It is essential, as with any treatment planning, that the final outcome is taken into account at the outset of the planning process. Consideration of the final restoration and the expectations of the patient must be taken into account at the outset so that the treatment plan can achieve the most desirable outcome.

INDICATIONS

Implants are primarily indicated when there is partial or total loss of the dentition and/or the supporting tissues or where there are teeth that are considered to have a hopeless prognosis that will require replacement. Teeth may be missing due to developmental problems, or the loss of teeth and supporting tissues may be a consequence of dental caries and periodontitis, resorptive lesions, or due to trauma, advanced tooth-wear or treatment for jaw pathology, such as neoplasia. Implants provide retention and support for a dental restoration that may take the form of a single tooth, groups of teeth or the entire dentition in one or both jaws. As well as replacement of missing teeth, each type of prosthesis can also include missing periodontium and alveolar tissue, or even facial appendages, such as the nose, orbit or auricle. Implants destined for future use as foundations for dental restorations can also be used in the interim as anchors for orthodontic treatment.

CONTRAINDICATIONS AND RELATIVE CONTRAINDICATIONS

There are few absolute contraindications for implant treatment. The surgery to insert implants may be considered an elective oral surgical procedure, and therefore any absolute or relative contraindications for surgery will also be applicable to surgery involved in the insertion of dental implants. In general terms, local or systemic conditions that impact upon wound healing would be expected to have the same effect upon healing at the implant site and may impact on the process of osseointegration and long-term success of implant treatment. As well as surgery, patients need to be able to tolerate the prosthodontic and maintenance stages of implant dentistry such as having impressions. A sufficient mandibular opening range is required to allow safe and effective use of instruments such as screwdrivers.

Absence of sufficient bone in which to place implants may rule out implant restorations unless bone can be augmented by some means. Patients who have a history of periodontal disease and associated risk factors such as smoking and diabetes are likely to be at higher risk of complications, and the presence of these factors can be regarded as relative contraindications.

CASE SELECTION

The selection of patients for implant treatment begins with thorough history and examination. It is important to determine why the patient is seeking implant treatment and to ascertain their understanding of what is involved, as well as finding out their expectations of the likely outcome in terms of function and aesthetics. It should then be possible to balance the patient's expectations with what is clinically achievable to ensure that both the patient and the clinical team are likely to be satisfied with the outcome.

A detailed discussion of the care pathway should be undertaken with the patient to ensure that they understand the extent of the procedures, timescales, side effects, risks, possible complications and long-term maintenance implications. For example, during the healing phase, it is sometimes necessary to ask the patient not to wear an interim prosthesis for a short period to aid healing. This may not be acceptable to some patients.

For fee-paying patients, the cost of delivering implant treatment (and long-term maintenance) must be clearly laid out in writing along with payment schedules and terms and conditions.

PROSTHODONTICALLY DRIVEN (OR REVERSE) PLANNING

Implant planning commences by establishing the features of the teeth and any missing alveolus that are to become the implant-borne restoration. In today's implant dentistry, it is not acceptable to simply place an implant where bone is available, on the assumption it can be effectively restored. A decision needs to be made as to whether it is appropriate to use the features of the patient's remaining dentition or current prosthesis as a basis for planning implant positions, or whether any modifications to the current situation need to be made to improve aesthetic features or occlusion before planning implant positions in detail.

For partially dentate patients, accurate preoperative study casts, mounted on a semi-adjustable articulator, will support the planning process and enable simulation of the final restoration using a diagnostic wax-up or try-in prosthesis.

When planning implant restorations in the aesthetic zone, particular attention needs to be given to planning how the mucosal (pink) supporting tissues around a final restoration will appear. For example, in cases where there is a high level to the animated upper lip, it may be unacceptable to restore an implant which, though stable, exhibits un-natural supporting tissues.

SPECIAL INVESTIGATIONS AND DETAILED PLANNING

Once the prosthodontic arrangement has been envisaged, it is necessary to find out whether there is sufficient bone present to accommodate implant(s) in the ideal position(s) to support the proposed restoration. Each type of implant restoration has particular requirements in this regard, and details are beyond the scope of this text.

An approximate estimation of the dimension of the alveolus may be made using callipers that penetrate the overlying soft tissues to estimate bone width along an edentulous space (ridge mapping). In all cases though, a detailed clinical examination needs to be supplemented with additional radiographic assessment such as plain film radiography, and computed tomography, such as coned beam computed tomography (CBCT). CBCT provides detailed three-dimensional (3-D) information about bone volume and adjacent structures which must not be violated during surgery to insert implant(s). It is usual to gain further information from CBCT scans by using software applications that enable the proposed prosthesis to be visualised and to carry out virtual implant insertion tailored to the requirements of the prosthesis (Fig. 5.2). The ways this can be achieved include:

- Creating virtual tooth replacements within the planning software itself
- Obtaining the CBCT whilst the patient has a radio-opaque replica of the intended prosthesis in place
- Using the planning software to combine a 3-D optical scan of the intended prosthesis with the CBCT data.

At this point in planning, it should be possible to determine if there is sufficient bone volume to house implant(s), or if not, whether additional bone can be generated using a bone augmentation technique such as bone grafting. Occasionally, radiographic investigations may show that insertion of implant(s) in prosthodontically driven positions is not possible.

If it is decided that there is sufficient bone to insert the implants in the required positions, it is usual to use the information to generate an implant insertion guide (often called a surgical stent), either using a digital workflow directly from the simulated planning environment or by traditional 'analogue' means in a dental production laboratory. It is also possible to use digital planning information with so-called dynamic guidance systems that allow visualisation of the bone-drilling instruments in relation to the 3-D plan in real-time, thereby avoiding the need for a surgical guide. Planning information can also be used to prefabricate restorations ready for immediate use following implant insertion.

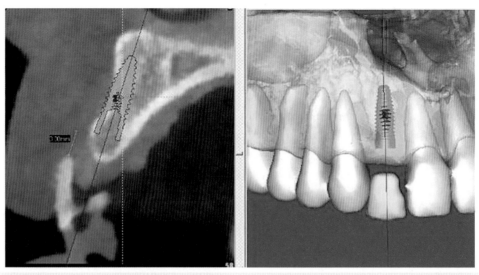

Fig. 5.2 Virtual placement of an implant to replace a missing maxillary lateral incisor. The figure on the left shows a cross section, and the figure on the right, a transparent 3D image of a virtually placed implant in a position to support the proposed prosthetic tooth (shown in yellow in the right hand figure).

TYPES OF RESTORATION

Restorations supported by dental implants may be classified into two broad groups:

- Those that replace only the lost dental hard tissues (teeth themselves) and are therefore directly comparable to conventional single crowns or bridges, with the dental implants acting as the 'roots' of the teeth (Fig. 5.3).
- Restorations that replace both the teeth and the supporting alveolar tissues to a greater or lesser extent. Such prostheses include implant-assisted removable dentures and fixed implant-assisted bridges that incorporate pink-coloured prosthetic material (Fig. 5.4).

Single tooth and tooth-only bridge restorations are retained on the implant abutments using either a cement lute or via screw retention. The access hole for the screw is restored using a directly placed restoration such as composite resin after first applying a layer of soft protection over the abutment screw head. Implant-assisted removable dentures achieve greater support and retention than their conventional counterparts because the implants with their abutments act to support and retain the overdenture. Abutments for implant-assisted dentures may incorporate various kinds of precision attachment, magnet or a bar and clip (Fig. 5.5).

The fixed implant-assisted bridge that incorporates pink-coloured prosthetic material to replace both teeth and pink tissues (periodontium and alveolus) is sometimes called a *hybrid prosthesis*. For added strength, it usually incorporates a titanium framework that is customised to be screwed either directly to the implants themselves or to transmucosal abutments.

TIMING OF PROCEDURES

Multidisciplinary treatment planning for implant cases is helpful to allow the clinical team to generate a customised

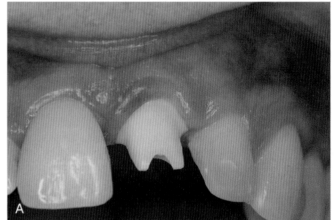
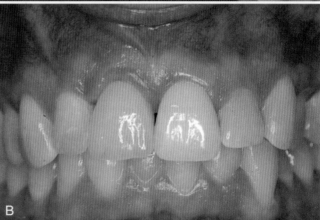

Fig. 5.3 (A) Screw-retained zirconium dioxide abutment and (B) cement-retained implant-supported crown.

care pathway for each patient. For example, surgery may be carried out by a different person from the person who plans and delivers the restoration. The different stages in the management pathway should be identified and any contingency plans that may need to be incorporated into the care

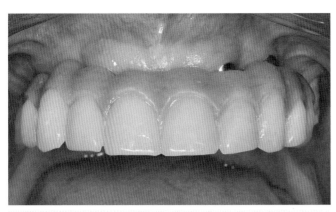

Fig. 5.4 Fixed implant maxillary bridge that incorporates pink-coloured prosthetic material.

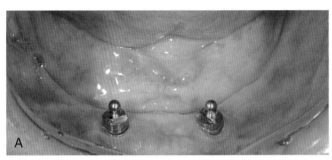

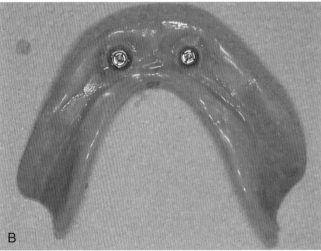

Fig. 5.5 Abutments as stud attachments (A) to provide retention for a mandibular implant-assisted overdenture (B).

pathway should be highlighted. Fig. 5.6 shows a flow chart of the potential care pathways that a patient may follow during implant management.

5.3 Surgical Phases

LEARNING OBJECTIVES

You should:
- be aware of the basic surgical principles for dental implant placement
- be aware of the restorative/surgical interface associated with the provision of dental implants.

A detailed description of the surgical aspects of implant treatment is outwith the scope of this text. What follows is a brief overview of implant placement and abutment connection with specific reference to the involvement of the restorative dentistry clinician.

PRE-IMPLANT PLACEMENT

The treatment plan should specify the precise positions for implants that will support the implant-borne superstructure that should already have been envisaged.

Should a failing tooth or root remnant be present at a potential implant site, the decision needs to be made as to whether the implant will be placed immediately after tooth extraction or following a delay to allow gingival healing. Details about decision-making in this situation are beyond the scope of this text.

IMPLANT PLACEMENT

The following description assumes the patient is able to tolerate minor oral surgery and the restorative dentistry procedures to complete treatment, has been deemed suitable in all other respects to embark on implant treatment and has given informed consent to proceed with treatment.

Once implant positions have been determined, and if sufficient bone exists to allow implants to be inserted with the likelihood of good stability, then surgery can proceed. Local anaesthesia, sometimes in conjunction with intra-venous sedation, is usually sufficient. Precise positioning of implants is essential if the goals of the treatment plan are to be achieved. Whilst it *may* be possible for the experienced implant dentist to insert implants accurately using local anatomical landmarks, the procedure is facilitated using a surgical guide that can precisely constrain the instruments used for making the osteotomy in bone. Implant insertion often involves making incisions to elevate a full thickness mucoperiosteal flap, although it may sometimes be possible to insert implants without flap elevation.

Once the implant is in place, a decision is made whether to attach the transmucosal section with adaptation of the mucoperiosteal flap around the transmucosal abutment or whether to close the mucosa over the implant to leave it to osseointegrate totally submerged.

An interim restoration is usually required before the implant is ready for restoration or further surgery to attach an abutment. Where implants are totally submerged or where only a healing abutment has been attached, either a removable denture or tooth-borne provisional bridge can be provided. It is important that interim restorations do not impart loads onto implants that could interfere with osseointegration.

ABUTMENT CONNECTION

If an implant is submerged beneath mucosa after insertion in order to assist osseointegration, then it will be necessary to uncover it, by means of a minor surgical procedure, in order to attach a transmucosal part (often a healing abutment – hence *abutment connection surgery*). This is achieved either by raising a mucoperiosteal flap or, in some cases, through a localised excision of the overlying mucosa using a tissue punch or laser. Abutment connection surgery also offers the

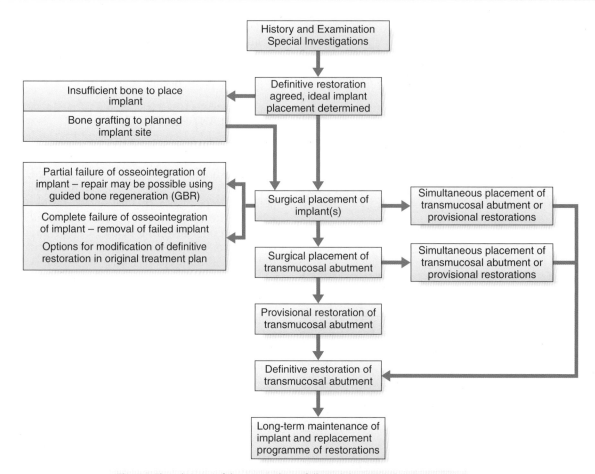

Fig. 5.6 Flow diagram of the care pathway followed during implant treatment.

opportunity to manipulate the peri-implant mucosal condition for optimal aesthetics and long-term resilience.

5.4 Provisional and Definitive Restoration of Dental Implants

LEARNING OBJECTIVES

You should:
- understand how dental implants are provisionally and definitively restored
- recognise the options available for restoring dental implants.

The numerous dental implant companies offer a plethora of components and tools to allow dentists to restore their implants. The practicing implant dentist must be intimately familiar with the relevant components and instruments. This section describes the basic stages during implant restoration.

IMMEDIATE RESTORATION OF IMPLANTS

Immediate restoration of implants describes attachment of either provisional or definitive transmucosal sections (abutments), which in turn carry the restoration. This approach requires implants tightly inserted into bone (i.e. have good

primary stability) that also benefit from being linked together (splinted) to share mechanical load. For fixed implant crowns and bridges, there are numerous ways of attaching the overlying restoration either directly to implants themselves by means of attachment (abutment) screws or to intermediary abutments by means of attachment (prosthetic) screws or cement. Immediate delivery of fixed restorations is most often by means of a provisional restoration which can either be developed at the chairside immediately following implant insertion or made ready prior to surgery via a digital workflow. Immediate restoration can also be achieved by fitting abutments onto implants immediately following implant insertion that enable a removable denture (an implant-assisted overdenture) to be attached. Typical attachment systems consist of ball-and-socket-type arrangements.

DELAYED RESTORATION OF IMPLANTS

Implants can be restored at the time of abutment connection surgery in the same way as for immediate restoration at the time of implant insertion, the difference being that the implants would now be expected to have osseointegrated. If records were obtained at the time of implant insertion, then restorations can be fabricated in readiness for attachment at the time of abutment connection.

Implants replacing teeth in the aesthetic zone usually benefit from being initially restored with provisional restorations. This approach, which may well be applicable to other parts of the mouth, allows trial and conformation of aesthetic, occlusal and phonetic qualities, as well as ensuring superstructures are as accessible to home and professional cleaning as possible. The provisional restoration can also be used to create a transmucosal emergence form that makes a suitable transition from round implant head to the natural cervical form of the tooth to be replaced.

Definitive restoration requires accurate capture of the implant position, the surrounding soft tissues and remaining teeth. This is achieved using transfer impression copings which are incorporated into either a physical impression or transfer copings which are recorded as part of a digital intraoral scan.

5.5 Maintenance Phase

LEARNING OBJECTIVES

You should:
- understand the requirement for long-term maintenance and follow-up of dental implants
- be familiar with potential complications associated with dental implants.

The long-term follow-up and maintenance of implant restorations is an essential requirement to help ensure long-term stability and success. The provision and maintenance of implants should be considered in conjunction with the long-term dental care and maintenance of the remaining dentition.

After delivery of implant treatment, the importance of long-term care must be emphasised to the patient. Patients must be instructed in the use of appropriate oral hygiene techniques using suitable aids such as floss or mini-interdental brushes.

Radiographs of completed restorations can be used as a baseline record of the implant–bone interface and allow the clinician to check that restorations have been seated correctly onto the implant or abutment with no gaps or excess cement seen at the interfaces.

LONG-TERM FOLLOW-UP

Implant, abutments and implant-supported restorations are susceptible to plaque accumulation, which can induce mucosal inflammation (peri-implant mucositis) that can lead to inflammatory processes that result in loss of peri-implant bone (peri-implantitis), eventually resulting in total loss of osseointegration: implant failure. It is essential that a long-term review and maintenance regime is established that is tailored to the risk profile of the individual patient, which needs to take account of factors such as:

- Susceptibility to peri-implantitis (e.g. smoking, diabetes, previous history of periodontal disease)
- Likelihood of mechanical overload (e.g. a patient with a history of bruxing)
- Complexity of the implant restoration where, for example, access for home hygiene is challenging
- Predictable wear and tear where overdenture attachments are present.

In practice, this means patients will benefit from review at least once per year. At follow-up appointments, the health of the peri-implant mucosa must be carefully assessed by observation and palpation. At the time of writing, peri-implant pocket depth measurement is controversial, partly because accurate pocket depth measurements are difficult to record, are not directly commensurate with disease in the same way as they are for teeth and also because there is concern that peri-implant probing might cause damage to the delicate peri-implant mucosal attachment. Percussion of an osseointegrated implant gives a high pitch/bright sound and provides a crude test for osseointegration. Percussion of a fixed implant restoration that produces a dull sound or mobility should alert the clinician to the possibility of implant failure or some other problem such as a loose abutment screw. Reassessment of the occlusal contacts on implant restorations must be made at follow-up appointments to ensure that they remain as planned.

Sequential radiographs (ideally long cone periapical) provide an assessment of supporting bone levels compared to baseline records taken at or soon after completion of treatment. Progressive loss of peri-implant bone is a cardinal sign of peri-implantitis. The frequency of radiographic follow-up should be a patient-based decision and should conform to best practice with respect to regulations for the use of ionising radiation.

COMPLICATIONS

Whilst the long-term survival rates of implants is high, complications of various sorts are relatively frequent and are categorised as biological or mechanical. Long-term, longitudinal clinical studies have reported success rates of nearly 90% 10 years following placement of fixed, implant bridges, although this success rate falls to 70% after 15 years. The success for single-tooth restorations supported by dental implants is higher, with a reported 10-year survival being in excess of 95%.

Biological complications are not at all uncommon and include peri-implant mucositis and peri-implantitis as described above. Peri-implant mucositis and peri-implantitis broadly correspond to gingivitis and periodontitis, respectively. Peri-implant mucositis is a reversible condition directly related to plaque accumulation and should prompt efforts to motivate and instruct the patient to achieve improved and sustained plaque control. Professional debridement may be required to remove plaque and calculus, and care must be taken to keep scalers and other instruments from damaging delicate surfaces. It may be necessary to periodically detach implant-borne superstructures to facilitate assessment and cleaning. Peri-implantitis usually commences as peri-implant mucositis and causes peri-implant bone loss. It may present with symptoms of discomfort or unsightly mucosal recession, but often it is symptomless until the implant loses osseointegration, at which point, it is not amenable to reparative treatment. Vigilance and radiographic follow-up is required to detect peri-implantitis. Unfortunately, peri-implantitis is difficult to treat: various surgical and non-surgical approaches are advocated.

Mechanical complications present in a variety of ways, probably the most common in fixed implant restorations being abutment screw loosening causing a loose restoration and fracture/delamination of prosthetic tooth material. For implant-assisted overdentures, wear and deterioration of detachable components is common.

Soft tissue recession around abutments and along implants may occur over time and lead to problems with aesthetics. Implant-supported restorations are not immune to the effects of trauma in the maxillofacial region. With the union between implant and bone being direct, there may be potentially more risk of bony fractures as compared to avulsion of a natural tooth.

Self-Assessment: Questions

EXTENDED MATCHING ITEMS QUESTIONS

Theme: Components of the implant system
The list below (1–10) comprises different components of the generic implant system together with restorations and prostheses that may be implant retained. For each of the statements (a–e), which describe an implant component or restoration that is often used in implant-retained units, select from the list the single most appropriate item that applies to that statement. Each item may be used once, more than once or not at all:

1. Implant.
2. Abutment.
3. Screw-retained crown.
4. Screw-retained bridge.
5. Cement-retained crown.
6. Cement-retained bridge.
7. Screw-retained metal/acrylic hybrid bridge.
8. Overdenture.
9. Abutment screw.
10. Impression coping.
    a. The section of an implant system that provides retention and stability to a restoration.
    b. The section of an implant system which traverses the epithelial lining of the oral cavity.
    c. A restoration which replaces the hard and soft tissues of the oral cavity and cannot be removed by the patient.
    d. A device which allows the accurate transfer of an implant's position and orientation within the oral cavity to the laboratory.
    e. A restoration that is retained by stud, magnetic or bar and clip precision attachments and that may be removed by the patient.

SHORT NOTES QUESTION

Write short notes on the steps taken to plan for a single tooth implant to replace a missing upper central incisor.

SINGLE BEST ANSWER QUESTIONS

1. Primary stability of a dental implant
   A. has no relationship to implant insertion torque
   B. is unrelated to implant thread design
   C. is unrelated to bone quality
   D. should be as low as possible if immediate loading is to be contemplated
   E. is related to the density of the bone surrounding it
2. For use in implant planning, a scan appliance that the patient wears at the time of having a cone beam volumetric tomography (CBCT) scan
   A. must contain radiolucent teeth
   B. should ideally contain discrete markers made with temporary acrylic
   C. should allow visualisation of the entire prosthetic volume
   D. prevents the prosthetic plan from being visualised in relation to alveolar bone
   E. can only be made by copying a removable denture
3. Peri-implant mucositis
   A. implies loss of attachment of bone from an implant surface
   B. is a reversible condition
   C. is a rare condition
   D. is best treated surgically
   E. has no similarities to gingivitis around teeth

Self-Assessment: Answers

EXTENDED MATCHING ITEMS ANSWERS

a. 1
b. 2
c. 7
d. 10
e. 8

SHORT NOTES ANSWER

A comprehensive list of notes would include:

Patient factors
  ▪ Willingness to undergo surgery.
  ▪ Willingness to leave restorations/prostheses out during immediate, postoperative healing periods.
  ▪ Lip/smile line.
Risk factors
  ▪ Systemic.
  ▪ Surgical.
  ▪ Environmental (further trauma to area; e.g. through contact sports).
  ▪ Sufficient funding.
  ▪ Other options for restoration (removable or fixed prostheses).
Site factors
  ▪ Sufficient space between adjacent teeth, the need for presurgical orthodontics.

■ Sufficient space/clearance interaction with occlusion.
■ Sufficient bone to implant into:
  ▫ Ridge mapping
  ▫ Computer simulation.
■ Available site to harvest bone and willingness to undergo grafting procedures if there is insufficient bone.
■ Relationship of ideal tooth position to the potential underlying implant placement:
  ▫ Diagnostic wax-up
  ▫ Production of custom surgical guides.
Restoration factors:
■ Relative dimensions of the restoration to the remaining dentition:
  ▫ Loss of space
  ▫ Drifting/tipping/rotation of teeth.
■ Choice of abutments:
  ▫ 'off-the-shelf'; prefabricated

  ▫ Bespoke custom
  ▫ Type of material.
■ Use of screw- or cement-retained definitive restorations.
■ Excessive spacing between teeth, therefore no support for papilla creation/augmentation.
■ Emergence of profile of restoration and soft tissue aesthetic consideration.
■ Thickness of tissue and impact of abutment materials (titanium will show through thin biotype gingival tissue).

SINGLE BEST ANSWER QUESTIONS ANSWERS

1. E
2. C
3. B

6 Conscious Sedation in Dentistry

Introduction

The use of drugs to help in the management of patients' anxieties regarding dental care is not new. The use of alcohol predates the invention of local analgesia, and a perusal of many art galleries will show travelling tooth pullers where patients sedate themselves prior to treatment.

The use of sedative techniques in dentistry has fluctuated in popularity since Horace Wells first discovered the potential of nitrous oxide in 1844. The administration of centrally acting drugs by dentists has attracted some concerns over safety; however, dentistry has an excellent record in this regard when compared with other medical specialties. The excellent safety record is built on the twin foundations of good quality education and adherence to appropriate clinical guidelines and standards of practice.

The techniques described in this chapter are safe and amenable to use by suitably trained dentists working in a clinical setting that is suitably equipped and meets the required standards.

6.1 Conscious Sedation

LEARNING OBJECTIVES

You should:

- understand what conscious sedation means
- know the indications for conscious sedation
- know when not to use conscious sedation
- be able to assess a patient's suitability to receive conscious sedation.

There have been many definitions of conscious sedation put forward over the years. The current definition that must be accepted in the United Kingdom is found in the Intercollegiate Advisory Committee for Sedation in Dentistry's report 'Standards for Conscious Sedation in the Provision of Dental Care' and the Scottish Dental Clinical Effectiveness Programme's document 'Conscious Sedation in Dentistry'. The definition is: 'Conscious Sedation is a technique in which the use of a drug or drugs produces a state of depression of the central nervous system enabling treatment to be carried out, but during which verbal contact with the patient is maintained throughout the period of sedation. The drugs and techniques used to provide conscious sedation for dental treatment should carry a margin of safety wide enough to render loss of consciousness unlikely'.

Techniques for producing conscious sedation are frequently considered as falling into two groups – basic and advanced. The basic techniques are:

- inhalation sedation using nitrous oxide/oxygen
- intravenous sedation using midazolam alone
- oral/transmucosal benzodiazepine, which has been demonstrated to provide adequate competence in intravenous techniques.

The advanced techniques are:

- any form of conscious sedation for patients under the age of 12 years other than nitrous oxide/oxygen inhalation sedation
- benzodiazepine + any other agent, for example, opioid, propofol and ketamine
- propofol either alone or with any other agent, for example, benzodiazepine, opioid and ketamine
- inhalation sedation using any agent other than nitrous oxide/oxygen alone
- combined (non-sequential) routes, for example, intravenous + inhalation agent (except for the use of nitrous oxide/oxygen during cannulation, which is discontinued prior to the administration of the intravenous agent).

This definition was published in 2007 by the Standing Committee on Sedation for Dentistry of the Faculty of Dental Surgery, The Royal College of Surgeons of England.

INDICATIONS FOR SEDATION

The indications for sedation can be considered under three main headings: psychosocial, medical and dental.

Psychosocial Indications

Indications relating to anxieties regarding dental treatment include:

- phobias
  - specific: drills, needles, extractions
  - general: things in mouth, all dental procedures

- gagging: inability to tolerate objects intraorally without retching
- persistent fainting during procedures, often associated with the administration of local analgesics
- idiosyncrasy to local analgesics: patients who have a problem where local analgesics appear not to work; the cause of the failure is psychological rather than anatomical or pharmacological.

Medical Indications

Some conditions may be aggravated by the stress of undergoing dental treatment. These include:

- ischaemic heart disease
- hypertension
- asthma
- epilepsy
- psychosomatic illnesses.

Many patients with these conditions can be treated quite 'normally' with local analgesic injections and tender loving care on the part of a sympathetic dentist. There are, however, a group of patients who, in addition to having a medical condition, also become quite anxious about dental treatment. A history of aggravation of the pre-existing condition in the dental environment may be the only clue as to the patient's concerns.

Some conditions affect the patient's ability to co-operate with dental treatment including:

- mild-to-moderate mental and physical disability
- spasticity disorders
- Parkinson's disease.

The use of sedation aids the management of these patients. The most important requirement is that the patient is able to understand what is being done. Lack of understanding will lead to failure of the technique. The assessment of a patient's understanding is extremely difficult.

Dental Indications

Sedation may be required for difficult or unpleasant procedures (e.g. extraction of wisdom teeth) or for orthodontic extractions, particularly in patients with limited previous dental care experience. The proper prescribing of sedation for these indications can help to prevent many patients having to suffer unpleasant experiences. It is well recognised that patients who have had a wisdom tooth surgically removed are more likely to fail to attend the appointment for the second surgical removal.

CONTRAINDICATIONS TO SEDATION

Contraindications can be grouped in a similar manner as indications.

Psychosocial Contraindications

Patients must be willing and co-operative. A failure to consent for treatment is an absolute contraindication to the provision of care under sedation. Similarly, patients must co-operate to allow the administration of the sedative agents by a given route. Failure to do so will prevent the dentist from being able to treat the patient.

Unaccompanied Patients

A responsible adult, who will remain with them until their recovery is complete, must accompany patients who are receiving sedation. The only exception to this rule is for adult patients receiving inhalation sedation with nitrous oxide and oxygen, who may be allowed to attend without an escort, provided that the dentist feels it is appropriate. Normally such patients will be asked to bring an escort to the first appointment so their response and recovery can be assessed. A responsible adult must accompany children receiving inhalation sedation.

Medical Contraindications

Severe or Uncontrolled Systemic Disease

Patients who are to receive sedation should have any general medical problems controlled prior to the commencement of their dental treatment. The administration of sedative drugs masks the patient's ability to detect if they are becoming unwell. It is recommended that patients who would be considered as grade III or worse in the American Society of Anesthesiologists' (ASA) classification of anaesthetic risk (Table 6.1) should not receive sedation outside an environment where the staff are trained to deal with the potential problems. This generally will mean these patients should not be treated outside a hospital setting.

Severe Learning or Movement Difficulties

The key to success in sedation is that the patient understands the procedure. If this understanding is lacking, then sedation is prone to failure.

Chronic Obstructive Pulmonary Disease

Chronic bronchitis causes a severe upset in respiratory physiology. It results in the respiratory drive being dictated by hypoxia rather than by changes in carbon dioxide levels. The clinical importance of this is, first, that the patient is significantly more sensitive to respiratory depressant drugs (including the benzodiazepines used in intravenous sedation) and, second, that high levels of oxygen, as used in inhalation sedation, in theory, may also cause the patient to stop breathing as hypoxic drive is reduced.

Severe Psychological/Psychiatric Problems

Patients suffering from delusional states, such as psychoses or schizophrenia are notoriously difficult and unpredictable

Table 6.1 American Society of Anesthesiologists' Classification of Anaesthetic Risk.

Grade	Description
I	Fit and well patient, no intercurrent disease
II	Patient with mild intercurrent disease that is well controlled and does not affect lifestyle
III	Patient with moderate intercurrent disease that does affect lifestyle
IV	Patient with severe intercurrent disease that is a constant threat to life
V	Patient who is unlikely to survive 24 hours with or without medical intervention
VI	A clinically brain-dead patient awaiting organ harvest

in their response to sedation. This relates to the frequently unpredictable reaction of the patient to the feelings of being sedated. Most of these patients are also taking heavy-duty antipsychotic drugs, which may interact with the sedatives that they are being given as part of their dental treatment. Consequently, only experienced sedationists should treat these patients.

Thyroid Dysfunction
Individuals who suffer from hypothyroidism are significantly more susceptible to the effects of central nervous system depressant drugs. Sedation should be avoided in this group.

Hyperthyroid patients may be difficult to sedate, and care has to be taken with the use of vasoconstrictors in local analgesic solutions.

Pregnancy and Lactation
It is wise to carry out as little treatment as possible for pregnant patients. Almost any drug that is given to the mother will cross the placenta and enter the fetal circulation. While the effects on the mother are easily observed, the effects on the fetus are masked from direct observation. The use of sedation during pregnancy should be restricted to a minimum. It is, however, permissible to use sedation to provide emergency dental care, perhaps in the situation where the fetus would be at greater risk from the repeated administration of antibiotics than from a single visit for treatment under sedation.

Inhalation sedation should be avoided during the first 3 months of pregnancy when there is the greatest risk of damage to the fetus. After this point, there is no evidence of any problem in the use of inhalation sedation with nitrous oxide. Common sense indicates that this will be the case, given the regular use of nitrous oxide as an obstetric analgesic.

There is no evidence that intravenous midazolam causes any fetal abnormalities. It can be used during the first 6 months of pregnancy if required. There is evidence that intravenous midazolam can cause hypotonia in the older fetus and, therefore, it should not be used during the last 3 months of pregnancy.

There is a balance to be reached between ensuring that the patient receives appropriate dental care, including the prevention of complications such as pregnancy gingivitis and management of risk to the fetus. Each patient must be individually assessed, and an individual-specific treatment plan devised.

Contraindications to Inhalation Sedation With Nitrous Oxide
In addition to the general contraindications above, a blocked nasal airway is a specific contraindication for the use of nitrous oxide sedation. Inhalation sedation will not work when a patient cannot breathe through the nose. Some blockages are temporary, such as hay fever or the common cold, and treatment may merely have to be postponed. Other blockages of the nasal airway are permanent. These could include enlarged adenoids or a deviated nasal septum. Alternative means of anxiety control may have to be used unless surgical correction is successful. In such cases, patients may have become so accustomed to mouth-breathing that it is difficult to re-establish nasal breathing,

Contraindications to Intravenous Sedation With Midazolam
The following conditions are contraindications to the use of benzodiazepine sedation (in addition to those described in the general section earlier).

Needle phobia. Siting an intravenous cannula is a prerequisite for intravenous sedation. If the patient cannot consent to and accept intravenous cannulation (with or without inhalation sedation or premedication), intravenous sedation cannot be carried out.

Hepatic insufficiency. Midazolam is detoxified in the liver. If hepatic function is greatly reduced, then its metabolism is also reduced. Because there is considerable extrahepatic metabolism of midazolam, it is generally accepted that a clinically significant decrease in the metabolism of midazolam would only occur when other hepatic functions, such as the production of blood clotting factors, are also significantly reduced, precluding many types of dental treatment.

Porphyria. In this condition, the use of certain drugs sensitises the sufferer to the effects of sunlight. The most notable drugs that cause these effects are barbiturates, although the benzodiazepines have also been implicated.

Myasthenia gravis. This autoimmune condition causes impairment of transmission at the neuromuscular junction. The resultant decrease in impulse transmission makes the sufferer very susceptible to the effects of other muscle relaxant drugs, including the benzodiazepines. Administration of benzodiazepine can lead to the patient being paralysed but awake.

Allergy to the benzodiazepine group of drugs. Although very rare, this must be considered as an absolute contraindication to the use of intravenous midazolam.

Dental Contraindications
The dental contraindications to sedation fall into two groups:

- those procedures considered too long or too difficult to be carried out under local analgesia
- where the presence of spreading infection in the floor of the mouth threatens the airway; in such cases, the airway must be secured under general anaesthesia (GA).

All forms of dental treatment may be carried out under sedation. The judgement as to whether it is appropriate to carry out any particular treatment must be made on a patient-to-patient basis.

PATIENT ASSESSMENT

This section will cover the areas of assessment which are specific to assessing patients for sedation.

The aim of patient assessment is to discover what sedation is required and suitable.

Patient's psychological ability to tolerate dental treatment. There are many patients who find dentistry difficult to cope with. Some of those are so phobic of dental treatment that they avoid attending at all costs, unless driven by intractable pain. It is important to find out what the patient's specific fears are, and what their previous experiences of dental treatment have been.

This also ensures that basic mistakes, such as suggesting that claustrophobic patients have inhalational sedation, are avoided.

Patient's physiological ability to tolerate dental treatment. If a patient suffers from any of the medical conditions highlighted above, it is important to establish how well they have tolerated receiving dental treatment previously. A history of aggravation of the medical condition in the dental setting should be taken as an indication for sedation.

The type and amount of dental treatment required. It is important to establish that the patient actually requires dental treatment prior to the administration of sedation. It is also impossible for the patient to give informed consent (see below) if the dental treatment has not been explained.

Is the treatment practical under sedation? It must be established that the treatment needed can be carried out under sedation.

Will any treatment provided be maintained? In many cases, patients attending for sedation may have a poor attendance record. The author has seen many patients who have had extensive treatment carried out under sedation and not returned until many restorations have been lost or there is extensive caries and periodontal disease. As with all patients, advanced treatment should not be provided unless the patient demonstrates the ability and motivation to maintain their oral health.

Does the patient need sedation? Information in the above areas will allow an informed decision as to whether or not the patient requires sedation. As in all areas, the provision of treatment should not be complicated unnecessarily. Sedation should only be used where there is a definite indication.

Are there any contraindications to sedation? It is important to ensure that there are no reasons to avoid sedation prior to offering it to a patient.

The Assessment Process

The assessment process follows similar lines to the history taking and examination of all dental patients.

Dental History

In addition to the current dental history, it is important to establish the patient's pattern of attendance and any specific fears. This will aid in treatment planning and will also give an indication of the potential co-operation once sedated. Those who are phobic of anything in their mouths tend to co-operate less well than those with a specific fear (e.g. needles or drills). There are specially designed questionnaires available for this purpose, but many tend to pose their questions in a threatening way. It is often better to ask the patient to say in their own words what they find difficult to cope with.

Medical History

In addition to the standard questions, it is important to establish if there has been a previous history of sedation, and how the patient coped. This may include sedation for medical procedures. Other factors that are of importance in sedation terms are:

- current drug history
- past drug history
- allergies (including to sticking plaster).

Dental Examination

It is frequently not possible to carry out a full dental examination. Anxious patients do not tolerate the use of probes (even periodontal) well. The reaction to the examination helps in the assessment of the level of anxiety. It also allows appropriate radiographs to be prescribed.

Physical Examination

All adult patients should have their blood pressure recorded as part of the assessment for sedation. Patients who are found to be hypertensive (systolic pressure more than 160 mmHg or diastolic more than 100 mmHg) should be referred for investigation. The airway should also be assessed to determine if there are likely to be problems maintaining patency during dental treatment under sedation.

If inhalational sedation is proposed, then the patency of the nasal airway and patient's nasal breathing should be confirmed. If intravenous sedation is proposed, it is important to establish if there are visible veins, along with ascertaining if there have been previous problems with having cannulae sited.

Establish Rapport With the Patient and Deal With Misconceptions

The importance of this process cannot be overstated. Most patients needing sedation will relate tales of a previous bad experience at the dentist. The most important part of building a rapport is to try (difficult as it is) to persuade the patient that you are different from the previous dentists. It is also important to deal with any misconceptions such as the difference between amnesia, as induced by sedation, and unconsciousness.

The patient should also give a written informed consent form at the assessment appointment.

6.2 Pharmacology of Sedative Agents

LEARNING OBJECTIVES

You should:

- understand the clinical effects of the sedative agents used in dentistry
- understand the side-effects of the sedative agents used in dentistry
- appreciate the hazards of occupational exposure to nitrous oxide.

The main drugs used for sedation are considered here. A number of other agents are known to be used, but their use is rare, and thus they are not included here.

NITROUS OXIDE

Nitrous oxide is the oldest sedative currently in use in clinical dentistry. It is the only drug that is in general use for inhalational sedation in dentistry.

Physical Properties of Nitrous Oxide

Nitrous oxide is a gas at room temperature and pressure. It is colourless and is sometimes described as having a sweet odour. It is 1.5 times as heavy as air and tends to collect at floor level. Pressurised nitrous oxide will liquefy, as its critical temperature (the temperature above which it cannot exist as a liquid) is 36.5 degrees Celsius. Nitrous oxide cylinders contain a mixture of gaseous and liquid nitrous oxide at a pressure of approximately 640 psi.

Anaesthetic and Analgesic Properties

Nitrous oxide is a weak anaesthetic agent. The MAC_{50} value (i.e. the theoretical value that would provide surgical anaesthesia for 50% of the population) is 110%. This can be contrasted with isoflurane at 1.15%. Nitrous oxide is insoluble in blood (blood:gas partition 0.47), which means that there is a rapid equilibration between the concentration of nitrous oxide in the alveoli and that in the blood, and induction of and recovery from sedation is extremely rapid.

The main effects of nitrous oxide are mood alteration, particularly euphoria, and analgesia. An inspired concentration of 50% nitrous oxide equates to approximately 15 mg of morphine, particularly when considering ischaemic muscle pain.

Effects of Chronic Exposure to Nitrous Oxide

It should be emphasised that there are virtually no problems of acute exposure for patients, provided that physiological concentrations of oxygen are administered with the nitrous oxide. There are, however, a number of potential problems with chronic exposure:

- decreased fertility in female staff
- increased rate of miscarriage in staff and partners of staff
- combination with cobalt-containing vitamins
  - oxidation of vitamin B_{12}
  - impairment of DNA synthesis
  - depression of haematopoiesis
- neurological effects: central nervous system (CNS) degeneration
- liver disease
- malignancy, especially cervical carcinoma.

All these effects tend only to be seen when there is no active scavenging of waste gases.

THE BENZODIAZEPINES

The benzodiazepines form a large group of drugs comprising over 50 marketed preparations. All of the group have basically the same effects on the body system (they are pharmacodynamically the same). Differences between the drugs primarily relate to the potency of the drug, which is a measure of affinity the drug has for its receptor, the strength of effect that it has on the receptor and also the length of time required to eliminate the drug from the body (pharmacokinetic properties). The pharmacokinetic differences relate to two areas:

- the length of time it takes to eliminate the parent drug (the elimination half-life)
- whether the elimination process produces metabolites that are themselves pharmacologically active.

The principal pharmacological effects of the benzodiazepines, listed as seen with increasing dose (with anxiolysis occurring with the lowest dose), are as follows:

- anxiolysis
- anticonvulsive
- mild sedation
- decreased attention
- amnesia
- more profound sedation
- muscle relaxation
- anaesthesia or hypnosis.

Mechanism of Action

Benzodiazepines have two distinct mechanisms of action. In higher centres of the brain, benzodiazepines bind to a receptor that controls sodium ion movement. The receptor is closely associated with a receptor for the endogenous, inhibitory neurotransmitter gamma-aminobutyric acid (GABA). The action of GABA allows chloride ions from the extracellular fluid to enter the cell. This makes the cell more negatively charged and, therefore, less likely to fire. The benzodiazepines increase the affinity of the GABA receptor for its transmitter and, thus, increase the inhibitory action of GABA. This action of the benzodiazepines is responsible for the sedative and anticonvulsant properties of this group of drugs.

The second mechanism of action is seen at lower centres in the brain stem and spinal cord. Here, the benzodiazepines mimic the action of another inhibitory neurotransmitter, glycine. This action of the benzodiazepines is responsible for the anxiolytic and muscle relaxant actions.

Repeated administration of benzodiazepines (e.g. when used as oral anxiolytic agents) produces tolerance to the effects that are mediated via GABA. The effects produced by mimicking glycine are, however, largely unaltered.

The amnesic actions of benzodiazepines are poorly understood. The administration causes anterograde amnesia (i.e. from the point of administration forwards in time). Long-term memory is affected more than short-term memory, and therefore patients remember less the week after the appointment than at the point of discharge.

Side-Effects of Intravenous Benzodiazepines

The principal side-effect of intravenous benzodiazepine administration is respiratory depression. This is produced by two mechanisms. First, the muscle relaxant actions of the drugs affect the respiratory muscles, namely, the intercostal muscles and the diaphragm. This reduces the efficiency of the contractions. Second, as with all drugs that depress the CNS, the carbon dioxide receptors in the brain are affected, resulting in a lesser response to changes in blood carbon dioxide. Consequently, although the patient can breathe and will take deep breaths with suitable encouragement, they do not feel the need to breathe.

The second notable side-effect is that of sexual fantasy production. Such fantasies have been described in the literature, although again the mechanism is unclear. It is also unclear why patients may remember the fantasy but have no memory of any treatment that has been carried out. The incidence is unknown, but it appears to be dose related with a threshold for midazolam of 0.1 mg/kg body weight. No member of the dental team must ever be left alone with a sedated patient, in case this should result in an allegation being made.

Available Benzodiazepines for Sedation

Midazolam

Midazolam is a water-soluble imiadazobenzodiazepine, which is painless on intravenous injection. It is available in three concentrations: 5 mg in 5 mL, 10 mg in 5 mL or 10 mg in 2 mL. The lowest concentration (5 mg in 5 mL) is the standard preparation for intravenous sedation. The 10 mg in 2 mL preparation is still used for oral sedation.

Pharmacokinetic properties. Midazolam is a short-acting drug with an elimination half-life of about 90 minutes. Its metabolites are largely inactive.

The metabolism of midazolam occurs both in the liver and extrahepatically. The half-life of midazolam is less affected by liver disease than any of the other benzodiazepines.

The effects of a single titrated dose are not prolonged by renal disease.

Midazolam is the first choice of oral and transmucosal sedative, despite the lack of a product licence for its use in the United Kingdom or the availability of an oral preparation. Midazolam tablets are available in other countries.

Other Benzodiazepines

Although there are in excess of 50 benzodiazepines currently available, no others are commonly used for dental sedation.

The future

Remimiazolam

Remimiazolam is related to midazolam but has a significantly shorter duration of action, as it is broken down by tissue esterases rather than cytochrome-dependent hepatic pathways. As such, this agent is administered by continuous intravenous infusion rather than titration. Currently, this agent is at the clinical trial stage of development. Initial results indicate that it has significant advantages in terms of increased flexibility of treatment time and decreased recovery time.

Benzodiazepine Antagonist Drugs

Flumazenil

Flumazenil was the first benzodiazepine antagonist drug to be marketed commercially. It is an imiadazobenzodiazepine that has a structure very similar to that of midazolam.

Flumazenil acts competitively to displace the active benzodiazepine molecule from the receptor site, thus blocking any potential action.

Pharmacokinetics. Flumazenil is a very short-acting drug. Its elimination half-life is 53 minutes, which is significantly shorter than that of any of the sedatives it may be used to reverse.

Contraindications to the administration of flumazenil. Flumazenil is a non-selective antagonist that will block the effects of all benzodiazepines. It should not be given to patients who are taking protracted courses of oral benzodiazepines as it may produce an acute withdrawal reaction. Where oral benzodiazepines are used to control epilepsy, the administration of the antagonist will antagonise the anticonvulsant action of the benzodiazepine, potentially leading to fitting.

Flumazenil is a benzodiazepine and must not be administered if an allergic reaction to the sedative is suspected.

OPIOIDS

Opioids are used in combination with other agents where single agents fail to produce an adequate level of anxiolysis to allow dental treatment to proceed. Opioids are centrally acting analgesics, which in addition produce other clinical effects including euphoria and sedation. Opioids have a number of side-effects. The most relevant to conscious sedation are respiratory depression, nausea and vomiting and depression of the cardiovascular system.

Fentanyl is the most commonly used opioid in the practice of sedation. It is presented as a 0.05 mg/mL solution. The standard adult dose of conscious sedation is 0.05 mg, and thus the 2-mL ampule is the most appropriate of the available preparations. A rare side-effect of fentanyl is chest wall rigidity. This is described at anaesthetic rather than sedative doses. The clinical effect of intravenous fentanyl is almost instantaneous and lasts for between 30 and 60 minutes. Nausea and vomiting are most likely if the patient is moved prior to the effects of fentanyl wearing off.

Shorter acting agents, such as remifentanil, have been described for use by infusion, usually in combination with propofol.

Opioid Antagonist Drugs

Naloxone

Naloxone is an opioid antagonist. It reverses the clinical effects of the opioids including sedation, analgesia, respiratory depression and nausea and vomiting.

Naloxone acts by competitively displacing opioid agonists. It is an opioid.

There are marked parallels with flumazenil:

- both are competitive antagonists
- shorter duration of action than the agonist leading to the possibility of residual sedation
- structurally similar to the agonists, so allergy to agonist likely to mean allergy to antagonist
- must be readily available in the dental environment where agonists are used for sedation.

PROPOFOL

Propofol (2,6-diisopropylenol) is a synthetic sedative hypnotic, which was introduced for the induction and maintenance of general anaesthesia. In common with other anaesthetic agents, it will produce sedation when given in lower doses.

Propofol is lipid soluble and thus is presented in a 1% (10 mg/mL) emulsion.

Clinical Effects of Propofol

The action of propofol is to enhance the effect of GABA. This is accomplished via a different mechanism from the benzodiazepines, allowing its use in regular benzodiazepine users.

Sedative doses of propofol produce a different quality of sedation from benzodiazepines. The effect is closer to a pure anxiolysis. This can be associated with patients becoming more talkative.

The amnesic actions of propofol are less predictable than those of benzodiazepines.

Side-Effects of Propofol

Propofol causes depressant effects on the cardiovascular system. It will cause a fall in arterial blood pressure and heart rate. Falls of 25–35% in systolic blood pressure have been recorded but are of little clinical significance to young, fit and healthy patients treated in the supine position.

Although propofol does produce profound respiratory depression in anaesthetic doses, it would appear that in sedative doses, less respiratory depression is seen with propofol than with midazolam.

Pain on injection (especially when small veins are used) is the most common cause of complaint from patients. Mixing a small amount of plain lignocaine with the solution can prevent this.

As with the other sedatives described, sexual fantasies have been described by patients receiving propofol sedation.

The Distribution and Elimination of Propofol

Propofol has an extremely short redistribution half-life. This accounts for the rapid patient recovery from sedation. The elimination from the body takes longer, and thus patients may have residual effects that they fail to appreciate.

KETAMINE

Ketamine is described as a dissociative anaesthetic agent. It produces effective analgesia, amnesia and sedation in sub-anaesthetic doses. Unlike all other sedative agents, ketamine stimulates the cardiovascular system and may stimulate the respiratory system.

The main disadvantage of ketamine is that it is associated with hallucinations in about 25% of patients. The incidence is said to be reduced when midazolam is used in combination with ketamine.

There is emerging evidence that ketamine may be more effective for paediatric sedation than midazolam, but it is not currently in general use.

6.3 Current Conscious Sedation Techniques

LEARNING OBJECTIVES

You should:
- know the advantages and disadvantages of each type of sedation
- be aware of the techniques involved
- appreciate the need for postgraduate training prior to independent practice of sedation
- appreciate the differences between basic and advanced sedation techniques
- understand the principles of monitoring patients under sedation
- understand clinical and electromechanical monitoring.

BASIC SEDATION TECHNIQUES

Inhalation Sedation

Techniques of inhalation sedation tend to fluctuate in popularity. It has also been described by a number of names, such as relative analgesia, inhalational sedation or inhalation psychosedation. All the widely available techniques involve the use of mixtures of nitrous oxide and oxygen.

Advantages of Inhalation Sedation

Rapid onset of sedation. The relative insolubility of nitrous oxide in blood results in the peak levels of nitrous oxide being attained within 3–5 minutes of inhalation.

Rapid recovery. There is effectively no metabolism of nitrous oxide, recovery being effected by exhalation of the gas via the lungs. The same factors that produce rapid induction of sedation lead to rapid recovery.

Recovery is independent of treatment time. Once a stable level of sedation is achieved, the continued administration of nitrous oxide merely maintains the equilibrium of blood:alveolar concentration. Consequently, patients recover as rapidly whether they have been treated for 10 minutes or 2 hours.

Absence of metabolism. Only 0.0004% of the inspired nitrous oxide is absorbed. The almost total absence of metabolism accounts for the safety of nitrous oxide and its ability to be used in a wide range of patients.

The technique does not involve an injection. Many patients are frightened of needles, and the fact that nitrous oxide administration does not require an invasive technique is an advantage.

A degree of analgesia is produced. Although the use of inhalation sedation will not provide sufficient analgesia to allow dental treatment to be carried out, it will make the administration of local anaesthetic injections easier.

Inhalation sedation can be used on virtually all patients. Inhalation sedation has very few contraindications and is the only technique currently recommended for patients of all ages.

Disadvantages of Inhalation Sedation

Bulk of equipment. The equipment required for the administration of inhalational sedation is bulky and can cause problems in a small surgery.

Expense of equipment. The equipment that is to be used must be a dedicated inhalational sedation machine. It is not acceptable to have a general anaesthetic machine that is used for both types of treatment. This is because general anaesthetic machines do not have the same safety features as relative analgesia machines. In addition to the equipment for drug administration, a scavenging system to remove expired gases is required. Finally, once in use, the costs of the gases must be taken into account.

Intrusion of nosepiece into the operating field. This can be a problem when treating upper anterior teeth (Fig. 6.1).

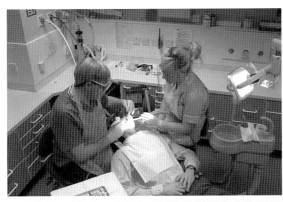

Fig. 6.1 The nosepiece of the MAC1 Inhalation Sedation Machine adapts against the upper lip, impairing access to the upper anterior teeth.

Disruption of the seal in this area will result in both a decrease in the effectiveness of sedation and an increase in chronic exposure of staff.

Patient's perception of equipment. Patients who have had a previous bad experience associated with general anaesthesia may find that the nosepiece reminds them of the GA mask.

Chronic exposure of staff. The major health problems that may be associated with the use of nitrous oxide will affect staff, not patients. Measures must be taken to ensure that occupational exposure is kept to a minimum.

Potential addiction. Nitrous oxide is an addictive drug; dentists should be aware of the risks to both their staff and themselves.

Technique for Inhalation Sedation

The technique described (Box 6.1) is based on the use of the McKesson MAC1 Inhalation Sedation Machine, which is one of the most widely used machines for this type of sedation (Fig. 6.2).

Signs and Symptoms of Adequate Sedation With Nitrous Oxide

Signs. The signs are what the operator sees:

- The patient is awake.
- The patient is relaxed and comfortable.
- Vital signs are within normal limits: heart rate, respiration rate and blood pressure (if measured) will all be normal.
- Blink rate is reduced.
- Mouth remains open on request: in this respect, inhalational sedation is very different from intravenous sedation.
- Protective reflexes are normal.
- Hyperactive gag reflexes are reduced, allowing dental treatment.
- Decreased response to painful stimuli.

Symptoms. The symptoms are what the patient feels:

- Relaxed and comfortable.
- Lessened awareness of pain.
- Paraesthesia/tingling.
- Mild intoxication.
- Euphoria.

Box 6.1   Technique for Inhalation Sedation.

1. Preprocedural machine checks. It is vital for the patient's well-being that all equipment is in working order and that there is a sufficient supply of nitrous oxide and, more importantly, oxygen for the session. The manufacturer's instructions for checking and servicing equipment should be followed.
2. The correct size of nosepiece for the patient should be selected. This is often best done at an assessment appointment as part of introducing the patient to the process of sedation.
3. The patient is brought into the surgery, and pre-treatment discussions completed.
4. The relative analgesia machine is turned on, with 100% oxygen at a flow rate of 6 L/min.
5. The nosepiece is fitted to the patient, and the flow rate titrated until the reservoir bag on the machine can be seen to move with each breath but does not fully collapse when the patient breathes in.
6. Nitrous oxide is introduced. The initial introduction is 10% increments at 1-minute intervals. After an inspired concentration of 20% has been reached, the increments are reduced to 5%. Throughout the process, the patient must be reassured and encouraged. The most important part of sedation is the patient management. Inhalational sedation will not work without the hypnotic suggestions of the operator.
7. Once adequate sedation has been achieved, dental treatment can commence.
8. The patient's level of sedation and breathing pattern should be monitored during treatment. The concentration of nitrous oxide and flow rate of gases should be adjusted as required to maintain patient comfort.
9. Reassurance and positive suggestions should be maintained throughout the procedure.
10. Once the treatment has been completed, the nitrous oxide should be reduced to 0%.
11. The patient should be encouraged to breathe 100% oxygen for a minimum of 2 minutes, or until recovered prior to removal of the nosepiece.
12. Turn off the flow of oxygen.
13. Reinforce postoperative instructions and discharge the patient.

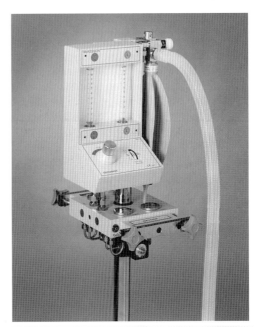

Fig. 6.2 The McKesson MC1 RA Machine. (Image courtesy of Cestradent McKesson.)

- Detachment.
- Warmth.
- Indifference to the passage of time.
- Dreaming.

Patients will not necessarily show all the signs, or experience all the symptoms of sedation that are listed here. It is a matter of judgement as to when adequate sedation has been achieved. The majority of patients will require between 25% and 40% nitrous oxide to achieve sedation. It is very important to avoid oversedation, as patients find overdoses of nitrous oxide unpleasant.

Signs and Symptoms of Oversedation
Oversedation can cause:

- persistent mouth closing
- spontaneous mouth-breathing
- complaints of unpleasant feelings
- lack of co-operation
- nausea and vomiting.

The treatment of a patient who is oversedated involves reducing the concentration of inspired nitrous oxide by 5–10% and reassuring the patient that things will improve.

Recovery From Sedation
Once dental treatment has been completed, the patient is allowed to breathe 100% oxygen for 2 minutes. This allows the nitrous oxide to be exhaled via the scavenging system rather than into the surgery. It can also prevent a phenomenon called diffusion hypoxia, which may arise owing to the rapid release of nitrous oxide from blood when it is removed from the inspired air.

After recovery, a child patient must be discharged into the care of a responsible adult. Adults may be discharged alone, and it is the dentist's responsibility to decide if the patient needs to be accompanied or not.

Dental Professionals Who Can Administer Inhalation Sedation
In addition to appropriately trained dentists, dental hygienists and therapists who have undergone postregistration training in inhalation sedation are able to administer this type of sedation. All who administer inhalation sedation must be assisted by an appropriately trained dental nurse. In addition, for hygienists and therapists, there must be a dentist on the premises, but not necessarily in the surgery (treatment room) in case the dental treatment unexpectedly moves beyond the competence of the treating Dental Care Professional (DCP).

Intravenous Sedation

Intravenous sedation is normally used for anxious adult patients. It is particularly useful for the extremely anxious or for those who feel claustrophobic when undergoing dental treatment. The basic technique for intravenous sedation involves a titrated dose of midazolam.

Advantages of Intravenous Sedation
Speed of onset of sedation. The hand-to-brain circulation time is of the order of 20 seconds; as a result, the onset of sedation is very rapid. This prevents an increase in anxiety while waiting in the dental environment.

The dose of sedative can be titrated against the patient's response. The patient receives the correct dose of sedative for their needs.

Administration is comfortable. Once venous access is achieved, the patient is not troubled (unlike intramuscular or subcutaneous injections).

Intravenous access is preserved. This allows the administration of other agents if required (as in the case of a medical incident).

Recovery. This is shorter than for drugs administered via the oral or intramuscular route.

Disadvantages of Intravenous Sedation
The establishment of intravenous access. Many patients find the process of having an intravenous cannula sited unpleasant. It is, however, amazing how many patients find that it is acceptable to have an injection in the hand but will not tolerate intraoral injections.

Rapid onset. The rapid onset of the effects of intravenous drugs means that care must be taken to ensure that patients are not oversedated.

Adverse reactions. Any adverse reactions to the drugs tend to be more severe if the drugs are administered by injection rather than orally.

No easy reversal is possible. There is no way to recover the drug once it has been administered. The only way to reverse sedation is by the use of antagonist drugs.

Technique of Intravenous Sedation
The primary prerequisite for the use of intravenous sedation is that all those involved in the patient's treatment have received the appropriate training and the surgery is equipped with the appropriate scale of equipment for administering the sedation, monitoring the patient and dealing with any emergencies. Both dentist and dental nurse should have attended relevant postgraduate/postcertification courses.

Equipment Required for Intravenous Sedation
Administration
- Surgical wipe to disinfect skin
- Gauge intravenous cannula
- Surgical tape to fix cannula
- Syringes
  - 10 mL to administer the sedative
  - 20 mL for the saline flush
- Gauge needle to draw up drug
- Labels to distinguish syringes
- Tourniquet
- Disposable tray

Monitoring equipment
- Stop watch
- Non-invasive blood pressure recording facility
- Pulse oximeter

Emergency equipment
  As for all dental surgeries and
- Flumazenil
- Facility to give supplemental oxygen at a flow of 2 L/min (most emergency cylinders are set to a minimum of 5 L/min)

Special dental equipment
- Mouth props
- Dental chair with a fast prone facility that will work in the event of power failure

Preparation of the Drugs

All drugs to be used for sedation (including normal saline) must be drawn up by the dentist administering the sedation. This task must not be delegated to a dental nurse.

As with all agents to be administered to patients (including local anaesthetics), agents must be checked to ensure that they have not passed their expiry date and that there are no signs of damage to the containers in which they are supplied. Once drawn up, drugs must be clearly labelled as there are many clear solutions, which can easily be confused.

Preparation of the Patient

It is important to ensure that all the formalities have been completed before the patient is sedated. This will include checking that the patient has signed a consent form and that their blood pressure has been recorded. It is also good practice to ensure that the patient has visited the toilet before embarking on a procedure that will keep the patient in the dental chair for about an hour or so. The patient's medical and dental histories should also be checked to ensure that nothing has happened since the previous appointment either to change the dental treatment plan or to modify the choice of sedation technique.

Intravenous Cannulation

Cannulation is a prerequisite for carrying out intravenous sedation. It is important to select a site that is accessible to the dentist, acceptable to the patient, away from structures that might be damaged in the process but where there are adequately sized superficial veins present. The dorsum of the hand is the usual choice in this situation. The process of cannulation is shown in Fig. 6.3.

Once the cannula has been sited, its correct location is confirmed using a dose of saline. The sedative agent can then be administered. The usual choice is midazolam (5 mg in 5-mL formulation). The dose should be titrated according to the patient's response. A small dose is administered, allowed to have its effect and then a decision made as to whether or not a sufficient dose has been administered. If not, the cycle is repeated. The usually recommended regimen is:

1. Slow bolus of 2 mg (2 mL).
2. Wait for 90 seconds.
3. Administration of 1-mg (1 mL) increments at 1-minute intervals until the patient is adequately sedated.

Signs of Adequate Sedation

A depth of sedation that will allow the patient to have treatment is often referred to as the 'endpoint', implying that it is discrete and apparent. This is not the case. There is a plane of sedation within which the patient needs to be to allow treatment to be undertaken. Different patients will require to be at different levels within this plane of sedation; indeed, the same patient may require to be at different levels of sedation depending on the type of treatment proposed, and how they are feeling in general.

The judgement of the correct depth of sedation largely comes down to clinical experience. An adjunct to assessing the adequacy of sedation is to ask the patient if they are ready to have dental treatment. A slow, ponderous answer is usually indicative of the correct level of sedation. Tests of co-ordination, such as asking the patient to touch their nose (and watching them miss), tend to embarrass patients and have the added disadvantage of being of little clinical use.

In general, once an adequate level of sedation has been achieved, the duration of the dental treatment should be tailored to the duration of the sedation, and no further increments of sedative given.

The dosage of midazolam required to produce sedation is extremely variable. Given that the ethos of sedation is that the dose of sedative is judged according to the patient's response, it is difficult to justify setting maximum doses. However, well over 95% of patients will be adequately sedated on a dose of 10 mg of midazolam or less. Doses in excess of this should only be given after careful assessment and consideration.

Dental Treatment Under Intravenous Sedation

Patients recover from the effects of intravenous sedation while they are being treated. Consequently, the longer the appointment progresses, the less sedated the patient will become. The pattern of dental treatment must be tailored to suit. The most invasive treatment (the administration of local anaesthetic and use of rotary cutting instruments) should be confined to the first 25 minutes of treatment. The remaining treatment (placement of restorations) can take place during the next 20 minutes or so. It should, however, be emphasised that all patients are different, and each patient should be treated for the amount of time that they are happy to receive treatment.

Recovery From Intravenous Sedation

Patients recover much more slowly from intravenous sedation than from inhalational sedation. It is impossible to set strict time limits on when patients should be discharged. It is more important to assess the patient's state of mind and ability to leave the surgery premises. A useful test is to ask the patient to walk across the room, turn and walk back. If they can negotiate that test without undue loss of balance, they are probably fit to be discharged. It is also worth checking that the patient is happy to leave, and that the escort is happy to take them.

All patients receiving intravenous sedation *must* be charged into the care of a responsible adult.

Complications of Intravenous Sedation

COMPLICATIONS ASSOCIATED WITH INTRAVENOUS CANNULATION. All of the following responses are difficult to cope with, and patients in these categories should be treated by those who are experienced in using sedation.

Venospasm. This is a condition, probably anxiety related, where the veins collapse at attempted cannulation. It is difficult to prevent even for those skilled at cannulation.

Extravascular injection. This results from an incorrectly sited cannula. The main thing is to prevent the extravascular injection of any pharmacologically active agent by testing that the cannula is correctly sited.

Intra-arterial injection. Injection of drugs into an artery is a potentially serious event. Once again it should be prevented by careful technique, particularly by checking that any vessel that is selected as a potential cannulation site does not pulsate.

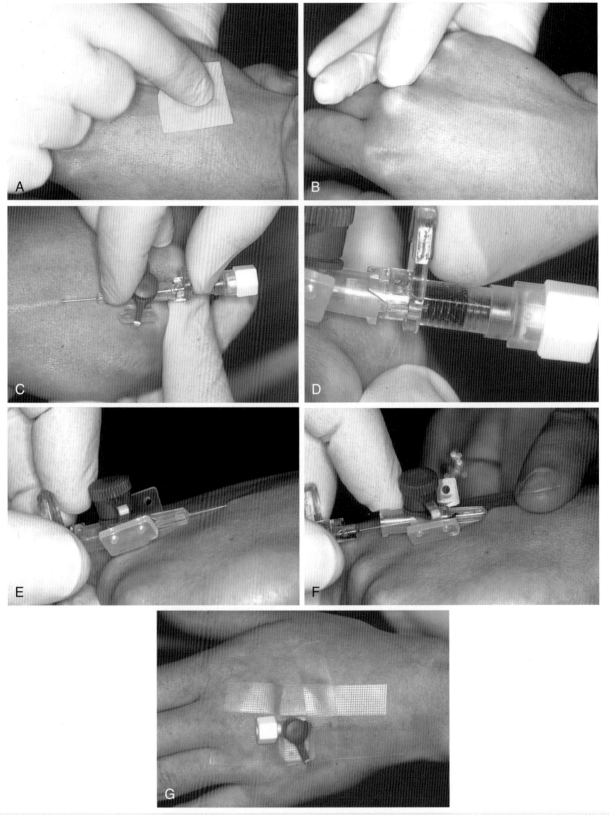

Fig. 6.3 The cannulation sequence. (A) Site for venepuncture disinfected with alcohol-containing wipe. (B) Vein immobilised with skin traction from operator's left hand. (C) Cannula inserted into vein. (D) Correct position confirmed by seeing flashback of blood. (E) Cannula slid down needle to site completely. (F) Vein occluded by assistant while needle removed. (G) Cap placed on end of cannula and wings secured with tape.

Haematoma formation. Haematomata form as a result of blood leaking from a blood vessel into the subcutaneous tissues. Formation may occur at cannulation, as a result of multiple vein wall punctures or when the cannula is removed as a result of insufficient pressure being applied to the site.

Pain on cannulation. Venous cannulation is uncomfortable, but for most patients it can be overcome with the use of distraction techniques.

PROBLEMS ASSOCIATED WITH SEDATION.

Oversedation. The most likely sign of a patient being oversedated is respiratory depression. In the majority of patients, this can be managed by encouraging the patient to breathe and by support until the overdose wears off. In more severe cases, supplemental oxygen may be required; should that fail, the sedation should be reversed with the benzodiazepine antagonist.

Hyporesponse. The patient fails to sedate despite the use of large doses of sedative.

Paradoxical reaction. The patient appears to have sedated normally but reacts in an uncontrolled fashion when treatment is attempted.

Hyper-response. The patient sedates very deeply on a very small dose of sedative.

Sexual fantasy. It appears that some patients who are sedated feel that they have been sexually assaulted. Such allegations are potentially distressing to the dentist, not to mention legally difficult as they may result in imprisonment. Consequently, no member of the dental team should be left alone with a sedated patient. Dentist and dental nurse act as each other's chaperone.

Reversal of Intravenous Sedation

The advent of flumazenil raised the possibility of being able to reverse a patient's sedation. This is, however, not recommended as a routine practice.

INDICATIONS FOR REVERSAL
- Oversedation
- Patients with a difficult journey home
- Patients who will be difficult to manage either because of a learning difficulty or who are much larger than their escorts.

CONTRAINDICATIONS TO REVERSAL
- Patients taking concurrent oral benzodiazepines (especially if used to control epilepsy)
- Patients who have had a suspected allergic reaction to the sedative.

Oral Sedation and Transmucosal Sedation

The administration of oral or transmucosal drugs is an attractive way of producing sedation. This is largely because of the simplicity of the techniques as far as the dentist is concerned and the acceptability for patients, particularly in the United Kingdom, of orally administered drugs. These are techniques that are gaining in popularity in the United Kingdom. These techniques still represent the third choice of sedation technique, as the drugs are given as bolus doses rather than titrated. In general, these techniques are not used when either intravenous or inhalation sedation can be used. The most commonly used transmucosal sedation technique is intranasal sedation.

Disadvantages

There are significant disadvantages to this type of sedation.

Prolonged latent period. Drugs taken orally will take a long time to act. It will usually be at least 20–30 minutes until there is a significant degree of sedation. The main problem is that patients who require sedation do not enjoy being in the dental environment and waiting for the sedation to act can be traumatic. The lag time with intranasal sedation is significantly less, but often up to 10–15 minutes.

Untitratable dose. The other techniques that are recommended for sedation involve titrating the dose of sedative drug to the patient's response. The long latent period involved with these techniques means that the dose has to be given on an mg/kg dose up to a set maximum. The only variation in dose that is possible is by judging the effect at one appointment and changing it for future appointments.

Unpredictable absorption. There are many factors that affect the absorption of drugs from the gastrointestinal tract. Elixirs and gelatin-filled capsules tend to be absorbed more rapidly than tablet formulations. Other factors include the amount, timing and constituents of any food in the stomach. Consequently, it cannot be predicted exactly when the drug that has been administered will have its effect. This only affects oral sedation.

First-pass metabolism. All drugs that are administered orally and are absorbed from the upper part of the gastrointestinal tract pass to the liver via the portal circulation. A significant proportion of the dose is metabolised as it passes through the liver prior to reaching the systemic circulation (first-pass metabolism). As a result, a higher dose must be used for oral drugs to achieve the desired effect. This only affects oral sedation.

Technique for Oral Sedation

Midazolam is administered mixed in a drink. The dose for children is 0.5 mg/kg body weight up to a maximum of 20 mg. The adult dose is 20 mg.

The onset of sedation is more rapid than with other benzodiazepines, with the patient being adequately sedated 20–30 minutes after administration. A suitably trained member of the dental team must supervise the patient once the sedative has been administered.

Once sedation is achieved, careful consideration should be given to siting an intravenous cannula to give intravenous access as when intravenous sedation is undertaken. The patient should be either sedated in the dental surgery or, if this is not possible, moved to the surgery as soon as sufficiently relaxed to allow this. Electromechanical monitoring should ideally be commenced before administration of the sedative.

Discharge after sedation depends on the patient being sufficiently recovered to walk unaided and being sufficiently co-ordinated to be discharged into the care of a responsible adult.

Monitoring of sedated patients is discussed later.

Technique for Intranasal Sedation

A concentrated version of midazolam (normally 10 mg/mL) is used. A dose of 0.3 mg/kg up to a maximum of 12 mg is administered. The dose is squirted up one nostril. The drug stings significantly, and thus it is advisable not to try to use divided doses. The onset of sedation is more rapid than with oral sedation, but significantly slower than intravenous or inhalation sedation.

Once sedation is achieved, careful consideration should be given to siting an intravenous cannula to give intravenous access as when intravenous sedation is undertaken. The patient should be either sedated in the dental surgery or, if this is not possible, moved to the surgery as soon as sufficiently relaxed to allow this. Electromechanical monitoring should ideally be commenced before administration of the sedative.

Discharge after sedation depends on the patient being sufficiently recovered to walk unaided and being sufficiently co-ordinated to be discharged into the care of a responsible adult.

ADVANCED SEDATION TECHNIQUES

The advanced sedation techniques have a role to play in the management of patients for whom the basic techniques are unsuitable or ineffective. As the techniques are more complicated, additional training is required after competence in the basic techniques has been gained. A brief summary of the types of advanced techniques used in dentistry is given here. For more details, readers should consult specialist sedation textbooks.

Intravenous Sedation With Combinations of Drugs

There are a number of techniques for producing conscious sedation using two or more drugs. Advantages cited for their use are that the drugs acting synergistically produce a better quality of sedation; however, the synergistic reactions also apply to the side-effects of the drugs. The most commonly used combination is an opioid (usually fentanyl) and midazolam.

Intravenous Sedation With Propofol

There are a number of techniques described using propofol for intravenous sedation. All involve using a syringe pump to deliver the solution to the patient. The techniques fall into two groups.

In the first group, the sedationist controls the level of sedation by altering the rate of infusion. The second group of techniques allows the patient to control the depth of sedation with the use of sophisticated technology. Currently, these techniques are used predominantly in hospital settings and are unsuitable for the operator–sedationist.

Inhalation Sedation Using Any Agent Other Than Nitrous Oxide/Oxygen Alone

Techniques using anaesthetic volatile agents such as sevoflurane or isoflurane either alone or in combination with nitrous oxide have been described. Currently there is no dedicated inhalation sedation equipment available to deliver this type of sedation. Thus, its use is restricted to a few 'specialist' centres, and these techniques are thus largely of academic interest only.

Combined (Non-Sequential) Routes, For Example: Intravenous + Inhalation Agent (Except for the Use of Nitrous Oxide/Oxygen During Cannulation)

When drugs are administered by different routes, they have different pharmacokinetic properties. Thus, using multiple routes makes the process of achieving a sedation endpoint more difficult. The use of oral followed by intravenous sedation can be an effective method of managing profoundly needle phobic patients. This technique has the drug or drugs administered by the two routes exerting a clinical effect at the same time and is pharmacokinetically more challenging than either technique alone.

MONITORING OF SEDATED PATIENTS

All patients who are having any form of dental treatment should be monitored by those who are providing that treatment. The importance of monitoring is greater when patients have been sedated, as they are less aware of their surroundings, and any changes that are occurring within their own bodies.

Clinical Monitoring

The cornerstone of all monitoring is the clinical observation of the patient.

Is the patient conscious? In this context, consciousness is defined as the ability to respond to verbal command.

Does the patient look relaxed and comfortable? This will show that they are tolerating treatment without undue distress. The patient's facial expression and general demeanour in the dental chair are good indications of their level of comfort.

Skin colour. Any changes in skin colour should be noted, as they may be indicative of an impending medical incident, for example, a bluish tinge may result from hypoxia secondary to respiratory depression. Reddening, particularly in an area where there has been contact with surgical gloves or rubber dam, may indicate an allergy.

Pattern and depth of respiration. Given that respiratory depression can occur with benzodiazepine sedation, patients should have the rate and depth of breathing monitored. Patients who are receiving inhalational sedation should also be monitored, as mouth-breathing is an early sign of overdose.

Electromechanical Monitoring

The clinical monitoring is complemented by the use of electromechanical devices.

Non-Invasive Blood Pressure Recording During Sedation

Adult patients should have their blood pressure recorded both as part of the assessment process and immediately prior to sedation. This allows the establishment of a baseline reading. Patients receiving sedation with nitrous oxide or midazolam alone do no need to have their blood pressure recorded regularly throughout the sedation period unless there is a medical issue that makes this advisable. Such patients would normally be categorised as ASA III (American Society of Anesthesiologists) or IV and thus tend to be seen in specialist facilities, by an experienced sedationist.

Any patient receiving multiple agent sedation or drugs by continuous infusion should have their blood pressure recorded at 5-minute intervals.

All adult patients should have a recording of their blood pressure taken immediately prior to discharge.

It is not normal to measure blood pressure for fit and well children prior to sedation.

Pulse Oximetry

The use of a pulse oximeter, which will pick up falls in arterial oxygen saturation before they are clinically evident, provides an early warning of respiratory depression. Falls of 4–5% must be corrected, and any fall below 90% saturation must be treated as potentially serious. The reasons for this will become apparent when the oxygen–haemoglobin dissociation curve is studied (Fig. 6.4). The oximeter should be attached to the patient and be switched on prior to the administration of any sedative so that the normal saturation can be noted. The pulse oximeter also displays a reading of the patient's pulse. Changes (particularly increases) may indicate distress or pain during treatment.

Pulse oximetry is not routinely used with inhalational sedation, as high concentrations of oxygen are always administered (the minimum is 30%), but should be considered as mandatory for intravenous, oral and transmucosal sedation.

Reservoir Bag on a Relative Analgesia Machine

In addition to the aforementioned, when inhalational sedation is used, observation of the movements of the reservoir bag allow an assessment of the patient's pattern of breathing. Increases in rate or depth may indicate anxiety, whereas a decrease in the amount of movement of the bag while the chest movements remain the same may indicate that the patient is mouth-breathing.

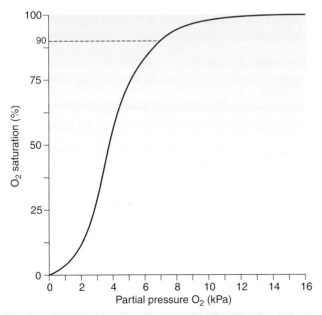

Fig. 6.4 The oxygen–haemoglobin dissociation curve; 90% saturation is at the top of the steep portion of the curve. Further respiratory depression will result in rapid falls in saturation.

As most sedation is carried out by an operator sedationist, the main burden of monitoring tends to fall on the dental nurse. The issue of training for the dental team is covered later.

The Future

Capnography

Monitoring exhaled carbon dioxide is a significantly more sensitive measure of respiratory depression than measuring oxygen saturation. It is not used routinely, as currently the technology is expensive and for the conscious patient produces a significant number of false alarms. Currently, sidestream capnography (diverting a portion of expired air through a sensor) is the recommended technique. It is sensitive to a patient's breath holding or mouth-breathing. An alternative technique is transcutaneous monitoring via electrodes placed on the skin.

The Academy of Medical Royal Colleges report in 2013 described capnography as a 'developmental standard' and the Intercollegiate Advisory Committee for Sedation in Dentistry indicated that there is little evidence to justify its use in ASA I or II patients. In the future, it is likely to become the 'go to' monitor of respirator function.

Bispectral Index Monitoring

The Bispectral Index (BIS) monitoring uses an electroencephalogram (EEG) to monitor brainwave activity and produce a numerical reading between 0 and 100. BIS scores of 90–100 equate to being fully conscious, 70–90 conscious sedation and 40–60 general anaesthesia. Currently, this monitor has been used largely for research, with applications including using the BIS reading to provide feedback to control infusion pumps administering agents such as propofol.

6.4 Dental Treatment Planning

LEARNING OBJECTIVES

You should:
- appreciate which procedures benefit from the use of sedation
- understand how to encourage patients to complete and maintain treatment.

All dental procedures that might be carried out under local anaesthesia can be performed under sedation and local anaesthesia. Some procedures are more easily carried out under one form of sedation than another (e.g. apicectomies on upper incisors are difficult under inhalational sedation, as the nosepiece tends to interfere with the operating field).

The main decision rests on what treatment is advisable to carry out for patients. As in all other areas of dentistry, these decisions depend much on the patient's co-operation.

Patients requiring sedation often have very poor attendance records, largely because they are terrified of being in the dental environment. Previous non-attendance means that they have not been exposed to oral health education, such as diet advice and oral hygiene instruction. In these patients, poor oral hygiene at first attendance should not be taken as an indication of lack of will to co-operate.

The ideal for dental treatment planning is to deal with any periodontal problems, manage the routine conservative work and provide advanced conservation (fixed prosthodontics and endodontics) with removable prosthodontics as the final stage. Berating an anxious patient on the merits of good oral hygiene and forcing them to have all hard and soft deposits removed from their teeth as a first stage will result in the patient failing to return for treatment. It is important to engage the patient in treatment first to show them that they can attend and cope with receiving treatment.

The decision of what treatment to provide will then depend on the patient's ability to cope with treatment under sedation, as well as their response to the health education message. It is inappropriate to promise patients advanced treatment prior to the initial sedation appointment, as it may well be that even with sedation, co-operation may be limited.

Treatment such as molar endodontics, multiple crowns and bridges and technique-sensitive procedures should be reserved for only the very co-operative and compliant patients who are likely to maintain good oral health in the future.

6.5 Medicolegal Aspects

LEARNING OBJECTIVES

You should:
- appreciate the obligations on the dental profession using sedation
- know the importance of compliance with current standards.

Sadly, all aspects of medical and dental practice are being affected by the need to consider the possibility of legal action for negligence.

The current standards for practice are found in the Intercollegiate Advisory Committee for Sedation in Dentistry's 2015 report. In Scotland, the Scottish Dental Clinical Effectiveness Programme produced guidance, which was updated in 2016. The principal recommendations are broadly similar, and the gist of the requirements is reproduced as follows:

- The definition of conscious sedation is as given at the beginning of this chapter. Although it allows latitude in the techniques that may be used for sedation, it does go on to say that 'No one technique is suitable for all patients. However, adopting the principle of minimum intervention, the simplest and safest technique that is likely to be effective, based on robust patient assessment and clinical need, should be used'.
- Dentists are entitled to act as operator/sedationist, with the proviso that they must have undertaken the relevant postgraduate training.
- If a dentist is to exercise this right, then the appropriate assistance must be available. This may be from a suitably trained dental nurse. Such a dental nurse should be registered with the General Dental Council and must have undertaken the relevant postcertification course.

- Courses providing training in sedation must be accredited by the Sedation Training Accreditation Committee based at the Royal College of Surgeons in London unless run by a university or postgraduate deanery.
- Those providing conscious sedation must undertake 12 hours of sedation-related continuing professional development (CPD) in every 5-year period.
- Sedation activity, including complication rates, must be audited.
- All centres providing conscious sedation for the delivery of dental care should be inspected to determine that the necessary standards are in place.
- All patients who are to have sedation must be assessed to ensure that the most appropriate management plan is devised.
- All patients having any treatment under sedation of any sort must give consent in writing. This consent should be informed; that is, that the dentist who is to administer the sedation explains the procedure to the patient and any alternative treatments that may be possible. This allows the patient to give their consent based on knowledge of the treatment options.
- Patients should be given age-appropriate written information regarding the sedative technique to be used including pre- and postoperative instructions. These instructions must include advice as to whether fasting is required prior to sedation. This is not normally required for sedation for dentistry, but the advice must be tailored to the individual patient.
- All patients should be carefully monitored during sedation (Section 6.3).
- Patients who are recovering from sedation must be protected and monitored in adequate facilities. They should only be discharged when the person administering the sedation is satisfied that they have recovered sufficiently. Patients receiving intravenous or oral sedation must be discharged into the care of a responsible adult, as must children receiving inhalational sedation. Adults receiving inhalational sedation with nitrous oxide and oxygen may be discharged alone at the dentist's discretion. This will largely depend on the patient's response to sedation and, therefore, can only really be suggested once the dentist has assessed the patient's reaction to having dental treatment in this manner.
- All of those who practise dentistry must be capable of dealing with a patient collapse. There are, however, no additional requirements on those practising sedation in terms of resuscitation skills from those required of all dentists. All who provide dental treatment should practise their emergency skills regularly in simulated emergency situations.
- Children and adolescents aged between 12 and 16 years should only receive sedation with midazolam or nitrous oxide unless treated in a specialist environment.
- Children aged under 12 years should only receive sedation with nitrous oxide unless treated in a specialist environment.

Intercollegiate Advisory Committee for Sedation in Dentistry's 2015 report was reviewed in 2019. The result of the review was that the committee felt that there was no reason to change the current standards.

It is each professional's responsibility to ensure that they are familiar with and comply with the required standards of practice. Although any discussion of medicolegal issues tends to cause panic, it should be remembered that those who practise ethically in accordance with guidelines have little to fear.

Self-Assessment: Questions

MULTIPLE CHOICE QUESTIONS

1. Assessment for sedation involves:
   a. Dental examination
   b. A trial attempt at dental treatment
   c. Recording the patient's blood pressure
   d. Taking a full medical history
   e. Obtaining verbal consent for treatment
2. Nitrous oxide is:
   a. A colourless gas with a pungent odour
   b. Is lighter than air
   c. Is highly soluble in blood
   d. Is a weak anaesthetic with a MAC_{50} value of about 110%
   e. Can only be used to sedate children
3. Flumazenil:
   a. Is recommended for routine use in order to hasten recovery
   b. Is not a benzodiazepine
   c. Antagonises the action of all benzodiazepines
   d. Is useful for managing allergic reactions to benzodiazepines
   e. Has a shorter half-life than midazolam
4. The following are contraindications to intravenous sedation:
   a. Myasthenia gravis
   b. Chronic bronchitis
   c. Liver failure
   d. Well-controlled angina
   e. Mild learning difficulty
5. The pharmacodynamic properties of the benzodiazepine group of drugs include:
   a. Anxiolysis
   b. Analgesia
   c. Antiemetic effect
   d. Sedation
   e. Anaesthesia
6. Nitrous oxide cylinders:
   a. Contain gaseous nitrous oxide at high pressure
   b. The pressure of the cylinder contents is directly proportional to the volume of gas remaining
   c. Are light blue with a white quartered top
   d. Must be stored vertically
   e. Can be connected to the same mounts as Entonox cylinders
7. Nitrous oxide sedation:
   a. Can only be used for children
   b. Is the only technique that can be used in general dental practices for children and adolescents aged 12–16 years
   c. Produces sufficient analgesia for soft tissue surgery
   d. Relies heavily on the operator's ability to use suggestion
   e. Is useful in patients with gagging problems

8. Oral sedation:
   a. Is less predictable than intravenous sedation
   b. Drugs may be subject to first-pass metabolism
   c. May be achieved with midazolam
   d. Means that the patient can attend without an escort
   e. Should be titrated against the patient's response
9. An overdose of intravenous benzodiazepine:
   a. Will most often present as respiratory depression
   b. May result in loss of consciousness
   c. May produce severe systemic effects including liver damage
   d. Always requires treatment with flumazenil
   e. Will result in the dental treatment having to be postponed until a future occasion
10. An overdose of nitrous oxide:
    a. Can lead to the patient laughing uncontrollably
    b. Reduces patient co-operation
    c. Occurs at the start of treatment but is unlikely later
    d. Can lead to vomiting
    e. Results in the patient's mouth becoming fixed in an open position
11. Midazolam:
    a. Is water soluble at all pH values
    b. Is half as potent as diazepam
    c. Has an elimination half-life of about 2 hours
    d. Metabolism is reduced by erythromycin
    e. Causes thrombophlebitis on injection
12. Scavenging must be used with relative analgesia sedation because nitrous oxide:
    a. Reacts with cobalt-containing enzymes
    b. Reduces the sperm count of male dentists
    c. Can cause vitamin B_{12} deficiency
    d. Makes female staff less fertile
    e. May increase incidence of cervical carcinoma in female staff.

EXTENDED MATCHING ITEMS QUESTIONS

Theme: Assessment for sedation

For each of the descriptions of patients who might be referred for conscious sedation for dental treatment (a–e), select from the list below (1–10) the **most appropriate option** for their management (more than one may be correct). Each option may be used once, more than once or not at all:

1. Provide treatment at a general dental practice with intravenous conscious sedation
2. Provide treatment at a general dental practice with inhalation sedation
3. Provide treatment at a 'Specialist Setting' with intravenous conscious sedation
4. Provide treatment at a 'Specialist Setting' with inhalation sedation
5. Provide treatment under local anaesthesia in a general dental practice

6. Provide treatment under local anaesthesia in a 'Specialist Setting'
7. Postpone treatment until the medical condition is controlled
8. Provide treatment with oral sedation
9. Provide dental treatment under general anaesthesia
    a. A 65-year-old man with hypertension and ischaemic heart disease taking aspirin, atenolol and ramipril. He has regular episodes of ischaemic chest after moderate exertion.
    b. A 58-year-old woman with untreated hypothyroidism who attends with multiple carious teeth requiring restoration but gives a history of a longstanding dental anxiety.
    c. An anxious 10-year-old requiring a lower first deciduous molar extracted. There is a history of previous failure of inhalation sedation.
    d. A 20-year-old student with a history of pericoronitis who requires both lower wisdom teeth extracted but has little experience of dental treatment.
    e. A 45-year-old patient who requires impressions taken to construct an acid-etch bridge but cannot tolerate these as they make him feel sick.

CASE HISTORY QUESTION

Case history

A 14-year-old female is referred for the extraction of four first premolars for orthodontic reasons. She is a pleasant but anxious child who attends a local boarding school.

Medical history

The patient says she faints easily but has not been investigated. She has an allergy to elastoplast.

Dental history

Although a regular attender for as long as she can remember, the patient has previously only had one small filling that did not require local analgesia.

Intraoral examination

The patient has good oral hygiene, with all teeth bar the third molars fully erupted. There is crowding evident in both arches.

1. What are the treatment options?
2. Which is the best option and why?
3. What is the major problem with providing treatment for this girl?

PICTURE QUESTIONS

Picture 1

1. What is the piece of equipment shown in Fig. 6.5?
2. What are the features labelled a–g?

Picture 2

1. What are the pieces of equipment in Fig. 6.6?
2. Given the choice, which would be used for dental sedation and why?

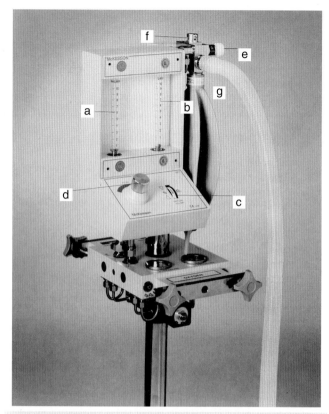

Fig. 6.5 Equipment used in sedation. (Image courtesy of Cestradent McKesson.)

SHORT NOTE QUESTIONS

Write short notes on:
1. the advantages of midazolam over propofol as an intravenous sedative
2. the disadvantages of oral sedation
3. the signs and symptoms of oversedation with nitrous oxide
4. factors that could cause the arterial saturation reading on a pulse oximeter to fall to 85% during sedation with intravenous midazolam
5. the principal clinical effects of the benzodiazepine group of drugs
6. factors observed during the clinical monitoring of a sedated patient.

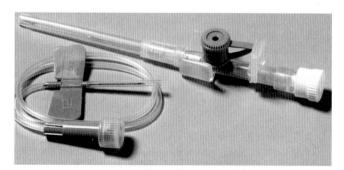

Fig. 6.6 Equipment for venous access.

VIVA QUESTIONS

1. How would you assess a patient who attends asking to be referred for intravenous sedation?

2. Describe how you would explain inhalational sedation to a 10-year-old child who is referred for treatment.

Self-Assessment: Answers

MULTIPLE CHOICE ANSWERS

1. a. True. It is important to at least have a look in the patient's mouth to establish that there is a treatment need and give the patient an idea of the amount of time required. If the patient is very anxious, then probing cavities and restoration margins or doing a periodontal assessment will tend to distress the patient.
    b. False. It is cruel and heartless to imply that patients must be shown to be unable to tolerate treatment before offering sedation.
    c. True. The only exception to this rule is that fit children who are to receive relative analgesia do not normally have their blood pressure recorded. It may also be that with some patients with moderate learning difficulties, there may be insufficient co-operation for what is an uncomfortable procedure.
    d. True. All patients undergoing any dental intervention should have a full medical history recorded.
    e. False. Written informed consent is required for all treatment under any form of sedation.

2. a. False. Although colourless, nitrous oxide has a sweet odour.
    b. False. Nitrous oxide is about 1.5 times as dense as air.
    c. False. Nitrous oxide is very insoluble in blood, a fact in the rapid onset of and recovery from sedation.
    d. True.
    e. False. Nitrous oxide is suitable for just about all ages of patients. It is vastly underused in adult patients.

3. a. False. It is currently recommended that flumazenil is only used in an emergency.
    b. False. Flumazenil is a benzodiazepine. In fact, it is very closely related to midazolam in chemical structure.
    c. True.
    d. False. If a patient is allergic to any other benzodiazepine, they will almost certainly be allergic to flumazenil. Giving it in this situation will make things worse, not better.
    e. True. The shorter half-life has been used as an argument against its routine use.

4. a. True. The muscle-relaxant properties of the benzodiazepines coupled with the poor transmission of motor impulses to muscles can lead to paralysis.
    b. True. The altered respiratory drive associated with chronic hypoxia in severe chronic bronchitis makes patients extremely sensitive to the respiratory depressant effects of the sedative agents.
    c. True. Midazolam is principally broken down in the liver. There is, however, significant extrahepatic breakdown. Consequently, liver failure will only be a problem when the function is sufficiently severe to cause problems with breakdown of local anaesthetics and a failure of clotting.
    d. False. If the angina is well controlled, sedation may be used. It may also be of great value if the patient normally has few problems but gives a history of exacerbation of the problem during dental treatment.
    e. False. Sedation may help such patients to cope with treatment.

5. a. True.
    b. False. Relief of anxiety may influence the patient's perception of stimuli or reaction to chronic pain, but benzodiazepines have no analgesic properties.
    c. False.
    d. True.
    e. True. Large enough doses of benzodiazepines, particularly if given rapidly intravenously, will produce loss of consciousness.

6. a. False. The cylinders contain both gas and liquid under pressure.
    b. False. The pressure remains constant until all the liquid has vaporised. This occurs when only one-eighth of the contents are left.
    c. False. The cylinders are light blue. The white quartered top denotes an Entonox cylinder.
    d. True. This prevents liquid entering the gas outlet.
    e. False. The pin index system is gas specific.

7. a. False. This technique is useful for a wide range of patients. Adults can be managed extremely well with inhalational sedation.
    b. False. Patients of this age can also be sedated with midazolam if it is assessed as the technique of choice for the dental treatment required.
    c. False. There is some analgesia, but insufficient for surgical procedures.
    d. True.
    e. True.

8. a. True. The pattern of drug absorption is unpredictable and, therefore, the effects of the dose and the time to onset of sedation are unpredictable.
    b. True. The drug once absorbed from the gastrointestinal tract passes via the portal circulation to the liver. Here, a significant proportion is metabolised.
    c. True.
    d. False. The effects may persist longer than intravenous agents. Temazepam has a significantly longer half-life than midazolam.
    e. False. The long latent period for the absorption of oral drugs means that the dose has to be given on a best guess basis.

9. a. True.
   b. True.
   c. False. There are no toxic effects to systems. The effects are of respiratory depression and anaesthesia. If the patient is supported until the drugs are eliminated, they will make an uneventful recovery.
   d. False. Minor overdose can be managed by encouraging the patient to breathe and supporting them until they recover to a normal level of sedation.
   e. False. Once the patient has returned to a normal level of sedation (if managed as in [d]), treatment can be carried out.
10. a. True. Hence the name laughing gas.
   b. True. It feels unpleasant to the patient, and they often become disorientated.
   c. False. Overdose often occurs later in treatment, when the part of the procedure that the patient dislikes most is past and their requirement for anxiolysis reduces.
   d. True. This is a relatively late sign of overdose, and one would hope that remedial action would be taken before this stage was reached.
   e. False. Spontaneous mouth closing is an early sign of overdose. Mouth props should not be used with inhalation sedation, as they mask this important sign.
11. a. False. It is lipid soluble at physiological pH and can cross the blood–brain barrier.
   b. False. It is about two to five times as potent as diazepam.
   c. True.
   d. True.
   e. False. This is one of midazolam's great advantages over diazepam.
12. a. True.
   b. False.
   c. True.
   d. True.
   e. True.

EXTENDED MATCHING ITEMS ANSWERS

a. **3, 4.** If the patient is assessed as needing sedation, then either 3 or 4 would be correct. In theory, the use of inhalation sedation has advantages, as it provides an increased amount of oxygen. Nitrous oxide also produces some vasodilatation, which may also improve the blood supply to the myocardium. Intravenous sedation can be used, but care should be taken to avoid hypoxia. This patient is ASA III, and therefore the treatment should be provided in a 'specialist' environment (i.e. one where the staff are used to providing sedation for medically compromised patients). If the patient can cope with treatment under local anaesthesia alone, then treatment could be provided in the primary care setting.

b. **7.** Patients with untreated hypothyroidism are unduly sensitive to both local anaesthetics and central nervous system depressant drugs. Once an appropriate level of thyroxine replacement is started, then the patient can be treated under the type of sedation that is assessed as being the most appropriate. There would then be no contraindication to sedation in the primary care environment.

c. **3 or 2.** If at assessment it is felt that inhalation sedation will fail again, then intravenous sedation is a possible option. General anaesthesia can be considered, but at the age of 10 years, the extraction will be relatively straightforward due to physiological root resorption. Thus GA is best avoided if possible. This patient cannot be treated in the primary care setting. If the patient is assessed, and it is felt that there has been a significant change in the patient since inhalation sedation failed, it could be considered.

d. **1, 3.** Many patients cope with the surgical extraction of wisdom teeth under local anaesthesia alone. There is, however, little doubt that it is a stressful procedure. The use of intravenous sedation is useful as the amnesia prevents the patient remembering the treatment. The choice between 1 and 3 will depend on the clinician's surgical ability. The sedation could be carried out in primary care.

e. **2.** Inhalation sedation is very good at controlling problems with gagging. Consideration should also be given to altering the impression technique (e.g. using a lower tray in the upper arch so that contact between the impression material and the palate is reduced).

CASE HISTORY ANSWER

1. The treatment options are:
   - local anaesthesia
   - inhalation sedation
   - intravenous sedation if child appears mature for her years
   - oral sedation
   - general anaesthesia.
2. Inhalation sedation is the best option, although all are potentially possible. Local anaesthesia alone is asking a child with little experience of dental treatment to tolerate a total of eight local anaesthetic injections (including two palatal) and cope with four extractions. In an attempt to avoid using gas, many dentists tried to persuade children in this category to have treatment under local anaesthesia, and the result was an increase in the number of children referred to have three first premolars out under general anaesthesia. Intravenous, oral and transmucosal sedation are all possible. At the age of 14 years, the patient is still considered a child in legal terms, but there is a wide range of variation in the maturity of individuals of the same age. Oral or transmucosal sedation would only be considered if it was felt that a greater level of sedation than could be produced by inhalation sedation was required, but the patient could not tolerate intravenous cannulation. General anaesthesia should be avoided if at all possible. Its use for a minor cosmetic procedure cannot be justified, particularly in the light of recent publicity.
3. The major problem in this case is medicolegal, not clinical. Obtaining consent for treatment for this patient is a problem, as the parents presumably live a long way from the school. The head teacher will have the power to act as guardian and give medical consent in an emergency situation, but this would not be the case for orthodontic treatment. The parents must at least be spoken to on the telephone and be sent a consent form to sign if they cannot be seen face to face.

PICTURE ANSWERS

Picture 1

1. This is the head of a MAC1 Inhalation Sedation Machine.

2. Features are:
   a. nitrous oxide flow rotameter
   b. oxygen flow rotameter
   c. gas mixture control
   d. gas flow rate control
   e. oxygen flush button
   f. air entrainment value
   g. common gas outlet.

Picture 2

1. These are (a) an intravenous cannula and (b) a butterfly needle.
2. The cannula is used in preference to the butterfly. The use of the butterfly leaves a needle in the patient's vein. This can cut out of the vein if the site is subject to movement. The cannula is soft, blunt ended and flexible and so once sited will not tend to cut out. The cannula is Teflon-coated and does not encourage the clotting of blood, whereas cells can coagulate around the steel of the butterfly. The cannula is more likely to give intravenous access for the duration of the appointment.

SHORT NOTE ANSWERS

1. Midazolam is water soluble and, therefore, does not cause pain on intravascular injection, whereas propofol causes pain on injection (particularly in small veins). Propofol should be administered by continuous infusion using a syringe pump, whereas midazolam is titrated to effect. The equipment costs for the administration of propofol are greater and a separate sedationist is required. All patients requiring sedation with propofol must have their blood pressure recorded every 5 minutes, which is uncomfortable and can cause patient movement, whereas fit and healthy patients sedated with midazolam need to only have recordings taken pre - and postsedation.
2. The disadvantages of oral sedation are:
   - prolonged latent period
   - unpredictable dose
   - unpredictable absorption
   - first-pass metabolism.
3. The signs of oversedation with nitrous oxide are:
   - persistent mouth closing
   - spontaneous mouth-breathing
   - disorientation
   - irrational or sluggish response to command
   - poor co-operation
   - unconsciousness.
   The five symptoms of oversedation with nitrous oxide are:
   - loss of control
   - unpleasant sensations
   - anxiety
   - headache
   - nausea.
4. Technical causes of fall in arterial oxygen saturation recorded by the pulse oximeter are:
   - probe loose or misplaced
   - cuff partially inflated on same limb.
   Patient causes of fall in arterial oxygen saturation are:
   - obstruction owing to oversedation
   - obstruction by foreign body

   - obstruction because of treating dentist's activity
   - respiratory depression caused by sedative agent
   - pre-existing respiratory or cardiovascular disease
   - collapse (e.g. faint).
5. The clinical effects of the benzodiazepines are:
   - anxiolysis
   - anticonvulsion
   - sedation
   - reduced attention
   - amnesia
   - muscle relaxation
   - anaesthesia
   - respiratory depression
   - fall in blood pressure (minimal)
   - increase in heart rate (slight)
   - potential sexual fantasy.
6. Factors monitored clinically during sedation:
   - level of consciousness (response to verbal command)
   - level of relaxation
   - response to treatment (effectiveness of sedation)
   - respiration
   - rate
   - depth
   - signs of obstruction
   - pulse
   - heart rate
   - rhythm
   - volume
   - colour: skin and mucosa.

VIVA ANSWERS

1. You should describe assessment in terms of:
   - medical history: any problems or contraindications to a particular type of sedation
   - dental history: current pain, previous care, particular fears, particular wishes regarding current treatment, previous management – what was successful and what was not
   - social history: alcohol or drug abuse; availability of an escort
   - physical evaluation: blood pressure measurement, assessment of the airway and assessment of potential intravenous cannulation sites
   - dental examination
   - radiographic examination
   - explanation of the likely treatment options
   - provision of written and verbal information including pre- and postoperative instructions
   - obtaining verbal and written consent to the sedation and dental treatment.
2. It is important in answering this type of question to use words that a 10-year-old child would understand. Thus, terms like 'tingly' should be used, not paraesthesia. In all events, it is important to emphasise that it will feel pleasant, warm etc. but always use phrases like 'you may feel' as not everyone has all of the symptoms described in the section on inhalational sedation. It is also wise to talk about a nosepiece rather than a mask in case the child has had a previous bad experience with general anaesthesia.

7 *Paediatric Dentistry I*

Overview

Successfully treating younger patients requires knowledge of normal child and adolescent development and behaviour, as well as the technical and clinical skills necessary to work in small and changing mouths. The clinicians' aim for this cohort of patients is to deliver them to young adulthood with good oral health and a positive attitude towards dental care. A focus on prevention and behaviour management is paramount if this aim is to be achieved.

7.1 Tooth Development and Eruption

LEARNING OBJECTIVES

You should:
- know at what age primary teeth begin to mineralise, at what age their root formation is complete and at what age they erupt
- know at what age permanent teeth begin to mineralise, at what age their root formation is complete and at what age they erupt.

TOOTH DEVELOPMENT

Tooth germs develop from the dental lamina, and the dental lamina develops from the primary epithelial band. The dental lamina forms a series of epithelial buds that grow into surrounding connective tissue. The buds become associated with a condensation of mesenchyme, and together they represent a tooth germ at its early 'cap' stage of development. The epithelial bud becomes the enamel organ and the mesenchymal cells the dental papilla and follicle. The cells at the margin of the enamel organ grow to enclose some mesenchymal cells, the 'bell' stage of development. Histo-differentiation of the enamel organ now forms the external and internal enamel epithelia, stratum intermedium and stellate reticulum.

On the lingual aspect of each primary tooth germ, the dental lamina proliferates to produce the permanent successor tooth germ. Permanent tooth germs with no primary precursors are produced by distal extension of the dental lamina.

Dentine formation occurs after differentiation of dental papilla cells into odontoblasts, which is induced by the internal enamel epithelium. Once dentine formation has begun, the adjacent cells of the internal enamel epithelium differentiate into ameloblasts and produce enamel. The dentine of the roots of teeth is produced in a similar fashion by differentiation of odontoblasts induced by the internal enamel epithelium, and root growth is controlled by the epithelial cells at the margins of the enamel organ – the root sheath of Hertwig. Root growth is not complete until 1–2 years in the primary dentition and 3–5 years in the permanent dentition after eruption of the crowns of the teeth. The beginning of mineralisation for both dentitions is given in Tables 7.1 and 7.2.

Eruption

The exact controlling mechanism of eruption has not yet been identified. It is likely that the dental follicle has a major part to play, as the connective tissue of the follicle is a rich source of factors responsible for the local mediation of bone deposition and resorption. Typical eruption times are given in Tables 7.1 and 7.2.

7.2 Management of the Child Patient

LEARNING OBJECTIVES

You should:
- know the milestones of child development
- be able to relate milestones to what an individual child can be expected to cope with in the dental surgery
- know the strategies that a dentist could employ to help children to cope
- appreciate the importance of an accurate and comprehensive history and examination.

Table 7.1 Typical Times for Calcification and Eruption of Deciduous Teeth.

	Calcification Begins (Weeks in Utero)	Eruption (Months)
UPPER		
Central incisor (a)	12–16	6–7
Lateral incisor (b)	13–16	7–8
Canine (c)	15–18	18–20
First molar (d)	14–17	12–15
Second molar (e)	16–23	24–36
LOWER		
Central incisor (a)	12–16	6–7
Lateral incisor (b)	13–16	7–8
Canine (c)	15–18	18–20
First molar (d)	14–17	12–15
Second molar (e)	16–23	24–36

Root calcification is complete 1–1.5 years after eruption.
Typical eruption sequence is a, b, d, c and e.

Table 7.2 Typical Times for Calcification and Eruption of Permanent Teeth.

	Calcification Begins (Months)	Eruption (Years)
UPPER		
Central incisor	3–4	7–8
Lateral incisor	10–12	8–9
Canine	4–5	11–12
First premolar	18–21	10–11
Second premolar	24–27	10–12
First molar	At birth	6–7
Second molar	30–36	12–13
Third molar	84–108	17–21
LOWER		
Central incisor	3–4	6–7
Lateral incisor	3–4	7–8
Canine	4–5	9–10
First premolar	21–24	10–12
Second premolar	27–30	11–12
First molar	At birth	5–6
Second molar	30–36	12–13
Third molar	96–120	17–21

Root calcification is complete 2–3 years after eruption.
Typical eruption sequence: upper 6 1 2 4 5 3 7 8; lower 6 1 2 3 4 5 7 8.

PSYCHOLOGICAL ASPECTS

Child Development

Development should be regarded as a continuum, as it differs from child to child. It is an uneven process and is influenced by periods of rapid bodily change. There are certain 'psychological signposts' that are important for the dentist and their staff to recognise.

Motor Development

Motor development occurs in a predictable order, and identification of failure to attain 'motor milestones' enables remedial intervention to help improve motor skills. The environment can influence general motor development, and this type of development is completed in early life. Skills or changes that follow walking are refinements rather than new skills. Dominance of one hand emerges early. Motor retardation in a child may be manifested by no specific handed dominance. At 6–7 years of age, a child may have sufficient co-ordination to brush their teeth reasonably well. Below 6–7 years, many areas of the mouth will be inaccessible without parental help.

Cognitive Development

Sensorimotor at 0–2 years. The infant can think of things as permanent without having to see them directly.
Preoperational at 2–7 years. Thought patterns are not well developed; the child is egocentric and inflexible.
Concrete operations at 7–11 years. The child can apply logical reasoning and consider another person's point of view.
Formal operations at 11 years or older. Transition to adult thinking results in the development of logical abstract thinking and different possibilities for action can be considered.

Perceptual Development

By age 7 years, children do develop selective attention and can determine which advice merits attention and which can be ignored. Concentration skills also improve. By age 9 years, children achieve adult proficiency.

Language Development

Language and thought are inter-related and lack of stimulation will delay both. Keep dental jargon to a minimum and always assess patients before offering advice.

Social Development

Separation anxiety is high until age 5 years, and then declines rapidly, so do not expect a child younger than this to enter the surgery on their own.

Adolescence

Increasing independency and self-sufficiency develop in adolescence. Young people can be moody, oversensitive to criticism and often feel miserable for no apparent reason. Therefore, do not criticise adolescents excessively, and try to give them support and reassurance.

Parental Influence and Dental Treatment

Parents are vital for positive reinforcement as regards how a child copes with dental intervention. Parents should be encouraged not to transfer any negative thoughts they may have regarding dentistry to their child. Treatment plans should be designed to accommodate the social dynamics of the family with regard to appointment times and number. Treatment plans should allow goals to be achieved one by one, never overloading parent or child.

Dentist–Patient Relationship

Each patient is a unique individual and should be treated as such. Overall, it is fair to conclude that while the technical skill of a dentist is of concern, the most important factors for a patient are gentle, friendly manner, explanation of treatment procedures and the ability to keep pain to a minimum.

Anxious and Uncooperative Children

The extent of dental fear and anxiety (DFA) does not relate to dental knowledge but is an amalgam of personal experiences, family concerns, disease levels and general personality traits. It is, therefore, not easy to pinpoint aetiological agents and measure anxiety. While there is no standard measure of anxiety, self-reported DFA measures such as the Modified Child Dental Anxiety Scale, suitable for completion by children aged 8–15 years, can be useful.

Helping Anxious Patients Cope

There are a number of non-pharmacological behaviour management approaches available which can help to reduce coping problems:

- Reducing uncertainty – tell, show, do.
- Pre-visit preparation, for example, send letter home explaining details of proposed visit.
- Modelling – this can incorporate videos or a relaxed and co-operative 'live' model.
- Enhancing control – for example, introduction of an agreed signal the child can use to indicate treatment should stop.
- Distraction – attempts to shift attention from dental setting towards another kind of situation (e.g. videos, headphones with music or stories). A patient can also be distracted during difficult procedures such as local anaesthetic by firmly rubbing their cheek and talking loudly to them, thus stimulating other senses.
- Guided imagery – helping the patient to 'daydream' promoting a state of relaxation. This involves three stages: relaxation, visualisation and positive suggestion.
- Behaviour shaping and positive reinforcement – this involves rewarding children when desired behaviour is displayed. Reinforcement can be verbal, for example, 'great mouth opening'! or with a small present, for example, a sticker.
- Negative reinforcement – removal of a stimulus the child finds unpleasant when desired behaviour is displayed, for example, a parent leaving the surgery when behaviour is inappropriate and returning when the desired behaviour is displayed.
- Relaxation – this is useful for high levels of tension and aims to bring about deep muscular relaxation; several simple techniques are available for use by dentists.
- Systematic desensitisation – gradually working through various levels of feared situations from those which cause 'least anxiety' to 'most anxiety'.
- Other options such as cognitive behavioural therapy (CBT) or hypnosis can be considered, but these can require further training before use.

Where non-pharmacological behaviour techniques are insufficient in allowing the child to cope with treatment, or where the complexity of the operative procedure demands it, pharmacological methods may need to be employed. These include:

- Inhalation sedation: usually for ages 5 years and over
- Intravenous sedation: usually for ages 12 and over
- General anaesthetic.

7.3 History, Examination and Treatment Planning

Entering the dental surgery can be a daunting experience for any child and/or their family. The initial meeting with a child and their family allows information to be collected which will help direct any care required. In addition, examination visits allow the dental team to gain a rapport with the family and set the scene for any future treatment requirements. Children should be addressed by name, and the dental staff should introduce themselves and explain who they are. At the beginning of the appointment, it can be useful to outline what it will involve, for example, today we are just going to have a chat about your teeth, and then if you are happy, we will have a look at your mouth with the mirror.

Patient/parent concerns. Depending on the age of the child, it may be appropriate to ask either the child themselves or the accompanying adult to outline and provide a history of any dental concerns.

Medical history. This should be updated at each examination appointment. Apart from allowing safe delivery of dental care, two additional factors can be gleaned: children with medical conditions may have a negative attitude to treatment because of the time they have spent in hospitals; they may also be more likely to fail dental appointments owing to the disruption in education that the medical problem has already caused.

Dental history. Past dental experiences may give an indication of how the child will cope with proposed treatment. Parental attitude to treatment is important. A treatment plan must be modified to accommodate this. Establish exactly why they have come. The answers from child and parent may be different!

Prevention. Ask about toothbrushing habits, for example, how often and when teeth are brushed, who brushes the child's teeth, concentration of fluoride toothpaste used, enrolment in school fluoride varnish programmes (e.g. Childsmile in Scotland). Ask about dietary habits including what the child eats between meals, what drinks are normally consumed, whether the child takes a bottle or a drink to bed and if so what is consumed.

Social history. Information should be collected on the school attended, who lives in the child's household, who has parental rights and responsibilities for the child and whether the family has an assigned social worker. This information can be helpful to assess social background, knowledge of dentistry and the family's expectations.

EXAMINATION

Clinical Examination

The clinical examination need not involve sitting in the dental chair at the first visit, and it may take some time before a child allows the dental examination to take place. It can be helpful to involve the child in the process and allow them an element of control, for example, the child could hold the dental mirror while handwashing takes place and a hand signal could be introduced allowing the child to stop if needed at any time. Where children attend with their family, it can be helpful to let them watch other (relaxed and co-operative) family members have a dental examination before it is their turn.

Extraoral

General appearance is noted; percentile charts are a useful way of monitoring height and weight. The head and neck are examined, making a sketch of any lesions/marks.

Intraoral

Teeth must be clean and dry to allow a thorough examination. It can be helpful to carry out a toothbrushing demonstration at the beginning of the appointment so teeth are cleaned prior to the examination.

Soft tissues. These may be an indicator of systemic disease.

Teeth. Teeth present should be confirmed to that expected for a patient's age. Any disturbance in the sequence of permanent tooth eruption, for example, a lateral incisor which erupts prior to the permanent incisor warrants further investigation. Teeth condition, for example, presence of caries or defects such as hypomineralisation should be recorded.

Occlusion. Assessment of incisor relationship, molar relationship, overjet, overbite, crowding, crossbite, mandibular deviations and the ability to palpate unerupted maxillary canines.

Periodontal condition. A modified Basic Periodontal Examination (BPE) should be completed in children aged 7–17 years. This assesses six index teeth (UR6, UR1, UL6, LL6, LL1 and LR6). BPE codes 0–2 are used for 7- to 11-year-olds (mixed dentition stage) to screen for bleeding and the presence of local plaque retentive factors. The full range of codes, including any furcation involvement, can be used in 12- to 17-year-olds (permanent teeth erupted).

Periodontal condition not consistent with oral hygiene may indicate an underlying condition and warrant further investigation.

SPECIAL TESTS

Radiographic Examination

There are three general indications for taking radiographs in children:

Caries Diagnosis

At least 50% more approximal lesions can be diagnosed by bitewing radiographs than with clinical examination. High-resolution digital orthopantomogram (OPT) films at the appropriate setting (that which will separate the interproximal contacts) are efficient at diagnosing occlusal and approximal caries. Many standard OPT films are, however, still inadequate for caries diagnosis and, in this case, intraoral bitewing radiographs remain the method of choice. Intervals for bitewing radiographs depend on caries risk. Intervals suggested by the European guideline on radiation protection in dental radiology 2004 are outlined as follows:

- High caries risk: radiographs should be repeated at 6 monthly intervals until no new or active lesions are apparent and the individual has entered a lower risk category.

- Moderate caries risk: radiographs should be repeated annually until no new or active lesions are apparent and the individual has entered a lower risk category.
- Low caries risk: intervals of 12–18 months (deciduous dentition) or 24 months (permanent dentition) may be used, although longer intervals may be appropriate where there is continuing low caries risk.

If extraction of permanent teeth is considered owing to caries, an OPT should be taken to assess the presence of dental anomalies (e.g. hypodontia), which may influence treatment decisions and also allow assessment of the stage of development of surrounding teeth, which can influence the timing of permanent tooth removal. For example, the ideal time to remove poor prognosis first permanent molars (FPMs), in the absence of orthodontic requirements, is when the furcation of the second permanent molar is developing.

Abnormalities in Dental Development

OPT views can be used to identify disturbances in development of the dentition in terms of the number, position and form of the teeth. Precise location of maxillary canines, if required, can then be achieved by intraoral parallax technique.

Detection of Bony or Dental Pathology

Periapical radiographs for individual teeth; OPT views for larger pathology or bony trauma.

Cone Beam Computed Tomography (CBCT)

CBCT has been available since the early 2000s and can provide three-dimensional imaging. This may be helpful, in selected cases. Evidence-based guidelines produced by the SEDENTEXCT project in 2012 outline justification, optimisation, referral criteria and training requirements for users of dental CBCT.

Radiation doses to patients from CBCT, although lower than from medical computed tomography (CT) equipment, can be significantly higher than those from conventional dental X-ray equipment.

Other Investigations

There are a number of other special tests that may be indicated:

- Sensitivity/sensibility testing: tests the nerve supply to a tooth. Hot and cold stimuli can be evoked using hot gutta-percha or ethyl chloride and electrical stimulation can be applied using an electric pulp tester. These tests are not suitable for the primary dentition, however, and are not completely reliable in the permanent dentition.
- Culture and sensitivity: bacterial, fungal and viral infections.
- Blood tests: haematological, biochemical, bacteriological and virological examination.
- Salivary flow rate tests are rarely required in children.

TREATMENT PLANNING

Planning should incorporate:

- management of pain: consider all teeth of poor prognosis
- long-term treatment planning: to include attitudes and motivation

- consideration of required behaviour management techniques
- preventive care: tailored to each individual
- restorative care: realistic aims are important
- aesthetic considerations: children can be under considerable peer pressure over their appearance Orthodontic needs.

7.4 Caries

LEARNING OBJECTIVES

You should:
- be able to explain the development of caries to any patient/parent
- know how to carry out a caries risk assessment
- know how to tailor a preventive plan in accordance with a child's caries risk
- know the current materials in use for the restoration of primary and permanent teeth and their respective advantages and disadvantages.

DEVELOPMENT OF CARIES

Fermentation of dietary sugars by micro-organisms in plaque on the tooth surface produces organic acids. This rapid acid formation lowers the pH at the enamel surface below the level (critical pH 5.5) at which enamel will dissolve, a process known as demineralisation. When sugar is no longer available to the plaque micro-organisms, the pH within plaque will rise through the outward diffusion of acids and their metabolites. As a result, remineralisation of enamel can occur.

Dental caries progresses only when demineralisation is greater than remineralisation. The early caries lesion is subsurface with white surface demineralisation (precavitation). This may be because a layer of dental plaque on the tooth acts as a partial barrier to diffusion. Plaque forms on tooth surfaces that are not cleaned and is visually obvious within 2–3 days of ceasing toothbrushing. Plaque composition is 70% micro-organisms. Diet influences plaque flora composition; in diets rich in carbohydrate, *Streptococcus mutans* predominates and is very efficient at metabolising sugars to acids. Precavitated carious lesions can be reversed by remineralisation if the plaque pH is high (alkaline). This can occur during the periods where there is no sugar intake. The concentrations of calcium, phosphate and fluoride in plaque are very important in the remineralisation process.

Once cavitation has occurred and the thin white surface layer has collapsed, it is necessary to restore the tooth surface with a restoration, treat with biological methods or pragmatically via enhanced prevention depending on individual patient assessment. It is not possible to reverse a cavitated lesion.

EPIDEMIOLOGY OF CARIES

The size of the problem of caries in the population has changed over time. Prevalence and extent have fallen markedly since the late 1970s in many countries, and this fall can largely be attributed to fluoridated toothpaste. The 2013 Child Dental Health Survey in England, Wales and Northern Ireland found that 34% of 12-year-olds and 46% of 15-years-olds had obvious decay experience in the permanent dentition, while 31% of 5-year-olds and 46% of 8-year-olds had obvious decay experience in the primary dentition. In the permanent dentition, there had been a continued improvement in dental health compared to results from 1993 and 2003. Results in the primary dentition could not be directly compared to previous years given a change in methodology. In Scotland, the National Dental Inspection Program found 20% of 12-year-old children had caries in the permanent dentition (2019 data), and that 29% of 5-year-old children had obvious decay experience in the primary dentition (2018 data). Results for both dentitions revealed a continuing improvement in dental health.

Assessing Dental Caries

The best method to assess caries is visual inspection on clean, dry teeth with good lighting. This can be supplemented by radiographs as outlined in section 7.3. The use of orthodontic separators to separate teeth and allow visual assessment of cavitation can be considered if enamel-only proximal lesions are identified radiographically.

CARIES RISK ASSESSMENT

Each child should undergo a caries risk assessment which will assist in future planning, particularly in relation to the preventive regime offered.

An effective caries risk assessment comprises seven elements:

1. Clinical evidence: this takes account of the past and present caries experience and the rate at which new lesions are developing. A child may be caries free at the time of examination, but if they have recently had carious teeth removed or repaired, they would remain as high risk. Other areas of clinical evidence adding to a child's risk include the wearing of orthodontic appliances.
2. Dietary habits: especially frequency of sugar intake is important in the development of caries.
3. Social history: main factors to look at are socioeconomic status and parental attitudes to oral health. Cost and availability of toothpaste and toothbrushes should also be explored as well as access to and cost of fresh fruit and vegetables. Children from more deprived areas or who have eligibility for free school meals are more likely to have obvious decay experience in both the primary and permanent dentition.
4. Fluoride use: ask about toothbrushing habits and toothpaste strength and as to whether or not any other sources of fluoride are used.
5. Plaque control: amounts of plaque in the mouth are dependent on oral hygiene practices and sugars in the diet.
6. Saliva: some children may have specific problems in relation to the amount or composition of their saliva, making them at higher risk of developing caries.
7. Medical history: some children are at greater risk of developing caries due to their medications, prescribed diet or ability to practise oral hygiene effectively. Other children are classified as high risk if poor oral health could have a considerable detrimental effect on their current medical condition, for example, patients with cardiac conditions or who are immunocompromised.

There is no consensus on which factors are more effective in determining caries risk, although previous caries experience appears to be the more reliable predictor of caries risk.

DENTAL CARIES PREVENTION

The preventive regime offered will relate directly to the child's caries risk assessment. A full preventive plan contains eight elements:

1. Regular dental visits: parents/carers should be encouraged to register their child with a dentist as soon as the first tooth erupts or by the age of 1 year at the latest and to visit regularly.
2. Toothbrushing instruction: brushing should commence as soon as the first primary tooth erupts. Teeth should be brushed at least twice daily with a fluoridated toothpaste. After brushing, excess toothpaste should be spit out rather than rinsed out. It is important to offer child and/or their parent a lesson on effective toothbrushing, as many will never have been shown how to brush their teeth properly. Children should be assisted with toothbrushing until they have the manual dexterity and motivation to brush well themselves. Disclosing solution or tablets can be useful in showing the child areas that they have missed. It is important to emphasise a systematic approach so that no surfaces are left unclean. Powered toothbrushes, timers toothbrushing apps and/or sticker charts can all be good motivational tools. Caries reduction cannot be achieved by toothbrushing alone. However, brushing will control gingivitis and periodontal disease and is an important way of conveying fluoride to the tooth surface.
3. Toothpaste strength advice: fluoride has the ability to increase enamel resistance to demineralisation as well as decreasing acid production in plaque and increasing remineralisation. Although it has a pre-eruptive effect, its major role is post-eruptive.

All children should use a toothpaste containing fluoride between 1000 and 1500 ppm. Children at increased risk of developing dental caries should use a higher strength of toothpaste when compared with those aged 10+ prescribed 2800 ppm fluoride toothpaste.

Toothpaste amount should be restricted to a smear under the age of 2 and a small pea size for 2–6 years. In this younger age group, supervision and assistance during brushing are needed for efficiency and to prevent excess swallowing of paste as this may lead to fluorosis.

4. Fluoride varnish frequency: professionally applied fluoride varnishes have been shown to be very effective. For children at high risk of caries, 22,600 ppm fluoride varnish can be placed 3 monthly from the age of 2 years. Care should be taken to follow manufacturers guidance for use of the varnish. Varnishes containing Colophony are not suitable for children with severe asthma or allergies.
5. Supplemental fluoride: fluoride mouthrinses for children over the age of 6 years could be considered. Fluoride drops and tablets for systemic use are now increasingly difficult to source and have been largely superseded by increased toothpaste strengths and regular professional application of fluoride varnish. Although each individual method of fluoride application is effective, a combination of methods may achieve greater benefit.
6. Dietary advice: non-milk extrinsic sugars (NME) are most cariogenic – sucrose, glucose, fructose maltose. While Intrinsic sugars (lactose in milk and sugars in fruit and vegetables) are generally less harmful, this depends on the form and timing of their consumption e.g. fruit becomes cariogenic if dried or pureed/juiced.

A 3- or 4-day diet diary is more effective than simply asking a child and parent about their diet. The diet diary, if filled out correctly, will provide information about frequency and time of day with regard to sugar intake. It is also good practice for the diary to include toothbrushing times and bedtime, which will increase the accuracy of your dietary analysis.

The general advice is to restrict foods and drinks to mealtimes and not to consume them within 20 minutes of bedtime. Dietary counselling should be personal, practical and positive and realistic targets for change/improvement should be agreed. Where complete restriction of cariogenic food/drink is not realistic focus should be on appropriate times for their intake. Suitable alternatives to cariogenic food/drinks should be suggested. Diet advice should focus on overall health of the child. Suggested diet advice is outlined below:

Drinks:
- Plain water or plain milk are safe choices to drink.
- If a drink is taken at bedtime, it must only be water. While milk is a safe drink during the day, it can cause decay if taken during the night.
- Tea and coffee are not suitable drinks for young children.
- All other drinks contain sugar and/or acid and should be avoided in between meals.
- Use of a feeder cup or bottle overnight with milk or juice should be strongly discouraged. If a child wants to drink throughout the night, the only safe liquid is plain water. In general, bottle-fed babies should not require overnight milk after 4–6 months old, and on-demand breastfeeding overnight should also be discouraged from this time.

Foods:
- Foods that contain sugar should be **avoided in between meals**. If taken at all, they should be restricted to a mealtime. Examples of tooth-friendly snacks are provided in Box 7.1.
- Many foods including those aimed at children and babies contain sugar. Be aware that statements on food packaging such as 'organic', 'no added sugar', 'natural ingredients' or 'no junk promise' DO NOT mean the food is sugar free.
- Checking the list of ingredients on food packaging can help to identify whether a food contains sugar. There are many different names for sugar which are listed in Box 7.2.

Non-sugar sweeteners allowed for use in food and drinks can be considered for practical purposes as non-cariogenic. There are two groups of non-sugar sweeteners:
1. Bulk: sorbitol, mannitol, isomalt, xylitol, lactitol and hydrogenated glucose syrup.
2. Intense: saccharin, acesulphame K, aspartame, thaumatin.

Bulk sweeteners have a laxative effect and should not be given to children under the age of 3 years.

Box 7.1   Examples of Tooth-Friendly Snacks.

- Whole fruit (not juiced or dried)
- Vegetables
- Reduced fat cheese
- Unsweetened natural yoghurt/plain fromage frais (could add fruit to these)
- Plain bread, for example, wholemeal, brown, granary, white, high fibre and rye bread, pitta, chapatti, rolls, baguettes and bagels
- Sandwiches fillings such as salad, fish, banana, oily fish (fresh or canned in water), egg
- Soft cheese
- Cheese spread
- Unsweetened breakfast cereals – plain unflavoured Ready Brek, porridge and Shredded Wheat have no added sugar
- Small portions of plain breadsticks
- Plain rice cakes
- Oatcakes occasionally (check labels as some contain added sugars)
- Savoury scones, for example, potato scone
- Homemade soup.

Box 7.2   Dietary Sugars.

If any of the following types of sugar are on the list of ingredients, the food is harmful for teeth and should be avoided in between meals:

- Sugar
- Dextrose
- Fruit juice concentrate
- Fructose
- Glucose
- Syrup
- Hydrolysed starch
- Isoglucose
- Levulose
- Maltose
- Molasses
- Sucrose
- Honey
- Treacle
- Dried fruit
- Corn sweetener

---

7. Fissure sealants: the most effective sealant is bisphenol-α-glycidyl methacrylate (bis-GMA) resin. At least 50% of sealants are retained for 5 years, and their effectiveness in reducing and delaying the onset of caries is not in doubt. Both unfilled and filled resins and clear and opaque resins have been used to equal effect. Isolation after etching and drying is essential to success (Box 7.3).

Indications or patient and tooth selection include: high caries risk; special needs (medical, physical, intellectual, social disability); occlusal surfaces of permanent molars, cingulum pits of upper incisors; seal as soon as moisture control permits; continue to monitor sealed teeth clinically and radiographically.

Glass ionomer fissure sealants may be used as a temporary measure in high-risk children when the tooth is partially erupted or in nervous children who cannot tolerate the acid-etch procedure. Use of glass ionomer

---

Box 7.3   Technique for Placement of a Resin Sealant.

1. Clean, wash and dry the tooth surface.
2. Etch with gel or liquid as per the manufacturer's instructions.
3. Apply thin coat of sealant to the pits and fissures, making sure to include the buccal extension in lower molars and the palatal groove in upper molars.
4. Light polymerise for 20 seconds.
5. Check occlusion.

Box 7.4   Technique for Placement of a GIC Sealant.

1. Clean, wash and dry the tooth surface.
2. Run/flow GIC into the fissures.
3. Compress using a gloved finger for 3 minutes.
4. Remove excess GIC with excavator.
5. Cover with petroleum jelly.

GIC, Glass ionomer cement.

---

fissure sealant may also be useful for its fluoride leaching properties and can be very useful for sensitive hypomineralised molars; however, they have poor bonding properties and require regular replacement (Box 7.4).

8. Sugar-free medicines: many children are on long-term medication, which is often supplied to them in a sweetened elixir form. Where sugar-free formulations of the medicine are available, it is important to liaise with the patient's general medical practitioner to ensure the child is prescribed the sugar-free version. In some cases, it is not possible to have a sugar-free alternative, such as lactulose, which is prescribed to many children for constipation. If sugared medicine is required, it is prudent to explore whether the child can take their medications at mealtimes to lessen its cariogenic effect. If this is not possible, it can be helpful for the child to rinse their mouth with water after taking their medication.

MANAGEMENT OF DENTAL CARIES

The treatment of carious teeth should be based on the needs of the child; the long-term objective should be to help the child to reach adulthood with an intact permanent dentition, no active caries, as few teeth restored as possible and a positive attitude towards their future dental health.

Restorative Materials

Amalgam. In July 2018, new environmental restrictions on dental amalgam use became applicable by law in the United Kingdom. Since then, the use of dental amalgam for treatment in patients under 15 years old, in pregnant or breastfeeding patients or for primary teeth in any patient is only allowed where deemed strictly necessary by the dental practitioner. These restrictions specified in Article 10(2) of Regulation (EU) 2017/852 on mercury were introduced to fulfil the requirements of the global Minamata Convention, which aims to phase-down the use of mercury on environmental grounds. The Scottish Dental Clinical Effectiveness Programme (SDCEP) has provided advice to support professionals in implementing these restrictions.

Glass ionomer cements (GIC). These consist of basic glass and acidic water-soluble powder; they set by an acid–base reaction between the two components. The cement bonds to enamel and dentine and releases fluoride to the surrounding tissues. This should be used as a temporary filling material only or for stabilisation of caries.

Resin-modified GIC. A hybrid of GIC/resin retains significant acid–base reaction in its overall curing process to set in the dark. There are two setting reactions: the acid–base reaction between glass and polyacid and a light-activated, free radical polymerisation of methacrylate groups of the polymer. This material has some physical advantages over conventional GIC, together with its ability to 'command set'. Again, this should be considered as a temporary or intermediate restorative material.

Polyacid-modified composite resin (compomer). This contains either or both essential components of a resin-modified GIC, but it is not water based and, therefore, no acid–base reaction can occur. It will not set in the dark. This technique is very sensitive to moisture contamination and should be placed under rubber dam isolation.

Resin-based composite. Their introduction revolutionised clinical dentistry, and their aesthetic benefits especially for the anterior teeth are unquestioned. Posterior resin-based composites have overcome initial problems of wear resistance, water absorption and polymerisation contraction. This technique is very sensitive to moisture contamination and should be placed under rubber dam isolation.

Preformed crowns. These preformed extra-coronal restorations are invaluable for in the restoration primary molars that have undergone pulp therapy, hypoplastic primary and permanent teeth and teeth in those children at high risk of caries, particularly those having treatment under general anaesthesia. The Hall technique of sealing caries into primary molars with a preformed metal crown has rapidly gained popularity.

Isolation

Adequate isolation is necessary for any restorative material to have a chance of success. Rubber dam isolation is the optimum but may necessitate local anaesthesia for the gingival tissues. Clamps should be secured individually with floss ligatures. Additional advantages of the rubber dam include airway protection, soft tissue protection and increased patient comfort. In the absence of rubber dam, good moisture control can be achieved with cotton wool rolls, dry tips and saliva ejector. When placing a preformed metal crown without the aid of rubber dam, it is prudent to have the child in an upright position using a sponge or gauze for airway protection and a pick-up stick or other sticky device to ensure you do not drop the crown once it has been delivered to the mouth.

Management of Caries affecting Primary Teeth

The first decision to be made is whether teeth can be retained or should be extracted. In general, teeth which have caused spontaneous or prolonged pain or where there are clinical or radiographic signs of infection require removal.

Recent developments in the restorative management of primary caries have moved away from traditional techniques of caries removal and restoration towards more conservative techniques which aim to seal caries from the oral environment. These techniques can be advantageous, given that these reduce the risk of pulpal exposure and normally avoid the use of local anaesthetic. They are currently described as the preferred option for the management of teeth with no clinical or radiographic signs of pulpal involvement and in the absence of medical complications.

SDCEP guidance suggests that the principle strategies for managing caries in the primary dentition are:

- No caries removal, seal with a crown (The Hall technique)
- No caries removal and fissure seal
- Selective caries removal and restoration (i.e. walls prepared to hard dentine with adequate depth for restorative material, previously known as partial caries removal)
- Pulpotomy

In addition to these techniques, other options for managing caries in the primary dentition include:

- Site-specific prevention (no caries removal, active prevention)
- Non-restorative cavity control (i.e. no caries removal, make cavity and lesion cleansable and apply fluoride)
- Complete caries removal and restoration
- Extraction, or review with extraction if pain or infection develops

In addition to techniques described above other new emerging techniques including the use of Silver Diamine Fluoride (SDF), which aims to arrest carious lesions may be of increasing use in practice.

Management options should be discussed with the parent/carer and child. It is important that all carious lesions are actively managed.

SDCEP guidelines suggest that:

"For a child with a carious lesion in a primary tooth, choose the least invasive, feasible caries management strategy, taking into account: the time to exfoliation, the site and extent of the lesion, the risk of pain or infection, the absence or presence of infection, preservation of tooth structure, the number of teeth affected, avoidance of treatment-induced anxiety"

The above techniques and their indications are described in detail in the SDCEP guideline 'Prevention and Management of Dental Caries in Primary Teeth Children'.

Management of Caries affecting Permanent Teeth

There is increasing evidence that less invasive approaches to caries management in permanent teeth (as in the primary dentition) are effective in reducing pulpal exposure and maintaining tooth structure. However, in the developing dentition, there can be advantages in conventional restoration techniques which can allow the extent of caries and therefore the prognosis of the tooth to be more fully assessed. This allows consideration to be given to removing teeth of guarded long-term prognosis either when there still exists potential for movement of unerupted adjacent teeth into the resultant space or to recommend removal of teeth for orthodontic purposes.

A thorough clinical and radiographic examination should be completed prior to any instrumentation of a tooth surface.

OCCLUSAL CARIES. A stained but non-cavitated fissure in a molar with no radiographic evidence of caries, a fissure sealant is the treatment of choice.

Where clinical or radiographic examination reveals dentinal caries, then a restoration will be required. Composite resin is the material of choice, and any remaining fissure pattern should also be sealed with fissure sealant.

Where caries is deep, and the tooth is to be retained, consideration should be given to using a step-wise technique. This involves a two-step process. Step 1 involves access to caries and removal of enough caries to allow an effective marginal seal. Caries should be removed to leave firm dentine on the cavity walls, while softer dentine can be left on the base. A bonded restoration, for example, GIC is placed. The provisional restoration is removed 6–12 months later. Any remaining soft dentine is removed until hard dentine is reached. A definitive restoration with resin-based composite can then be placed.

APPROXIMAL CARIES. Early, non-cavitated lesions with potential to remineralise can be initially managed with site-specific prevention and careful monitoring. Once cavitation occurs, the potential to remineralise is lost, and the tooth needs to be managed in an alternative way.

Composite resin is the material of choice for approximal caries in children under 15 years old following recent enforced restrictions upon the use of amalgam. It should be placed under rubber dam isolation. Dental amalgam can still be considered, however, where the dental practitioner deems this strictly necessary. This decision needs to be justified, communicated to the patient/parent and valid consent obtained. The justification should be recorded in the patient's dental record.

Anterior Teeth

Composite resin is the material of choice. Incisal edge restorations require careful design to maximise the surface area of normal enamel for bonding.

7.5 Tooth Discolouration

LEARNING OBJECTIVES

You should:
- know which treatments are appropriate for each type of discolouration.

The colour of a young person's teeth is of great importance. Peer group pressure can be significant, and teasing about size, position and colour of teeth can be distressing. Options to manage discolouration should be considered if/when the child (rather than the family) becomes concerned about their appearance.

Causes of intrinsic and extrinsic tooth discolouration are outlined in Table 7.3. Molar-incisor hypomineralisation (MIH) is covered in more detail in Section 7.8. Amelogenesis imperfecta, fluorosis, chronological disturbances, dentinogenesis imperfecta, dentine dysplasia and environmentally determined defects are considered further in Chapter 8.

Table 7.3 The Aetiology of Tooth Discolouration.

Staining Type	Cause
Extrinsic staining	Beverages/food Smoking Poor oral hygiene (chromogenic bacteria give a green/orange stain) Drugs: iron supplements (black stain), minocycline (black stain), chlorhexidine (brown/black stain)
INTRINSIC DISCOLOURATION OF ENAMEL	
Local causes	Caries Idiopathic Injury/infection of primary predecessor Internal resorption
Systemic causes	Amelogenesis imperfecta Drugs (e.g. tetracyclines) Fluorosis Idiopathic Systemic illness during tooth formation
INTRINSIC DISCOLOURATION OF DENTINE	
Local causes	Caries Internal resorption Metallic restorative materials Necrotic pulp tissue Root canal filling materials
Systemic causes	Bilirubin (haemolytic disease of newborn) Congenital porphyria Dentinogenesis imperfecta Drugs (e.g. tetracyclines)

Once the aetiology of the discolouration has been identified, the most appropriate method(s) of treatment can be chosen. Treatment emphasis should be on minimal tooth preparation.

TREATMENTS

Treatments for discoloured anterior teeth are listed as follows:

1. Microabrasion
2. Tooth whitening
3. Resin infiltration
4. Direct composite restoration
5. Veneer
6. Full coverage restoration

Microabrasion

Microabrasion is a controlled removal of surface enamel in order to improve discolourations that are *limited* to the outer enamel layer.

As hypomineralised enamel can appear whiter than surrounding teeth, the patient should understand that teeth may look slightly darker following treatment.

The technique is described in Box 7.5. It is achieved by a combination of abrasion and erosion, and the term 'abrosion' is sometimes used. Normally, no more than 100 μm of enamel is removed, although care should be taken when preforming the technique on larger hypomineralised areas which may be more susceptible to wear.

Box 7.5   Microabrasion Technique.

Armamentarium

- Bicarbonate of soda/water
- Fluoridated toothpaste
- 500 ppm fluoride mouthwash
- Pumice
- Rubber dam
- Rubber prophylaxis cup
- 3M Sof-LexTM Contouring and polishing discs
- Hydrochloric acid 6% or 37% phosphoric acid (etch)

Technique

1. Take preoperative vitality tests, photographs +/– radiographs.
2. Isolate teeth to be treated with rubber dam.
3. Place a mixture of sodium bicarbonate and water on the dam behind the teeth to protect in case of spillage.
4. Mix hydrochloric acid or phosphoric acid with pumice into a slurry.
5. Apply a small amount to the labial surface on either a rubber cup rotating slowly for 5 seconds or a wooden stick/flat plastic instrument rubbed over the surface for 5 seconds before washing for 5 seconds directly into an aspirator tip. Repeat until the stain has reduced, up to a maximum of ten 5-second applications per tooth. Any improvement that is going to occur will have done so by this time.
6. Apply 500 ppm fluoride mouthwash to the teeth for 3 minutes.
7. Remove the rubber dam.
8. Polish the teeth with the finest Soflex discs.
9. Polish the teeth with fluoridated toothpaste for 1 minute.
10. Review in 1 month for vitality tests and clinical photographs.
11. Review biannually, checking pulpal status.

Once completed, the procedure should not be repeated. Too much enamel removal is potentially damaging to the pulp and, cosmetically, the underlying dentine colour will become more evident.

Indications

- Fluorosis
- Molar-incisor hypomineralisation
- Idiopathic speckling
- Postorthodontic demineralisation
- Prior to veneer placement for well-demarcated stains
- White/brown surface staining (e.g. secondary to primary predecessor infection or trauma; Turner teeth)

Effectiveness

Critical analysis of the effectiveness of the technique should not be made immediately but delayed for at least 1 month, as the appearance of the teeth will continue to improve over this time. Experience has shown that although white mottling is often incompletely removed, it does become less perceptible. This phenomenon has been attributed to the relatively prismless layer of compacted surface enamel produced by the 'abrosion' technique, which alters the optical properties of the tooth surface.

Long-term studies of the technique have found no association with pulpal damage, increased caries susceptibility or significant prolonged thermal sensitivity. Patient compliance and satisfaction are good, and any dissatisfaction is usually a result of inadequate preoperative explanation.

The technique is easy to perform for operator and patient and is not time-consuming. Removal of any mottled area is permanent and is achieved with an insignificant loss of surface enamel. Failure to improve the appearance by the microabrasion technique does not have any harmful effects and may make it easier to mask some lesions with veneers.

Tooth Whitening for Vital Teeth

Tooth whitening involves the chemical use of oxidation agents to lighten tooth colour. Several bleaching agents have been described in the past; however, 10% carbamide peroxide is currently recommended for all techniques.

Carbamide peroxide gel (10%) breaks down in the mouth into 3% hydrogen peroxide and 7% urea. Both urea and hydrogen peroxide have low molecular weights, which allow them to diffuse rapidly through enamel and dentine. This explains the transient pulpal sensitivity occasionally experienced with bleaching systems for use at home.

The advantages of the home bleaching technique are:

- easy for operator and patient
- conserving of tooth tissue
- maintenance of the original crown morphology.

Disadvantages are as follows:

- There are strict regulations around the use of tooth whitening products in the United Kingdom. The legal position of tooth whitening must be taken into consideration when discussing these techniques with patients. This may preclude the use of bleaching agents on patients under 18 years old.
- The colour of restorations will remain unchanged after bleaching and therefore these may need to be replaced.
- Clinical studies have demonstrated that colour regression can be expected with this technique.

Side effects:
- Sensitivity is the most common side effect reported. Sensitivity is transient and resolves once treatment is complete. Application of products containing casein phosphopeptide-amorphous calcium phosphate (CPP-ACP, as found in GC Tooth Mousse) used within the bleaching tray on alternative nights to bleaching can help reduce this.
- There is no evidence that bleaching itself significantly affects the hardness of enamel; however, repeated access to the root canal system for non-vital bleaching techniques could weaken the tooth structure.
- Cervical resorption has been described as a side effect when high concentrations of hydrogen peroxide or heat are used for non-vital bleaching.
- Reduction in the bond strength to composite occurs for 2 weeks after bleaching. Use of composite resin should therefore be delayed over this period.

Non-Vital Tooth Bleaching

Non-vital bleaching is used for teeth that have become discoloured by the diffusion into the dentinal tubules of haemoglobin breakdown products from necrotic pulp tissue. Prior to bleaching, radiographs should be taken to ensure adequate root canal obturation and no sign of periapical disease.

Indication

- Discoloured non-vital teeth with a well-condensed gutta-percha root filling and no clinical or radiographical signs of periapical disease.

Contraindications

- Heavily restored teeth
- Staining from amalgam.

The following techniques can be considered to manage non-vital discoloured teeth.

1. External bleaching
2. Internal bleaching – walking bleach technique
3. Combination of internal and external bleaching
   a. Inside–outside open bleaching technique
   b. Inside–outside closed bleaching technique

1. External bleaching

Bleaching agents have the ability to diffuse rapidly through teeth when applied from the external surface. It has recently been suggested that external bleaching should be considered as the first line of treatment where the tooth has discoloured despite adequate endodontic treatment, thorough debridement and restoration (Greenwal-Cohen and Greenwall 2019). This can avoid repeated access to the pulp chamber. Carbamide peroxide 10% should be applied to the affected tooth via a specially constructed single tooth bleaching tray.

2. Internal bleaching – non-vital walking bleach technique

This technique is described in Box 7.6. In this technique, bleach is sealed into the pulp chamber following preparation. The bleach may need to be replaced over several visits to reach the desired tooth shade. Once the correct colour is established, the bleach is removed and the tooth initially sealed with a temporary dressing prior to definitive restoration with composite after a period of > 2 weeks.

3. Inside–outside non-vital bleaching techniques

The inside–outside bleaching techniques involve construction of a single tooth bleaching tray to bleach the external tooth surface, while also bleaching internally from the pulp chamber. 10% carbamide peroxide can be used for each technique described.

The open inside–outside bleaching technique (IOO) is described in Box 7.7. The access cavity is left open between visits. Patients apply 10% carbamide peroxide into both the open access cavity and the bleaching tray using the supplied syringe before seating the tray. Bleaching agent can be worn overnight or alternatively replaced every 4–6 hours. This is continued until the desired colour change is obtained.

For the closed inside–outside bleaching (IOC) technique, 10% carbamide peroxide is sealed into the pulp chamber, as for the walking bleach technique (Box 7.6). The patient then applies carbamide peroxide externally via the bleaching tray each night until the tooth reaches the desired colour change.

In comparison with the walking bleach technique, these techniques allow the patient more control over the colour of the tooth. The closed technique avoids leaving an open access cavity which risks food packing.

Box 7.6   Non-Vital Walking Bleach Technique.

Armamentarium

- Rubber dam
- Glass ionomer lining cement
- 10% carbamide peroxide gel
- Cotton wool
- White gutta-percha
- Resin composite

Technique

1. Preoperative periapical radiographs are essential to check for an adequate root filling.
2. Clean teeth with pumice, and make a note of the shade of the discoloured tooth.
3. Place rubber dam isolating the single tooth. Ensure adequate eye and clothing protection for the patient, operator and dental nurse.
4. Remove palatal restoration and pulp chamber restoration.
5. Carefully remove root filling 2 mm below the level of the dentogingival junction.
6. Place 1-mm glass ionomer cement over the gutta-percha.
7. Freshen dentine with a round bur. Do not remove excessively.
9. Fill the pulp chamber with 10% carbamide peroxide gel.
10. Place cotton wool roll over the caramide peroxide gel, and seal the cavity with glass ionomer cement.
11. Repeat process at weekly intervals until the desired tooth colour is established.
12. Place non-setting calcium hydroxide into the pulp chamber for 2 weeks. Seal with glass ionomer cement.
13. Finally, restore the tooth with white gutta-percha (to facilitate reopening pulp chamber again if necessary at a later date) and resin composite.

Vital Bleaching

NIGHTGUARD VITAL BLEACHING. The nightguard vital bleaching technique involves the daily replacement of carbamide peroxide gel into a custom-fitted tray of either the upper and/or lower arch (Box 7.8). It demands a high degree of patient compliance and motivation. Ideally, this technique should be avoided in the mixed dentition, as teeth unerupted at the time of bleaching will remain darker in colour. Its main remit is in the older patient to treat the yellowing of teeth.

Indications in Paediatric Dentistry

- Mild fluorosis/MIH
- Moderate fluorosis/MIH as an adjunct to microabrasion.

Recall

Patients should be recalled regularly (at least every week) to monitor the success of the technique. For techniques where bleach application is fully controlled by the patient (vital bleaching, external bleaching and open inside–outside bleaching), the patient should review tooth colour each morning and cease bleaching once the desired colour is achieved. Where bleach is sealed into the pulp chamber (walking bleach and closed inside–outside bleaching), the patient should be advised to contact the dental surgery if they feel the desired colour has been reached before the next scheduled review, to avoid overbleaching.

Box 7.7 Non-Vital Inside–Outside Open Bleaching Technique.

Armamentarium

- Alginate impression compound
- Rubber dam
- Glass ionomer lining cement
- 10% carbamide peroxide gel
- Cotton wool
- White gutta-percha
- Resin composite

Technique

1. Preoperative periapical radiographs are essential to check for an adequate root filling.
2. Clean teeth with pumice, and make a note of the shade of the discoloured tooth.
3. Take an alginate impression of the arch to be treated, and cast a working model in stone.
4. Request a soft pulldown, vacuum-formed, non-reservoir bleaching tray, no more than 2 mm in thickness which does not cover the gingivae.
5. Place rubber dam isolating the single tooth. Ensure adequate eye and clothing protection for the patient, operator and dental nurse.
6. Remove palatal restoration and pulp chamber restoration.
7. Carefully remove root filling 2 mm below the level of the dentogingival junction.
8. Place 1-mm glass ionomer cement over the gutta-percha.
9. Freshen dentine with a round bur. Do not remove excessively.
10. Instruct the patient how to apply the gel into the back of their tooth and into their mouthguard.
11. The bleach should be applied each evening. The length of time the guard should be worn depends on the product used. The patient should check the colour of their teeth each day and stop bleaching once the desired colour has been established.
12. Review the patient every 2 weeks. Once the desired colour has been reached, place non-setting calcium hydroxide into the pulp chamber for 2 weeks. Seal with glass ionomer cement.
13. Finally, restore the tooth with white gutta-percha (to facilitate reopening pulp chamber again if necessary at a later date) and resin composite.

Box 7.8 Nightguard Vital Bleaching Technique.

Armamentarium

- Alginate impression compound
- Carbamide peroxide gel 10%

Technique

1. Take an alginate impression of the arch to be treated, and cast a working model in stone.
2. Request a soft pulldown, vacuum-formed, non-reservoir bleaching tray, no more than 2 mm in thickness which does not cover the gingivae.
3. Instruct the patient on how to floss their teeth. Perform a full mouth prophylaxis, and instruct the patient how to apply the gel into the mouthguard.
4. The length of time the guard should be worn depends on the product used.
5. Review the patient about 2 weeks later to check that they are not experiencing any sensitivity, and then at 6 weeks, by which time 80% of any colour change should have occurred.

Effectiveness

Effectiveness can vary by the initial degree of discolouration with bleaching generally being less successful for teeth which are more severely discolored.

For non-vital bleaching techniques, failure of a tooth to bleach could be caused by inadequate removal of filling materials from the pulp chamber. This should be checked before abandoning a procedure.

Resin Infiltration

Resin infiltration is a minimally invasive restorative treatment, which may have a role in the management of hypomineralised/decalcified lesions. Further research in this area is required (Borges et al 2017).

Localised Composite Resin Restorations

Defective enamel can be replaced with a tooth-coloured restoration that bonds to, and blends with, enamel (Box 7.9). It is indicated for well-demarcated white, yellow or brown patches.

The localised restoration is quick and easy to complete. Advances in bonding and resin technology make these restorations simple and obviate the need for a full labial veneer. Disadvantages are removal of tooth structure, marginal staining and difficulty in achieving an accurate colour match.

Composite Resin Veneers

Although some form of porcelain restoration may be the most satisfactory long-term restoration for a severely hypoplastic or discoloured tooth, it is not an appropriate

Box 7.9 Localised Resin Composite Restorations for Defective Enamel.

Armamentarium

- Rubber dam/contoured matrix strips
- Round and fissure diamond burs
- Enamel/dentine bonding kit
- Hybrid resin composite
- 3M Sof-LexTM Contouring and polishing discs and interproximal polishing strips

Technique

1. Take preoperative photographs, and make shade selection.
2. Apply rubber dam and contoured matrix strips.
3. Remove demarcated lesion with round diamond fissure bur.
4. Etch enamel margins, wash and dry as per the manufacturer's instructions.
5. Apply enamel and dentine bonding agent, and light-cure as per the manufacturer's instructions.
6. Apply chosen shade of composite using a brush lubricated with the bonding agent to smooth and shape. Light-cure for the recommended time.
7. Remove matrix strip/rubber dam.
8. Polish with graded Soflex discs (3M), finishing burs and interproximal strips if required. Add characterisation to surface of composite.
9. Take postoperative photographs.

solution for children for two reasons: the large size of the young pulp horns and chamber and the immature gingival contour.

Composite veneers may be direct (placed at initial appointment) or indirect (placed at a subsequent appointment having been fabricated in the laboratory). Composite veneers are durable enough to last through adolescence (Box 7.10).

Indications
- Discolouration
- Enamel defects
- Diastemata
- Malpositioned teeth
- Large restorations

Contraindications
- Insufficient available enamel for bonding
- Beware patients who play woodwind instruments!

Porcelain Veneers

Normally, porcelain veneers can be considered from 18 years of age when the gingival margin is at an adult level and the standard of oral hygiene is acceptable. Note, however, that gingival changes can continue into the early 20s.

Box 7.10   Technique for Placement of Resin Composite Veneers.

Armamentarium
- Rubber dam/contoured matrix strips
- Preparation and finishing burs
- Polishable hybrid resin composite
- 3M Sof-LexTM Contouring and polishing discs and interproximal polishing strips

Technique
1. Clean teeth with a slurry of pumice in water. Wash and dry, and select shade.
2. Isolate the tooth with rubber dam, and place a contoured matrix strip.
4. Etch the enamel as per the manufacturer's instructions.
5. Where dentine is exposed, apply dentine primer.
6. Apply a thin layer of bonding resin to the labial surface with a brush, and cure as per the manufacturer's instructions. It may be necessary to use an opaquer at this stage if the discolouration is intense.
7. Apply resin composite of the desired shade to the labial surface, and roughly shape it into all areas with a plastic instrument before using a brush lubricated with unfilled resin to 'paddle' and smooth it into the desired shape. Cure 60 seconds gingivally, 60 seconds mesio-incisally, 60 seconds disto-incisally and 60 seconds from the palatal aspect if incisal coverage has been used. Different shades of composite can be combined to achieve good matches with adjacent teeth and a transition from a relatively dark gingival area to a lighter, more translucent incisal region.
8. Flick away the unfilled resin.
9. Finish the margins with diamond finishing burs and interproximal strips and the labial surface with graded sandpaper discs. Care should be taken to ensure composite at the gingival margin is smooth with no overhang. Characterisation should be added to improve light reflection properties.

7.6 Tooth Surface Loss (Wear)

LEARNING OBJECTIVES

You should:
- be able to give accurate advice to patients/parents about which foods and drinks can be harmful to the teeth
- be able to suggest suitable alternatives to the above
- know the medical causes of tooth surface loss (TSL)
- know the main treatment objectives for tooth surface loss
- know the appropriate materials to treat tooth surface loss.

Dentists have been aware of the problem of tooth wear or non-carious loss of tooth tissue for a long time. However, it is only more recently that it has been associated increasingly with our younger population. There are three processes that make up the phenomenon of tooth wear:

1. *Attrition*: wear of tooth as a result of tooth-to-tooth contact.
2. *Erosion*: irreversible loss of tooth substance brought about by a chemical process that does not involve bacterial action.
3. *Abrasion*: physical wear of tooth substance produced by something other than tooth-to-tooth contact.

In children, abrasion is relatively uncommon. The most frequent cause of abrasion is overzealous toothbrushing, which tends to develop with increasing age. Attrition during mastication is common, particularly in the primary dentition, where almost all upper incisors show some signs of attrition by the time they exfoliate. However, in the 1990s, the contribution of erosion to the overall process of tooth wear in the younger population was highlighted.

While erosion may be the predominant process, attrition and abrasion may be compounding factors (e.g. toothbrush abrasion may be increased if brushing is carried out immediately after the consumption of erosive foodstuffs or drinks). It is often difficult to identify a single causative agent in a case of tooth wear, so the general term *tooth surface loss* may be more appropriate.

PREVALENCE

There is very little published evidence on the prevalence or severity of tooth wear in children. In 2013, the National Child Dental Health Survey reported that 57% of 5-year-old children had tooth surface loss of the palatal surfaces of their primary incisors, with 16% showing progression into the dentine or pulp. The prevalence of tooth surface loss affecting the palatal surfaces of permanent incisors was also alarmingly high, affecting 38% of 12-year-olds and 44% of 15-year-olds. This progressed into dentine or pulp in 2% of 12-year-olds and 4% of 15-year-olds.

AETIOLOGY

In young patients, there are three main causes of tooth surface loss:

1. Dietary
2. Gastric regurgitation
3. Parafunctional activity

In addition to these, certain environmental factors have been linked to tooth wear. With the exception of frequent use of chlorinated swimming pools, most environmental and occupational hazards do not apply to children.

Dietary Causes of Tooth Surface Loss

The most common cause of erosive surface loss is excessive intake of acidic food or drink. Food and drink implicated in erosive tooth surface loss in young patients include:

- acidic drinks (diluting juice, carbonated drinks, fruit juice)
- citrus fruits (e.g. lemons, oranges, grapefruits)
- tart apples
- vinegar and pickles
- yoghurt
- fruit juices
- vitamin C tablets.

Acidic drinks, in particular, are available to all age groups of children. Pure 'baby' fruit juices are marketed for consumption by infants, and these have been shown to have pH values below the critical pH for the dissolution of enamel (pH 5.5). Many of these drinks are given to infants in a feeding bottle, and the combination of the highly acidic nature of the drink and the prolonged exposure of the teeth to the acidic substrate may result in excessive tooth surface loss as well as dental caries. While a wide range of foods and drinks is implicated in the aetiology of tooth surface loss, soft drinks make up the bulk of the problem. Both normal and so-called 'diet' carbonated drinks have very low pH values and are associated with tooth surface loss, as are other fruit juices and diluting juices. While there is no *direct* relationship between the pH of a substrate and the degree of tooth surface loss, pH does give a useful indication as to the potential to cause damage. Other factors, such as titratable acidity, the effect on plaque pH and the buffering capacity of saliva, will influence the erosive potential of a given substrate. In addition, it has been shown that erosive tooth surface loss tends to be more severe if the frequency and volume of drink consumed is high or if the intake occurs at bedtime or during the night.

The pattern of dietary erosive tooth surface loss depends on the manner in which the substrate is consumed. Carbonated drinks are commonly held in the mouth for some time as the child 'enjoys' the sensation of the bubbles. This habit may result in a generalised loss of surface enamel. Generalised loss of surface enamel of posterior teeth is often evident, particularly on the first permanent molars. Characteristic saucer-shaped lesions develop on the cusps of the molars. This phenomenon is known as *perimolysis*.

Gastric Regurgitation and Tooth Surface Loss

The acidity of the stomach contents is below pH 1.0; therefore, any regurgitation or vomiting is potentially damaging to the teeth. As many as 50% of adults with signs of tooth surface loss have a history of gastric reflux. The aetiology of gastric regurgitation may be divided into those with upper gastrointestinal disorders and those with eating disorders.

In young patients, long-term regurgitation is associated with a variety of underlying problems:

- Gastro-oesophageal reflux
- Oesophageal strictures

- Chronic respiratory disease
- Disease of the liver/pancreas/biliary tree
- Overfeeding
- Feeding problems/failure to thrive conditions
- Reye's syndrome
- Rumination.

In addition, there is a group of patients that suffer from gastro-oesophageal reflux disease (GORD). This may be either symptomatic, in which case the individual knows what provokes the reflux, or the more insidiously asymptomatic GORD, in which the patient is unaware of the problem and continues to ingest reflux-provoking foods.

Parafunctional Activity

Localised tooth surface loss frequently occurs in patients who exhibit abnormal parafunctional habits. The excessive grinding that is a feature of this problem is not always apparent to the patient. However, apart from the marked tooth tissue loss, other signs of bruxism may be evident including hypertrophy of the muscles of mastication, cheek biting and tongue faceting. An example of erosion and parafunction having a disastrous effect on the dentition may be seen (and heard) in children who have cerebral palsy. These children often have chronic gastric regurgitation and also severe bruxism, resulting in excessive tooth surface loss.

MANAGEMENT

Immediate Management

- *Early recognition*
- *Prevention advice*
- *Monitoring*
- *Temporary restoration*

The most important part of management is early recognition and prevention. It is important to establish the aetiology and, where possible, eliminate the cause.

Children with TSL should have a targeted prevention regime as outlined in Section 7.4. In addition, particular advice should be given relating to the consumption of dietary acids and use of sugar-free chewing gum to stimulate salivary flow. 'Enamel care' toothpastes and age-appropriate high-fluoride toothpastes can be considered.

Dietary counselling should be personal, practical and positive. Suitable alternatives should be suggested, with the most appropriate times for their intake:

- Inform patients of types of foods and drinks that have greatest erosive potential.
- Suggest plain water or milk as an alternative to acidic drinks.
- Limit the intake of acidic foods/drinks to meal times.
- Use of a wide bore reusable straw held towards the back of the mouth may help acidic drinks to bypass teeth. However, paper straws which become saturated with fluid on use are unlikely to be helpful.
- Toothbrushing should be avoided immediately after consuming acidic food or drink.

Immediate temporary coverage of sensitive teeth with GIC or composite resin can relieve symptoms and act as a diagnostic aid.

Study models and clinical photographs can help monitor progression of TSL. These should be taken at initial diagnosis and at periodic intervals to monitor progress.

Definitive Management in the Primary or Mixed Dentition

The main treatment objectives are to:

- resolve sensitivity
- restore missing tooth structure
- prevent further tooth tissue loss
- maintain a balanced occlusion.

Ideally, aetiological factors should be identified and controlled prior to treatment.

In the primary dentition, if the child has experienced no symptoms, the teeth can be monitored. If there are associated symptoms, small areas of TSL can be restored with composite, while larger areas can be restored with composite crowns anteriorly and preformed metal crowns posteriorly. Teeth with severe TSL, if associated with spontaneous pain or signs of infection, may require extraction.

The permanent dentition should also be managed conservatively where possible with composite addition to areas of TSL. This can include placement of fissure sealants or resin composite. Where resin composite is used, it can be helpful to clean surfaces with pumice/water or gently freshen the surface with a slow-speed rosehead bur to enhance resin infiltration into the sclerotic dentine and also to use a dentine bonding agent to improve adhesion. During growth, these restorations are well tolerated. Alternative options may need to be considered where TSL is extensive. Table 7.4 outlines treatment options for TSL in the primary and permanent dentition.

Long-Term Review

Long-term review is necessary to:

- reinforce prevention messages
- monitor future tooth surface loss
- maintain the existing restorations
- provide support for the patient.

Table 7.4 Treatment Technique for Tooth Surface Loss.

Dentition	Anterior	Posterior
Primary dentition	No treatment Resin composite restoration Composite crowns Extraction	No treatment Resin composite restoration Preformed metal crowns Extraction
Permanent dentition	Long-term monitoring Fissure seal palatal surface Resin composite restoration	Long-term monitoring Resin composite restoration Preformed metal crown Metal/composite onlay Extraction

7.7 Endodontics

LEARNING OBJECTIVES

You should:
- know the indications and contraindications for primary molar pulp treatment
- know the medicaments used in primary molar pulp treatment
- know the treatment for vital and non-vital immature permanent incisors
- know the initiating factors in the different types of resorption.

PRIMARY TEETH

The question of whether to retain primary teeth should be based on three factors: medical, behavioural and dental.

Medical, which *may* be contraindications to extraction of primary teeth
- Bleeding disorders and coagulopathies.
- Hypodontia associated with syndrome (e.g. ectodermal dysplasia).

Medical indications for extraction of primary teeth
- Congenital cardiac disease.
- Immunosuppression.
- Poor healing potential (e.g. unstable diabetes).

Behavioural reason for retention of primary teeth
- Poor co-operation makes extraction difficult.

Behavioural reason for extraction of primary teeth
- Need for dental general anaesthetic – depending on available services.

Dental contraindications to extraction of primary teeth
- Well-maintained arch.
- Orthodontic considerations.
- Hypodontia: lack of permanent successor.

Dental indications for extraction of primary teeth
- Extensive caries with gross coronal breakdown, and caries penetrating pulpal floor.
- Acute infection.
- Excessive tooth mobility.
- Poorly maintained mouth.

Pulpal Treatment Options for Primary Teeth

Vital Pulp Therapy for Primary Teeth:
  Direct pulp capping
  (Indirect pulp treatment)
  Pulpotomy.
Non-Vital Pulp Therapy for Primary Teeth:
  Pulpectomy.

Vital Pulp Therapy for Primary Teeth

Indications

- Symptom-free tooth or transient pain of short duration, suggesting reversible pulpitis
- No sign of peri-radicular pathology
- No clear radiographic barrier between caries and dental pulp – precluding the use of the Hall technique.

Isolation

Rubber dam should be used to aid isolation of teeth for pulp therapy.

Direct Pulp Capping for Primary Teeth:

Indications

A small mechanical exposure on a vital symptom-free tooth that is well isolated is the only situation where direct capping should be applied. If direct capping is applied in other situations, pulp inflammation usually persists and results in total pulp necrosis. In the majority of children, pulpotomy is the preferred treatment, with a high rate of success.

Indirect Pulp Treatment for Primary Teeth:

The aim of this treatment is to remove caries from the cavity wall, leaving softened dentine over the pulp and avoiding pulpal exposure. The remaining softened dentine is covered with setting calcium hydroxide to destroy any remaining micro-organisms and to promote the deposition of reparative secondary dentine. This is then covered with a glass ionomer lining and the tooth restored at the same visit with a preformed metal crown.

Pulpotomy of Primary Teeth:

Pulpotomy involves the amputation of vital inflamed pulp from the coronal chamber as a means of preserving the vitality and function of the remaining portion of radicular pulp (Fig. 7.1 and Box 7.11).

There remains some controversy over the most appropriate medicaments for use in vital primary molar pulpotomies. Currently, ferric sulphate or mineral trioxide aggregate are materials of choice. It is postulated that ferric sulphate works by controlling pulpal bleeding and promotes formation of a 'protective' metal/protein clot over the underlying

| Box 7.11 | **Technique for Vital Pulpotomy of a Primary Molar.** |

1. A preoperative radiograph is taken of the affected tooth.
2. Use local anaesthesia and isolation.
3. Removal of caries and formation of an endodontic access cavity.
4. Excavation of coronal pulp with slow-speed 6 or 8 bur or a spoon excavator (see Fig. 7.1B).
5. Haemorrhage control. Place a cotton wool pellet soaked with ferric sulphate into the excavated coronal pulp chamber. Remove after 20 seconds: if bleeding persists, then repeat. If bleeding is still a problem, it is likely that the radicular pulp is inflamed and hyperaemic. At this point, pulpectomy or extraction should be considered instead.
6. Restore pulp chamber with reinforced zinc oxide/eugenol cement and reinforced glass ionomer cement (see Fig. 7.1D).
7. Restore the tooth with a preformed crown (see Fig. 7.1E).
8. MTA can be used as an alternative to ferric sulphate. If MTA is to be used, bleeding in step 5 should be with a cotton wool pellet soaked in saline. Once haemorrhage is controlled, MTA can be placed to fill the pulp chamber. This is then lined with glass ionomer cement and the tooth restored with a preformed metal crown.

MTA, Mineral trioxide aggregate.

vital radicular pulp. Mineral trioxide aggregate (MTA) has excellent bioactive properties and essentially stimulates cytokine release from pulpal fibroblasts, which in turn stimulates dental hard tissue formation. If successful, the treated tooth should be asymptomatic. Failure will result in pain, swelling, increased mobility, fistulae and radiographic signs of either radiolucency at the furcation or apex or internal/external resorption of the root.

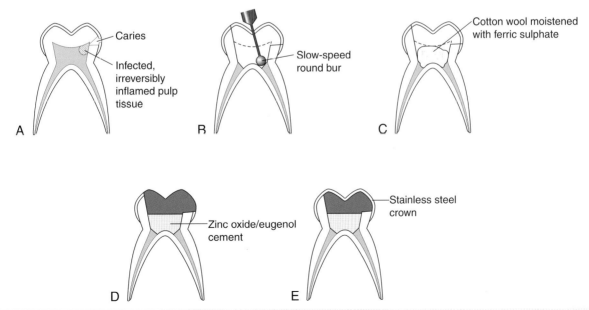

Fig. 7.1 Primary molar pulp amputation (vital pulpotomy). (From Whitworth JM, Nunn JH. In: Welbury RR, ed. *Paediatric Dentistry*. Oxford University Press; 2001:171, Fig. 9.11. By permission of Oxford University Press, www.oup.com.)

Radiographic assessment every 12 months is necessary to check the above and the developing underlying permanent successor.

Non-Vital Pulp
Therapy for Primary Teeth:

Indications
- Irreversible pulpitis.

Pulpectomy for Primary Teeth:
Pulpectomy involves the chemomechanical preparation of primary root canals with endodontic hand instruments and irrigants. Because of the anatomy of the root canals and the presence of the permanent successor, greater emphasis is often placed on the use of the antimicrobial properties of the obturating material, especially in primary posterior teeth. Given the risk to the permanent successor and the complex anatomy of the root canal system, pulpectomy is rarely indicated in general practice.

PERMANENT MOLAR TEETH WITH IMMATURE APICES

The treatment of choice for the cariously exposed young permanent tooth is dependent on:

- stage of root development
- status of the crown
- orthodontic considerations for the tooth and the arch
- The condition and presence of the remaining dentition.
- psychological and behavioural factors.

The final decision has to balance the long-term advisability of retaining the tooth and the practicality of restoring the crown. Consideration should be given to removal of teeth with extensive caries and a guarded long term prognosis, particularly when there is potential for movement of unerupted teeth into the resultant space or a tooth removal is required for orthodontic purposes.
Options include:

Vital Pulp Therapy Immature Permanent Molars:
- Indirect pulp treatment/step-wise caries removal
- Direct pulp cap
- Partial pulpotomy
Non-Vital Pulp Therapy for Immature Permanent Teeth:
- Pulpectomy.

Vital Pulp Therapy Immature Permanent Molars:

For vital teeth with immature roots, the aim of therapy is to preserve vitality to ensure completion of root development. As in the primary dentition, the tooth should be symptom free or have transient pain of short duration, suggesting reversible pulpitis, and there should be no sign of periapical pathology. The need for pulp therapy can indicate a guarded long-term prognosis, and therefore, as mentioned above, the benefits and disadvantages of removal versus restoration should be considered.

Indirect Pulp Cap
An indirect pulp cap is indicated in teeth with minimal symptoms. A thin layer of carious dentine is left over the pulp because its removal would create an exposure.

Calcium hydroxide cement is usually placed over the softened dentine but glass ionomer cement has also been advocated. The 'step-wise technique' is described in more detail in Section 7.4.

Direct Pulp Cap
Permanent teeth respond well to direct pulp capping procedures, unlike primary teeth. Selection of appropriate cases is important.

Indications
- Small carious exposures
- Teeth with no history of swelling or spontaneous pain
- No radiographic changes
- Controllable bleeding at exposure site.

Setting calcium hydroxide, MTA or biodentine can be placed directly onto the exposed pulp, covered with a glass ionomer cement and a definitive restoration placed.

Partial Pulpotomy
The aim of this treatment is removal of 1–3 mm inflamed pulp tissue, with a clean round diamond high-speed bur, beneath the site of a pulpal exposure leaving underlying healthy pulp. Calcium hydroxide, MTA (at least 1.5 mm) and biodentine are suitable materials for this technique to promote bridge formation at the exposure site. These should be lined with a glass ionomer liner prior to restoration of the tooth, ideally at the same visit.

Non-Vital Permanent Teeth with Immature Roots

Non-vital teeth with immature roots often require to be removed, although short-term retention for orthodontic reasons may be desirable. After root canal instrumentation and cleaning, a medicament such as non-setting calcium hydroxide should be placed and the crown restored.

PERMANENT INCISOR TEETH WITH IMMATURE APICES

Vital

Permanent vital incisors can be treated with calcium hydroxide pulpotomy or Partial (Cvek) pulpotomy (apexogenesis). The aim is removal of contaminated pulp tissue with a clean, round, high-speed diamond bur in order to allow continued root development and apical closure. (Fig. 7.2 and Box 7.12).
Success rate is 80–96%. Prognosis is best if the procedure is completed within 24 hours of exposure.

Non-Vital Incisors with Immature Apices

Non-vital immature incisors with an open apex have no apical barrier against which to condense conventional obturation materials. Creation of an apical barrier (apexification) is therefore required prior to obturation. The most appropriate way to achieve this is with MTA (Figure 7.3 and Box 7.13). Use of non-setting Calcium Hydroxide to stimulate calcific barrier formation, was popular in the past but is now rarely used given its long-term use makes the tooth root brittle and liable to fracture.

Endodontic Treatment of Root Fractured Teeth:
Root canal therapy can often be confined to the non-vital coronal portion of the canal. Instrumentation using hand

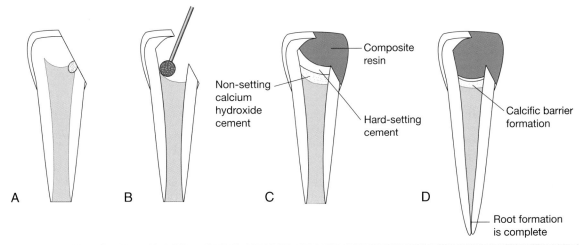

Fig. 7.2 Permanent incisor pulpotomy (apexogenesis). (From Whitworth JM, Nunn JH. In: Welbury RR, ed. *Paediatric Dentistry*. 2nd edn. Oxford University Press; 2001:173, Fig. 9.14, By permission of Oxford University Press, www.oup.com.)

Box 7.12   Pulpotomy of Vital Permanent Incisors.

1. Clinical examination (see Fig. 7.2A) shows a complicated fracture with microbial invasion of the coronal pulp. The pulp has been exposed to the mouth for longer than 24 hours.
2. Use local anaesthesia.
3. Place rubber dam.
4. The coronal pulp is accessed with a diamond bur running at high speed with constant water cooling (see Fig. 7.2B), and pulp tissue excised with a slow-speed bur until healthy bleeding pulp is found. If there is excessive bleeding or no bleeding, then continue to excise pulp tissue until all the coronal pulp is removed.
5. Wash pulp with saline until haemorrhage stops. Remove any clots with gentle saline washing. If pulp is either hyperaemic or not bleeding once all coronal pulp has been removed, then a pulpectomy and not a pulpotomy is required.
6. Non-setting calcium hydroxide is placed over pulp remnant. Cover with setting calcium hydroxide and semipermanent restorative material (see Fig. 7.2C).
7. Review at 6 weeks. If there is no evidence of pulp pathosis, review at a further 6 weeks, and then 6 monthly for clinical evaluation of pulp vitality and assessment of calcific bridge formation, further root formation and signs of pathosis radiographically. Fig. 7.2D shows a calcific barrier with healthy pulp at 12 months.
8. If vitality is lost, non-vital pulp therapy should be undertaken through the calcific bridge.
9. Pulpectomy when root development is complete may be required if the root canal is required for restorative purposes. A modified Cvek pulpotomy, where the surface 1–2 mm of exposed pulp tissue is removed by a slow bur, is also used with equal success.

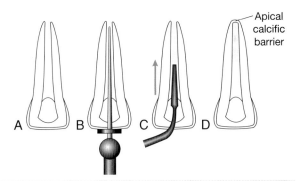

Fig. 7.3 Permanent incisor root-end closure (apexification). (From Whitworth JM, Nunn JH. In: Welbury RR, ed. *Paediatric Dentistry*. 2nd edn. Oxford University Press; 2001: 178, Fig. 9.18, By permission of Oxford University Press, www.oup.com.)

Box 7.13   Permanent Root-End Closure for Non-Vital Incisors.

1. Use local anaesthesia.
2. Place rubber dam.
3. Access cavity (see Fig. 7.3A).
4. Extirpate necrotic pulp tissue.
5. Prepare canal 1 mm short of radiographic apex.
6. Gentle instrumentation and irrigation with 1% sodium hypochlorite solution to remove and dissolve organic debris and kill micro-organisms. Use gentle debridement in a crown–apex direction and determine working length (see Fig. 7.3B).
7. Fill canal with calcium hydroxide as inter-visit medication if required.
8. Place 5–6 mm of MTA (7.3C) at apex using specialised carriers and pluggers, take check of periapical. Allow to set (time required dependent on the material used), then obturate canal with gutta-percha, and restore tooth with composite.
9. If MTA placement not possible, can redress with non-setting calcium hydroxide after 1–2 weeks, then 3 monthly (see Fig. 7.3C). Via this method, the average time to barrier formation is 1 year.

files and placement of MTA or biodentine at the fracture line aims to produce a stop at the coronal side of the fracture line. The coronal portion can then be obturated with gutta-percha and sealer.

If the apical portion is non-vital, it may be possible to instrument across the fracture line, although it can be very difficult to prevent bleeding into the canal. Failure to instrument a non-vital apical fragment necessitates surgical removal of the fragment. Splinting across fracture lines with a post is a radical temporary solution with a poor long-term prognosis.

Root Resorption of Permanent Teeth

Infection related: Infection-related resorption can affect the external or internal root surface.

External. Resorption is initiated by damage to the periodontal ligament, and then propagated by necrotic pulp tissue via dentinal tubules. Diagnosis is by asymmetrical radiolucent shape of surface of root with intact root canal walls (Fig. 7.4).

Internal. Resorption is initiated by cells of the pulp within the root canal. Diagnosis is as a ballooning of the root canal with intact root surface (Fig. 7.5).

Treatment of both types is by thorough mechanical and chemical debridement, followed by non-setting calcium hydroxide paste for 4 weeks. Obturation is then completed, although if resorption continues, the tooth will eventually be lost.

Cervical. This is an unusual form of external infection-related resorption initiated by damage to the root surface in the cervical region and propagated either by infected root canal contents or by periodontal microflora. Treatment is usually by obturation of the root canal, followed by surgical external repair and restoration.

Ankylosis-related resorption (replacement resorption):

Ankylosis-related resorption is progressive resorption of tooth structure and its replacement with bone as part of continued bone remodelling. It occurs after trauma in which there is significant periodontal ligament injury (i.e. luxation, intrusion and avulsion). It cannot be

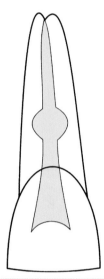

Fig. 7.5 Ballooning of the root canal caused by internal resorption. (From Whitworth JM, Nunn JH. In: Welbury RR, ed. *Paediatric Dentistry*. Oxford University Press; 1997. By permission of Oxford University Press, www.oup.com.)

treated. The tooth should be maintained in the mouth for as long as possible which will avoid early need for prosthetic tooth replacement and maintain adjacent bone. Patients should be informed that Ankylosis-related resorption will continue and the tooth will eventually be lost. Consideration should be given to tooth removal or decoronation when infra-occlusion is noted.

7.8. Molar-Incisor Hypomineralisation

MIH is defined as a developmentally derived dental defect that involves hypomineralisation of between 1 and 4 FPMs, frequently associated with similarly affected permanent incisors.

Second primary molars, which form at a similar time as the FPMs, can also be affected. This is defined as hypomineralised second primary molar (HSPM). It has been suggested that the presence of hypomineralised second primary molars can be an early predicator of MIH, given these children are 4.6 times more likely to have MIH (Garot et al 2018).

Teeth affected with MIH present with well-demarcated areas of enamel hypomineralisation, which can vary in size, position and colour. White opacities represent a milder form, while yellow/brown lesions have more extensive hypomineralisation. The affected teeth initially erupt with a normal thickness of enamel; however, hypomineralised areas, particularly yellow/brown lesions affecting the posterior dentition, can be subject to rapid deterioration following eruption known as post-eruptive breakdown (PEB). This leads to irregular cavitation and increases susceptibility to plaque accumulation and dental caries. In more severely affected teeth, it can lead to destruction of the crown shortly after eruption.

Teeth affected by MIH can be acutely sensitive and uncomfortable when performing toothbrushing or consuming cold or sweet food/drink.

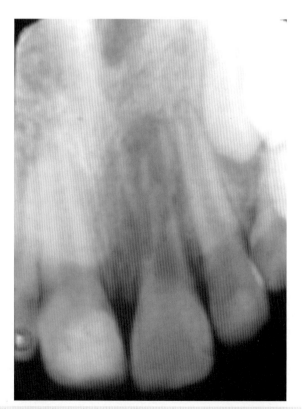

Fig. 7.4 Radiograph showing the radiolucent shape of external root resorption.

The global prevalence of MIH is 14.2%. There is no difference in prevalence between males and females (Zhao et al 2018).

The aetiology of MIH is not fully understood. Several causes relating to disturbances during development of the incisors and FPM, in the prenatal, perinatal or postnatal period have been described. Recent literature review suggests early childhood illnesses, for example, fever, asthma and pneumonia are likely to be associated with the development of MIH.

DIAGNOSIS OF MIH

Ghanim et al (2017) described key features in identifying teeth affected by MIH, (shown in Box 7.14).

During clinical examination, the presence and extent of any hypomineralised lesions should be recorded. For each individual tooth affected, it is helpful to record:

- The presence, position and colour of any demarcated lesions
- Presence of post-eruptive breakdown
- Presence of an atypical restoration
- Presence of atypical carious lesions.

The extent of any lesion should then be measured according to the surface area of the enamel affected:

1. Less than one-third of a tooth surface
2. At least one-third but less than two-thirds
3. At least two-thirds of the tooth surface.

MIH can be mistaken for other conditions including amelogenesis imperfecta, fluorosis and enamel hypoplasia.

Table 7.5 Differences Between MIH and Other Enamel Defects.

Table 7.7	MIH
Fluorosis	Fluorosis tends to present as diffuse opacities, which have a symmetrical distribution bilaterally, while MIH is more likely to have more demarcated lesions with a non-symmetrical distribution. In addition, opacities relating to fluorosis tend to be more resistant to dental caries.
Amelogenesis imperfect (AI)	AI presents with generalised involvement of the dentition, while MIH tends to affect the FPM, incisors ± SPM.
Enamel hypoplasia	The margins of hypoplastic defects tend to be smooth, while the margins of post-eruptive breakdown areas are irregular.
Demineralisation associated with caries	Occur in areas of plaque stagnation, while MIH lesions can occur on surfaces not normally associated with dental caries.

FPM, First permanent molar; *MIH*, molar-incisor hypomineralisation; *SPM*, second primary molar.

These conditions are outlined further in Chapter 8; however, Table 7.5 outlines differences between conditions which might assist differential diagnosis.

Severity of MIH (Ghanim et al 2017)

A tooth diagnosed with colour changes only (i.e. creamy, white, yellow, orange or brown) is considered as 'Mildly affected'. A tooth diagnosed with post-eruptive enamel breakdown and/or atypical restoration/caries/missing is considered as 'Severely affected'.

Management of MIH

1. Prevention
Any child diagnosed with MIH/HSPM should have an intensive prevention regime as outlined in section 7.4.
2. Management of sensitivity
   - Casein phosphopeptide and amorphous calcium phosphate paste (e.g. GC Tooth Mousse) can help decrease sensitivity (Ozgul et al 2013).
   - Desensitising toothpaste can be helpful in reducing mild sensitivity.
   - Fissure sealants can help protect posterior teeth against progression of dental caries and help decrease sensitivity. Glass ionomer cement can be used to seal teeth which are partially erupted, have porous enamel/areas of PEB or where sensitivity precludes the use of resin sealants. Where resin sealants can be used, the use of a dental bonding agent after etching can improve retention to hypomineralised enamel.

Management of Anterior Teeth

The aims of treatment to manage affected anterior teeth are:

- Manage aesthetic concerns
- Relief of symptoms
- Protect remaining tooth structure.

Management options for discoloured anterior teeth are discussed in section 7.5.

Box 7.14 Key Features in Identifying Teeth Affected by MIH.

Demarcated opacities

- Having a clearly defined boundary from adjacent healthy enamel.
- Alteration in enamel translucency.
- Normal thickness of enamel.
- Colour ranges white–cream–orange–yellow–brown.

Post-eruptive enamel breakdown

- Loss of enamel from an initially formed surface after tooth eruption.
- The loss is often associated with a pre-existing demarcated opacity.
- Is characterised by sharp and irregular borders.

Atypical restoration

- Frequently extends to the buccal and palatal/lingual surfaces.
- Frequently associated with an opacity at the restoration margin.
- For incisors, there may be a buccal restoration not related to trauma.
- Often seen in otherwise caries-free mouths.

Atypical carious lesions

- The size and form of the carious lesion do not match the present carious lesion distribution in the child's mouth.
- The existing carious lesion is usually associated with demarcated opacities.

Management of Posterior Dentition

1. Hypomineralised Second Primary Molars
   - Fissure sealants can be used to protect teeth without post-eruptive enamel breakdown.
   - Glass ionomer cement or resin composite can be used to restore small areas of post-eruptive breakdown.
   - Preformed metal crowns are the restoration of choice where there has been significant post-eruptive breakdown. These will also protect the remaining tooth structure against further deterioration.
2. Hypomineralised First Permanent Molars

The aims of treatment to manage affected posterior teeth are:
   - Relief of symptoms
   - Protect remaining tooth structure
   - Restore function.

Where affected permanent teeth have a guarded long-term prognosis, extraction should be considered. The decision to extract is based on a number of factors including:
   - The stage of dental development
   - Presence/absence of the remaining dentition including third permanent molars
   - Severity of symptoms
   - Condition of surrounding teeth
   - Medical history
   - Occlusion
   - Co-operation for treatment.

The ideal time to consider tooth removal would either be when the furcation of the second permanent molars is beginning to develop or later as part of an orthodontic treatment plan. A thorough clinical, orthodontic and radiographic evaluation around the age of 8.5 years is helpful to identify if removal should be considered.

Where a decision is made to restore the hypomineralised teeth (either definitively or to maintain until extraction), the following techniques can be considered:

- GIC – this is appropriate as a provisional restoration to decrease sensitivity and maintain the tooth until it can be definitively restored or extracted.
- Resin composite can be used as a definitive restorative material. Amalgam is not appropriate for hypomineralised teeth. When preparing the cavity, all porous enamel should be removed, leaving cavity margins on a firmer enamel surface which is resistant to removal with a slow-speed bur.
- Preformed metal crowns (PMC) can be used to restore severely affected molars temporarily prior to future extractions. These can be placed with minimal or no reduction of the molar. PMCs can provide more robust protection and reduction of sensitivity than other options, such as placement of GIC. It can be more comfortable to use local anaesthetic prior to placement of PMC on FPM, and therefore they can be more demanding of patient co-operation than GIC.
- Indirect adhesive onlay restorations (Gold/NiCr) can be considered for older children. These can be placed with minimal tooth preparation, given the increased vertical dimension normally re-establishes after a short time (Harley and Ibbetson 1993).

Self-Assessment: Questions

MULTIPLE CHOICE QUESTIONS (TRUE/FALSE)

1. The mineralisation of these teeth may be affected by maternal illness during pregnancy:
   a. Primary molars
   b. Primary incisors
   c. Permanent incisors
   d. Primary canines
   e. First permanent first molars
2. With regard to childhood development and dental treatment:
   a. Separation from parents is possible after age 5 years
   b. Adequate manual dexterity for good oral hygiene is possible at age 5 years
   c. Parental influence is important
   d. By age 5 years, children have developed selective attention
   e. Teenagers respond well to criticism
3. Bitewing radiographs should be taken every 6 months for:
   a. Primary dentition with high caries risk
   b. Primary dentition with low caries risk
   c. Mixed dentition with low caries risk
   d. Mixed dentition with high caries risk
   e. Permanent dentition with low caries risk
4. Conventional orthopantograms:
   a. Diagnose occlusal caries accurately
   b. Diagnose interproximal caries accurately
   c. Identify abnormalities in dental development of number, position or form
   d. Can precisely localise teeth
   e. Identify larger areas of pathology
5. In caries development:
   a. Plaque consists mainly of food debris
   b. Precavitation lesions are reversible
   c. Cavitated lesions are reversible
   d. In the United Kingdom, most of the domestic water supply
   e. Dietary advice should be the same for everyone
6. In caries epidemiology:
   a. The fall in caries prevalence since the 1970s is largely a consequence of toothbrushing
   b. Preschool caries is related to maternal *Streptococcus mutans* levels
   c. Nursing caries is associated with frequent use of sugared drinks
   d. Nursing caries can be prevented by correct advice
   e. Caries prevention can be maximised by professional application of fluoride varnish

7. With regard to molar-incisor hypomineralisation (MIH)
   a. Patients with hypomineralised second primary molars are more likely to have MIH
   b. All four first permanent molars will be affected
   c. White marks represent a more severe form of MIH than yellow/brown lesions
   d. Teeth with MIH have a reduced enamel thickness
   e. The aetiology of MIH is poorly understood
8. With regard to the restoration of permanent posterior teeth in children:
   a. Composite can be placed in pit and fissure location as long as good moisture control is possible
   b. Amalgam is the preferred material to restore approximal cavities
   c. Regular bitewing radiographs are required for fissure-sealed teeth
   d. Fissure sealant is the restoration of choice for a stained but non-cavitated fissure in a molar with no radiographic evidence of caries
   e. 'Occult' caries is easy to diagnose clinically
9. In extrinsic tooth discolouration:
   a. Stains can be removed by polishing
   b. Bleaching is an accepted treatment
   c. Mouthwashes can be an important factor
   d. Liquid oral medicines are never involved
   e. Food and beverages are a common cause
10. Intrinsic discolouration:
   a. May be caused by internal resorption
   b. Is caused by some drugs
   c. If caused by fluorosis, it can be treated by micro-abrasion
   d. May be caused by previous trauma to primary teeth
   e. In non-vital teeth, can be treated by bleaching
11. In primary molar endodontics:
   a. Vital pulpotomy has a low success rate
   b. Calcium hydroxide can be used over the pulp stumps
   c. Teeth with furcation caries should be extracted
   d. Treatment is indicated in children with cardiac defects
   e. Treatment is indicated in children with bleeding coagulopathies
12. In permanent incisors with open apices:
   a. Pulpotomy is preferred to pulp cap for pulpal exposures over 1 mm in size
   b. Pulpotomy medicament of choice is non-setting calcium hydroxide
   c. Pulpotomy enables radicular development with vital pulp tissue
   d. Pulpectomy with non-setting calcium hydroxide can allow continued root-end growth
   e. MTA is the material of choice for apical barrier formation.

EXTENDED MATCHING ITEMS QUESTIONS

1. Theme: Dental diagnosis in children
   For each of the case scenarios (a–e), select from the list below (1–14) the single most appropriate diagnosis for the signs and symptoms given. Each diagnosis may be used once, more than once or not at all:
   1. Reversible pulpitis.
   2. External inflammatory resorption.
   3. Erosion.
   4. Tooth discolouration.
   5. Molar-incisor hypomineralisation.
   6. Attrition.
   7. Bruxism.
   8. Irreversible pulpitis.
   9. Fluorosis.
   10. Abrasion.
   11. Enamel caries.
   12. Nursing/early childhood caries.
   13. Internal inflammatory resorption.
   14. Replacement resorption.
      a. A 3-year-old child attends your surgery with caries affecting the upper incisors and first primary molars.
      b. An 8-year-old boy suffers from GORD, and you notice the enamel on the palatal surface of his upper incisors has a glass-like surface.
      c. You take a radiograph of an immature permanent incisor tooth with a history of lateral luxation. The root outline differs from previous radiograph with asymmetrical areas of radiolucency noted.
      d. You decide to provide hydrochloric acid micro-abrasion for a 10-year-old boy with a previous history of eating toothpaste.
      e. A 9-year-old patient attends your surgery for a dental examination. He reports his back teeth are sore when they are brushed. There are white marks on his maxillary central incisors and the first permanent molars are yellow/brown in colour.
2. Theme: Endodontic treatment in children
   For each of the case scenarios (a–e), select from the list below (1–6) the appropriate endodontic options. There may be more than one answer for each scenario.
   1. Direct pulp cap
   2. Primary tooth pulpotomy
   3. Partial pulpotomy (Cvek pulpotomy)
   4. Primary tooth pulpectomy
   5. Indirect pulp treatment
   6. Pulpectomy
      a. Permanent maxillary central incisor with an immature root following an enamel dentine pulp fracture?
      b. Symptom-free primary molar with a carious pulpal exposure during restoration.
      c. Symptom-free carious second primary molar with a mesial occlusal cavity. Radiograph shows no obvious barrier between caries and the dental pulp.
      d. Non-vital maxillary permanent lateral incisor.
      e. Mandibular first premolar following a small pulpal exposure during restoration.

CASE HISTORY QUESTIONS

Question 1

An 8-year-old child who was previously caries free suddenly develops early interproximal lesions noted radiographically.

1. What investigations would you carry out?
2. What treatment would you advise?

Question 2

A 9-year-old patient attends your surgery. Examination reveals severe hypomineralisation of the maxillary first permanent molars and mild hypomineralisation of the mandibular first permanent molars and maxillary central incisors.

1. What additional information may be useful to collect when taking a history?
2. What is the likely diagnosis?
3. The patient's mother asks why this has developed. What would you suggest?

Question 3

Possible adverse sequelae following an incidence of dental trauma include pulpal necrosis or resorption. What management is advised for each of the following occurring in a permanent incisor?

1. Pulpal necrosis
2. Infection-related resorption
3. Ankylosis-related resorption (replacement resorption)

PICTURE QUESTIONS

Picture 1

Fig. 7.6 shows teeth that erupted 12 days after birth.

1. What is the name given to these teeth?
2. Are these teeth usually part of the normal dentition?
3. What problems can arise with these teeth?
4. How should they be treated?

Picture 2

Fig. 7.7 shows stained teeth.

1. What type of staining is shown?
2. What is the likely cause of the staining?

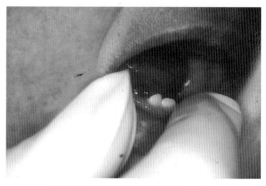

Fig. 7.6 Oblique view of mouth.

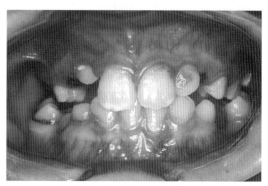

Fig. 7.7 Front view of mouth.

SHORT NOTE QUESTIONS

Write short notes on:

1. Drinks to avoid for a patient with tooth surface loss of dietary origin.
2. The main clinical features and risk factors for 'nursing' caries.
3. Indications and contraindications for inhalation sedation.

Self-Assessment: Answers

MULTIPLE CHOICE QUESTIONS

1. a. True. Primary molars begin mineralising at 3.5–6 months of pregnancy.
   b. True. Primary incisors begin mineralising at 3–4 months of pregnancy.
   c. False. Permanent incisors do not begin mineralising until 3–4 months after birth.
   d. True. Primary canines begin mineralising at 3.5–4.5 months of pregnancy.
   e. True. First permanent molars begin mineralising at 7–8 months of pregnancy. They are the only permanent teeth for which mineralisation can be affected by events during pregnancy.

2. a. True. Separation anxiety is high until the age of 5 years.
   b. False. Co-ordination is normally sufficiently developed at age 6–7 years.
   c. True. Absolutely vital for positive reinforcement.

   d. False. By age 7 years, children have developed selective attention and can determine which advice is important.
   e. False. Teenagers require support and reassurance.
3. a. True. This is the correct frequency.
   b. False. Bitewings should only be taken every 12–18 months.
   c. False. Bitewings should only be taken every 12–18 months.
   d. True. This is the correct frequency.
   e. False. Bitewings should be taken every 24 months.

4. a. False. They may suggest that caries is present, but bitewings give a more accurate diagnosis.
   b. False. They may suggest that caries is present, but bitewings give an accurate diagnosis.
   c. True. They are invaluable in this regard.
   d. False. Only in conjunction with intraoral radiographs can they be used to localise teeth.
   e. True. They are excellent for the diagnosis of larger pathological lesions.

5. a. False. Plaque is 70% micro-organisms.
   b. True. These lesions can undergo remineralisation.
   c. False. Once the surface layer is broken and cavitated, they need to be restored.
   d. False. Very few areas in the United Kingdom have fluoridated water.
   e. False. It requires time and thought. It must be personal, practical and positive.
6. a. False. It is linked to fluoridated toothpaste.
   b. True. Levels of maternal *S. mutans* have been shown to correlate with caries levels in preschool children.
   c. True. Especially if the sugared drinks are taken on demand throughout the night.
   d. True. Advice at birth to the new mother by the health visitor is probably the most important factor in establishing correct habits.
   e. True. 22,600 ppm fluoride varnish application four times per year will reduce caries experience.
7. a. True. It has been suggested that the presence of hypomineralised second primary molars can be an early predicator of MIH, given these children are 4.6 times more likely to have MIH.
   b. False. Between one and four first permanent molars are affected.
   c. False. White opacities represent a milder form, while yellow/brown lesions have more extensive hypomineralisation.
   d. False. The affected teeth initially erupt with a normal thickness of enamel; however, hypomineralised areas, particularly yellow/brown lesions affecting the posterior dentition, can be subject to rapid deterioration following eruption known as post-eruptive breakdown.
   e. True. The aetiology of MIH is not fully understood. Several causes relating to disturbances during development of the incisors and FPM in the prenatal, perinatal or postnatal period have been described.
8. a. True. Any remaining fissure should be sealed.
   b. False. Amalgam is not routinely used for patients aged 15 years and under. Composite can be used as an alternative.
   c. True. A macroscopically intact sealant is not necessarily microscopically intact.
   d. True.
   e. False. By definition, it is difficult and requires bite-wing radiography.
9. a. True. Polishing should be completed on all discoloured teeth to allow accurate assessment, diagnosis and treatment planning.
   b. False. Bleaching is a treatment for intrinsic discolouration.
   c. True. Chlorhexidine mouthwash binds tannin to produce black staining around the gingival margin.
   d. False. Iron supplements will produce a black stain and some antituberculosis drugs a red–brown stain.
   e. True. Especially in the presence of poor oral hygiene.
10. a. True. This gives a characteristic 'pink spot' appearance to the overlying enamel.
    b. True. Tetracyclines are the most notorious offenders, producing a yellow–grey discolouration with intensification of the colour and banding in the cervical third of the crown.
    c. True. The majority of fluorotic stains involve the outer 100–300 μm enamel. Controlled microabrasion removes approximately 100 μm enamel and changes the optical properties of enamel to render residual stains less perceptible.
    d. True. Previous trauma to primary teeth can produce localised hypoplasia of permanent crowns.
    e. True. However, the legal position of bleaching must be taken into consideration.
11. a. False. Ferric sulphate has a success rate of around 95%.
    b. True. Calcium hydroxide, zinc oxide eugenol and mineral trioxide aggregate are all acceptable medicaments.
    c. True. These cannot be restored.
    d. False. Absolutely contraindicated. Extract.
    e. True. This avoids extraction, which would have bleeding complications.
12. a. True. Its chance of success and hence its ability to retain vital radicular pulp is superior to pulp capping.
    b. True.
    c. True. This is the important factor in choosing pulpotomy as opposed to pulpectomy.
    d. False - following complete removal of the pulp further dental development will cease.
    e. True. Apexification with calcium hydroxide can lead to brittle roots and a prolonged number of treatment visits.

EXTENDED MATCHING ITEMS ANSWERS

Question 1

a. 12
b. 3
c. 2
d. 9
e. 5

Question 2

a. 1 or 3
b. 2
c. 5 or 2
d. 6
e. 1 or 3

CASE HISTORY ANSWERS

Question 1

1. It is essential to establish the cause of the caries. A 3-day diet analysis is very important. The family circumstances may have recently changed, and there may have been an increased exposure to sugared sweets and snacks. Use of separators may be considered to allow direct visualisation of interproximal surfaces where cavitation is suspected.

2. Dietary advice, suggesting that sugars are kept to main meal times with savoury snacks between meals. Drinks should not contain sugar, and no food or drink should be taken within 20 minutes of going to bed. Additional therapy could include topical fluoride application, toothbrush and flossing instruction, toothpaste strength advice and fissure sealant placement on first permanent molars.

Question 2

1. It would be useful to enquire about whether anyone else in the family has similar dental issues, fluoride history, any prenatal, perinatal illness or complications and any history of early childhood illnesses such as asthma, fever or pneumonia.
2. Given the asymmetrical distribution of the hypomineralisation, this is likely to be molar-incisor hypomineralisation. It is important to consider/exclude other possible causes such as amelogenesis imperfecta, fluorosis or enamel hypoplasia.
3. The aetiology of MIH is poorly understood, and therefore it is difficult to provide a definitive answer. Several causes relating to a disturbance during the development of the incisors and first permanent molars have been described.

Question 3

1. Pulp extirpation and completion of root canal treatment.
2. Infection-related resorption is caused by damage to the periodontal ligament, which is then propagated by necrotic pulp tissue via the dentinal tubules. Treatment involves controlling pulpal infection. The canal should be extirpated promptly and the tooth dressed with calcium hydroxide for up to 4 weeks prior to obturation. This is best referred for specialist care.
3. This occurs following significant periodontal ligament damage. It cannot be treated. The tooth should be maintained in the mouth for as long as possible while plans are made for long-term prosthetic replacement. Interceptive management of infraocclusion may be required. Endodontic treatment is not appropriate in the absence of pulpal necrosis. This is best referred for specialist care.

PICTURE ANSWERS

Picture 1

1. Neonatal teeth. If these teeth are present at birth, they are called natal teeth.
2. Yes. Lower incisors are the commonest teeth involved.
3. Ulceration of the infant's tongue or the mother's breast and a danger to the airway if they are excessively mobile.
4. If they fulfil any of the above or if they are supernumeraries, then they should be extracted. If they are part of the normal dentition, then retention is beneficial.

Picture 2

1. Extrinsic staining.
2. Foods and beverages, chlorhexidine mouthwash, oral drug suspensions (e.g. iron preparations).

SHORT NOTE ANSWERS

1. The acidogenic potential is a term that takes into account a liquid's resistance to changes in its pH (i.e. its inherent buffering capacity – natural juices have a very high acidogenic potential), followed by fruit-flavoured carbonated waters and drinks, and then carbonated cola drinks. Patients should be advised to try and eradicate all carbonated beverages except on special occasions, and at these times to try to take them at a main meal with a straw. Natural fruit juices should be advised only at meal times.
2. The main clinical features are rapidity of onset, surfaces affected (characteristically, the smooth labial and/or palatal surfaces of upper incisors); teeth affected (characteristically teeth are affected in the order they erupt - however lower incisor teeth are usually spared). The risk factors include prolonged consumption of milk through a bottle at night, use of a pacifier dipped in a sugar solution, prolonged on-demand sugary drink feeding.
3. Indications for inhalation sedation include:
   - mild to moderate dental anxiety
   - marked gag reflex
   - unpleasant dental treatment
   - needle phobia
   - medical conditions precluding use of alternative techniques

   Contraindications include:
   - blocked nasal airway
   - tonsillar and adenoidal enlargement
   - severe pulmonary conditions
   - chronic bronchitis
   - lack of sufficient co-operation with the technique
   - myasthenia gravis
   - first trimester of pregnancy.

References

Borges AB, Caneppele TM, Masterson D, Maia LC. Is resin infiltration an effective esthetic treatment for enamel development defects and white spot lesions? A systematic review. *J Dent.* 2017;56:11–18.

Garot E, Denis A, Delbos Y, Manton D, Silva M, Rouas P. Are hypomineralised lesions on second primary molars (HSPM) a predictive sign of molar incisor hypomineralisation (MIH)? A systematic review and a meta-analysis. *J Dent.* 2018;72:8–13

Ghanim A, Silva MJ, Elfrink MEC, Lygidakis NA, Marin RJ, Weerheijm KL and Manton DJ. Molar incisor hypomineralisation (MIH) training manual for clinical field surveys and practice. *Eur Arch Paediatr Dent.* 2017;18:225–242.

Greenwall-Cohen J, Greenwall LH. The single discoloured tooth: vital and non-vital bleaching techniques. *Br Dent J.* 2019;226:11.

Harley KE, Ibbetson RJ. Dental anomalies—are adhesive castings the solution? *Br Dent J.* 1993;174(1):15–22.

Ozgül BM, Saat S, Sönmez H, Oz FT. Clinical evaluation of desensitizing treatment for incisor teeth affected by molar-incisor hypomineralization. *J Clin Pediatr Dent.* 2013;38(2):101–105.

Zhao D, Dong B, Yu D, Ren Q, Sun Y. The prevalence of molar incisor hypomineralization: evidence from 70 studies. *Int J Paediatr Dent.* 2018;28(2):170–179.

8 Paediatric Dentistry II

Overview

This chapter covers dental trauma, dental anomalies and the special needs of medical, physical and intellectual disability.

Increased knowledge of the pathophysiology of dental trauma has resulted in development of the standard of care for traumatised teeth and an improvement in their prognosis. Teeth that would have been previously extracted can now often be maintained in function during adolescence and early adulthood. The category of special needs has increased with successful scientific advances in paediatric medicine and surgery. More children now survive previously fatal illnesses. However, they often do so with either direct oral and dental side-effects of the original illness or its treatment or with significant risk of morbidity or mortality from oral or dental infection.

8.1 Traumatic Injuries

LEARNING OBJECTIVES

You should:
- know the most common injuries in the primary and the permanent dentitions
- be able to classify crown/root fractures and periodontal ligament (displacement) injuries
- know the appropriate treatments for each classification of injury
- appreciate the importance of a high index of suspicion in child physical abuse, know what actions to take and where to go to for help.

Traumatic injuries to teeth and jaws can occur at any age. They are, however, very common in children. Boys have twice as many injuries as girls in both the primary and permanent dentitions. The majority of injuries affect the maxillary incisors. The most common types of injury are:

- primary dentition: subluxation, luxation
- permanent dentition: crown fractures.

Peak injury times occur at 2–4 years in the primary dentition when a young child is exploring and becoming adventurous and 7–10 years in the permanent dentition owing to falls when playing. At age 5 years, 31–40% of boys and 16–30% of girls will have injured their teeth. The respective figures at age 12 years are 12–33% and 19%.

ASSESSMENT

Classification

Table 8.1 summarises the classification of dento-alveolar injuries based on the World Health Organization (WHO) system.

History

Dental History

When did injury occur?
   The time interval between injury and treatment significantly influences the prognosis of avulsion, luxations, crown fractures (with or without pulpal exposures) and dento-alveolar fractures.
Where did the injury occur?
   May indicate the need for tetanus prophylaxis.
How did the injury occur?
   The nature of the accident can yield information on the type of injury expected. Discrepancy between history and clinical findings raises suspicion of non-accidental injury (NAI).
Lost teeth/fragments?
   When a tooth or fragment is missing, efforts should be made to account for it. Locations to investigate include: the tooth not retrieved at the scene of the injury, imbedded in the soft tissues if a laceration is present or swallowed by the patient.
If a tooth or fractured crown portion cannot be accounted for when there has been a history of loss of consciousness, then a chest radiograph should be obtained to exclude inhalation.
Concussion, headache, vomiting or amnesia?
   The dentist assessing the patient must be vigilant for other non-dental injuries, which may take precedence over the dental injuries.
   Brain damage must be excluded and referral to a hospital for further investigation organised.
Previous dental history?
   Previous trauma can affect pulpal sensibility tests and the recuperative capacity of the pulp and/or periodontium. In addition, is the child injury prone or are there

Table 8.1 Classification of Dento-alveolar Injuries.

Injury	Description
INJURIES TO THE HARD DENTAL TISSUES AND THE PULP	
Enamel infraction	Incomplete fracture crack of enamel without loss of tooth substance
Enamel fracture	Loss of tooth substance confined to enamel
Enamel–dentine fracture	Loss of tooth substance confined to enamel and dentine, not involving the pulp
Complicated crown fracture	Fracture of enamel and dentine exposing the pulp
Uncomplicated crown root fracture	Fracture of enamel, dentine and cementum but not involving the pulp
Complicated crown root fracture	Fracture of enamel, dentine, cementum and exposing the pulp
Root fracture	Fracture involving dentine, cementum and pulp; can be subclassified into apical, middle and coronal third
INJURIES TO THE PERIODONTAL TISSUES	
Concussion	No abnormal loosening or displacement but marked reaction to percussion
Subluxation (loosening)	Abnormal loosening but no displacement
Extrusive luxation (partial avulsion)	Partial displacement of tooth from socket
Lateral luxation	Displacement other than axially with comminution or fracture of alveolar socket
Intrusive luxation	Displacement into alveolar bone with comminution or fracture of alveolar socket
Avulsion	Complete displacement of tooth from socket
INJURIES TO SUPPORTING BONE	
Comminution of mandibular or maxillary alveolar socket wall	Crushing and compression of alveolar socket; found in intrusive and lateral luxation injuries
Fracture of mandibular or maxillary alveolar socket wall	Fracture confined to facial or lingual/palatal socket wall
Fracture of mandibular or maxillary alveolar process	Fracture of the alveolar process; may or may not involve the tooth sockets
Fracture of mandible or maxilla	May or may not involve the alveolar socket
INJURIES TO GINGIVA OR ORAL MUCOSA	
Laceration of gingiva or oral mucosa	Wound in mucosa resulting from a tear
Contusion of gingiva or oral mucosa	Bruise not accompanied by a break in the mucosa, usually causing submucosal haemorrhage
Abrasion of gingiva or oral mucosa	Superficial wound produced by rubbing or scraping the mucosal surface

suspicions of NAI? Previous treatment experience, age and parental/child attitude will affect the choice of treatment.

Medical History

Congenital heart disease, rheumatic fever or *severe immunosuppression* are contraindications for prolonged endodontic treatment with a persistent necrotic focus. Reimplantation of avulsed teeth may be contraindicated in these patients, and their relevant medical team should be consulted, including whether antibiotic cover is required as part of their dental management.

Bleeding disorders must be of prime concern if there is soft tissue laceration, avulsion or luxation, or if extractions are required.

Allergies require a suitable alternative antibiotic if necessary.

Tetanus status may require a referral for tetanus toxoid booster (if no previous immunisation in the last 5 years).

Extraoral Examination

Swelling, bruising or lacerations may indicate underlying bony and tooth injury. Lacerations require careful debridement to remove foreign bodies. Crown fracture with associated lip swelling and a penetrating wound may suggest fragment retention in the lip.

Intraoral Examination

Examination must be systematic and include recording of lacerations, haemorrhage and bruising as well as abnormalities of tooth occlusion, displacement, fractures or cracks. Tooth examination should include:

- mobility assessment: possible root fracture, displacement, dento-alveolar fracture
- percussion: duller note may indicate root fracture
- colour: early change seen on palatal or gingival third of crown
- sensibility tests:
  - thermal with warm gutta-percha or ethyl chloride
  - electric pulp tester notoriously unreliable, and not recommended for primary teeth. Never use in isolation from other clinical and radiographic data.
  - always test contralateral teeth and compare.

Special clinical investigations for dental trauma can be conveniently grouped into a 'trauma stamp' table layout – this is useful as an aide-mémoire and for quick reference and comparison over time. Table 8.2 shows pulpal survival at 5 years after injuries involving the periodontal ligament.

Radiographic Examination

Periapical Radiographs

Periapical radiographs are the best view for accurate diagnosis and clinical audit. Two radiographs at different angles may be essential to detect a root fracture. However, if access and co-operation are difficult, one anterior occlusal radiograph rarely misses a root fracture.

Occlusal Radiographs

To detect fractures and foreign bodies within the soft tissues:

- Upper lip: lateral view using an occlusal film held by patient/helper at side of mouth.
- Lower lip: occlusal view using an 'occlusal' film held between teeth.

Orthopantogram

An orthopantogram is essential where a bony injury is suspected. Other views include:

- lateral oblique
- lateral skull:
- specialist views for maxillofacial fractures
- anteroposterior skull
- occipitomental.

Photography

Photographs are useful for clinical records and for medicolegal use.

PRIMARY DENTITION

During its early development, the permanent incisor is located palatally to, and in close proximity with, the apex of the primary incisor. With any injury to a primary tooth, there is risk of damage to the underlying permanent successor.

The most accident prone time is between 2 and 4 years of age. Realistically, this means that few restorative procedures will be possible, and in the majority of children, the decision is between extraction and maintenance without extensive treatment. A primary incisor should always be removed if its maintenance will jeopardise the developing tooth bud.

A traumatised primary tooth that is retained should be assessed regularly for clinical and radiographic signs of pulpal or periodontal complications. Radiographs may detect damage to the permanent successor. Soft tissue injuries in children should be assessed weekly until healed. Tooth injuries should be reviewed every 3–4 months for the first year, and then annually until the primary tooth exfoliates and the permanent successor is in place.

Crown Fractures

Uncomplicated Crown Fracture

This is treated either by smoothing sharp edges or by restoring with an acid-etch restoration if co-operation is satisfactory.

Complicated Crown Fracture

Normally, extraction is the treatment of choice. However, pulp extirpation and canal obturation with zinc oxide cement, followed by an acid-etch restoration, is possible with reasonable co-operation.

Crown Root Fracture

The pulp is usually exposed and any restorative treatment is very difficult. The tooth is best extracted.

Root Fracture

A root fracture without displacement and with only a small amount of mobility should be treated initially by keeping the tooth under observation. If the coronal fragment becomes non-vital and symptomatic, it should be removed. The apical portion usually remains vital and undergoes normal resorption. Similarly, with marked displacement and mobility, only the coronal portion should be removed.

Concussion, Subluxation and Luxation Injuries

Associated soft tissue damage should be cleaned by the parent twice daily with 0.2% chlorhexidine using cotton buds or gauze swabs until healing is completed.

Concussion

Concussion is often not brought to a dentist until a tooth discolours.

Subluxation

If the tooth has slight mobility, a soft diet for 1–2 weeks is advised, with the traumatised area kept as clean as possible. Marked mobility requires extraction.

Extrusive Luxation

Marked mobility requires extraction.

Lateral Luxation

If the crown is displaced palatally, the apex moves buccally and hence away from the permanent tooth germ. If there is no occlusal interference present, monitoring for spontaneous realignment is possible. If the crown is displaced buccally, the apex will be displaced towards the permanent tooth bud and extraction is indicated in order to minimise further damage to the permanent successor.

Intrusive Luxation

This is the most common type of injury. The aim of investigation is to establish the direction of displacement through radiographical examination. If the root is displaced palatally towards the permanent successor, then the primary

Table 8.2 Pulpal Survival at 5 Years After Injuries Involving the Periodontal Ligament.

Injury	Open Apex (%)	Closed Apex (%)
Concussion	100	96
Subluxation	100	85
Extrusive luxation	95	45
Lateral luxation	95	25
Intrusive luxation	40	0
Replantation	30	0

tooth should be extracted to minimise possible damage to the successor. If the root is displaced buccally, monitoring for spontaneous re-eruption should be allowed. Review should be weekly for a month, then monthly for a maximum of 6 months. Most re-eruption occurs between 1 and 6 months. If this does not occur, then ankylosis is likely and extraction is necessary to prevent ectopic eruption of the permanent successor.

Avulsion

Replantation of avulsed primary incisors is not recommended because of the risk of damage to the permanent tooth germs. Space maintenance is not necessary following the loss of a primary incisor as only minor drifting of adjacent teeth occurs. The eruption of the permanent successor may be delayed for about 1 year as a result of abnormal thickening of connective tissue overlying the tooth germ.

Sequelae of Injuries to the Primary Dentition

Pulpal Necrosis

Necrosis is the most common complication of primary trauma. Teeth of a normal colour rarely develop periapical inflammation; conversely, mildly discoloured teeth may be vital. A mild pink colour occurring soon after trauma may represent intrapulpal bleeding with a pulp that is still vital. This colour may recede; if it persists, then necrosis should be suspected. Radiographic examination should be 3-monthly to check for periapical inflammation. Failure of the pulp cavity to reduce in size is an indicator of pulpal death. Teeth should be extracted whenever there is evidence of periapical inflammation to prevent possible damage to the permanent successor. It is important to council the patient's parents about the possibility of necrosis and the signs to monitor for at home, including sinus formation – which often occurs in the absence of pain symptoms.

Pulpal Obliteration

Obliteration of the pulp chambers and canals is a common reaction to trauma. Clinically, the tooth becomes yellow/opaque. Normal exfoliation is usual, but occasionally periapical inflammation may intervene and, therefore, annual radiography is advisable.

Root Resorption

External inflammatory resorption is usually seen after intrusive injuries and internal resorption with subluxation and other luxation injuries. Extraction is advised for all types of root resorption.

Injuries to Developing Permanent Teeth

Injuries to the permanent successor tooth can be expected in 12–69% of primary tooth trauma and 19–68% of jaw fractures. Intrusive luxation causes most disturbances; avulsion of a primary incisor will also cause damage if the apex moves towards the permanent tooth bud before the avulsion. Most damage to the permanent tooth bud occurs under 3 years of age, during its developmental stage. However, the type and severity of disturbance are closely related to age at the time of injury. Changes in the morphology and mineralisation of the crown of the permanent incisor are most common but later injuries can cause radicular anomalies. Injuries to developing teeth can be classified as:

- white or yellow–brown discolouration   of enamel: injury at 2–7 years
- white or yellow–brown discolouration of enamel with circular enamel hypoplasia: injury at 2–7 years
- crown dilaceration: injury at about 2 years
- odontoma-like malformation: injury at <1–3 years
- root duplication: injury at 2–5 years
- vestibular or lateral root angulation and dilaceration: injury at 2–5 years
- partial or complete arrest of root formation: injury at 5–7 years
- sequestration of permanent tooth germs
- disturbance in eruption.

Most enamel defects can be treated with a combination of microabrasion and/or composite restoration. Most dilacerations and eruption abnormalities require surgical exposure and orthodontic alignment.

PERMANENT DENTITION

The aims and principles of treatment are considered as emergency, intermediate and definitive actions.

1. Emergency:
   - retain vitality of fractured or displaced tooth
   - treat exposed pulp tissue
   - reduction and immobilisation of displaced teeth
   - antiseptic mouthwash, analgesia, antibiotics and tetanus prophylaxis.
2. Intermediate:
   - with or without pulp therapy
   - minimally invasive crown restoration.
3. Definitive:
   - apexification
   - root filling with or without root extrusion
   - with or without gingival and alveolar collar modification
   - semi or permanent coronal restoration.

Trauma cases require regular follow-up to identify any complications early and instigate the correct treatment. The intervals between examinations depend on the severity of trauma, but the following schedule is a guide: 1, 3 and 6 weeks, then at 3, 6 and 12 months with annual checks for 4–5 years. The 'Dental Trauma Guide' is a useful online resource for clinicians, which outlines the management of dental trauma and the follow-up protocols required for each injury. At these reviews, the 'trauma stamp' can be utilised to collate the findings from special investigations and appropriate radiographs are examined for periodical pathology, resorption, continued development of the immature root and changes within the pulp cavity. An example of 'trauma stamp' is shown in Fig. 8.1.

Injuries to the Hard Dental Tissues and the Pulp

Enamel Infraction

These are incomplete fractures and without proper illumination are easily overlooked. Periodic recalls are necessary to review pulpal status.

Tooth	E.g. 12	11	21	22
Sinus/swelling				
Colour				
Mobility				
TTP				
Percussive note				
EC				
EPT				

Fig. 8.1 A 'trauma stamp' with clinical aide-mémoire.

Apex	Intrusion severity	Repositioning		
		Spontaneous	Orthodontic	Surgical
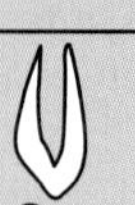 **Open**	Up to 7 mm	★		
	More than 7 mm		★	★
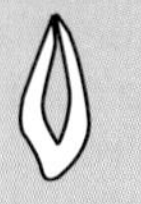 **Closed**	Up to 3 mm	★		
	3–7 mm		★	★
	More than 7 mm			★

Figure reproduced with permission from Andreasen JO et al. "The Dental Trauma Guide–Your interactive tool to evidence based trauma treatment." www.dentaltraumaguide.org

Enamel Fracture

Treatment is usually limited to smoothing any rough edges. Periodic review is necessary.

Enamel–dentine Fracture

Immediate treatment is necessary because of the involvement of dentine. The pulp requires protection against thermal irritation and from bacteria via the dentinal tubules. Restoration of crown morphology also stabilises the position of the tooth in the arch. Emergency protection of the fractured tooth is via an adhesive bandage of resin composite or glass ionomer, ensuring all exposed dentine is covered.

These will serve as temporary retainers until further eruption occurs.

Intermediate restoration of most enamel–dentine fractures can be achieved by:

- acid-etched composite applied either freehand or utilising a celluloid crown former
- reattachment of crown fragment: using etch, bond and flowable composite to adhere the fractured crown portion. There is a tendency for the distal fragment to become opaque or require further restorative intervention in the future.

If the fracture line through dentine is not very close to the pulp, the fragment may be reattached immediately.

If, however, it runs close to the pulp, it is advisable to place a suitably protected calcium hydroxide dressing over the exposed dentine for at least 1 month while storing the fragment in saline, which should be renewed weekly (Box 8.1).

Box 8.1   Technique for Refitting a Fragment of Tooth.

1. Check the fit of the fragment and the vitality of the tooth.
2. Clean fragment and tooth with pumice-water slurry.
3. Isolate the tooth with rubber dam.
4. Attach fragment to a piece of gutta-percha to facilitate handling.
5. Etch enamel for 30 seconds on both fracture surfaces and extend for 2 mm from fracture line on tooth and fragment. Wash for 15 seconds and dry for 15 seconds.
6. Apply enamel–dentine bonding agent to both surfaces, then lightly blow away any excess. Light-cure for 10 seconds.
7. Place appropriate shade of flowable composite resin over both surfaces and position fragment. Remove gross excess and cure 60 seconds labially and palatally.
8. Remove any excess composite resin with sandpaper discs.
9. Remove a 1 mm gutter of enamel on each side of fracture line both labially and palatally to a depth of 0.5 mm using a small round or pear-shaped bur. The finishing line should be irregular in outline.
10. Etch the newly prepared enamel, wash, dry, apply composite, cure and finish.

Complicated Crown Fracture

The major concern after pulpal exposures in immature teeth is the preservation of pulpal vitality in order to allow continued root growth. The injured pulp must be sealed from bacteria so that it is not infected during the period of repair. Partial pulpotomy or pulpotomy is often the treatment of choice.

Uncomplicated Crown Root Fracture

After removal of the fractured piece of tooth, these vertical fractures are commonly a few millimetres incisal to the gingival margin on the labial surface but down to the cementoenamel junction palatally. Prior to placement of a restoration, the fracture margin has to be brought supragingival either by gingivoplasty or extrusion (orthodontically or surgically) of the root portion.

Complicated Crown Root Fracture

Follow the same management principles as for uncomplicated crown root fracture, with the addition of endodontic treatment. If extrusion is planned, then the final root length must be no shorter than the final crown length, otherwise the result will be unstable. Root extrusion can be successful in a motivated patient and leads to a stable periodontal condition.

Root Fracture

Root fractures occur most frequently in the middle or the apical third of the root. The coronal fragment may be extruded or luxated. Luxation is usually in a lingual or palatal direction.

If displacement has occurred, the coronal fragment should be repositioned as soon as possible by gentle digital manipulation and the position checked radiographically. Mobile root fractures need to be splinted to encourage repair of the fracture. Apical third fractures, in the absence of concomitant periodontal ligament injury, are often firm and may not require splinting. They do need to be regularly reviewed to check pulpal status and to be treated endodontically if necessary.

Splinting of apical and middle third fractures aims to repair the fracture for long-term stability and prognosis of the tooth. A flexible splint with one abutment tooth on either side of the fractured tooth should remain in place for 4 weeks. If the fracture is in the coronal third of the root, splinting should be for at least 4 months. The splint should allow colour observations, sensibility testing and access to the root canal if endodontic treatment is required. The splint design and placement techniques are discussed below. In about 80% of all root-fractured teeth, the pulp remains viable and repair occurs in the fracture area. Three main categories of repair are recognised:

1. Repair with calcified tissue: invisible or hardly discernible fracture line.
2. Repair with connective tissue: narrow radiolucent fracture line with peripheral rounding of the fracture edges.
3. Repair with bone and connective tissue: a bony bridge separates the two fragments.

In addition to these changes in the fracture area, pulp canal obliteration is commonly seen. Fractures in the cervical third of the root will repair as well as those in the middle or apical thirds as long as no communication exists between the fracture line and the gingival crevice. If such a communication exists, splinting is not recommended and a decision must be made to extract the coronal fragment and retain the remaining root, to extract the two fragments or to splint the root fracture internally. The latter can only be regarded as a temporary solution.

If the root is retained, the remaining radicular pulp should be removed and the canal temporarily dressed prior to obturating with gutta-percha. Three options are now available for the root-treated radicular portion:

1. Post, core and crown restoration if access is adequate.
2. Extrusion of root either surgically or orthodontically if the fracture extends too far subgingivally for adequate access.
3. Cover the root with a mucoperiosteal flap; this will maintain the height and width of the arch and will facilitate later placement of a single tooth implant.

Pulpal necrosis occurs in about 20% of root fractures and is the main obstacle to adequate repair. Most instances of necrosis are diagnosed within 3 months of a root fracture. A persistent negative response to electric stimulation is usually confirmed on radiography by radiolucencies adjacent to the fracture line.

Splinting

Trauma may loosen a tooth either by damaging the periodontal ligament or by fracturing the root. Flexible splinting stabilises the tooth in the correct anatomical position so that further trauma is prevented and healing can occur. Different injuries require different splinting regimens; the 'Dental Trauma Guide' should be consulted to confirm the splinting period required for each injury (https://dentaltraumaguide.org).

Periodontal Ligament Injuries

Approximately 60% of periodontal ligament healing has occurred after 10 days and it is complete within a month. The splinting period should be as short as possible, and the splint should allow some functional movement to prevent replacement root resorption (ankylosis); this is why the term flexible splint is used to indicate that teeth are not completely immobilised. As a general rule, avulsion injuries require 2 weeks, luxation injuries 4 weeks.

Apical and Middle Third Root Fractures

These require 4 weeks of flexible splinting to encourage repair. A connective tissue repair may be satisfactory, but if mobility persists, the fracture site becomes filled with granulation tissue and the tooth remains mobile.

Dento-alveolar Fractures

These require 4 weeks of flexible splinting.

Coronal Third Root Fractures

These require 4 or more months of flexible splinting to repair.

Splint Construction

The composite resin and wire splint technique is the preferred option for splinting (Box 8.2). Generally, flexible splints should have one abutment tooth each side of the injured tooth.

Box 8.2   Technique for Flexible Splint.

1. Bend a flexible orthodontic wire to fit the middle third of the labial surface of the injured tooth/teeth and one abutment tooth either side.
2. Stabilise the injured tooth in the correct position with red wax palatally or composite over the incisal edges of the traumatised tooth and its adjacent tooth.
3. Clean the labial surfaces. Isolate, dry and etch middle of crown of teeth with 37% phosphoric acid for 30 seconds, wash and dry.
4. Apply 3-mm diameter circle of composite resin to the centre of the crowns.
5. Position the wire into the filling material, then apply more resin.
6. Use a brush lubricated with unfilled composite resin to mould and smooth the composite.
7. Cure the composite for 60 seconds.
8. Smooth any sharp edges with sandpaper discs. Ensure the composite does not encroach on the gingival tissues to aid good oral hygiene.

Other types of flexible splint include orthodontic brackets and wire, upper removable orthodontic-like appliances with an extended baseplate, interdental wiring, foil/cement splint (temporary) and Essix Retainer-like thermoplastic splints.

Injuries to the Periodontal Tissues

Figures for pulp survival 5 years after periodontal ligament injuries are shown in Table 8.2.

Concussion

The impact force causes oedema and haemorrhage in the periodontal ligament and the tooth is tender to percussion (TTP). There is no rupture of periodontal ligament fibres, and the tooth is firm in the socket.

Subluxation

In addition to the above, in subluxation, there is rupture of some periodontal ligament fibres and the tooth is mobile in the socket, although not displaced. The treatment for both these injuries is:

- occlusal relief
- soft diet for 7 days
- stabilisation with a splint for 2 weeks if TTP is significant
- chlorhexidine 0.2% mouthwash, twice daily.
  There is little risk of pulp necrosis or resorption.

Extrusive Luxation

In extrusive luxation, there is rupture of the periodontal ligament and pulp. These injuries should have a flexible splint for 2 weeks.

Lateral Luxation

Lateral luxation involves rupture of periodontal ligament and pulp and compression injury of the alveolar plate. The treatment for lateral luxation is:

- local anaesthesia (buccal and palatal)
- atraumatic repositioning of tooth with gentle firm digital pressure
- flexible splint 4 weeks
- chlorhexidine mouthwash
- soft diet 2–3 weeks.

The decision to progress to endodontic treatment depends on subsequent regular clinical and radiographic examination.

With more significant damage to the periodontal ligament, there is an increased risk of root resorption (up to 35% of injuries).

Orthodontic appliances should be used to reduce firm older injuries, as digital pressure could further damage the periodontal ligament.

Intrusive Luxation

Intrusive luxation injuries are the result of an axial, apical impact. There is extensive damage to the periodontal ligament and alveolar plate(s). Two distinct categories exist: the open and closed apex. At the outset, both categories should receive chlorhexidine mouthwash and a soft diet as previously described. The risk of pulpal necrosis in these injuries is high, especially with a closed apex. The incidence of resorption and ankylosis sequelae is also high.

The different management approaches for these injuries depend on two factors:

1. Maturity of root
2. Severity of intrusion.

The treatment options are summarised in the following table. Following repositioning, an intruded tooth should have a flexible splint placed for 2 weeks.

Teeth with closed apices will frequently undergo loss of vitality after an intrusive injury. Endodontic treatment should be commenced after 2–3 weeks following repositioning, and calcium hydroxide is an appropriate inter-visit canal dressing.

Ongoing endodontic treatment does not preclude orthodontic movement. Immature apex endodontic treatment includes mineral trioxide aggregate (MTA) apical plug placement and obturation with a thermoplastic gutta-percha technique.

Avulsion and Replantation

Replantation of an avulsed permanent tooth should nearly always be attempted even though it may offer only a temporary solution because of the frequent occurrence of external inflammatory and replacement (ankylosis) resorption. Even when resorption occurs, the tooth may be retained for years, acting as a natural space maintainer and preserving the height and width of the alveolus to facilitate later implant placement. When replacement resorption occurs, the tooth must be closely monitored for the development of infraocclusion, this can progress rapidly during growth spurts. Poorly managed infraoccluded teeth can result in a significant vertical bony and soft tissue defect; this has a detrimental impact on future implant treatment. The treatment of choice for infraoccluded teeth is de-coronation and root burial, and this allows further vertical alveolar bone deposition.

Successful healing after replantation can only occur if there is minimal damage to the pulp and the periodontal ligament. The type of extra-alveolar storage medium and the extra-alveolar time (i.e. the time the tooth has been out of the mouth) are critical factors. The suggested protocol for replantation can be divided into advice on the telephone, immediate treatment in surgery and review (Box 8.3). The immature tooth with an extra-alveolar time

Box 8.3 Technique for Replantation of a Tooth.

Advice on Phone (To Teacher, Parent etc.)

1. Do not touch the root, hold by the crown.
2. Wash gently under cold tap water.
3. Replace into socket or transport in milk to surgery.
4. If replaced, bite gently on a handkerchief and come to surgery.

The best transport medium is the tooth's own socket. Understandably, non-dentists may be unhappy to replant the tooth, and milk is an effective iso-osmolar medium. Saliva, the patient's buccal sulcus, or normal saline are alternatives.

Immediate Surgery Treatment

1. Do not handle root. If replanted, remove tooth from socket.
2. Rinse tooth with normal saline. Note state of root development. Store in saline.
3. Local anaesthesia.
4. Irrigate socket with saline and remove clot and any foreign material.
5. Push tooth gently but firmly into socket.
6. Place a flexible splint for 2 or 4 weeks dependent on the tooth's maturity and extra-alveolar time.
7. Check occlusion.
8. Take baseline radiographs: periapical or anterior occlusal. Any other teeth injured?
9. Consider if antibiotics are required.

10. Give patient and parents home care advice including analgesics, chlorhexidine mouthwash and soft diet as previously mentioned.
11. Check tetanus immunisation status.

Review

1. Take radiograph prior to splint removal at 2 weeks.
2. Remove splint at 2 weeks.
3. For open apex with an extra-alveolar time of less than 45 minutes, simply observe the tooth.
4. For open apex with an extra-alveolar time greater than 45 minutes or a closed apex, endodontics is commenced prior to splint removal.
5. Initial intracanal dressing with polyantibiotic or antibiotic/steroid (Ledermix, Lederle) paste.
6. Subsequent intracanal dressing with non-setting calcium hydroxide.
7. Treatment then differs for open and closed apex:
   a. For open apex, carry out immature apex endodontics treatment with mineral trioxide aggregate plug placement and thermoplastic obturation.
   b. For closed apex, obturate with gutta-percha at 12 months as long as there is no progressive resorption.
8. Review radiographically at 1 and 3 months, then 6-monthly for 2 years and, finally, annually.
9. If resorption is progressing unhalted, keep non-setting calcium hydroxide in the tooth until exfoliation, changing it 6-monthly.

---

of less than 45 minutes may undergo pulp revascularisation. However, these teeth require regular clinical and radiographic review because once external inflammatory resorption occurs, it progresses rapidly.

REPLANTATION OF TEETH WITH A DRY STORAGE TIME OF GREATER THAN 1 HOUR. Mature teeth with a dry storage time of greater than 1 hour will have a non-vital periodontal ligament. The periodontal ligament and the pulp should be removed at the chair side and the tooth placed for 20 minutes in 2.4% sodium fluoride solution at pH 5.5. The root canal is then obturated with gutta-percha, and the tooth replanted and splinted for 4 weeks. The aim of this treatment is to maintain the tooth as a natural space maintainer, perhaps for a limited period only. The sodium fluoride is believed to slow down resorptive processes, but pragmatically this solution is problematic to get hold of and has a very limited shelf life.

Each individual case should be considered on its own merits, but it is probably not prudent to reimplant very immature lower incisors with an extra-alveolar dry time of greater than 1 hour. Conversely, even a very poor prognosis immature upper central incisor can act as an important guide for the positioning of an erupting lateral which will drift/erupt into an unfavourable position without its presence. Once the lateral has fully erupted, it will be possible to maintain it in a good position with an upper removable appliance.

Injuries to Supporting Alveolar Bone

The extent and position of the alveolar fracture should be verified clinically and radiographically. If there is displacement of the teeth to the extent that their apices have risen up and are now positioned over the labial or lingual/palatal alveolar plates ('apical lock'), they will first require extruding to free the apices prior to repositioning.

The segment of alveolus with teeth requires 4 weeks of splinting with one abutment tooth either side of the fracture, together with antibiotics, chlorhexidine, soft diet and tetanus prophylaxis if necessary.

Pulp survival is more likely if repositioning occurs within 1 hour of the injury. Root resorption is rare.

CHILD SAFEGUARDING

Safeguarding a child's welfare is an important part of the dentist's role. Child welfare is a concern when aspects of a child's life deviate from the normal and acceptable social parameters of our culture. Organisations such as health, social services, teaching and policing are all empowered to act as advocates for child safety and wellbeing.

There are different forms of child maltreatment, categorised into physical, sexual and emotional abuse along with neglect, which may be physical and/or emotional. Most perpetrators of child maltreatment are known to the child and rarely strangers. Emerging problems in child safeguarding include online abuse and child trafficking.

Safeguarding itself is the action that is taken to promote the welfare of all children and protect them from harm. It is defined as protecting children from maltreatment, preventing impairment of children's health or development, ensuring that children are growing up in circumstances consistent with the provision of safe and effective care and, importantly, acting to enable all children to have the best outcomes (HM Government 2018).

Child protection is part of safeguarding and includes activities undertaken to protect children who have been harmed or are at significant risk of being harmed. It can be defined as preventing and responding to violence, exploitation, neglect and abuse against children (UNICEF).

Child wellbeing refers to the quality of a child's life including how well the child is and how their lives are going. It is generally poorly defined, but there is some emerging consensus that childhood wellbeing is multi-dimensional; should include dimensions of physical, emotional and social wellbeing; should focus on the immediate lives of children but also consider their future lives and should incorporate some subjective as well as objective measures (Statham and Chase 2010).

Approximately 60% of UK child physical abuse cases have signs of injury on their head, neck, face or inside the mouth (Cairns et al 2004). These areas are all accessible to the dental team, and we should always ask about how injuries occurred to exclude suspicions of maltreatment. The incidences of common orofacial injuries are shown in Table 8.3.

The following points should be considered whenever doubts and suspicions are aroused:

1. Could the injury have been caused accidentally and, if so, how?
2. Does the explanation for the injury fit the age and the clinical findings?
3. If the explanation of cause is consistent with the injury, is this itself within normally acceptable limits of behaviour?
4. If there has been any delay seeking advice, are there good reasons for this?
5. Does the story of the accident vary?
6. The nature of the relationship between parent and child.
7. The child's reaction to other people.
8. The child's reaction to any medical/dental examinations.
9. The general demeanour of the child.
10. Any comments made by child and/or parent that give concern about the child's upbringing or lifestyle.
11. History of previous injury.

Dental neglect is defined as the persistent failure to meet a child's basic oral health needs, likely to result in the serious impairment of a child's oral or general health

or development (Harris et al 2009). Dental disease impacts a child's general health, development and wellbeing. Episodes of pain and uncontrolled infection are of particular concern. Where families have been informed of the presence of oral disease and offered appropriate management including social support but fail to access treatment, this is dental neglect. Multiple missed or rescheduled appointments, frequent emergency visits when in pain and repeated requirements for general anaesthetic are all indicators for dental neglect.

More advice on the responsibility of the dental team in child protection, recognition of abuse and neglect, responding to that recognition and reorganising a practice to be child friendly can be found in 'Child protection and the dental team' (https://bda.org/childprotection).

8.2 Dental Anomalies

LEARNING OBJECTIVES

You should:
- know the types of number and form (morphology) of anomaly and their incidence
- know the types of inherited enamel defect and their incidence
- know the types of inherited dentine defect and their incidence
- know the causes of premature and delayed eruption and exfoliation.

NUMBER AND MORPHOLOGY

Hypodontia

Congenital absence of some teeth is common. This can occur sporadically or be inherited. The most common teeth to be absent are the last teeth in each series (i.e. lateral incisor, second premolar and third molar). The presence of conical teeth is often associated with the absence of the same teeth on the opposite side of the arch. Hypodontia arises because of an abnormality in the induction of oral ectoderm by ectomesenchyme.

Anodontia is the term used for the total lack of one or both dentitions. Oligodontia is an older term that has been replaced by hypodontia.

Incidence

Hypodontia in the primary dentition has an incidence of 0.1–0.9%; the gender ratio is not known.

The incidence in the permanent dentition is 3.5–6.5% (excluding wisdom teeth, 9–37%). There is a 1:1.4 male:female ratio.

Permanent anomalies occur in 30–50% of those with hypodontia in the primary dentition.

Hypodontia may be seen in a number of syndromes:

- Ectodermal dysplasia
- Clefting
- Down syndrome
- Chondro-ectodermal dysplasia (Ellis–van Creveld syndrome)

Table 8.3 The Incidence of Common Orofacial Injuries in Non-Accidental Injury.

Type of Injury	Incidence (%)
EXTRAORAL	
Contusions and ecchymoses	66
Abrasions and lacerations	28
Burns and bites	4
Fractures	2
INTRAORAL	
Contusions and ecchymoses	43
Abrasions and lacerations (including frenal tears)	29
Dental trauma	29

- Reiger syndrome
- Incontinentia pigmenti
- Orofacial digital syndrome (types I and II).

Management

Management can be complex and requires co-ordination between a number of specialties including paediatric dentistry, orthodontics, restorative dentistry and oral surgery.

Supernumerary Teeth

Supernumerary teeth can be inherited as an autosomal dominant or X-linked trait and occurs by budding of the dental lamina. The extra tooth can resemble the normal series (supplemental tooth) or, more commonly, it may be conical or tuberculate. Almost all (98%) occur in the maxilla, mostly in the anterior palate.

Incidence

The incidence of supernumerary teeth in the primary dentition is 0.2–0.8%, with the male:female ratio unknown. In the permanent dentition, it is 1.5–3.5% with a male:female ratio of 2:1.

Diagnosis

- Failed or ectopic tooth eruption.
- Routine radiography.
- Part of a syndrome: cleidocranial dysplasia, Gardner's syndrome, orofacial digital syndrome (type I), clefting.

Management

Conical supernumeraries often erupt and are extracted easily. Tuberculate or inverted conical forms usually require surgical removal.

Macrodontia

Any tooth (or teeth) that is larger than normal for that particular tooth is macrodontic. True macrodontia affecting the whole dentition is rare. More commonly, single teeth are large owing to an isolated disturbance of morphodifferentiation.

True generalised macrodontia may occur in pituitary gigantism. Relative generalised macrodontia occurs in orthodontic skeletal base–tooth size discrepancy. True localised macrodontia may be associated with facial hemihyperplasia, hereditary gingival hyperplasia and hypertrichosis.

Incidence

The incidence of macrodontia in the primary dentition is unknown; in the permanent dentition it is 1%.

Management

- Judicious grinding to reduce mesiodistal width.
- Build-up of contralateral tooth to match if only one tooth is affected.
- Extraction and replacement with a prosthesis.

Microdontia

Any tooth (or teeth) that is smaller than normal for the tooth type. Most commonly, this affects one or two teeth, but it can be generalised in syndromes with hypodontia (see earlier) and in children who have undergone radio- and chemotherapy.

True generalised microdontia may occur in pituitary dwarfism and syndromes with hypodontia. The relative generalised form will occur in orthodontic skeletal base–tooth size discrepancy. True localised microdontia may occur after radio- and chemotherapy.

Incidence

The incidence of microdontia is <0.5% in the primary dentition, 2% in the permanent dentition and it is more common in females.

Management

Management involves build-ups with composite resin or porcelain. The mesiodistal width at the gingival margin will limit the size to which restoration is possible.

Double Teeth

Double teeth encompasses the terms fusion and gemination and describes a structure that resembles two teeth that have been joined together. Radiographs are required to determine if there are two pulp systems or if they are joined.

Incidence

The incidence of double teeth is 2.5% in the primary dentition and 0.2% in the permanent dentition. There is a male:female ratio of 1:1 in both. Permanent anomalies occur in 30–50% of those with primary anomalies.

Dens Invaginatus

Developmental invagination of the cingulum pit commonly occurs on the maxillary lateral incisors with only a thin layer of hard tissue between the pulp and oral cavity. Pulp necrosis may result in significant facial cellulitis.

Incidence

The incidence of dens invaginatus in the primary dentition is 0.1%, and in the permanent dentition it is 4%. It is more common in males than in females.

Management

- Fissure-seal newly erupted tooth.
- Root canal therapy if morphology is favourable.
- Extraction if internal anatomy is complex.

Dens Evaginatus

In dens evaginatus, an enamel-covered tubercle projects from the occlusal surface of usually a premolar or sometimes a canine or molar. It is usually bilateral and is more common in the mandible. The tubercle usually contains pulp tissue.

Incidence

The incidence in the primary dentition is unknown, but that of the permanent dentition is 4%.

Management

- Composite resin build-up to recontour occlusal surface incorporating the tubercle.
- Pulpotomy to allow continued radicular growth.
- Extraction may be required owing to the immaturity of the root if pulp necrosis occurs.

Talon Cusp

A talon cusp is a horn-like projection of the cingulum of maxillary incisor teeth. It may reach and contact the incisal edge.

Incidence

The incidence in the primary dentition is unknown; incidence in the permanent dentition is 1–2%.

Management

- No treatment if there is no occlusal interference
- Sequential enamel reduction +/− fissure sealant
- Pulpotomy/pulpectomy.

Taurodontism

Taurodontism is an enlarged pulp chamber where the distance from the cementoenamel junction to the bifurcation of the root is greater than the length of the roots. It is caused by a failure of Hertwig's root sheath to invaginate and may be inherited either in a normal individual or as part of a syndrome.

Incidence

The incidence is unknown.

Conditions with enlarged pulp chambers include:

- vitamin D-resistant rickets (hypophosphophataemic rickets)
- rickets (vitamin D-dependent)
- hypophosphatasia
- dentinogenesis imperfecta (some cases)
- regional odontodysplasia
- Klinefelter's syndrome
- shell teeth.

DEFECTS OF ENAMEL

Enamel defects may be inherited or acquired. Enamel can exhibit either hypoplasia owing to deficient matrix production or hypomineralisation from imperfect mineralisation of matrix proteins.

Chronological Disturbances

Any severe systemic event during the development of the teeth (from 3 months in utero to 20 years) will result in some dental abnormality. Different teeth will show defects at different levels of the crown depending on the stage of crown formation at the time of the disturbance. The enamel may be reduced in quantity or quality and may, therefore, show discoloration, opacities (hypomineralisation) and hypoplasia.

Chronological defects usually affect teeth of the same type on either side of the arch.

Fluorosis

In its mildest form, fluorosis appears as hypomineralisation of enamel causing opacities. These can range from diffuse flecks to confluent opaque patches that lack translucency. At higher fluoride concentrations, hypoplasia occurs with a defect in quantity of matrix. Fluorotic mottling affects the outer third of the enamel.

Amelogenesis Imperfecta

Amelogenesis imperfecta (AI) describes hereditary enamel defects resulting from single gene mutations; they follow autosomal dominant, autosomal recessive or X-linked patterns of inheritance.

Incidence

Incidence is 1 in 10,000.

There are three main types:

1. Hypoplastic
2. Hypomineralised: hypocalcified or hypomature
3. Mixed.

In most, but not all, types of AI, teeth in both the primary and the permanent dentitions are affected.

HYPOPLASTIC AI. There is deficient matrix production, but the enamel that is present is normally mineralised. Clinical variants range from the autosomal dominant thin and smooth type of AI to the pitting and grooving of X-linked dominant AI.

HYPOCALCIFIED AI. Teeth erupt with enamel that is dull, lustreless, opaque white or honey coloured. Distribution throughout the mouth is not usually even, although there is bilateral symmetry. Soft enamel may wear, leaving rough, discoloured, sensitive dentine exposed. The cervical regions of the crowns often have normal enamel.

HYPOMATURATION AI. This is very similar to hypocalcified AI but with no normal enamel in cervical regions.

Management

Management is discussed together with dentine defects, next.

DEFECTS OF DENTINE

Defects of dentine may be inherited or acquired. Genetic defects can be either limited to dentine or associated with a generalised disorder.

Defects limited to dentine:

- Dentinogenesis imperfecta type II (hereditary opalescent dentine)
- Dentine dysplasia type I (radicular dentine dysplasia)
- Dentine dysplasia type II (coronal dentine dysplasia)
- Fibrous dysplasia of dentine.

Defects associated with a generalised disorder:

- Osteogenesis imperfecta (dentinogenesis imperfecta type I)
- Ehlers–Danlos syndrome
- Brachio-skeleto-genital syndrome
- Vitamin D-resistant rickets
- Vitamin D-dependent rickets
- Hypophosphatasia.

Dentinogenesis Imperfecta Type II (Hereditary Opalescent Dentine)

In dentinogenesis imperfecta type II, both dentitions are usually affected. The teeth are opalescent and on transillumination appear bluish or brownish in colour. Sometimes, later-forming permanent teeth are less affected. There is early loss of enamel, exposing underlying dentine that undergoes rapid wear. This is usually most marked in the primary dentition. Radiographically, the crowns appear bulbous and the roots may be short and thin. The pulp chambers obliterate soon after eruption, and the root canals are progressively narrowed by deposition of abnormal dentine. Transmission is usually autosomal dominant.

Incidence

The incidence is 1 in 8000.

Dentine Dysplasia Type I (Radicular Dentine Dysplasia; Rootless Teeth)

In dentine dysplasia type I, crown colour ranges from normal to bluish or brownish tinge. Radiographs show normal crown morphology but excessively short or blunt roots. Pulp chambers may be small and root canals absent. Primary and permanent dentitions are affected and inheritance is probably autosomal dominant. It is rare.

Dentine Dysplasia Type II (Coronal Dentine Dysplasia)

Primary teeth in dentine dysplasia type II resemble those in dentinogenesis imperfecta type II, but permanent teeth are clinically normal and radiographs show thistle- or flame-shaped pulp chambers partially occluded by pulp stones and narrowing root canals. It is rare and probably autosomal dominant.

Dentinogenesis Imperfecta Type I With Osteogenesis Imperfecta

Osteogenesis imperfecta is a heterogeneous group of connective tissue disorders involving inherited abnormalities of type I collagen. Bone fragility, lax joints, blue sclerae, opalescent teeth, hearing loss and a variable degree of bone deformity are features.

Inheritance is autosomal recessive or dominant. Recessive varieties are frequently lethal at or shortly after birth.

Opalescent teeth are commonly observed in the dominant variety. Features are similar to dentinogenesis type II except that the permanent dentition is often less affected and the upper anterior teeth particularly may be clinically normal.

Environmentally Determined Dentine Defects

Local trauma may interfere with dentine formation, and a number of systemic influences can occur, such as nutritional deficiencies (minerals, proteins and vitamins), drugs such as tetracycline and the anticancer drugs (e.g. cyclophosphamide). There is increased formation of interglobular dentine, predentine and osteoid.

MANAGEMENT OF ENAMEL AND DENTINE DEFECTS

There are four main clinical problems associated with inherited enamel and dentine defects:

1. Poor aesthetics
2. Chipping and attrition of the enamel, which may cause reduced face height
3. Exposure and attrition of the dentine causing sensitivity
4. Poor oral hygiene, gingivitis and caries.

While it is not possible to draw up a definitive treatment plan for all patients, it is possible to define the principles of treatment planning for this group of patients. It is important to realise that not all children with amelogenesis imperfecta or dentinogenesis imperfecta are affected equally. Many will not have marked tooth wear or symptoms and will not require advanced intervention. Table 8.4 describes the principles of treatment in terms of the age of the child/adolescent and with regard to the three aspects of care: prevention, restoration and aesthetics.

ERUPTION AND EXFOLIATION DISORDERS

Premature Eruption

Premature eruption may be familial. There is a tendency to early eruption in children with a high birthweight. Excessively early eruption is seen in endocrine abnormalities (e.g. precocious puberty, increase of thyroid and growth hormone).

Natal and Neonatal Teeth

Natal (present at birth) and neonatal (erupts within 30 days of birth) teeth occur in about 1 in 2000–3000 births; the teeth are part of the normal series and development is consistent with age (no root present).

It may be familial but is also associated with some syndromes: pachyonychia congenita, Ellis–van Creveld, Hallermann–Streiff.

Management

Teeth are left if possible to allow normal root formation. Extraction may be necessary because of extreme mobility and airway danger, painful suckling or tongue ulceration.

Table 8.4 Principles of Treatment for Amelogenesis and Dentinogenesis Imperfecta.

	Prevention	Restoration	Aesthetics
Primary dentition (0–5 years)	Diet advice; fluoride varnish; oral hygiene instruction	Adhesive restorations; stainless steel crowns (SSCs) particularly on Es	Minimal intervention
Mixed dentition (6–16 years)	Diet advice; fluoride supplements; oral hygiene instruction ± chlorhexidine	SSCs on primary molars; adhesive castings or SSCs on first permanent molars; adhesive restorations	Direct or indirect composite veneers
Permanent dentition (16+ years)	Oral hygiene instruction; topical fluoride	Adhesive castings on premolars; full mouth rehabilitation	Porcelain or composite veneers; full crowns, over dentures, complete dentures

Delayed Eruption

In the primary dentition, delayed eruption tends to occur in preterm children or those of very low birthweights. It is also associated with a number of conditions:

- Down syndrome
- Turner syndrome
- Nutritional deficiency
- Endocrine disorders: hypothyroidism and hypopituitarism
- Cleidocranial dysostosis
- Hereditary gingival fibromatosis.

In the permanent dentition, localised causes are more frequent: ectopic crypt positions, supernumeraries, odontomes and impaction.

Premature Exfoliation

Apart from trauma (accidental or non-accidental), there are a number of rare conditions that may result in premature loss of primary teeth:

- Hypophosphatasia
- Immunological conditions causing neutropenia
- Histiocytosis X.

Delayed Exfoliation

Delay in normal exfoliation of primary teeth may be seen in association with:

- double primary teeth
- hypodontia affecting permanent successors
- ectopic permanent successors
- subsequent to trauma or severe periradicular infection of primary teeth
- infraocclusion (preferred term to 'submerged' or ankylosed teeth, which describes teeth that have failed to achieve or maintain their occlusal relationships to adjacent and opposing teeth); on occasion, teeth may be totally reincluded (covered) by surrounding tissues, which is thought to be caused by imbalance in the normal pattern of resorption and repair in primary teeth.

Incidence of Infraocclusion

Infraocclusion occurs in 1–9% with an equal incidence in males and females. It is more common in the primary dentition, but there is a higher incidence of absent permanent successors.

Treatment of Infraocclusion
- Onlays
- Extraction and space maintenance for permanent successor
- Extraction and orthodontic space closure
- Extraction and prosthetic restoration of space if successor absent.

8.3 Special Needs

LEARNING OBJECTIVES

You should:
- appreciate the impact of dental disease on patients with specific medical disorders
- understand the importance of enhanced dental prevention in specific medical disorders
- appreciate the role that the dental practitioner has to play in maintaining the 'whole' patient fit and healthy.

CONGENITAL CARDIAC DISEASE

Congenital cardiac disease occurs in 8–10 per 1000 live births and has an equal sex distribution. Multifactorial inheritance patterns are responsible, and the main types of congenital condition are shown in Table 8.5. The degree of morbidity is dependent on the haemodynamics of the lesion. Flow disturbances are caused by structural or obstructive defects. For convenience, defects are divided into cyanotic or acyanotic depending on clinical presentation.

Acyanotic defects with shunts. Connection between systemic and pulmonary circulation with a shunt from left to right occurs in:

- atrial septal defect
- ventricular septal defect
- patent ductus arteriosus
- anomalous pulmonary venous return
- atrioventricular canal.

Acyanotic defects with obstruction include:

- coarctation of aorta
- aortic stenosis
- pulmonary stenosis.

Cyanotic defects have right to left shunting of desaturated blood and include:

- tetralogy of Fallot
- Eisenmenger's syndrome (right to left shunt through a ventricular septal defect)
- tricuspid atresia
- transposition of great vessels.

Other cardiac diseases include:

- cardiomyopathies
- cardiac arrhythmias (accessory conduction pathways)
- rheumatic fever.

Dental Management

Antibiotic prophylaxis against infective endocarditis for patients with congenital cardiac defects is very much a 'hot

Table 8.5 Prevalence of Congenital Cardiac Disease.

Condition	Prevalence (%)
Ventricular septal defect	28
Atrial septal defect	10
Pulmonary stenosis	10
Patent ductus arteriosus	10
Tetralogy of Fallot	10
Aortic stenosis	7
Coarctation of the aorta	5
Transposition of great arteries	5
Rare/diverse conditions	15

topic' at present. Introduction of the word 'routinely' into the National Institute for health and Care Excellence (NICE) guidelines in 2016 has caused some confusion within the dental profession. It is often not clear what a 'routine' patient with a cardiac defect is, and expert opinion differs amongst our paediatric cardiology colleagues. Dentists should keep up to date with developments in this area, and guidelines developed by the Scottish Dental Clinical Effectiveness Group are a useful resource to consult. (http://www.sdcep.org.uk/published-guidance/antibiotic-prophylaxis/)

The following patients are considered to be at *increased risk* of infective endocarditis:

- Acquired valvular heart disease with stenosis or regurgitation
- Hypertrophic cardiomyopathy
- Previous infective endocarditis
- Structural congenital heart disease, including surgically corrected or palliated structural conditions but excluding isolated atrial septal defect, fully repaired ventricular septal defect or fully repaired patent ductus arteriosus, and closure devices that are judged to be endothelialised
- Valve replacement.

A sub-group of the above patients may be 'non-routine' and therefore require liaison with their cardiologist regarding the appropriateness of antibiotic prophylaxis for invasive dental procedures.

Dentists should be informed and confident in discussing infective endocarditis with their patients and be able to outline the risks and benefits of providing antibiotic prophylaxis or not.

Dentists should also provide advice on maintaining good oral health, ensure the patient and carer is aware of the symptoms of infective endocarditis and the importance of seeking medical advice. Patients and their parents should also be made aware of the risks of undergoing invasive procedures, including non-medical procedures such as tattooing and piercings.

Signs and symptoms that a person may be developing infective endocarditis include: fever; fatigue; aching joints and muscles; night sweats; shortness of breath; pallor; persistent cough; swelling of the legs, feet or abdomen; unexplained weight loss and tenderness of the spleen.

All invasive procedures carry a risk of bacteraemia; therefore maximising oral health is paramount.

If any doubt exists, the cardiologist should be consulted before invasive dental procedures are undertaken.

Other problems may include prolonged bleeding caused by thrombocytopenia and anticoagulant medicine. It is essential to check the platelet count and prothrombin time if dental extractions are planned. The patient's prothrombin time is compared with normal and called the international normalised ratio (INR).

BLEEDING DISORDERS

Primary haemostasis is initiated after injury to a blood vessel and results in the formation of a primary plug. This is mediated by interactions between platelets, plasma coagulation factors and the vessel wall. Secondary haemostasis, with fibrin as the end-product, is also triggered by the initial injury and reaches its greatest intensity after the primary platelet plug is formed. It provides the framework for the formation of a stable clot.

Clinical manifestations of a haemostatic disorder vary depending on the phase affected. Defects in primary haemostasis (platelet initiated) generally result in bleeding from skin or mucosal surfaces, while defects in secondary haemostasis (fibrin clot), for example, haemophilia, result in deep-seated muscle and joint bleeding. Classification of bleeding disorders is shown in Table 8.6.

Inherited Coagulation Disorders

The main inherited coagulation disorders are described in Table 8.7. The severity of haemophilia A depends on the levels of factor VIII: $<1\%$ is severe, $1–5\%$ is moderate-to-severe and >5 to 40% is mild disease.

Thrombocytopenia

In the thrombocytopenias, there is a reduction in numbers of circulatory platelets (normal is $150 \times 10^9/L$ to $400 \times 10^9/L$).

The minimum for invasive dental procedures is $50 \times 10^9/L$.

DENTAL MANAGEMENT. Good communication with the physician/haematologist is essential. Aggressive prevention should be employed from a very early age. Regional anaesthesia should be avoided. Pulp treatment of primary molar teeth may be required to avoid extractions.

Haemophilias

Treatment involves:

- replacement and monitoring of factor VIII and IX levels
- desmopressin (DDAVP) for mild-to-moderate haemophilia A instead of factor replacement
- antifibrinolytics, epsilon-aminocaproic acid (EACA) or tranexamic acid, to prevent clot lysis
- avoiding non-steroidal anti-inflammatory agents.

von Willebrand's Disease

Treatment involves:

- DDAVP in combination with EACA or tranexamic acid
- factor replacement in more severe disease.

Table 8.6   Classification of Bleeding Disorders.

Types	Examples
COAGULATION DEFECTS	
Inherited	Haemophilia A (factor VIII deficiency), haemophilia B (factor IX deficiency, Christmas disease)
Acquired	Liver disease, vitamin deficiency, anticoagulant drugs (heparin, warfarin), disseminated intravascular coagulation (DIC)
THROMBOCYTOPENIC PURPURAS	
Primary	Idiopathic thrombocytopenic purpura (ITP), pancytopenia, Fanconi syndrome
Secondary	Systemic disease (leukaemia), drug-induced, physical agents (radiation)
NON-THROMBOCYTOPENIC PURPURAS	
Vascular wall alteration	Scurvy, infections, allergy
Disorders of platelet function	Inherited (von Willebrand's disease), drugs (aspirin, non-steroidal anti-inflammatory drugs, alcohol, penicillin), allergy, autoimmune disease, uraemia

Table 8.7 Prevalence of Inherited Bleeding Disorders.

Type	Missing Factor	Inheritance	Prevalence (%)	Incidence
Haemophilia A	VIII	X-linked recessive	80	1:20 000
Haemophilia B	IX	X-linked recessive	13	1:1000
von Willebrand's disease	Abnormal VIII	Autosomal dominant		
Haemophilia C	XI	Autosomal	6	(1:1000 in Ashkenazi Jews in Israel)

RED AND WHITE CELL DISORDERS

Red Cell Disorders: Anaemias

Iron deficiency in children is usually caused by a dietary deficiency or malabsorption. Vitamin B_{12} and folic acid may also be reduced by either mechanism and both are needed for maturation of red blood cells in the marrow.

Glucose-6-phosphate dehydrogenase deficiency causes premature haemolysis of red blood cells; it is an X-linked condition.

Sickle cell anaemia is an autosomal recessive disease with substitution of a single amino acid in the haemoglobin chain to produce haemoglobin-sickle (HbS). Homozygotes have sickle cell disease; heterozygotes have sickle cell trait. Clumping together of red cells under conditions of lowered oxygen tension, such as general anaesthesia, can lead to blockage of small vessels causing pain and necrosis. This is known as a 'sickle crisis'. The trait is carried in 10% of American–Black children and 25% of central African–Black children.

Thalassaemia is a homozygous or heterozygous trait resulting in abnormal globin synthesis. It results in a progressive haemolytic anaemia.

Management

A full blood count should be obtained for all anaemic patients especially with reference to general anaesthesia.

Immunodeficiency

Immunodeficiency may be caused by quantitative or qualitative defects in neutrophils, primary deficiencies involving B or T cells or both or by acquired disorders.

Neutrophils

Qualitative neutrophil disorders include:

- chemotactic disorders: Chediak–Higashi syndrome, lazy leukocyte syndrome, leukocyte adhesion defect
- phagocyte disorders: agammaglobulinaemia
- defects in microbial killing: chronic granulomatous disease, recurrent skin infections with *Staphylococcus aureus*.

Quantitative neutrophil disorders include neutropenia, cyclic neutropenia, leukaemic infiltration of bone marrow by other cells, agranulocytosis, aplastic anaemia, drug induced (including induced by chemo- and radiotherapy for neoplasia).

Primary Immunodeficiencies

- B cell defects: selective IgA deficiency, agammaglobulinaemia
- T cell defects: DiGeorge syndrome with thymic aplasia, chronic mucocutaneous candidiasis

- Combined immunodeficiency: severe combined, Wiskott–Aldrich syndrome, ataxia telangiectasia
- Acquired immunodeficiency: HIV, drug induced (cytotoxics, steroids, ciclosporin).

Dental Problems in Blood Cell Deficiencies

NEUTROPHIL DEFICIENCIES AND T CELL DEFECTS

- Candidosis
- Severe gingivitis/prepubertal periodontitis
- Gingivostomatitis
- Recurrent aphthous ulceration
- Recurrent herpes simplex infection
- Premature exfoliation of primary teeth.

B CELL DEFICIENCIES

- Few oral complications
- Recurrent bacterial infections, especially pneumonia and skin lesions.

Dental Management

- Prevention and regular review
- Chlorhexidine 0.2% mouthwashes
- Antifungals
- Aciclovir
- Prophylactic antibiotics
- Extraction of pulpally involved teeth.

Leukaemia

Leukaemia is a malignant proliferation of white blood cells. It is the most common form of childhood cancer, accounting for about one-third of new cases of cancer diagnosed each year. Acute lymphocytic leukaemia accounts for 75% with a peak incidence at 4 years of age. The general clinical features of all types of leukaemia are similar as all involve a severe disruption of bone marrow functions. Specific clinical and laboratory features differ, however, and there are considerable differences in response to therapy and long-term prognosis.

Acute leukaemia has a sudden onset, but the initial symptoms are usually non-specific, with anorexia, irritability and lethargy. Progressive failure of the bone marrow leads to pallor, bleeding and fever, which are usually the symptoms that lead to diagnostic investigation. The bleeding tendency is often shown in the oral mucosa, and there may be infective lesions of the mouth and throat. The dental practitioner may, therefore, be the first to note the condition. Bone pain and arthralgia are also important presenting complaints in about one-quarter of children. On initial haematological examination, most patients will have anaemia and thrombocytopenia. The diagnosis of leukaemia can be suspected on seeing blast cells on the blood smear, confirmed by bone-marrow biopsy, which will show replacement by leukaemic lymphoblasts.

Treatment consists of specific phases:

1. Induction of remission: to remove abnormal cells from the blood and bone marrow; drugs used include vincristine and prednisone.
2. Prophylactic treatment to central nervous system; drugs used include intrathecal methotrexate plus irradiation of central nervous system.
3. Consolidation: drugs used include cytosine arabinoside plus asparaginase.
4. Maintenance: drugs used include methotrexate plus mercaptopurine for approximately 2 years.

On this regimen, over 70% of children now survive and can be regarded as cured.

Dental Management

All paediatric oncology patients should have a dental review and the opportunity to be made dentally fit before commencing chemo or radiotherapy. This will often involve rapid organisation of a dental general anaesthetic if the patient does not have sufficient co-operation for treatment. It is important to understand that a cancer diagnosis will have a significant impact on the patient's dental health, and all of these patients should be treated as high caries risk, regardless of their previous status. Unless there is a major dental emergency, no active dental treatment should be carried out until the child is in remission. Any dental pain should be treated conservatively by the use of antibiotics and analgesics. The drug regimen used to induce remission has numerous side-effects, including nausea and vomiting, reversible alopecia (hair loss), neuropathy and oral mucositis and ulceration. It can be extremely difficult to carry out normal mouth care for children at this stage, and many have difficulty with toothbrushing because of acute nausea. Swabbing the mouth with chlorhexidine mouthwash and routine use of antifungal agents are essential. Local anaesthesia preparations, such as 20% benzocaine gel or benzydamine hydrochloride (Difflam) applied before mealtimes can help to reduce pain from ulceration or mucositis.

Once the leukaemia is in remission and after consultation with the child's physician, routine dental care can be undertaken with the following adjustments:

- If invasive procedures are planned, current haematological information is required to assess bleeding risks.
- Prophylactic antibiotic therapy to prevent postoperative infection should be considered; it is given if the functional neutrophil count is depressed.
- Children who are immunosuppressed are also at risk of fungal and viral infections; fungal infections should be treated aggressively with amphotericin B or fluconazole, and herpetic infections with topical and/or systemic aciclovir.
- Regional block anaesthesia may be contraindicated because of the risk of deep haemorrhage.
- Long-term preventive dental care is important.
- An awareness of longer term sequelae of chemo- and radiotherapy to the patient's developing dentition.

RESPIRATORY DISEASE

Asthma

Asthma involves hyperactivity of the airway to a variety of stimuli, causing breathlessness, coughing and wheezing. It affects at least 10% of children in the United Kingdom.

Dental Management

- Stress may precipitate an attack in the dental surgery.
- Steroids may cause immunosuppression.
- Sugared medicines may have caused a high caries rate.
- No contraindications to nitrous oxide.
- General anaesthesia may require inpatient management.

Cystic Fibrosis

Cystic fibrosis is an autosomal recessive multisystem disorder of the mucus-secreting exocrine glands. A thick mucus is produced in the lungs, leading to chronic obstruction and recurrent chest infections. Pancreatic exocrine insufficiency will produce malabsorption and failure to thrive.

Dental Management

- Previous treatment with tetracyclines may have produced intrinsic staining of the dentition.
- Use of regional or general anaesthetics must be discussed with the physician.
- Avoid long appointments.

METABOLIC AND ENDOCRINE DISORDERS

Diabetes Mellitus

Type 1 or insulin-dependent diabetes is the most common form in children: 2 per 1000 school-age children will be affected. However, type 2 diabetes is increasing as a result of the increase in childhood obesity.

Periodontal disease is associated with poor diabetic control. Xerostomia and recurrent intraoral diseases may be present. Enamel hypocalcification and hypoplasia, together with reduced salivary flow, can predispose these patients to an increased frequency of caries. They also have altered flora, with an increase in *Candida albicans*.

Dental Management

- Well-controlled diabetics can have routine treatment under local anaesthesia as long as mealtimes are not interrupted. General anaesthesia, which requires fasting, will need inpatient management.
- Healing can be delayed and antibiotics may be indicated in surgical cases.

Adrenal Insufficiency

If a child has adrenal insufficiency and/or is receiving steroid therapy, any infection or stress may precipitate an adrenal crisis. For simple extractions and routine restorative care, no steroid supplementation is indicated. However, if more extensive oral surgery is indicated or the patient is particularly apprehensive, oral steroid dosage should be increased or parenteral supplementation given (Table 8.8).

Table 8.8 Corticosteroid Cover for Dental Procedures.

	No Steroids in Previous 12 Months	Steroids Given in Previous 12 Months	Steroids Taken Currently
Single extraction under local anaesthetic	No cover required	Hydrocortisone i.m. or i.v., preoperatively	Hydrocortisone orally, i.m. or i.v. preoperatively; normal steroid medication postoperatively
Multiple extractions, minor oral surgery or treatment under general anaesthesia	Consider cover if large doses given previously	Hydrocortisone i.v. preoperatively; oral or i.m. for 24 hours postoperatively	Hydrocortisone i.v. preoperatively; oral or i.m. for normal steroid medication

Doses of hydrocortisone: under 12 years, 50 mg; 12–16 years, 100 mg. Oral doses given 2 hours preoperatively. Intramuscular (i.m.) and intravascular (i.v.) doses given 30 minutes preoperatively.

Hypopituitarism

Anterior pituitary insufficiency (dwarfism) gives rise to potential risks related to adrenal gland activity and steroid production.

Hyperpituitarism (Gigantism)

In hyperpituitarism, there is accelerated dental development and eruption.

Thyroid Disorders

Hypothyroidism results in delayed eruption and increased spacing of teeth. Hyperthyroidism is often associated with other immunological deficiencies and results in precocious eruption of teeth, periodontal destruction and osteoporosis.

Dental Management
- Principal risks are related to general anaesthesia.
- Oral infections should be treated aggressively as they may exaggerate hyperthyroidism.
- Antithyroid drugs may produce parotitis and agranulocytosis.

Parathyroid Disorders

Hypoparathyroidism gives rise to:

- hypoplasia of enamel, hypodontia and root anomalies
- delayed or arrested tooth eruption
- acute and chronic oral candidiasis
- circumoral paraesthesia and spasm of facial muscles.

Hyperparathyroidism results in bony lesions (brown lesions) containing areas of haemorrhage with multinucleated giant cells, fibroblasts and haemosiderin. Generalised osteoporosis with cortical resorption is the most common bone lesion. The dental effects include:

- increasing mobility and drifting of teeth with no apparent periodontal pocketing
- malocclusion
- metastatic soft tissue calcification
- periapical radiolucencies and root resorption
- loss of lamina dura and generalised loss of radiodensity.

NEOPLASTIC DISEASE

In the United Kingdom, 1 in 600 children under the age of 15 years of age develop cancer. There are 1200–1500 new cases each year. Leukaemia is the most common form of cancer (31%); tumours of the central nervous system (26%), lymphomas (10%), neuroblastomas (6%) and nephroblastomas (5%) are the most common solid tumours.

Prognosis varies with the type of tumour, the stage at which it was diagnosed and the adequacy of treatment. The side-effects of treatment have been discussed previously and good oral care is essential.

Dental Management

Dental management is similar to that as for all immunocompromised children:

- Extraction of teeth with dubious prognosis
- Meticulous oral hygiene and 0.2% chlorhexidine mouthwash four times a day
- Topical analgesics: 20% benzocaine gel (flavoured) or 2% xylocaine (plain) for mucositis ulceration
- Topical fluoride
- Topical and systemic antifungals
- Prophylactic antibiotics
- Systemic antivirals.

ORGAN TRANSPLANTATION

Kidney, Heart, Liver and Pancreas Transplantation

Renal transplantation is the result of end-stage renal disease. Heart transplantation is commonly required because of congenital heart disease, and myopathy and liver transplantation is commonly required for biliary atresia. Transplantation recipients are prone to infection, bleeding and delayed healing owing to leucopenia and thrombocytopenia.

Dental Management

PRETRANSPLANT PLANNING. Remove any teeth of doubtful prognosis, treat active caries and institute a full preventive regimen.

IMMEDIATE POST-TRANSPLANT. Supportive dental care includes careful oral hygiene utilising chlorhexidine as a mouthwash or spray and a disposable sponge if the mouth is too sore for a toothbrush.

STABLE POST-TRANSPLANT PERIOD. Reinforce all preventive advice. Antifungal prophylaxis is needed for a few months after transplant. Delayed eruption and exfoliation of primary teeth and ectopic eruption of permanent teeth are related to gingival overgrowth associated with treatment with ciclosporin and nifedipine.

Bone Marrow Transplantation

Bone marrow transplantation is used to treat first or second relapse of acute lymphoblastic leukaemia, acute myeloid leukaemia in first remission, aplastic anaemia, grade IV neuroblastoma and immunological deficiencies.

Dental Management

If possible, all treatment should be completed 2 weeks prior to induction chemotherapy or total body irradiation. Following transplant:

- chlorhexidine 0.2% mouthwashes or gels four times a day
- prophylactic systemic aciclovir and antifungals during immunosuppression
- topical fluoride application
- artificial saliva if significant xerostomia
- antibiotic coverage for all procedures.

Graft-versus-host Disease

Transplanted T cells recognise host tissues as foreign, a reaction known as graft-versus-host disease (GVHD). Significant manifestations are present in 50% of patients. Acute GVHD produces fever, rash, diarrhoea, abnormal liver function and jaundice. Chronic GVHD may occur months after transplantation and is characterised by lichenoid or scleroderma-like changes to skin and mucosa, keratoconjunctivitis, pulmonary insufficiency, abnormal liver function and intestinal problems. Oral manifestations often include mild mucosal erythema, painful desquamative gingivitis, angular cheilitis, loss of lingual papillae, lichenoid maculae and striae, and xerostomia.

Diagnosis

A biopsy is taken of the lower lip to include minor salivary glands. Histological changes will be evident in stratified squamous epithelium with chronic lymphocytic inflammatory infiltrate and in the minor salivary glands with chronic sialadenitis.

ORAL DISEASE ASSOCIATED WITH HIV

Oral diseases are often early warning signs of HIV. Children commonly manifest candidosis, gingivitis and parotid swelling.

Herpes simplex infections occur intraorally and circumorally; recurrences are frequent. Treatment is with aciclovir.

Aphthous-type ulcers are persistent and common. Treatment is palliative.

Salivary gland enlargement is unilateral and bilateral, resulting in xerostomia and pain. Xerostomia can result in candidosis and dental caries. Treatment involves the use of saliva replacements, mouth sprays and salivary stimulants.

Hairy leukoplakia occurs in adults but is rare in children. It occurs on the lateral border of the tongue and, occasionally, the buccal mucosa and soft palate. No treatment is required.

Oral candidosis. Acute pseudomembranous candidosis is an early sign and suggests other opportunistic infections. It responds well to treatment with systemic antifungals and oral hygiene improvement.

Necrotising periodontal diseases, as defined in the 2017 classification of periodontal diseases, may present in patients who have a diagnosis of HIV/AIDS. *Necrotising gingivitis* may present with red erythematous gingival tissues extending to free gingival margin. There is often spontaneous gingival haemorrhage and petechia at gingival margin, either localised or generalised. *Necrositing periodontitis* gives rise to deep pain, spontaneous bleeding, interproximal necrosis and cratering and intense erythema. Treatment is similar to that for these acute conditions that involve improved oral hygiene and 0.2% chlorhexidine mouthwash or gel four times a day, with the use of systemic antimicrobials (metronidazole).

Kaposi's sarcoma is uncommon in children and adolescents. It affects the palate particularly but can occur on gingivae and tongue. Treatment is by chemotherapy, radiotherapy or laser excision.

RENAL DISEASE

End-stage renal failure leads to a fall in the glomerular filtration rate, which results in progressive hypertension, fluid retention and a build-up of metabolites, which are not excreted normally. Conditions affecting kidney functions include ureteric reflux, obstructive uropathy, glomerulonephritis and glomerulosclerosis, medullary cystic disease, systemic lupus erythematosus and cystinosis. Renal patients may be anaemic and have a bleeding tendency because of capillary fragility and thrombocytopenia. Those on dialysis will be taking anticoagulants. Caries rates may be lower, probably because of the ammonia released in saliva. Uraemic stomatitis may develop, with high serum urea. Teeth that are mineralising during renal failure will exhibit chronological hypoplasia or hypomineralisation.

Dental Management

Dental problems should be minimised by aggressive prevention; otherwise:

- pulpally involved teeth should be extracted; patients on haemodialysis can have extractions 1 day after dialysis under DDAVP cover; sockets should be packed and sutured
- consult with nephrologist regarding antibiotic prophylaxis requirements
- inpatient facilities required for general anaesthesia.

Drug Interactions in Renal Disease

End-stage renal failure is managed with antihypertensives and steroids, and these patients are anaemic and immunocompromised. Metabolism of drugs by the kidney, as well as renal excretion of drugs, is impaired. The following drugs should be avoided:

- Paracetamol
- Penicillin
- Tetracycline.

HEPATIC DISEASE

Hepatic disease can affect the metabolism of many drugs. Biliary atresia is congenital obliteration or hypoplasia of bile ducts, resulting in biliary cirrhosis and portal hypertension. It is the most common cause of transplantation in children. Deficiency of α_1-antitrypsin leads to progressive hepatomegaly and cirrhosis. It is treated by transplantation.

Dental Management

Coagulation problems may occur in hepatic failure because the vitamin K-dependent factors II, VII, IX and X are produced in the liver. Patients will be immunocompromised because of the high dosage of steroids used and will be mildly anaemic through destruction of red blood cells. High levels of unconjugated bilirubin causes a green intrinsic staining of the teeth. Treatment requires:

- aggressive preventive measures
- coagulation problems managed with fresh frozen plasma
- consult with hepatologist regarding antibiotic prophylaxis requirements.

Hepatitis A, B, C

Hepatitis A is an infectious condition with no carrier state. The transmission period is short (3 weeks). Treatment is delayed for 4 weeks in patients who are positive for hepatitis A. Hepatitis B is assessed through the hepatitis B antigen (HSsAg) test on serum. Those with a negative test are chronic healthy carriers, while those with a positive test are chronic active carriers. In the former, there may be some level of infectivity although less than that in chronic active carriers. Liver function is usually normal. A chronic active carrier has active viral replication and is very infective. They have active liver disease and liver function tests are abnormal.

Hepatitis C (non-A, non-B) is usually asymptomatic although liver function tests may be intermittently abnormal. It is transmitted by blood or blood products. Patients are chronic carriers and are potentially infectious.

Dental management requires close liaison with the physician.

NEUROLOGICAL DISEASE

Febrile Convulsions

Febrile convulsions affect 5% of children and are associated with illnesses that cause rapid high fevers up to the age of 3 years. It is important to eliminate CNS infection. Febrile convulsions do not commonly result in any permanent damage nor proceed to epilepsy.

Epilepsy

The term epilepsy is applied to recurrent seizures either of unknown origin (idiopathic) or caused by congenital or acquired brain lesions (secondary epilepsy). Epilepsy affects 0.5–1.0% of the population.

Dental Management

Phenytoin, used in epilepsy, is associated with gingival overgrowth, and a high standard of oral hygiene is necessary to minimise the development of overgrowth. Gingival surgery should not be contemplated if the oral hygiene is not excellent.

Cerebral Palsy

Many patients with cerebral palsy have no mental impairment, and it can take a long time in a patient to assess cognitive ability. Verbal communication requires patience or a communication aid. It is important not to change voice tone or level when speaking to these children.

Dental visits may trigger limb extension, especially if transfer to the dental chair occurs. It may be more appropriate to treat in their chair with appropriate pillow support for the head on a special moulded insert on the dental chair.

Gag, cough, bite and swallowing reflexes may be impaired, and the position of the child is crucial. They should be upright with slight neck flexion. Rubber dam is especially valuable to reduce the amount of water in the mouth from the air-rotor in those with swallowing problems. Mouth props may be used, but good suction must be available to prevent aspiration. Bite reflex to oral stimulation is difficult to overcome, but sometimes gentle finger pressure on the anterior border of the ascending ramus and retromolar area will help to open the mouth and instruments should be introduced from the side rather than the front.

Some patients who have hydrocephalus will have shunts from the ventricles of the brain to either the vasculature or the peritoneal cavity.

VISUAL IMPAIRMENT

A visually impaired person should be allowed to make full use of their tactile sense. Do not lead them roughly to the dental chair but merely guide if required. Allow them also to make full use of their sense of smell when familiarising them to the dental environment and procedures.

Give verbal and physical reassurance once rapport has been established. This is especially important as the patient cannot see your face or your smile.

Constantly describe procedures and the environment to help the patient to relax and feel comfortable in their surroundings.

Photophobia may be a problem in many visually impaired persons. Safety glasses in this situation should be tinted.

DEAFNESS

Establish how the patient communicates. A patient who lip reads will understand if you speak more slowly and make sure your lips and mouth are visible. Basic sign language will certainly improve your rapport with the patient and improve the patient's confidence.

Deaf people are often vibration sensitive; consequently, a full exploration of procedures and slow introduction of the different drill speeds is necessary.

A hearing-aid that is switched on during treatment may produce alarming feedback. It is better to turn it off or reduce the volume.

DEVELOPMENTAL DISABILITY

The initial consultation is not only important to allow the dentist (and parent) to establish what treatment is required but also to find what is possible. Find out the patient's likes, dislikes and behaviour patterns.

Children with a developmental disability often also have a mental disability, so a full history is important.

Dental Management

- Aggressive prevention is mandatory.
- Treatment when required is often under general anaesthesia, which in itself is not without risk especially in the multiple disability syndromic child.

- Assessment procedures for general anaesthesia require full documentation of all medical complications.

AUTISM

Autism is a lifelong developmental condition that affects how people perceive the world and interact with others. Patients with autism have difficulties with ways of thinking, social interaction and communication. It is a spectrum disorder, and individuals are affected to different degrees and in different ways. Approximately 1 in 100 people in the United Kingdom have autism.

Have a discussion with the child and their carers regarding their likes/dislikes – what may contribute to sensory overload for the patient, and what could be used to make them comfortable and less anxious in the new environment.

Bright lights, loud noises and strong smells may all be difficult for a patient with autism to cope with during a dental appointment.

'Social stories', welcome letters with photographs of the surgery and staff members and acclimatisation visits can all be very helpful in familiarising an autistic patient with the dental setting. It is often useful to have the dental chair semi-reclined before the patient enters the room, to avoid startling the patient by moving it when they sit down.

Use clear and concise language when communicating with an autistic patient – they may take what is said literally and therefore not understand idioms such as 'take a seat'. It is often helpful to use the 'first and then' approach – the autistic patient can then construct a timeline, e.g. 'first I am going to count your teeth, then I will use some special toothpaste and then you will go back to school'.

Self-Assessment: Questions

MULTIPLE CHOICE QUESTIONS (TRUE/FALSE)

1. In primary tooth trauma:
   a. Injuries are most common at age 6–7 years
   b. Luxation injuries are commonest
   c. A discoloured upper central without clinical or radiographic evidence of infection can be reviewed
   d. Palatal luxation injuries carry the highest risk to the developing permanent dentition
   e. Dilaceration of the permanent successor tooth is common
2. In permanent incisor trauma:
   a. Luxation injuries require rigid splinting
   b. Immature 'open' apex teeth have a better prognosis for pulp vitality compared with mature 'closed' apex teeth
   c. Avulsion injuries should be splinted for 2 weeks
   d. Open apex teeth replanted within 45 minutes may revascularise
   e. Resorption is greatest in subluxation injuries
3. In intrusion injuries:
   a. Closed apex teeth often retain their vitality
   b. Open apex teeth may re-erupt
   c. Closed apex teeth must be repositioned quickly
   d. Surgical repositioning may be necessary in severe injury
   e. Resorption is a rare complication
4. In avulsion and reimplantation:
   a. Mouthwash is an ideal tooth storage medium
   b. Closed apex teeth may revascularise
   c. Internal resorption is the commonest type of resorption
   d. Ankylosis leads to progressive intrusion of the tooth
   e. Telephone advice is crucial to long-term outcomes
5. Lateral luxation injuries:
   a. Should be left to reposition naturally
   b. May cause occlusal interference
   c. Involving open apex teeth have a better prognosis for pulp vitality than closed apex teeth
   d. Should be extirpated routinely at splint removal
   e. Involve fractures of the alveolar plates

6. Root fractures:
   a. Involving the middle third do not require splinting
   b. Involving the coronal third are easily treated
   c. Usually cause loss of vitality
   d. Can heal by firm union with cementum-like tissue
   e. Are easily diagnosed on radiographs
7. In child abuse:
   a. There are approximately 30,000 children on at-risk registers in England and Wales
   b. The Children Act of 1989 states five categories of abuse
   c. Most 'at-risk' children live in rural communities
   d. Males are the most common perpetrators
   e. Disability of a child may be a contributory factor
8. In child physical abuse:
   a. More than 50% of abused children have orofacial signs
   b. Facial fractures are common injuries
   c. Bruises can have a recognised shape or pattern
   d. Dental trauma has a characteristic appearance
   e. A damaged upper labial frenum can be caused by forcible feeding
9. In dental anomalies:
   a. Hypodontia is familial
   b. Supernumerary teeth may prevent eruption of permanent teeth
   c. Macrodontia occurs in Down syndrome
   d. 'Dens in dente' teeth are easily root filled
   e. Supernumerary teeth are more common than missing teeth
10. In dental anomalies:
    a. Amelogenesis imperfecta may look like fluorosis
    b. Amelogenesis imperfecta may be associated with osteogenesis imperfecta
    c. Teeth with dentinogenesis imperfecta usually undergo pulpal obliteration
    d. Hypoplasia infers deficient matrix with normal mineralisation
    e. Infraoccluded teeth have a higher incidence of absent permanent successors

11. In patients with coexisting disease:
    a. Congenital cardiac defects do not require antibiotic cover for scaling and polishing
    b. Penicillin is the antibiotic of choice for prophylaxis
    c. Mortality associated with infective endocarditis is about 5%
    d. Cystic fibrosis can result in decreased saliva formation
    e. A platelet count of 80×10^9/L is safe for invasive procedures in general dental practice
12. In patients with neoplasia or immunodeficiencies:
    a. Neuroblastoma is the most common childhood malignancy
    b. Bone marrow transplant is the preferred treatment for acute lymphoblastic leukaemia
    c. 5-year survival rates for acute lymphoblastic leukaemia are about 60–70%
    d. Candidal infections are common in immunosuppression
    e. Nifedipine and phenytoin can cause gingival overgrowth
13. In patients with renal or hepatic disease:
    a. Renal disease is associated with high caries rate
    b. Penicillin is contraindicated in renal disease
    c. Hepatic disorders can produce coagulation problems because of a deficiency of production of factors V and VIII
    d. Hepatitis C is potentially infective
    e. Renal patients on dialysis receive anticoagulants
14. In patients with coexisting disease or developmental disorders:
    a. 5% of childhood convulsions are associated with febrile illness
    b. Patients with cerebral palsy are always mentally impaired
    c. Photophobia occurs in the visually impaired
    d. Deafness can result in vibration sensitivity
    e. Developmental disability is not commonly associated with other medical problems

EXTENDED MATCHING ITEMS QUESTIONS

Theme: Traumatic dental injuries
It is important to classify dental trauma. This is essential for effective treatment planning. Below is a list of classifications for dental trauma (1–12). For each of the case scenarios (a–e), select from the list the single most appropriate diagnosis for the signs and symptoms given. Each classification may be used once, more than once or not at all:

1. Concussion.
2. Subluxation.
3. Enamel infraction.
4. Intrusive luxation.
5. Lateral luxation.
6. Crown root fracture.
7. Enamel–dentine fracture.
8. Avulsion.
9. Enamel–dentine–pulp fracture.
10. Root fracture.
11. Extrusive luxation.

12. Enamel fracture:
    a. A 4-year-old child falls off the new bicycle they got for their birthday. The parents bring you an upper primary incisor that was found lying on the road at the site of the accident.
    b. An 8-year-old boy hits his face on the side of a swimming pool when trying to climb out. His upper central incisors appear to be in original position, but there is evidence of bleeding from the periodontal ligament.
    c. A 12-year-old girl attends your surgery several days following a road traffic accident. She has a broken arm and a deep laceration on her chin. She has been complaining that her teeth are sore. When you percuss her upper right central incisor, you hear a different note compared to the adjacent teeth.
    d. A 10-year-old boy got his upper incisors caught in the protective netting round a trampoline. When you examine him, you notice that his left central incisor appears to be 3 mm in a more labial position compared to the right central incisor.
    e. A 15-year-old female has been hit in the face with a hockey stick during the county interschools final. She complains that the corner of her tooth is missing and she has some sensitivity when having cold drinks.

PICTURE QUESTIONS

Picture 1

The patient in Fig. 8.2 has had a heart transplant.

1. Which drugs may have caused his mandibular gingival hyperplasia?
2. What other drugs commonly cause the condition?
3. Why does hyperplasia occur?

Picture 2

This patient (Fig. 8.3) has severe wear and discoloration of her teeth.

1. What is the condition?
2. How common is the condition?
3. Will the permanent dentition be affected?
4. How would you treat her?

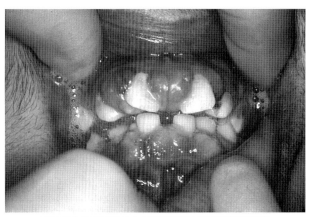

Fig. 8.2 A patient who has had a heart transplant.

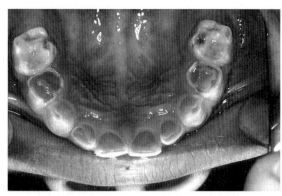

Fig. 8.3 Patient with severe wear and discoloration.

SHORT NOTE QUESTIONS

Write short notes on:

1. oral complications that might be expected in a patient undergoing cancer chemotherapy and their prevention
2. the management of an insulin-dependent diabetic who requires an extraction under (a) local and (b) general anaesthesia
3. immediate treatment for a palatally luxated central incisor without a root fracture but with an enamel–dentine fracture in a 9-year-old child with no medical illness
4. factors that would make you suspicious of child physical abuse (non-accidental injury).

SINGLE BEST ANSWER QUESTIONS

1. Which of the following dental injuries has the highest risk of root resorption in permanent teeth?
   A. Subluxation
   B. Enamel dentine fracture
   C. Intrusion
   D. Alveolar fracture
   E. Lateral luxation
2. Which of the following answers is incorrect.
   There are some situations in which a tooth should NOT be reimplanted. These include:
   A. Closed apex with an extra-alveolar time of >1 hour
   B. Primary tooth avulsion
   C. Very immature permanent tooth
   D. Significantly immunocompromised patient

3. Which of these aspects of a clinical 'trauma stamp' review are not indicated for traumatised primary teeth?
   A. Tenderness to percussion
   B. Electric pulp testing
   C. Mobility
   D. Sinus formation
   E. Colour
4. Which of these splinting regimens is correct for avulsion of a closed apex tooth with extra-alveolar dry time of >1 hour?
   A. Flexible splint for 2 weeks
   B. Rigid splint for 2 weeks
   C. Flexible splint for 4 weeks
   D. Rigid splint for 4 weeks
   E. Flexible splint for 4 months
5. Which of the following outlines the aim of placing a flexible splint in dental trauma management?
   A. To prevent loss of pulp vitality and avoid the need for endodontic treatment
   B. To prevent further trauma
   C. To use the tooth as a space maintainer
   D. To allow periodontal ligament healing via retaining some functional movement of the tooth, preventing ankylosis
6. Which of the following is a recognised permanent tooth sequelae of trauma to a primary predecessor?
   A. Enamel defect formation
   B. Root dilaceration
   C. Disturbance of eruption
   D. Odontome formation
   E. All of the above
7. Which of the following is not a stage of oncology treatment?
   A. Maintenance
   B. Consolidation
   C. Induction
   D. Initiation
8. 'An enlarged pulp chamber where the distance from the cementoenamel junction to the bifurcation of the root is greater than the length of the roots'. The term for this dental anomaly is:
   A. Talon cusp
   B. Microdont
   C. Taurodontism
   D. Dens invaginatus
   E. Double tooth

Self-Assessment: Answers

MULTIPLE CHOICE ANSWERS

1. a. False. Age 2–4 years is the peak age for injuries to the primary teeth.
   b. True. This is because of the relative elasticity of young alveolar bone.
   c. True. Extraction need only be contemplated if there is clinical or radiographic evidence of infection.
   d. False. Intrusion injuries carry the highest risk. Palatal luxation carries the root of the tooth away from the developing permanent tooth germ.
   e. False. Hypoplasias are the most common sequelae. Dilaceration is a rarer complication.

2. a. False. Functional splinting for 4 weeks is required.
   b. True. There is less chance of the neurovascular bundle being compressed by oedema around the developing apex.
   c. True. 60% of periodontal fibres are reunited within 10–14 days.
   d. True. Revascularisation proceeds at 0.5 mm a day. This is best assessed by new Doppler technology.
   e. False. Greatest in intrusion and avulsion injuries where the damage to the periodontal ligament is severest.

3. a. False. There is no evidence that any will retain vitality.

b. True. After initial disimpaction, a period of 2–3 months should be allowed for re-eruption.

c. True. These teeth will not re-erupt spontaneously, unlike open apex teeth.

d. True. This will often be the most practical option.

e. False. The incidence of resorption is high because of the severe damage to the periodontal ligament by tearing and crushing.

4. a. False. Saliva, normal saline or milk are the best storage media.

b. False. Only open apex teeth replanted within 45 minutes may revascularise.

c. False. External inflammatory resorption initiated within the damaged periodontal ligament occurs initially. This will be propagated if non-vital pulp tissue remains in the root canal.

d. True. Once the periodontal ligament is lost and bone is fused directly to the tooth tissue, there will not only be progressive loss of root as bone is remodelled but also progressive intrusion.

e. True. The immediate management will influence the extra-alveolar time that the tooth is out of the socket and the storage medium that a tooth is kept in.

5. a. False. Require immediate manual reduction if an injury is new, or orthodontic repositioning if an injury is over 2–4 days old.

b. True. This is corrected on repositioning.

c. True. Evidence after 5 years suggests that while 85% of open apex teeth will retain vitality, only 25% of closed apex teeth will.

d. False. This decision should be made after thorough clinical and radiographic examination at regular periods.

e. True. Crush fractures will occur on the side of the alveolus to which a portion of root is displaced.

6. a. False. Only apical fractures may not require splinting.

b. False. It is difficult to achieve a firm union over the fracture line because of proximity of the periodontal pocket.

c. False. 80% of root-fractured teeth retain their vitality.

d. True. This requires splinting within 24 hours of injury. Persistent mobility will allow growth of periodontal ligament cells across the fracture line.

e. False. Often requires two radiographs at different angles to detect.

7. a. True. Children will remain on registers for 1–2 years.

b. False. There are four categories: physical, emotional, neglect, sexual.

c. False. Abuse is mainly an urban or metropolitan phenomenon. However, there will be pockets of severe deprivation in some rural areas, where unemployment is high, which will have a high registration rate.

d. True. It is often the male member of a household who is responsible.

e. True. Crying, soiling of clothes, and unwanted pregnancy are also contributory factors on behalf of the child.

8. a. True. A more accurate figure is 60–80%.

b. False. Only 2% of orofacial injuries are fractures. This is because of elasticity of the young facial skeleton.

c. True. The pattern of grab marks, pinch marks and slap marks can be recognised.

d. False. It would be other factors or marks in association with the dental trauma that would raise suspicion.

e. True. This may be associated with a grab mark on the face.

9. a. True. Autosomal dominant inheritance.

b. True. In the upper anterior region especially. In clinical practice, if a permanent central incisor has not erupted within 6 months of its antimere, then a radiograph should be taken.

c. False. Microdontia is associated with Down syndrome.

d. False. Unless the invagination is limited to the coronal portion of the crown and can be totally removed with a bur, extraction is usually necessary.

e. False. In the permanent dentition, hypodontia (excluding wisdom teeth) occurs in 3.5–6% of the population, while supernumerary teeth occur in 1.5–3.5%.

10. a. True. The 'snow-capped' variety may resemble fluorosis.

b. False. Dentinogenesis imperfecta type I is associated with osteogenesis imperfecta.

c. True. They also have bulbous crowns and smaller roots.

d. True. Hypocalcification by comparison infers a normal matrix that is poorly calcified.

e. True. If successors are present, however, then infra-occluded teeth should exfoliate with normal time limits.

11. a. True. These are not recommended for the prevention of infective endocarditis.

b. False. Amoxicillin is the antibiotic of choice. If patients are allergic or have received amoxicillin during the previous month, then clindamycin is the choice.

c. False. The actual figure is 20–30%.

d. True. This can predispose the patient to caries.

e. True. Any injections, scaling or extractions below this at platelet levels should only be done in a hospital department.

12. a. False. Leukaemia accounts for 48% of childhood malignancies. Neuroblastoma occurs in only 7% of childhood malignancies.

b. False. Bone marrow transplant is used for relapses of acute lymphoblastic leukaemia and for acute myeloblastic leukaemia, aplastic anaemia and immunological deficiencies.

c. True. This is amazing when you consider the survival rate in 1950 was nil.

d. True. These can be treated with standard agents, such as nystatin and amphotericin.

e. True. However, why some patients are better 'responders' (i.e. produce more overgrowth) is not known.

13. a. False. A low caries rate is thought to be a result of ammonia in the saliva.

b. True. This is because the metabolism of the drug and its renal excretion are impaired. Paracetamol and tetracycline should also be avoided.

c. False. Factors II, VII, IX, X (Vitamin K-dependent) are reduced in hepatic disease.

d. True. Infectious and transmitted by blood and blood products.

e. True. Any dental treatment required needs to be discussed with the physicians involved in the renal care.

14. a. True. 'Febrile convulsions' rarely occur after age 3 years and any convulsions will be epileptic form.
    b. False. A large proportion of patients with cerebral palsy are of normal intelligence.
    c. True. Be very careful with bright surgery lights.
    d. True. Always explain what instruments you will be using.
    e. False. A large proportion have associated syndromes and multiple medical problems.

EXTENDED MATCHING ITEMS ANSWERS

a. 8
b. 2
c. 10
d. 5
e. 7

PICTURE ANSWERS

Picture 1

1. Ciclosporin, nifedipine.
2. Phenytoin.
3. The exact mechanism of drug interaction is unknown. There is proliferation of subgingival collagen, mainly of the interdental papillae, which become grossly swollen, pale and firm. Hyperplasia is more pronounced when oral hygiene is poor.

Picture 2

1. Dentinogenesis imperfecta.
2. Approximately 1 in 8000.
3. Yes, but teeth that develop later may be less affected.
4. Full preventive programme, establishment of posterior occlusion with stainless steel crowns, composite strip crowns or veneers to improve upper anterior aesthetics.

SHORT NOTE ANSWERS

1. These patients will be immunosuppressed and, therefore, will be specifically prone to oral mucosal disease (ulceration, mucositis), infection (leucopenia) and haemorrhage (thrombocytopenia). These could lead to significant morbidity and even mortality. Removal of teeth of dubious prognosis prior to treatment, restoration of other teeth and aggressive prevention are required. The prevention will include oral hygiene instruction, 0.2% chlorhexidine mouthwash four times a day, topical fluoride application, antifungals and modification of diet (realistic modifications for a child's condition).

2. a. An early morning or early afternoon appointment, which would be close to their last major meal intake.
   b. These patients need to be starved prior to a general anaesthetic and, therefore, are not suitable for treatment as outpatients. They need hospital admission to stabilise diabetic control by intravenous drip the night before the extractions, and then careful conversion back to their normal regimen postoperatively.

3. Reposition the tooth with gentle finger pressure under local anaesthesia. Splint with a functional splint – composite and ortho wire attached to one abutment tooth either side of the luxated tooth – for 4 weeks. Place a composite or compomer bandage over the enamel–dentine fracture. Record baseline clinical and radiographic data, including vitality tests and radiographs of all teeth in the upper labial segment. Prescribe antibiotics (commonly amoxicillin 250 mg twice daily) for 5 days, antibacterial mouthwash (chlorhexidine 0.2% four times a day) and a soft diet for the duration of the splint.

4. Any of the following factors:
   - delay in seeking advice or help
   - explanation does not fit the age and clinical findings
   - story of the accident varies
   - child may say something contradictory to parents
   - history of previous injury
   - history of violence in the family
   - child's reaction to any medical/dental examinations
   - child's reaction to other people
   - nature of the relationship between parent and child
   - parent's mood is abnormal and child's needs are not seen as a priority.

SINGLE BEST ANSWER QUESTION ANSWERS

1. C. Intrusion
2. B. Primary tooth avulsion
3. B. Electric pulp testing
4. C. Flexible splint for 4 weeks
5. D. To allow periodontal ligament healing via retaining some functional movement of the tooth, preventing ankylosis
6. E. All of the above
7. F. Initiation
8. C. Taurodontism

References

Cairns et al. An overview and pilot study of the dental practitioner's role in child protection. Child Abuse review 2004;13:65–72.

Harris et al. British Society of Paediatric Dentistry: a policy document on dental neglect in children. *Int J Paediatr Dent* 2009;28:e14–e21.

HM Government. Working together to Safeguard Children. July 2018.

Stratham and Chase. Childhood wellbeing: a brief overview. Department for Education UK 2010.

9 Orthodontics I: Development, Assessment and Treatment Planning

Overview

Orthodontics relates to facial and occlusal development as well as to the supervision, interception and correction of occlusal and dentofacial anomalies. The practice of orthodontics, therefore, spans from birth into adulthood, with current practice aiming to establish optimal and stable occlusal relationships with dentofacial harmony. An appreciation of facial and occlusal development is fundamental to understanding the possible aetiology of some orthodontic problems, as well as being critical for their assessment and the planning of any likely treatment.

This chapter commences with an account of the rudiments of facial and occlusal development. It then details the elements of comprehensive clinical and cephalometric orthodontic assessment. Finally, the principles of treatment planning are considered.

9.1 Craniofacial Growth and Occlusal Development

LEARNING OBJECTIVES

You should:
- understand the pattern of growth of the calvarium, cranial base, the nasomaxillary complex and the mandible
- be aware of what is meant by 'growth rotations' and their impact on the occlusion
- know how occlusal development proceeds in the 'average' child.

An understanding of both craniofacial growth and occlusal development is essential to orthodontic practice as the former has a significant impact on the latter.

CRANIOFACIAL GROWTH

Pattern of Craniofacial Growth

At birth, the face and jaws are underdeveloped compared with those in the adult. More growth, therefore, occurs of the facial skeleton than of the cranial structure postnatally. Growth patterns have been established for four major body tissue systems – lymphoid, neural, general or somatic, and genital – and it is important to have an appreciation of these as some patterns are followed by tissues involved in craniofacial growth (Fig. 9.1). Lymphoid growth is rapid up to about 10 years but undergoes involution as the genital growth is accelerating at puberty. Neural growth, however, is virtually complete by 6–7 years, while somatic growth increases in early childhood, then slows, before increasing dramatically at puberty.

The pattern of neural growth affects skeletal growth of the calvarium and orbit, whereas the somatic growth pattern is followed approximately by the mandible and maxilla. More precisely, the jaw growth pattern falls between that followed by the neural and general body tissues, with the mandible aligning itself more to the latter than the maxilla. The spurt in jaw growth at puberty almost coincides with the spurt in height, on average between 10 and 12 years in girls and 2 and 3 years later in boys, although considerable individual variation exists.

For both the maxilla and mandible, on average, growth in width is completed in advance of that in length, which ceases before growth in the vertical dimension. The transverse dimensions of the jaws and dental arches do not tend to alter during puberty, as growth in width is largely completed before the growth spurt. That is with the exception of a small increase in inter-condylar distance and across the terminal molar width in both arches to keep pace with growth in jaw length. Growth in length usually continues in girls until around 15 years in the maxilla and 17 years in the mandible with somewhat later in boys, around 17 years and 19 years, respectively. Vertical growth may extend into the late teens in girls and into the twenties in boys. For males and females, growth of the maxilla in all dimensions is completed before that of the mandible.

Growth continues into adult life, with vertical changes in the facial skeleton predominating over anteroposterior changes, and least change taking place laterally. In the twenties, growth tends to resume slightly in females who

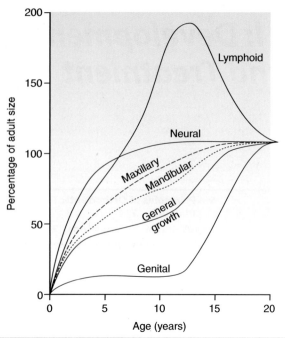

Fig. 9.1 Postnatal growth curves of various tissue types with superimposed maxillary and mandibular curves.

overall exhibit a backward mandibular rotation. In males, a forward rotation of the mandible is usual in adulthood. Irrespective of the direction of mandibular growth rotation, compensatory adjustment occurs in the occlusal relationships. Facial growth should, therefore, be seen as a process that continues well into adult life and not as one that is complete in the late teens.

Control of Facial Growth

Both genetic and environmental factors impact the regulation of craniofacial growth but the exact mechanisms are unclear. In theory, genetic control may be expressed primarily via bone, cartilage or the adjacent soft tissues ('functional matrix theory'); the current concept is a merging of these second and third theories, bone largely having being discounted. Sutures and periosteal tissues do not determine craniofacial growth primarily, as sutural growth is reactive rather than inherently programmed. The maxillary sutures are not growth centres, but rather growth sites. The synchondroses of the cranial base and the nasal septum, to a lesser degree, probably act as independent growth centres, but the cartilage of the mandibular condyle appears to react to, rather than initiate, growth. Both cartilaginous growth at the nasal septum and the mandibular condyle appear to be under strong genetic control in regard to growth of the maxilla and mandible, respectively; this is proposed to have greater impact on anteroposterior than on vertical growth.

Growth of the cranium and of the orbit in direct response to growth of the brain and of the eyes, respectively, lend support to the 'functional matrix theory'. Growth of the cranial base, although mainly by endochondral growth coupled with bony replacement at the synchondroses, may be influenced by growth of the brain. Cartilaginous growth of the nasal septum and growth of the surrounding soft tissues probably contribute to moving the maxillary position forward, but the amount apportioned to the former is unknown.

The soft tissues, including the masticatory muscles, are also contributors to spatial translation of the mandible and to addition of new bone at the condyle.

Growth Prediction

At present, no method is available to predict accurately the amount, direction and timing of facial growth. Instead, the assumption is usually made that for most patients whose direction and amount of facial growth are about average, the likelihood is that their growth pattern will follow the same pattern through orthodontic treatment.

Methods attempting to predict the pattern of facial growth or the likely timing of the pubertal growth spurt to assist orthodontic treatment planning include:

- superimposition of a template with average annual growth increments on the patient's cephalometric tracing
- digitisation of a cephalometric film followed by computer addition of average annual growth increments
- Cervical Vertebral Maturation (CVM) Index.

Six maturational stages based on the morphology of the bodies of the second, third and fourth cervical vertebrae have been identified and designated with respect to the pubertal growth spurt as follows: pre – stages CS1 and CS2, circum – stages CS3 and CS4, post – stages CS5 and CS6. With training, this classification system has been shown to be reliable. CS1 is advised as the optimal time for class III correction with maxillary protraction facemask treatment in conjunction with rapid maxillary expansion as maximal midfacial modification is possible (see Section 10.4). The mandibular growth spurt is likely to start within 1 year of observation of CS2, and at CS3 craniofacial growth is expected at its greatest pace.

As the amount and direction of growth may not be 'average' in an individual, there is a considerable amount of imprecision with regard to ascertaining clinically useful growth prediction. The assumption is often made, however, that the direction of mandibular growth rotation is likely to continue.

Growth of the Craniofacial Skeleton

Craniofacial growth can be considered conveniently in relation to the calvarium, the cranial base, the maxillary complex and the mandible.

Calvarium

The precursors to the skull bones develop in membrane, and six open spaces (fontanelles) that exist at birth are eliminated by 18 months. Contact between the bones is at sutures. Bone apposition occurs at these periosteum-lined sites in response to brain growth and they fuse eventually in adulthood. The contour of the cranial vault also changes by periosteal remodelling at the inner and outer surfaces. The growth in size of the calvarium is mostly complete by 7 years.

Cranial Base

The cranial base forms initially in cartilage, which is transformed to bone by endochondral ossification starting in the second trimester. Sutural growth and surface remodelling occur laterally in response to brain growth. Of greater significance are primary cartilaginous growth sites (synchondroses): sphenoethmoidal, intersphenoid and, most importantly, the spheno-occipital. The spheno-occipital synchondrosis grows until the early to mid-teens in females and somewhat later in males (15–17 years), having a profound impact on the anteroposterior skeletal pattern; it finally fuses at about 20 years. Because of its location in front of the temporomandibular joints (TMJ) but behind the anterior cranial base, both growth in length and in shape of the cranial base affect the maxillary–mandibular relationship. A long cranial base or large cranial base angle is associated with a class II skeletal pattern, while the converse is generally associated with a class III pattern (see Section 9.3 for definitions).

Maxillary Complex

The frontal process and a mesenchymal condensation in the maxillary processes of the first pharyngeal arch form the maxilla which then ossifies intramembraneously, starting in the lateral aspects of the cartilaginous nasal capsule. Growth of the maxilla occurs via:

- bone apposition at the circum-maxillary suture system
- passive displacement from its articulation with the cranial base
- surface remodelling.

Growth at the maxillary sutures assumes a greater role after age 7 years, when neural growth is complete and growth at the cranial base synchondroses lessens. As the maxilla moves downwards and forwards in response to growth of the surrounding soft tissues, the space opened at the superior and posterior sutures is obliterated by bone deposition on either side of the suture. Resorption of the anterior maxillary surface occurs simultaneously. Displacement of the maxilla inferiorly is accompanied by bone resorption from the nasal floor and deposition on the palate, while the alveolar process also develops vertically with tooth eruption. Bone is deposited also at the midline suture in response to lateral displacement of the maxillary halves, leading to an increase in midfacial width. The increase in maxillary dimensions lag behind those of the nasal structures, especially at puberty where a 25% differential is recorded. Maxillary growth is complete by about 17 years in males and on average 2 years earlier in females.

Mandible

Like the maxilla, the mandible is derived from the first pharyngeal arch. It begins development as a mesenchymal condensation just lateral to Meckel's cartilage. Ossification proceeds intramembraneously, spreading posteriorly along Meckel's cartilage without directly replacing it by newly formed bone. Condylar cartilages are formed distant to the mandibular body but fuse with it at about 4 months. These secondary cartilages are not primary instigators of mandibular growth but respond to other controlling influences. Endochondral ossification at the condyles accounts, in part, for mandibular growth. Elsewhere, bone apposition and remodelling are responsible for an increase in size and shape. As the mandible is translated downwards and forwards, largely in response to muscular forces, contact with the base of the skull is maintained by cartilaginous growth

at the condylar heads, which increases ramal height. The alveolar processes also increase in height with tooth eruption.

Mandibular length is increased by periosteal apposition along the posterior border and simultaneous bone removal from the anterior aspect of the ramus; the regular annual increase (2–3 mm) throughout childhood in mandibular body length is about half of what occurs during the pubertal years. An increase in mandibular width occurs principally by remodelling posteriorly. The chin is almost passive as a growth area but, by the late teenage years, it has become more prominent particularly in males due to resorption of bone between the chin and the alveolar process as the chin is moved forward with mandibular growth. On average, mandibular growth is complete by about 17 years in females and 2 years later in males, but it can proceed for longer.

Growth Rotations

The trend is for the facial skeleton to grow downwards and forwards away from the cranial base, although implant studies have indicated that rotations of both the maxilla and mandible occur during growth. These have more marked effects on the mandible than on the maxilla, where remodelling disguises their true impact. Mandibular growth rotations represent a growth imbalance in anterior and posterior facial heights. The direction of condylar growth and the vertical magnitude of growth at the spheno-occipital synchondrosis influence posterior facial height. Growth of the masticatory and suprahyoid musculature, including associated fascia and influenced partly by the vertical growth changes in the spinal column, affects the anterior facial height together with the eruption of teeth.

While mandibular growth rotations occur in all individuals, these are particularly different where the vertical facial proportions are markedly reduced or increased. A forward rotation, characterised by greater growth in posterior than in anterior facial height, is more common than a posterior growth rotation, where the change in facial height ratio is opposite to that observed in forward rotation (Fig. 9.2). Where forward rotation of the mandible is extreme:

- the lower border is convex with a reduced mandibular plane angle
- the lower anterior facial height is reduced
- the overbite is deep.

Conversely, a backward rotational pattern of mandibular growth results in:

- a concave lower border
- a pronounced antegonial notch with a high mandibular plane angle
- increased lower anterior facial height
- a reduced or anterior open bite.

The pattern of rotation has an impact on treatment. Whereas a forward rather than a backward rotation aids correction of a class II skeletal discrepancy, it also tends to increase overbite. Where the rotation is marked, overbite reduction is more difficult. Growth rotations also influence the inclination and anteroposterior position of the lower incisors. A forward growth rotation leads to retroclination of the lower incisors and an increase in lower labial segment

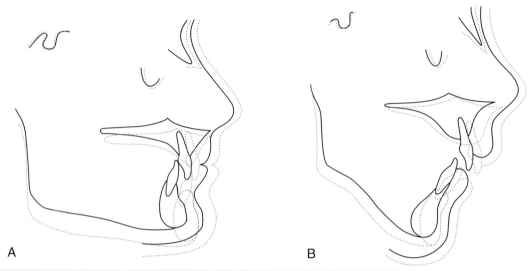

Fig. 9.2 Growth rotation. (A) Forward growth rotation owing to greater increase in posterior than in anterior facial height, resulting in an increased overbite. (B) Backward growth rotation owing to a greater increase in anterior than in posterior facial height, resulting in a reduced overbite.

crowding. With a posterior mandibular growth rotation, the incisors become upright, shortening the dental arch and producing crowding of the lower incisor area. Lower labial segment crowding is common in late teens particularly where mandibular growth continues after maxillary growth has ceased, but other factors are also likely contributors (see later).

Soft Tissue Growth

At birth, the orofacial musculature is well developed to allow suckling and breathing, and it soon responds to other functional demands of mastication, speech, facial expression and changes to the swallowing pattern. The light pressures from the lingual and buccolabial musculature affect tooth position, guiding the teeth towards a functional relationship and compensating, where possible, for any skeletal discrepancy. However, where a severe skeletal discrepancy or an unfavourable soft tissue behaviour exists (e.g. a lip trap with a class II division 1 malocclusion), the dento-alveolar compensatory mechanism will be insufficient.

Facial musculature lengthens with facial growth which increases the likelihood of lip competence. Nasal growth occurs to the greatest extent during teenage years, for girls maximally around 12 years and for boys 1–2 years later with completion in the former group generally by age 16 years, whereas in the latter it continues into the late teens and beyond. In adulthood, soft tissue profile changes take place in both sexes in concert with, but are much larger than, those of the facial skeleton. Notably, the nose tends to lengthen and the lips move down relative to the teeth so, over time, less of the maxillary and more of the mandibular incisors become exposed on smiling; the fullness of the lips also decreases. An increase in chin prominence is common in males, whereas in females, the chin may become more retrusive or show minor change.

OCCLUSAL DEVELOPMENT

What follows is an account of idealised occlusal development: the changes one would expect to see in the 'average' child. It is important to appreciate the range that exists within expected boundaries, so that developing problems may be recognised early and appropriate orthodontic intervention planned, if required. A thorough knowledge of the calcification and eruption dates of the 20 primary and 32 permanent teeth is essential (see Tables 7.1 and 7.2,). As well as allowing comparison of dental and chronologi-

Table 9.1   Dental Arch Development.

Characteristic	Measurement	Developmental Changes
Arch circumference	Line drawn through the buccal cusps and incisal edges of the teeth from the distal surface of second primary molars or second premolars	Maxilla: minimal Mandible: ~4 mm decrease
Intercanine width	Distance between the cusp tips of primary or permanent canines	Maxilla: ~1–2 mm increase from 3 to 6 years; ~3.5 mm increase from 6 to 13 years; then decreases Mandible: ~1–2 mm increase from 3 to 6 years; ~3 mm increase from 6 to 10 years; then decreases
Arch width	Distance from the palatal/lingual cusps of second primary molars or second premolars	Mostly determined in mixed dentition Maxilla: ~2–3 mm increase from 3 to 18 years Mandible: ~2–3 mm increase from 3 to 18 years

Table 9.2 Factors implicated in Late Lower Incisor Crowding.

FACTORS	
Skeletal	Increase in mandibular prognathism
	Mandibular growth rotations
	Minimal forward maxillary growth
Soft tissue	Increase in soft tissue tone of lips and cheeks
	Trans-septal fibre contraction
Dental/occlusal	Lack of approximal attrition
	Dento-alveolar disproportion
	Tooth size
	Mesial drift secondary to anterior component of occlusal force, eruptive force of third molars
	Uprighting of posterior teeth in response to increase in lower facial height
	Third molars prevent posterior teeth shifting distally relative to the mandibular body in late mandibular growth

cal age, this information also helps to identify the timing of any insult that has led to alterations in the enamel or dentine mineralisation and indicates if a tooth that is absent radiographically is likely to develop.

Development of the Primary Dentition

The gum pads, containing the primary teeth, enlarge and widen following birth, with the lower lying slightly behind the upper by the time the first primary teeth (lower incisors) start to erupt at about 6 months of age. These are followed closely by the other incisors. The first primary molars erupt 4–6 months later, followed by the primary canines and then the second primary molars. The incisors tend to be upright, and anterior spacing is common. Spacing is most common mesial to the upper canine and distal to the lower canine – the anthropoid or primate spaces. With a 1- to 2-mm increase in the intercanine distance, spacing between the incisors often increases as the child grows. In the absence of generalised spacing of the primary teeth, crowding of the permanent teeth is likely. The overbite, which is often initially 'deep' in terms of lower incisor crown coverage, reduces, and by 5 years of age an edge-to-edge occlusion with incisor attrition is common.

Development of the Permanent Dentition

At about 6 years, the eruption of the first permanent molars, followed by the permanent incisors, signifies the transition from the primary to the permanent dentition, commonly referred to as the 'mixed dentition phase'. The permanent successors are slightly larger than the primary teeth and the first permanent molars need to be accommodated. Existing space is present between the primary teeth. Additional space is provided by minor modifications in arch length, arch width and intercanine distance (Table 9.1). Once the primary dentition is fully erupted, however, the dental arch size remains more or less constant anteriorly apart from a modest change in shape with some growth in the intercanine distance. In addition, growth at the back of the arches is necessary to accommodate the permanent molars and to maintain the arch relationship while the face grows vertically.

The permanent lower incisors develop lingual to their predecessors and are frequently misaligned on eruption, but this usually resolves with intercanine growth. The upper anterior teeth develop palatal to their primary predecessors and are accommodated:

- by the existing spacing in the arch
- by erupting downwards and slightly forward so that they are placed on a wider arc
- by a small increase in intercanine distance (see Table 9.1).

The upper permanent lateral incisors usually move distally and labially with eruption of the central incisors, but they may be trapped palatally in crowded arches. The upper central incisors are often distally inclined when they first appear. An associated diastema tends to reduce as the lateral incisors erupt. At this time, the upper central and, to a greater extent, the lateral incisors are divergent, the latter because of pressure on their roots from the unerupted canines; this has been referred to as the 'ugly duckling' phase of dental development, terminology that is best avoided in the company of concerned parents.

The maxillary canines migrate from their palatal developmental position to lie labially and distally above the roots of the lateral incisors, leading to approximation of the incisor crowns as they erupt.

The combined mesiodistal widths of the primary canines and molars in each quadrant are slightly greater than those of the permanent canines and premolars. This difference in dimension is known as the 'leeway space' and is about 1 mm in the upper arch and 2.5 mm in the lower arch. The larger leeway space in the lower arch, probably in combination with mandibular growth, allows greater forward movement of the lower first permanent molar, converting a 'flush terminal plane' relationship of the primary molars to a class I occlusion (see later).

Six features (keys) of a good ('ideal') permanent occlusion have been described by Andrews:

- Molar relationship: the mesiobuccal cusp of the upper first molar lies in the groove between the mesiobuccal and middle cusp of the lower first molar; the distal surface of the distobuccal cusp of the upper first molar contacts the mesial surface of the mesiobuccal cusp of the lower second molar; the mesiolingual cusp of the upper first molar occludes in the central fossa of the lower first molar.
- Crown angulation: mesial for all teeth.
- Crown inclination: labially for incisors; lingually for canines through molars.
- No rotations.
- No spaces.
- Flat or mildly increased (≤ 1.5 mm) curve of Spee.

In addition, the following functional occlusal relations should exist:

- Centric relation should coincide with centric occlusion.
- A working side canine rise or group function should be present on lateral excursions with no occlusal contact on the non-working side; the incisors should only contact in protrusion.

Maturational Changes in the Occlusion

The occlusion of any child must be seen as dynamic and responding to changes in the facial skeleton. As the face continues to grow throughout the late teens and into adulthood, changes in the dentition and occlusion follow:

■ There is an increase in lower incisor crowding. This has been observed even in children with previously well aligned, spaced arches and can be regarded as expected. Factors implicated in its aetiology are listed in Table 9.2.
■ The interincisal angle increases, with uprighting of the incisors.
■ There is a tendency for the overbite to reduce.
■ A slight increase occurs in mandibular prognathism in males; in females there is a slight increase in mandibular retrusion.

9.2 Malocclusion: Classification and Aetiology

LEARNING OBJECTIVES

You should:
• be able to classify the first permanent molar and permanent incisor relationships
• know how to categorise malocclusion according to the Index of Orthodontic Treatment Need (IOTN)
• be aware of how the outcome of orthodontic treatment may be assessed.

Malocclusion is an unacceptable deviation either aesthetically or functionally from the ideal occlusion. Prevalence of malocclusion varies with age and racial origin as well as according to the assessment methods, but not all malocclusion requires treatment.

CLASSIFICATION OF MALOCCLUSION

Classification for Diagnosis

Angle's Classification
Angle's classification is based on the first permanent molar relationship (Fig. 9.3).

Class I (also referred to as neutrocclusion). The mesiobuccal cusp of the upper first permanent molar occludes in the buccal groove of the lower first permanent molar. Discrepancies no greater than half a cusp width were also regarded as class I by Angle.

Class II (also referred to as postnormal occlusion or distocclusion). The mesiobuccal cusp of the upper first permanent molar occludes anterior to the buccal groove of the lower first permanent molar.

Class III (also referred to as prenormal occlusion or mesiocclusion). The mesiobuccal cusp of the upper first permanent molar occludes posterior to the buccal groove of the lower first permanent molar.

Angle believed that the anteroposterior dental arch relationship could be assessed reliably from the first permanent molar relationship, as its position, he maintained remained constant following eruption. As this tenet is incorrect and difficulties arise in classification where mesial drift or loss of a first permanent molar has occurred, other classification systems are now used for that purpose.

British Standards Institute Classification
The British Standards Institute classification relates to the incisor relationship (Fig. 9.4).

Class I. The lower incisor edges occlude with, or lie immediately below, the cingulum plateau (middle third of the palatal surface) of the upper central incisors.
Class II. The lower incisor edges lie posterior to the cingulum plateau of the upper incisors.
　Division 1. The upper central incisors are proclined or of average inclination and there is an increase in overjet.
　Division 2. The upper central incisors are retroclined; the overjet is usually minimal but may be increased.
Class III. The lower incisor edges lie anterior to the cingulum plateau of the upper incisors. The overjet is reduced or reversed.

Permission to reproduce extracts from *British Standards Incisor Classification* is granted by British Standard Institute (BSI). British Standards can be obtained in PDF or hard copy formats from the BSI online shop: www.bsigroup.com/Shop or by contacting BSI Customer Services for hardcopies only: Tel: +44 (0)20 8996 9001, email: cservices@bsigroup.com.

Classification to Assess Treatment Need, Treatment Outcome and Treatment Complexity

Index of Orthodontic Treatment Need (IOTN)
The IOTN was developed to help to identify those malocclusions most likely to benefit in dental health and

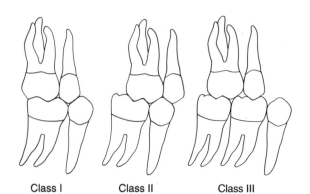

Class I   Class II   Class III

Fig. 9.3 Angle's classification based on the first permanent molar relationships.

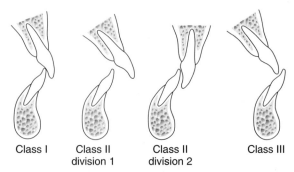

Class I   Class II division 1   Class II division 2   Class III

Fig. 9.4 British Standards Institute classification based on incisor relationship.

appearance from orthodontic treatment. It comprises two components.

The dental health component. Malocclusion is categorised into five grades (Table 9.3) based on the severity of occlusal characteristics that could increase the morbidity of the dentition and impair function. Grading, in relation to treatment need, is according to the single worst feature of a malocclusion.

To facilitate the grading process, a ruler (Fig. 9.5) has been developed. Occlusal features are assessed in the following order:
- missing teeth (M)
- overjet (O)
- crossbite (C)
- displacement of contact points (i.e. crowding) (D)
- overbite (O).

The order above gives rise to the acronym MOCDO. With practice, the treatment need category to a given malocclusion can be ascribed easily and reliably.

The aesthetic component. This consists of a set of 10 photographs of anterior teeth in occlusion with increasing aesthetic impairment (Fig. 9.6). These comprise class I and class II malocclusions; class III malocclusion and anterior open bite are not represented. Depending on whether the assessment is made clinically or from study models (with the anterior teeth in occlusion), colour or black and white photographs are used respectively. To categorise the treatment need, a score is given by

Table 9.3 The Index of Orthodontic Treatment Need: Dental Health Component.

Grade		Characteristics
5 (Very great)	5.i	Impeded eruption of teeth (with the exception of third molars) owing to crowding, displacement, the presence of supernumerary teeth, retained primary teeth and any pathological cause
	5.h	Extensive hypodontia with restorative implications (more than one tooth missing in any quadrant) requiring prerestorative orthodontics
	5.a	Increased overjet >9 mm
	5.m	Reverse overjet >3.5 mm with reported masticatory and speech difficulties
	5.p	Defects of cleft lip and palate
	5.s	Submerged primary teeth
4 (Great)	4.h	Less extensive hypodontia, requiring prerestorative orthodontics or orthodontic space closure to obviate the need for a prosthesis
	4.a	Increased overjet >6 mm but ≤9 mm
	4.b	Reverse overjet >3.5 mm with no masticatory or speech difficulties
	4.m	Reverse overjet >1 mm but <3.5 mm, with recorded masticatory and speech difficulties
	4.c	Anterior or posterior crossbites with >2 mm discrepancy between retruded contact position and intercuspal position
	4.l	Posterior lingual crossbite with no functional occlusal contact in one or both buccal segments
	4.d	Severe displacements of teeth >4 mm
	4.e	Extreme lateral or anterior open bites >4 mm
	4.f	Increased and complete overbite with gingival or palatal trauma
	4.t	Partially erupted teeth, tipped and impacted against adjacent teeth
	4.x	Supplemental teeth
3 (Moderate)	3.a	Increased overjet >3.5 mm but ≤6 mm with incompetent lips
	3.b	Reverse overjet >1 mm but ≤3.5 mm
	3.c	Anterior or posterior crossbites with >1 mm but ≤2 mm discrepancy between retruded contact position and intercuspal position
	3.d	Displacement of teeth >2 mm but ≤4 mm
	3.e	Lateral or anterior open bite >2 mm but ≤4 mm
	3.f	Increased and complete overbite without gingival or palatal trauma
2 (Little)	2.a	Increased overjet >3.5 mm but ≤6 mm with competent lips
	2.b	Reverse overjet >0 mm but ≤1 mm
	2.c	Anterior or posterior crossbite with ≤1 mm discrepancy between retruded contact position and intercuspal position
	2.d	Displacement of teeth >1 mm but ≤2 mm
	2.e	Anterior or posterior open bite >1 mm but ≤2 mm
	2.f	Increased overbite ≥3.5 mm without gingival contact
	2.g	Prenormal or postnormal occlusions with no other anomalies; includes up to half a unit discrepancy
1 (None)		Extremely minor malocclusions including displacements <1 mm

Reprinted from Brook PH, Shaw WC. The development of orthodontic treatment priority. *Eur J Orthodont.* 1989;11(3):309-320, by permission of Oxford University Press.

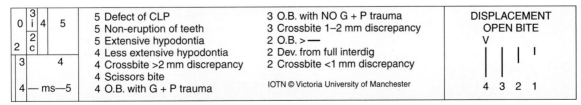

Fig. 9.5 The Index of Orthodontic Treatment Need (*IOTN*) ruler (not drawn to scale). Occlusal features are assessed in the order given by the acronym MOCDO. M = missing teeth; O = overjet; C = crossbite; D = displacement of contact point (i.e. crowding); O = overbite. (Reproduced by kind permission of Ortho-Care (UK) Ltd.)

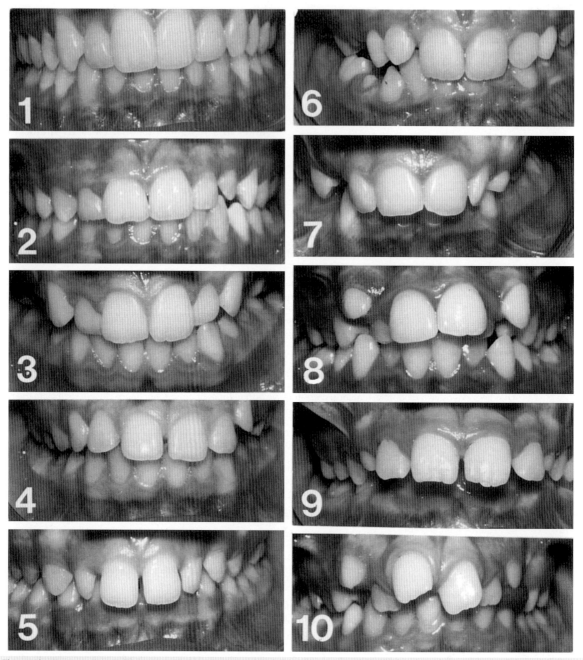

Fig. 9.6 The aesthetic component of the Index of Orthodontic Treatment Need. The need for treatment is categorised by subjective judgement based on the photographs: Score 1 or 2 = no need; 3 or 4 = slight need; 5–7 = moderate/borderline need; 8–10 = definite need. The aesthetic component was originally described as 'SCAN'. (Reprinted from Evans R, Shaw W. Preliminary evaluation of an illustrated scale for rating dental attractiveness, *Eur J Orthodont.* 1987;9(4):314-318, by permission of Oxford University Press.)

selecting the photograph thought to be of an equal aesthetic handicap (and likely psychological impact on the patient), but judgement is very subjective. For this reason, treatment need tends to be based primarily on the dental health component of IOTN.

Index of Orthognathic Functional Treatment Need (IOFTN)

The IOFTN arose from the IOTN and incorporates similar five grades. It includes, however, functional and other aspects pertinent to cases with marked dentofacial deformity

not recognised by IOTN, e.g. facial asymmetry, excessive gingival display and whole buccal segment(s) scissors bite with functional or occlusal trauma.

To assess treatment outcome. Assessment can be carried out objectively by applying the dental health component of IOTN and subjectively by application of the aesthetic component. In addition, the Peer Assessment Rating (PAR) may be recorded. A score is given to the pre- and post-treatment occlusion from the study models. The components and their weightings (by which the score is multiplied) are: crowding ($\times 1$); buccal segment relationship in anteroposterior, vertical and lateral planes ($\times 1$); overjet ($\times 6$); overbite ($\times 2$) and centrelines ($\times 4$). Measurement is facilitated by use of a specially designed ruler.

The percentage change in PAR score, obtained from the difference in pre- and post-treatment scores, is a measure of treatment success. A reduction of greater than 70% indicates a 'greatly improved' occlusion, while a 'worse/no different' assignment is indicated by less than or equal to 30%.

To assess treatment need and complexity of treatment.
The Index of Complexity, Outcome and Need (ICON) incorporates scores for: the aesthetic component of IOTN ($\times 7$); upper arch crowding/spacing ($\times 5$); crossbite ($\times 5$); overbite/open bite ($\times 4$) and buccal segment relationship ($\times 3$). A score in excess of 43 represents an evident treatment need. To indicate the improvement grade which reflects the outcome of treatment, $4\times$ the post-treatment score is subtracted from the pre-treatment score (intended to reflect need for and likely complexity of treatment).

AETIOLOGY OF MALOCCLUSION

A general overview of the aetiology of malocclusion is presented here while specific aspects related to the aetiology of each malocclusion type are considered in Chapter 10.

The aetiology of malocclusion is often the result of several interacting factors. These are principally genetic and environmental, although the precise role of inherited factors is not fully understood. Whereas the craniofacial dimensions and both size and number of teeth are largely determined genetically, the dental arch dimensions are influenced more by environmental factors.

Specific developmental defects with a genetic basis, which involve the maxilla or mandible, are rare, as is malocclusion caused primarily by trauma or pathology.

Skeletal Problems

The majority of anteroposterior skeletal problems are caused by inherited jaw proportions, which are strongly genetically determined. Inherited characteristics (e.g. mandibular deficiency) account for almost all of moderate class II malocclusion, while the added insult of environmental soft tissue influences is likely in more severe cases. For class III malocclusion, mandibular prognathism has a strong racial and familial tendency although mandibular posturing, possibly caused by tongue or pharyngeal size, may stimulate growth and influence jaw size secondarily. Maxillary deficiency is also most likely due to inherited jaw dimensions and a simple environmental factor seems unlikely, but its exact aetiology is almost completely unidentified.

Vertical jaw proportions are also inherited, but soft tissue postural effects (e.g. anterior tongue position or mandibular postural changes induced by partial nasal obstruction) may contribute in particular to anterior open bite. Other environmental influences, such as a high lower lip line, may contribute to deep overbite.

A unilateral crossbite with displacement is often caused by a functional alteration, but it is usual for a skeletal crossbite to have an additional genetic input.

Crowding

Crowding is the most common orthodontic problem, caused in part by a reduction in jaw and tooth size over the centuries, and experienced now by around two out of every three people in white populations. Interpopulation breeding has also been implied as arch width is influenced by jaw size, which is under tight genetic control.

Environmental influences, for example early loss of primary teeth due to caries or trauma or a digit-sucking habit, may likewise be instrumental in the aetiology of crowding. Also implicated is a softer, less abrasive modern diet which results in reduced interproximal tooth wear and smaller demands on jaw function; the latter may have added to a general tendency for smaller jaw size which was already happening. Soft tissue pressure of sufficient duration (more than 6 hours per day) in combination with the developmental tooth position may be responsible for a localised crossbite or malalignment.

9.3 Patient Assessment in Orthodontics

LEARNING OBJECTIVES

You should:
- know what to ask about in the orthodontic history and how to conduct an orthodontic assessment
- be able to carry out basic cephalometric analysis and interpretation.

Orthodontic diagnosis consists of a list of all aspects that deviate from what is ideal in relation to a particular occlusion, that is, a problem list. These problems may be categorised into pathological (e.g. caries or periodontal disease) and developmental (related to the malocclusion), the former needing to be dealt with before treatment starts. The diagnosis is a prelude to treatment planning as it allows the relationship between the various factors and their likely impact on treatment and prognosis to be considered. Diagnosis is based on the accurate gathering of information about the patient from a logical case assessment.

ASSESSMENT

Timing

At 7–8 years, an assessment of the developing occlusion should be undertaken to note, in particular, the form, position and presence of the permanent incisors and to plan appropriate intervention should an abnormality be detected that is likely to interfere with the expected eruption sequence. The prognosis of the first permanent molars should be assessed routinely from age 8 years, and palpation of the maxillary permanent canines is carried out on a regular basis from about 10 years. Early detection of a skeletal discrepancy will allow also for optimal timing of treatment to maximise growth potential but, in most children, assessment is delayed until the permanent dentition has erupted.

All general dentists should be able to carry out a basic orthodontic assessment for their patients and recognise when referral to a specialist is appropriate. When dental and/or occlusal development deviates from what is expected or when significant discrepancies in established dentofacial or occlusal relationships concern the patient and may compromise dental health over the long term, referral is indicated.

Apart from basic personal details, including relevant history with regard to medical, dental and social factors, the referral letter should give a brief summary of the salient features of the malocclusion incorporating the incisor and molar classifications (see Section 9.2). It should also include specific reference to:

- the patient's perception of the problem
- the attendance record
- the level of dental awareness including that of the parents (if appropriate)
- the oral hygiene status
- the likely prognosis of restored or traumatised teeth.

Any recent radiographs should be forwarded with the referral. Study models are also of great assistance with treatment planning.

Orthodontic assessment comprises three stages:

- A complete history
- A thorough and systematic clinical examination
- Collating relevant information from appropriate special investigations.

Demand for Treatment

The demand for orthodontic treatment is influenced by two main factors:

- **Patient/parent factors**, which include patient gender, age, level of self-esteem, self- and peer-perception of any occlusal or skeletal discrepancy, social class and parental desires
- **Awareness by dental professionals and the health care system.**

In general, demand for treatment is greatest when the **orthodontist:population and orthodontist:general dentist ratios are small**. Overall demand is increasing in adults, is higher in females, in those from better socioeconomic backgrounds and when a lower orthodontist:population ratio exists, as appliances become more common and their acceptance increases.

History

Initially the following must be identified:

- the patient's reason for attendance
- who raised the issue of treatment
- attitude, motivation and expectations regarding treatment (including that of parents)
- growth status (ongoing or complete) and habits (existing or previous).

Many children are unaware of why they attend for orthodontic assessment but commonly this relates to concerns regarding dental aesthetics although there may be dental health (e.g. gingival trauma) or on occasion functional problems (e.g. crossbite with mandibular displacement). Often attendance is prompted by parents. It is important to document whether the patient is unconcerned with the appearance of their teeth, particularly in the presence of obvious malocclusion, as any attempt to persuade the patient to undertake treatment is likely to be met with indifference. Attitude to treatment is best assessed from response to enquiries about their perception of orthodontic treatment for their peers, and by carefully observing their reaction when shown photographs or examples of appliances. Adults usually have a high level of dental awareness, are able to specify their concerns and motivation is high for treatment. Motivation to comply with treatment is central to a successful outcome and where this is doubtful treatment is best avoided. While treatment must deal with the patient's primary concern, the patient must also have realistic expectations as to what treatment can achieve. Whether growth is still ongoing is important for certain treatments (e.g. growth modification or surgical correction). The nature and frequency of habits such as thumb sucking or nail biting, which respectively influence incisor position and risk of root resorption, should also be ascertained.

Medical History

A health questionnaire should be completed by each patient or a parent, and the findings verified by a clinical interview. Several medical conditions may impact orthodontic treatment. Some are given below; where any uncertainty exists, liaison with the relevant medical specialist(s) is required.

Cardiac Defects with Infective Endocarditis Risk

Referral to up-to-date guidelines regarding the need for antibiotic prophylaxis is advised and where any doubt exists, the patient's medical practitioner or cardiologist should be consulted.

Recurrent Oral Ulceration

Appliance therapy should be avoided until this condition has been investigated thoroughly. Depending on the frequency and nature of ulceration, limited appliance treatment may be possible.

Epilepsy

Due to the risk of airway obstruction from appliance parts fractured during an epileptic attack and the difficulty with tooth movement in the presence of gingival hyperplasia, no orthodontic appliance should be fitted until the epilepsy is well controlled and the gingival condition healthy.

Diabetes

Patients with diabetes are more prone to periodontal breakdown, and active appliance therapy should be withheld until the periodontal condition is sound and the diabetes is stabilised.

Hay Fever/Asthma

Hay fever may interfere with the wearing of functional appliances over the summer months. An alternative approach to treating the malocclusion may be sought. Asthmatics using steroidal inhalers are liable to Candida infections where the palate is covered by an appliance necessitating extra vigilance with maintenance of a high standard of oral hygiene.

Nickel Allergies

In patients with a confirmed severe hypersensitivity to nickel, nickel-free brackets and wires should be used; in some cases, clear aligner therapy may be considered as an alternative.

Latex Allergy

Latex-free gloves, elastomeric separators, modules/chain, intraoral elastics and headgear components should be used.

Bleeding Diatheses

If extractions are necessary, special medical arrangements will need to be in place.

Behavioural/Learning Difficulties

These will influence the aims and scope of treatment possible. Extractions alone may produce an improvement in dental aesthetics and facilitate tooth-cleaning measures.

Arthritis or Osteoporosis/Bisphosphonates

Because juvenile or adult-onset rheumatoid arthritis often requires management with chronic steroid administration, lengthy orthodontic treatment is inadvisable due to the increased possibility of periodontal problems arising.

Oral doses of prostaglandin inhibitors or resorption-inhibiting agents (bisphosphonates) may be administered to adults being treated for arthritis or osteoporosis, respectively; as tooth movement may be affected, advice should be sought from the treating physician. Orthodontic treatment and extractions are contraindicated if bisphosphonates are given intravenously due to the osteonecrosis risk.

Dental History

The nature, extent and frequency of previous dental treatment together with the level of patient co-operation should be recorded, along with details of daily oral hygiene practices. A history of early loss of primary teeth, incisor trauma, enamel hypoplasia, absent teeth or TMJ problems should be noted. If orthodontic treatment has been carried out previously, details relating to extractions and appliance type should be recorded. If treatment was abandoned, the patient must be questioned carefully for the reasons.

Social History

The ease with which regular appointments can be attended and any forthcoming events that may influence attendance should be noted as both affect compliance with treatment.

CLINICAL EXAMINATION

Before the child patient takes a seat in the dental chair, it is often worthwhile to attempt to estimate their chronological age from their height and general level of physical maturity. This may give some indication of future growth potential. If the patient is accompanied by a parent, obvious familial malocclusion traits may be observed. The purpose of the clinical examination is to assess and record facial, dental, occlusal and related functional aspects of a patient in order to request appropriate diagnostic aids. An extraoral followed by an intraoral examination should be performed.

Extraoral Examination

The skeletal pattern, soft tissues of the lips, tongue position during swallowing, speech, temporomandibular joints and mandibular path of closure should be assessed and the presence of any habits noted.

The relationship of the mandible to the maxilla should be assessed in all three planes of space: anteroposteriorly, vertically and laterally. Before proceeding, it is important to ensure that:

- the patient is seated upright with the head in the natural postural position or with the Frankfort plane (a line joining the upper border of the external auditory meatus to the inferior aspect of the bony orbit) horizontal; natural head posture may be obtained by asking the patient to look straight ahead focusing on the horizon
- the lips are in repose
- the teeth are in centric occlusion.

Anteroposterior Plane

The relationship of the dento-alveolar parts of the mandible to those of the maxilla and their relationship to the cranial base in the anteroposterior plane is assessed by observing the patient in profile. Three means may be used.

- Drop a perpendicular from soft tissue nasion (zero-meridian line): the upper lip should lie on or slightly ahead and the chin point slightly behind where the skeletal pattern is class I.
- Palpate the soft tissue profile over the apices of the upper and lower incisors in the midline, which allows the following classification to be made (Fig. 9.7).
  Class I: the mandible lies 2–3 mm behind the maxilla.
  Class II: the mandible is retruded in relation to the maxilla.
  Class III: the mandible is protruded in relation to the maxilla.
  No indication is given as to where a skeletal discrepancy may lie as the classification reflects solely the position of the mandible and the maxilla relative to each other.
  As this method is not always reliable because of variation in lip thickness, palpation of the alveolar bases intraorally in the same locations has been claimed to give a better assessment. In essence, any significant discrepancy in the anteroposterior dental base relationship should be investigated more thoroughly by taking and analysing a lateral cephalometric film (see later).
- The angle of facial convexity (upper (mid-eyebrow to base of nose) to lower (base of nose to chin point); mean $12° + 4°$) may also be assessed allowing the following classification: average (class I or straight), increased (class II or convex) or decreased (class III or concave).

Vertical Plane

Two assessments of the vertical relationship of the face should be made (Fig. 9.8).

Assessment of lower facial height. In a well-balanced face, the face can be divided into equal thirds. The distance from the hairline to the mid-eyebrow height should be equal to that of the upper facial height (the mid-eyebrow level to the base of the nose) and the lower facial height (base of the nose to the inferior aspect of the chin). The lower facial height may, therefore, be assessed as average when the upper and lower facial heights are

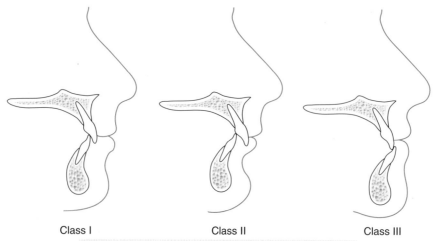

Class I   Class II   Class III

Fig. 9.7 Classification of the anteroposterior skeletal pattern.

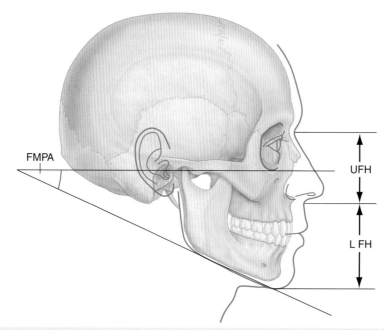

Fig. 9.8 Assessment of the vertical facial relationships. Lower facial height (*LFH*) compared with upper facial height (*UFH*) and Frankfort–mandibular planes angle (*FMPA*).

equal, reduced (when lower facial height is less than upper facial height) or increased (when lower facial height is greater than upper facial height).

Assessment of the Frankfort–mandibular planes angle (FMPA). With one hand, or the handle of a dental mirror, along the inferior aspect of the mandible and another hand along the Frankfort plane, these two lines can be projected backward in the imagination to give an estimate of the FMPA. Where the vertical dimensions of the face are as expected, both lines should meet at the back of the skull (occiput) and the FMPA is regarded as average. If the FMPA is reduced, the lines will meet beyond occiput, and if the FMPA is increased, they will meet anterior to it.

Transverse Plane

Obvious facial asymmetry may be assessed first from in front of the patient and then, if present, by standing directly behind the patient and looking down across the face, checking the coincidence of the midlines of the nose, upper and lower lips and midpoint of the chin. In most people, some degree of facial asymmetry is present and may be regarded as what is expected. Marked asymmetries, however, require further investigation. The location and extent of any marked asymmetry (e.g. upper, middle or lower facial third) should be recorded. As a general guide, eye width is a fifth of the facial width.

Soft Tissue Assessment

The following should be evaluated:

- Naso-labial angle: this may be classified as high, average (90–110°) or low and is affected by upper incisor inclination.
- Lip protrusion: using a line joining soft tissue chin and the upper lip (Rickett's E plane) as a reference, the lower

lip sits 2 mm (±2 mm) ahead of this with the upper lip slightly behind, but it is important to acknowledge differences, seen in diverse populations of people of colour and who are white. In the majority of people, some vermillion is visible and the lips everted at rest.

- Whether the lips are together (competent) or apart (incompetent) at rest: if lips are apart, it should be noted if they are slightly (potentially competent so capable of being brought together if required but incisor position stops this) or wide apart; markedly incompetent lips confer a poor prospect for stability of overjet correction with class II division 1 malocclusion.
- Lower lip position and coverage in relation to the upper incisors: the upper incisors may lie behind, on, or in front of the lower lip. At rest, on average, the lower lip should cover at least one-third to one-half of the upper incisor teeth.
- Upper lip level in relation to the upper incisors: the length of the upper lip and amount of exposure of the upper incisors at rest should be assessed; in males 1–2 mm display of the incisors is average, with slightly more in females.
- Tongue position at rest, during swallowing and speech: throughout the examination tongue position should be observed and particular note made if it lies in contact with the lower lip as this is likely to contribute to an incomplete overbite. How an anterior oral seal is achieved and atypical tongue activity on swallowing, or marked hyperactivity of the lower lip, should be noted. A tongue thrust may be adaptive especially where a thumb-sucking habit (see later) has produced an anterior open bite but in rare instances may be endogenous, the latter associated with an interincisal forward resting tongue position, marked circumoral contraction of the lips on swallowing, a lisp and proclined labial segments.
- Smiling: Typically a smile has the following components: symmetrical, upper dental midline in line with the facial midline, minimal buccal corridors (space between the furthest visible tooth and the corner of the mouth), full crown length of the upper incisors and related interproximal gingivae shown, gingival margins of the central incisors and canines level but lateral incisors about 1 mm more incisal, curvature of the upper incisors matches but does not touch the lower lip. In general, maxillary incisor exposure on smiling is greater in fe males than in males by about 1–2 mm.

Speech

Obvious impacts such as a lisp will be noticed during general questioning of the patient, and specific assessment by a speech therapist is rarely indicated in patients referred for orthodontic advice.

Habits

The tell-tale signs of finger- or digit-sucking habits are generally easy to ascertain:

- Proclination of maxillary incisors
- Retroclination of mandibular incisors
- Incomplete overbite or open bite, often asymmetric
- Increase in overjet

- Tendency to bilateral buccal segment crossbite, often resulting in a unilateral crossbite with displacement.

Effects vary depending on whether the finger or thumb is placed in a median or paramedian position and on whether one or more digits are sucked. An adaptive tongue thrust is common. Inspection of the hands will usually identify the offender. The patient and parent should be made aware of the effects of the habit on the dentition and occlusion. Note also if the patient is a nail biter or bruxist.

Temporomandibular Joints

Opening and lateral mandibular movements should be assessed by first observing the patient from in front and, second, by palpation of the condylar heads while listening for the presence of crepitus, or a joint click. Expected findings should be recorded as a baseline for future reference. Palpation of the masticatory muscles is not required unless symptoms are present. Referral to a specialist may be required in advance of any orthodontic treatment.

Mandibular Path of Closure

The path of closure from rest position to maximum interdigitation should be assessed, noting any anterior or lateral mandibular displacement. This may be difficult to detect in a young and anxious patient where a habitual posture has developed to avoid a premature contact, often from an instanding incisor. Applying gentle backward and upward pressure to the chin while instructing the patient to touch the back of the mouth with the tip of the tongue usually addresses this.

Intraoral Examination

The soft tissues of the buccal mucosa, floor of the mouth, tongue and the attachment of the maxillary labial frenum should be observed and any abnormality noted. A general dental examination should be carried out prior to assessing the individual arches of teeth and the occlusal relationships. The following should be charted:

- Standard of oral hygiene and caries rate.
- Gingival condition, paying particular attention to any area of gingival recession or attachment loss.
- All erupted teeth, noting those with atypical shape or size. A quick way to assess if an anterior tooth-size discrepancy exists is to compare the mesiodistal widths of the upper and lower lateral incisors. The upper laterals should be larger than the lower incisors, but only discrepancies of greater than 1.5 mm should be recorded as these are likely to affect treatment planning.
- Teeth with untreated caries, hypoplasia, large restorations or previous trauma. The condition of the first permanent molars should be examined, in particular, and a record made of any cervical decalcification (buccally on the uppers or lingually on the lowers), or large areas of hypoplasia, which may indicate a poor prognosis.
- The presence of erosion on the palatal surfaces of the upper incisors. In these cases, the patient should be questioned about frequency of intake of acidic or carbonated drinks.
- Marked attrition of the dentition. If present, enquiry should be made regarding bruxism.

The lower arch followed by the upper arch should then be assessed independently.

Assessment of the Upper and Lower Arches

LOWER ARCH

Symmetry and overall alignment. Include here the presence of rotations (classified by the surface furthest from the line of the arch).

Inclination of the lower labial segment to the mandibular plane. By placing the index finger of the right hand along the mandibular body and gently everting the lower lip, the inclination of the lower incisors may be assessed as average (if they appear to make almost a 90° angle with the mandibular plane), retroclined or proclined.

Angulation of the canines. These may be described as upright, mesially inclined or distally angulated.

Depth of curve of Spee. Measure the distance from the premolar cusps to a line joining the distal cusps of the first permanent molars and the tips of the incisors.

Presence and site of spacing or crowding including the magnitude of each. The degree of spacing/crowding may be assessed by performing a space analysis on the study models. This only takes account of any space discrepancy anterior to the first permanent molars and is usually carried out as described later.

For each quadrant. Measure with dividers the distance from the mesial surface of the first permanent molar to the distal surface of the permanent lateral incisor, and from there to the midline. Add these measurements for each arch to give the space available.

Measure the mesiodistal width of each tooth and add these together to calculate the space required. Where the canines and premolars have not erupted, on average 21 mm in each lower quadrant and 22 mm per quadrant in the upper arch is an estimate of their space requirements.

Quantify any surplus or deficit. Subtract the space available from the space required. Individual arches may then be classified as uncrowded, mildly crowded (<4 mm), moderately crowded (4–8 mm) or severely crowded (>8 mm).

UPPER ARCH

Symmetry and overall alignment. (As for the lower arch.)

Inclination of the upper incisors relative to the Frankfort plane. With the patient sitting upright and a finger or ruler placed along the Frankfort plane, the angulation of the upper incisors may be assessed as retroclined, average or proclined.

Angulation of the canines and presence and site of spacing or crowding including the magnitude of each. Assessed as for the lower arch.

Assessments With the Teeth in Occlusion

With the teeth in maximum intercuspation, the remaining aspects should be recorded.

Incisor relationship. This may be categorised according to the British Standards Institute classification (see Section 9.2).

Overjet (the horizontal overlap of the upper over the lower incisors). This is usually measured (in millimetres) from the mesial of the upper central incisors to the lower incisors. If there is a marked difference for each upper central incisor, both measurements should be noted.

Overbite (vertical overlap of the upper over the lower incisors). This is measured (in millimetres) – an indication should be given as to whether it is complete, incomplete or if there is an anterior open bite or traumatic overbite. The overbite is complete when the lower incisors occlude with the opposing maxillary teeth or with the palatal mucosa; it is incomplete if there is no contact with the opposing surfaces. The extent (in millimetres) of an anterior open bite should be noted and the site of mucosal ulceration recorded (either palatal to the upper incisors, labial to the lower incisors or in both locations) in the presence of a traumatic overbite.

Centrelines. Upper and lower centrelines should be coincident with the midline of the face and in line with each other; any centreline shift should be recorded (in millimetres) with a note to indicate the direction of the shift.

Molar relationship. Providing a corresponding molar is present in the opposing arch, the molar relationship may be categorised according to Angle's classification (see Section 9.2).

Where the first permanent molar is missing in either arch, the premolar or canine relationship may be assessed.

Canine relationship. This should be recorded in addition to the molar relationship, as although they are often the same, on occasion discrepancies are present.

The presence of anterior or posterior crossbite (buccolingual discrepancy in arch relationship). Is the crossbite buccal or lingual, bilateral or unilateral, anterior or posterior (Fig. 9.9)? For the premolar and/or molar teeth, a buccal crossbite exists when the buccal cusps of the lower tooth occlude buccally to the buccal cusps of the upper teeth. A lingual crossbite exists when the buccal cusps of the lower tooth occlude lingually to the palatal

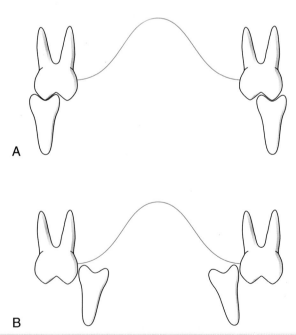

Fig. 9.9 Bucco-lingual discrepancies. (A) Bilateral buccal crossbite. (B) Bilateral lingual crossbite.

cusps of the upper teeth. A unilateral crossbite affects teeth on one side of the arch while teeth on both sides of the arch are affected with a bilateral crossbite. Often a unilateral crossbite is associated with an anterior or lateral mandibular displacement (Fig. 9.10).

Diagnostic Records

Study Models
These provide a record of the starting malocclusion and should include all erupted teeth and supporting areas. They may be produced traditionally in dental stone from alginate impressions or from intraoral scans of the arches or of the impressions, all of which may then be stored digitally.

Extra- and Intraoral Photographs
Facial views at rest and on smiling, as well as right and left buccal and occlusal views should be recorded. These may act as an incentive during treatment. Localised gingival recession, enamel defects or traumatised teeth may warrant a separate view.

Special Investigations

Sensibility Tests
Traumatised incisors or other teeth with suspect vitality should be sensibility tested, the most accurate of which is probably electric pulp testing, and their status recorded.

Radiography – Conventional or Digital
All radiographs should be justified on clinical grounds. Radiographs forwarded by a referring practitioner may provide sufficient information to supplement the clinical findings but often the following views are needed.

Dental Panoramic Tomograph (DPT)
The bony architecture of the maxillary and mandibular bases as well as that of the mandibular condyles (if included) should be checked first to exclude any dentally related, or other, pathology. All teeth should be identified and counted. It is a good routine to start in one area (e.g. upper right third molar area) and follow systematically through the upper left, lower left and finally lower right quadrants to ensure that nothing is missed. Then the condition of each tooth should be checked for caries, hypoplasia or resorption. All unerupted teeth should be charted, noting their developmental stage and position. Teeth previously extracted, those developmentally absent and any pathology should be recorded. Due to the narrow focal trough anteriorly, other views of the incisors are often required for those. Although large carious lesions will be obvious on a panoramic film, a more thorough assessment should be made from bitewing or periapical radiographs if required.

Upper Anterior Occlusal
This provides a good view of the upper anterior teeth and is useful to check root lengths of the incisors or to exclude the presence of a supernumerary or other pathology. Additionally, it may be used to locate ectopic maxillary canines when used in conjunction with another film taken at a different angle employing the parallax technique.

Periapical and Bitewing Radiographs
The former are indicated to check the position of unerupted teeth, root anatomy and pulpal pathology, whereas the latter are used for assessment of caries and restoration status.

Cone Beam Computed Tomography (CBCT)
Only where standard radiographs have not or are doubtful to provide sufficient information for diagnosis, should this be requested. It is particularly indicated with unerupted teeth to exclude resorption of adjacent teeth but is also indicated in cases requiring combined surgical-orthodontic management, cleft lip and palate cases particularly prior to alveolar bone grafting, and for implant planning with regard to width and volume of alveolar bone.

Lateral Cephalometric Radiograph
This film is indicated in the presence of anteroposterior and/or vertical skeletal discrepancies, particularly when incisor movement anteroposteriorly is planned.

CEPHALOMETRIC ANALYSIS

Cephalometric analysis involves the evaluation and subsequent interpretation of both lateral and posteroanterior views of the skull although, in practice, it is usually confined to the former because of difficulty in interpreting the posteroanterior view.

To allow comparison of measurements recorded for the same patient at different times, or between patients, a standardised technique is used. Originally developed by Broadbent and Hofrath independently in 1931, the radiograph is taken with the Frankfort plane horizontal or in natural head position, the latter achieved by looking straight ahead at the eyes in a mirror placed slightly

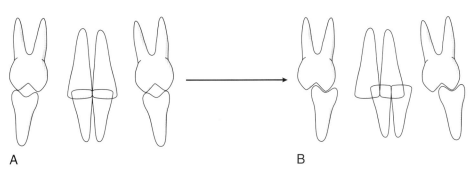

A   B

Fig. 9.10 Unilateral buccal crossbite with mandibular displacement and associated lower centreline shift. (A) Initial cusp-to-cusp molar contact. (B) Maximum intercuspal position.

further away. The ear posts are located in the external auditory meati and the teeth in centric occlusion. The central ray should pass through the ear posts. Importantly, the X-ray source to midsagittal plane distance (typically 150–180 cm) and the midsagittal plane-to-film distance (about 30 cm) should be standardised to facilitate reproducibility and to minimise magnification (7–8%). To allow accurate calculation of magnification, a steel rule of known length should be placed at the midsagittal plane and recorded on each film.

It is now common practice to collimate the X-ray beam, thereby avoiding radiation exposure to areas of the head not required for lateral cephalometric analysis. To enhance the soft tissue profile, the beam intensity can be reduced by placing an aluminium filter between the X-ray source and the patient, but this is less necessary with digital technology. Digital radiographs, whether taken using photostimulable phosphor plates or solid-state sensors, eliminate the need for developing and allow immediate viewing, rapid transfer and facilitate storage of images.

Uses of Lateral Cephalometric Analysis

Lateral cephalometric analysis is used:

- as a diagnostic aid and pre-treatment reference
- to check treatment progress
- to assess treatment and growth changes
- for dentofacial research.

A Diagnostic Aid and Pre-Treatment Reference

Lateral cephalometric analysis sheds light on the dental and skeletal characteristics of a malocclusion, thereby assisting in determining its aetiology and in planning correction. In some patients, particularly those with class III skeletal pattern, growth may be checked from serial radiographs and treatment considered at the appropriate time. Assessment of skeletal age, based on the characteristics of cervical vertebral maturation, has also been developed which indicates where an individual is with regard to the peak growth at adolescence. The image may also assist in identifying the position of unerupted teeth as well as soft or hard tissue pathology, including upper incisor root resorption. It provides a useful reference of pre-treatment incisor position, especially if anteroposterior movement is intended.

A Means of Checking Treatment Progress

During treatment with fixed or functional appliances, it is customary to check incisor inclinations and anchorage considerations. Any change in the position of unerupted teeth may be checked also.

A Means of Assessing Treatment and Growth Changes

A near end of treatment radiograph is useful to check that the treatment objectives have been achieved and to assist in planning retention. Where concern exists regarding the stability of treatment or unfavourable growth, a radiograph may be taken after treatment although this is rare.

If films are to be compared, they must be superimposed on some stable area or points. As orthodontic treatment is generally carried out during the growth period, no natural fixed points or planes exist. The following, however, are reasonably stable areas and are used commonly for superimposition:

- *Cranial base*: after 7 years of age, the anterior cranial base is found to be relatively stable. The S–N (sella–nasion) line is a close approximation to the anterior cranial base (N is not on the anterior cranial base), and holding at sella allows the general pattern of facial growth to be assessed; superimposition on de Coster's line (the anatomical outline of the anterior cranial base) reflects more accurately changes in facial pattern but requires greater skill to carry out.
- *Maxilla*: superimposition on the anterior vault of the palate, or on the easier recognised maxillary plane at posterior nasal spine (PNS), shows changes in maxillary tooth position.
- *Mandible*: changes in mandibular tooth position may be assessed by superimposition on Bjork's structures. These are the inner cortex of the symphysis, the tip of the chin, the mandibular canal outline and the third molar tooth germ before root development.

Dentofacial Research

The taking of serial images to assess longitudinal dentofacial growth changes, although practised formerly as part of data collection in several growth studies, is no longer ethical. Nonetheless, if ethically approved and informed consent obtained, growth and treatment data gleaned from radiographs routinely taken for diagnostic and treatment purposes may be used for research purposes.

Aim and Objective of Cephalometric Analysis

The aim of cephalometric analysis is to assess the anteroposterior and vertical relationships of the upper and lower teeth with supporting alveolar bone to their respective maxillary and mandibular bases, and to the cranial base. The objective is to compare the patient with expected population standards appropriate for his/her racial group, identifying any differences between the two. The technique used is outlined in Box 9.1.

It is important, however, to remember that irrespective of whether cephalometric measurements are made directly from a digitiser or indirectly from a tracing, the cephalometric technique and its subsequent analysis are open to error of projection, landmark identification and measurement. The technique relies on reducing the three-dimensional (3D) facial skeleton to a two-dimensional X-ray film. Bilateral landmarks, therefore, are superimposed. The validity of the analysis depends upon the ability of the operator to identify points accurately and reproducibly and make measurements which in turn is dependent on the film quality and operator experience.

Three-dimensional (3D) analysis of facial form is now possible with CBCT, having its greatest value in planning combined surgical-orthodontic management notably of asymmetry, but at present, no uniform means exists for 3D cephalometric analysis.

Cephalometric Interpretation

The following aspects may be assessed from the cephalometric analysis.

Box 9.1   Technique for Cephalometric Analysis.

1. First check the radiograph to ensure that the teeth are in occlusion and that the patient is not postured forward. It may be necessary to refer to clinical measurements to verify the overjet. It is advisable to scan the film for any pathology including resorption of the upper incisor roots, enlarged adenoids or degenerative changes in the cervical spine.
2. In a darkened room, attach tracing paper or tracing acetate (preferable due to better transparency) to the X-ray film and secure both to an illuminated viewer ensuring that the Frankfort plane is horizontal and parallel to the edge of the viewing screen.
3. With a sharp 4H pencil, identify the points (Fig. 9.11) and planes, the definitions of which are listed in Table 9.4. By convention, the most prominent incisor is traced and, for structures with two shadows (e.g. the mandibular outline), the average is selected for analyses. Alternatively, landmarks may be digitised using a cursor linked to a computer program that allocates *x* and *y* co-ordinates to each point. Angular and linear measurements are calculated automatically. A piece of cardboard with a cut-out area of about 5 cm × 5 cm is helpful in blocking out background light and aiding landmark identification.
4. Record the values for the measurements listed in Table 9.5.

Anteroposterior Skeletal Pattern

ANB (A point, nasion, B point) angle. This is determined by the difference between SNA (sella–nasion A) and SNB (sella–nasion B; the relative positions of the maxilla and mandible to the cranial base, respectively) and allows the following broad classification:

Class I skeletal pattern: $2° \leq ANB \leq 4°$
Class II skeletal pattern: $ANB > 4°$
Class III skeletal pattern: $ANB < 2°$

The ANB value should be considered along with the measurement for SNA, as ANB is affected by variation in the

Table 9.4   Definition of Commonly Used Cephalometric Points and Planes (Fig. 9.11).

Points and Planes	Definition
S	sella: midpoint of sella turcica
N	nasion: most anterior point of the fronto-nasal suture (may use the deepest point at the junction of the frontal and nasal bones instead)
Po	porion: uppermost, outermost point on the bony external auditory meatus (upper border of the condylar head is at the same level, which helps location)
Or	orbitale: most inferior anterior point on the margin of the orbit (use average of the left and right orbital shadows)
ANS	tip of the anterior nasal spine
PNS	tip of the posterior nasal spine (pterygo-maxillary fissure is directly above, which helps location)
A	A point: most posterior point of the concavity on the anterior surface of the premaxilla in the midline below ANS
B	B point: most posterior point of the concavity on the anterior surface of the mandible in the midline above pogonion
Pog	pogonion: most anterior point on the bony chin
Me	menton: lowermost point on mandibular symphysis in the midline
Go	gonion: most posteroinferior point at the angle of the mandible (bisect the angle between tangent to the posterior ramus and inferior body of the mandible to locate)
S–N line	line drawn through S and N
Frankfort plane	line connecting Po and Or
Maxillary plane	line joining PNS and ANS
Mandibular plane	line joining Go to Me
Functional occlusal plane	line drawn between the cusp tips of the first permanent molars and premolars/primary molars

Table 9.5   Eastman Cephalometric Values for White (Caucasian) populations.

Parameter	Value (±SD)
SNA	81 ± 3°
SNB	78 ± 3°
ANB	3 ± 2°
S–N/Max	8 ± 3°
1 to maxillary PL	109 ± 6°
1 to mandibular PL	93 ± 6°
Interincisal angle	135 ± 10°
MMPA	27 ± 4°
Facial proportion	55 ± 2%

SD, standard deviation; *SNA*, sella-nasion A; *SNB*, sella-nasion B; *ANB*, A point nasion, B point; *PL*, plane, *MMPA*, maxillary/mandibular planes angle.

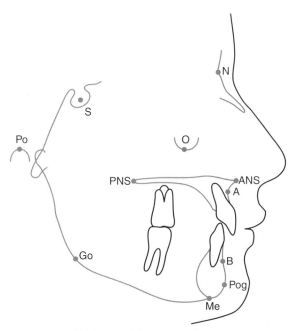

Fig. 9.11 Standard cephalometric points.

position of nasion. In cases where the SNA value is above or below the average value of 81° and provided the S–N/maxillary plane angle is within 8 ± 3°, a correction may be employed to the ANB value as follows: for every degree SNA is greater than 81°, subtract 0.5° from the ANB, and vice versa.

The Wits analysis and Ballard conversion. This is an alternative means of assessing the skeletal pattern in which the distance (in mm) is measured between perpendiculars from A and B point to the functional occlusal plane (a line joining the cusp tips of the permanent molars and premolars or primary molars). The average values for males and females are 1 ± 1.9 mm and 0 ± 1.77 mm, respectively. No indication is given, however, of the relation of the dental bases to the cranial base and the functional occlusal plane is difficult to locate. In some cases, however, it may be a useful check to complement that made from the ANB value.

With the Ballard conversion, the angles made by the upper and lower incisors to the maxillary and mandibular planes, respectively, are normalised by rotating around their centroids (one-third of the root length from the apex) taking into account any compensation necessary (for the lower incisor angle (LIA) with the maxillary/mandibular planes angle (MMPA); see later). The overjet is then measured as an indicator of the anteroposterior skeletal pattern.

Nasion perpendicular. Relative to a perpendicular to the Frankfort plane from nasion, A point should be 0–1 mm and pogonion –2 mm to 4 mm when assessed at 90° to this line.

Vertical Skeletal Pattern (MMPA and Facial Proportion) (Fig. 9.12)

Both anterior and posterior lower facial heights are considered in the MMPA whereas facial proportion assesses the contribution of lower anterior facial height to total facial height. The facial proportion should lend support to the value obtained for the MMPA; a reduced facial proportion is usually consistent with a low MMPA and vice versa. Where there is disagreement between these two assessments, the tracing should be checked to identify the cause.

Incisor Position

Angle of the upper incisor to the maxillary plane. The mean value for this angle is 109 ± 6°; the incisors may be classified as retroclined or proclined relative to the mean value. In class II division 1, it is often helpful to carry out a 'prognosis tracing' to indicate if correction of the incisor relationship may be undertaken by tipping or bodily movement (Fig. 9.13). An alternative method is to apply the following rule of thumb: for every 1 mm of overjet reduction, subtract 2.5° from the upper incisor to maxillary plane angle. Provided the final upper incisor angle is not likely to be less than 95° to the maxillary plane, tipping rather than bodily movement may be acceptable.

Angle of the lower incisor to the mandibular plane. This must be looked at in conjunction with the ANB and MMPA angles as the lower incisor angulation may compensate for discrepancies in the anteroposterior and vertical skeletal pattern. Under the influence of the soft tissues, the lower incisors may procline in class II malocclusion or retrocline in class III malocclusion. There is also an inverse relationship between the MMPA and the lower incisor angle (LIA); for every degree MMPA is greater than average (27°), the LIA is 1° less than the average (93°); the opposite holds true when the MMPA is less than average. Alternatively, the lower incisor angle is determined by subtracting the MMPA from 120°.

Lower incisor to A–pogonion line. This has been used as an aesthetic reference line for lower incisor positioning (average 0–2 mm) but it is unwise to lend too much credence to this measurement for treatment-planning purposes. Both point A and pogonion may shift with treatment or growth, and orientating the lower incisors correctly with respect to the A–pogonion line does not improve the prospect of a stable result.

Analysis of Soft Tissues

Various reference lines, regarded as indicators of pleasing facial appearance, have been suggested to assess the relationship of the soft tissues of the nose, lips and chin. These lines are more helpful in orthognathic surgical planning than in planning conventional orthodontic treatment. Aside from the facial plane which intersects the Frankfort plane at about 86°, joins soft tissue nasion and soft tissue chin, with A point lying on it, two other commonly used lines are shown in Fig. 9.14.

- *Holdaway line*: joins the upper lip and chin and, when extended, should bisect the nose if facial proportions are correct.
- *Rickett's E plane*: joins the nasal tip to the chin such that the lower lip is positioned 2 mm (±2 mm) in front of the E plane, the upper lip lying slightly further behind.

9.4 Principles of Orthodontic Treatment Planning

> **LEARNING OBJECTIVES**
>
> You should:
> - know the potential benefits and limitations of orthodontic treatment
> - know and understand the steps generally adopted in treatment planning
> - know what factors should be considered in presentation of the final treatment plan
> - know how space requirements may be assessed and how space may be created for desired tooth movement.

PROBLEM LIST AND TREATMENT NEED

The first stage in treatment planning is to summarise the features of a patient's malocclusion to produce a problem list of the pathological and developmental (orthodontic) problems; the latter should document what troubles the patient regarding their dentofacial appearance and level of enthusiasm for treatment, skeletal and dental relationships (anteroposterior, vertical and lateral) including appraisal of

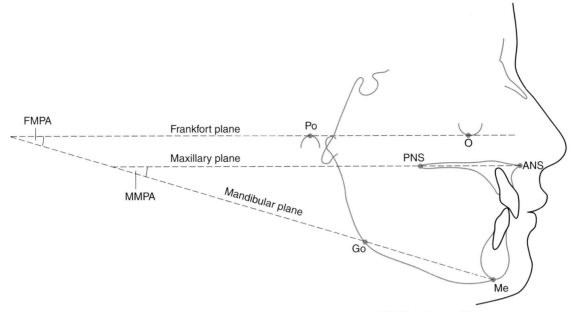

Although measurement of FMPA is favoured by some analyses, MMPA is preferable due to easier and more accurate location of the maxillary plane.

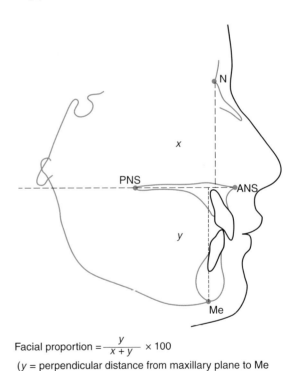

Facial proportion $= \dfrac{y}{x+y} \times 100$

(y = perpendicular distance from maxillary plane to Me
x = perpendicular distance from maxillary plane to N)

Fig. 9.12 Maxillary–mandibular planes angle (*MMPA*) and facial proportion.

the smile and profile, followed by the degree of upper and lower arch crowding and centreline discrepancies. The need for treatment on dental health and aesthetic grounds should then be considered (see Section 9.2). Only if appliance therapy and/or extractions can confer significant benefit to dental health and/or appearance of the dentition, should treatment be undertaken. If there is any doubt, treatment is best withheld.

Potential Benefits and Limitations of Orthodontic Treatment

Dental Health and Function

Overall, the oral health-related benefits of orthodontic treatment are rather limited.

Caries. No significant relationship has been found between dental caries experience and malocclusion. Orthodontic

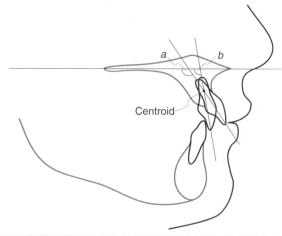

Fig. 9.13 Prognosis tracing to assess if correction of the incisor relationship can be achieved by tipping or bodily movement. a = presenting angle of 1 to maxillary plane; b = angulation of 1 to maxillary plane following rotation around the centroid to simulate tipping movement.

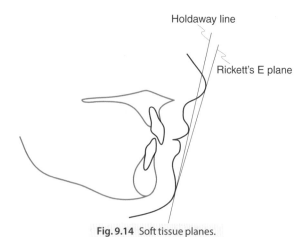

Fig. 9.14 Soft tissue planes.

treatment could not be claimed to prevent caries but in selected cases, extractions alone may allow greater access for tooth cleaning and potentially reduce the caries risk.

Periodontal disease. In general, crowding is weakly associated with periodontal disease and improvement in oral hygiene techniques/motivation are more likely than orthodontic treatment to reduce susceptibility to periodontal disease. Where an occlusal relationship is causing periodontal trauma, e.g. displacing occlusal contacts leading to gingival recession and mobility where one lower incisor or all of the lower incisors are in crossbite, or where a deep overbite produces palatal or labial gingival trauma, periodontal health is improved by corrective orthodontic treatment. Similarly, gingival recession may arise where teeth are markedly displaced from the arch due to crowding and orthodontic alignment may confer benefits to periodontal health.

Incisor trauma. The risk of trauma to the upper anterior teeth is twice as great when the overjet is increased more than 3 mm. Although trauma is more widespread in boys and when the lips are incompetent, of note is that overjet has a greater impact on girls. Where a higher propensity to upper incisor trauma is considered likely due to their prominence in the presence of markedly incompetent lips and particularly when previous trauma has occurred, early orthodontic treatment aimed at overjet reduction may be justified.

Tooth impaction. Unerupted teeth may cause resorption of the adjacent teeth or dentigerous cyst formation. In the case of a maxillary canine, timely surgical exposure and orthodontic traction may reduce the risk of resorption or arrest it by moving the tooth away from the adjacent incisors/premolars. Removal of supernumerary teeth may allow eruption of the related permanent tooth/teeth but surgical exposure is often required in advance of successful orthodontic alignment of maxillary incisors.

Speech. Speech is a complex process involving mutual compensation between the contributing organs (brain, lips, tongue and laryngeal muscles) so drawing firm conclusions regarding the correlation between a speech disorder and malocclusion is difficult although hypernasal speech is associated with a cleft of the soft palate. No guarantee could be made that correction of malocclusion (e.g. severe class II or class III malocclusion or anterior open bite which may be associated with lisping) would improve a speech impediment without accompanying speech therapy.

Masticatory function. In those with marked anterior open bite, increased or reverse overjet, incising food may be difficult or even impossible while marked hypodontia may compromise eating; each of these clinical features may impact quality of life. However, minimal evidence exists that dental health and masticatory function will be compromised long term if ideal occlusion is not achieved.

Temporomandibular joint dysfunction syndrome (TMJDS). Research has linked, although weakly, crossbites, class III malocclusion, asymmetry, class II mandibular retrusion and open bite with TMJDS. Orthodontic treatment, with or without extractions, will not lead to or resolve TMJDS. Due to the multifactorial aetiology, any initial treatment should be conventional and not irrevocable, but all symptoms should be addressed before starting any orthodontic treatment.

Social/psychological wellbeing. Malocclusion may have a negative impact on self-confidence and self-esteem resulting in poorer oral health-related quality of life (OHRQoL). The severity of malocclusion is not always commensurate with the psychosocial effect. In a UK study where almost 13% of adolescents reported being bullied, this was significantly associated with increased overjet and low self-esteem. Interceptive orthodontic treatment reduced the frequency of bullying and significantly improved OHRQoL but interestingly had no effect on self-esteem. In contrast, compared to controls, a North American study found short-term gain in self-concept with early treatment at 8–10 years for children with class II division 1 malocclusion. Could self-esteem perhaps be a factor influencing how one responds to malocclusion, rather than an effect? Furthermore, long-term longitudinal assessment in adulthood of orthodontic treatment undertaken during childhood has indicated only limited positive impact on psychological health or quality of life. This may be linked to personal differences regarding coping strategies, personality, values and societal issues. Additionally, occlusal status in adulthood appears to have limited association with psychological factors and quality of life.

Summary

Dental health is likely to benefit long term where any of the following exist: impacted teeth with a risk of resorption, increased overjet with a trauma risk, mandibular displacement in the presence of a crossbite, traumatic overbite and crossbite or crowding associated with gingival recession. Psychosocial wellbeing/quality of life is also likely to improve with early treatment for increased overjet. The impact of orthodontic treatment on long-term social/psychological wellbeing appears limited.

Limitations of Orthodontic Treatment

Orthodontic treatment, like all forms of dental treatment, has some limitations, and these should be borne in mind when the aims of treatment and treatment plan are being devised.

- Tooth movement is confined to cancellous bone.
- Limited differential eruption of anterior or posterior teeth may be used successfully to aid correction of malocclusion, but there is limited evidence on the permanency of any alteration in vertical skeletal pattern.
- Some small restraint or redirection of maxillary and/or mandibular growth is possible with headgear or functional appliance therapy; with rapid maxillary expansion, some orthopaedic increase in maxillary dental base width is possible.
- The effect of tooth movement on the facial profile is modest, with the growth of the nose and chin having a greater effect.
- Tooth movement is generally more efficient in a growing child but may still be undertaken in the adult.
- Growth may aid or hinder correction of a malocclusion and attempts to modify its expression, even though this is limited, may be considered on occasion in the early mixed dentition.
- Removable appliances tip teeth, whereas fixed appliances may bodily move, tip, intrude, extrude, rotate or torque teeth.
- Functional appliances alter arch relations through a combination of actions that involves tipping of teeth, differential eruption and possibly some restraint or stimulation of maxillary and/or mandibular growth, depending on the specifics of the design.
- Headgear restrains or redirects growth of the maxillary complex depending on the force magnitude and direction employed.
- Treatment success is dependent on:
  - correct diagnosis, treatment planning including assessment of anchorage, and proficiency in whatever appliance system is selected on the part of the operator
  - regular attendance, compliance with all instructions regarding appliance wear and maintenance of a high standard of oral hygiene by the patient
  - a stable result is only possible if the forces from the soft tissues, occlusion and periodontium are in equilibrium and facial growth is favourable.

Aims of Treatment

The aims of treatment should arise from the problem list arranged in the order of priority and outlines in a logical sequence the steps required to achieve the desired outcome. For example, in a patient with a class II division 1 malocclusion with moderate upper and lower arch crowding as well as a half unit class II molar relationship, these would often be as follows:

- Relief of crowding.
- Alignment within the arches.
- Overbite reduction.
- Overjet correction.
- Closure of residual spacing and correction of molar relationship to class I.

One should always aim for the ideal plan initially but keep an open mind, as sometimes this plan may require alteration (e.g. if the patient does not wish to wear a particular type of appliance). Importantly, where a limited objective plan is proposed, the patient must still benefit and not be compromised in the long term.

TREATMENT PLANNING

All pathological problems (e.g. caries and periodontal disease) must be addressed before any orthodontic treatment is considered. Treatment success requires a highly motivated patient and must satisfy the patients' concerns and expectations provided the latter are realistic.

In broad terms, the following series of steps will be useful for treatment-planning purposes in most malocclusions (refer to the sections covering management of each malocclusion).

Consider the Profile and Smile

While the influences of orthodontic treatment on the facial profile may be variable, nonetheless, upper lip support should not be compromised by incisor retraction which may increase an already obtuse nasolabial angle. Additionally, treatment mechanics that would extrude the upper labial segment and worsen smile aesthetics should be avoided in the presence of a gummy smile.

Plan the Lower Arch

In general, the lower arch form is to be accepted, particularly the anteroposterior position of the lower labial segment, which lies in a narrow zone of balance between the lips and tongue. Movement beyond this narrow zone is likely to lead to an unstable result apart from in certain circumstances (where thumb sucking has retroclined the lower incisors, class II division 2 malocclusion, class III camouflage treatment and bimaxillary proclination); these invariably require specialist management. In some cases where the lower incisors are mildly crowded, proclination may be apposite but this is often undertaken in combination with limited interproximal reduction (IPR). The general and local factors that govern the need for and choice of any extractions are described below.

Imagine the lower canine repositioned for alignment of the lower labial segment. If the canine is mesially angulated in a crowded arch, it will upright spontaneously following the extraction of a first premolar, thereby providing space for alignment of the lower labial segment. Most improvement occurs within the first 6 months following extraction, and if the premolars are removed as the canines are erupting. If the canine is upright or distally angulated, a fixed appliance will be necessary for its retraction.

Plan the Upper Arch

Mentally correct 3 position to a class I relationship with the aligned lower canine. This is done assuming that the lower labial segment is not spaced and that the upper incisor teeth are all of proportional size and not retroclined. The space needed may come from extractions, arch expansion or distal movement of the buccal segment. Importantly, if all of an extraction space is required to achieve a class I canine relationship, anchorage will need to be reinforced. The appliance type needed to achieve the desired canine relationship may be assessed also.

Consideration should be given as well to relief of upper labial segment crowding, reduction of the overjet and/or overbite and the appliance type necessary to achieve correction.

Plan the Final Buccal Segment Relationship and the Need for Closure of Any Residual Spaces

In most cases, if corresponding teeth have been extracted in each quadrant, the final buccal segment relationship should be class I; however, if only upper arch extractions or lower arch extractions have been undertaken, the final relationship will be class II or class III, respectively. The potential for spontaneous space closure depends on:

- the degree of initial crowding
- the age of the patient
- the vertical pattern of facial growth (space closure tends to occur more rapidly in patients with increased Frankfort–mandibular planes angle compared to those with a reduced angle).

Alternatively, space closure may be produced mechanically by applying intramaxillary (from within the same arch), intermaxillary (from the opposing arch) or extraoral traction.

Plan the Mechanics and Consider the Anchorage Demands

Removable appliances are limited to tipping movements, whereas bodily movement is possible with fixed appliances. Functional appliances are generally confined to correction of class II malocclusion in growing children and mostly produce tipping rather than bodily movement of teeth.

Tipping movements make only modest demands on the balance between the desired tooth movements and the space available (i.e. anchorage), whereas bodily movements place greater strain on anchorage. Where all the space available from extractions is required to relieve crowding, reduce an overjet or both, anchorage is at a premium and will need reinforcement.

Treatment Timing

Intervention in the mixed dentition is advisable in some circumstances (Section 9.3). Certain orthodontic treatments rely on growth for success. For example, overbite reduction and functional appliance therapy and treatment are usually best started in the late mixed dentition. However, where a severe skeletal problem exists that is likely to be exacerbated by growth, treatment is best deferred until the late teens when a combined orthodontic surgical approach can be considered.

Retention

A phase of retention is usually required following tooth movement with appliance therapy to allow consolidation of the new tooth positions through adaptation of the alveolar bone, gingival and periodontal tissues. Planning the retention phase of treatment requires an appraisal of the original features of the malocclusion as well as:

- the skeletal pattern and growth pattern
- soft tissue and periodontal factors
- the type and duration of treatment.

The likely retention regimen should be individualised for each patient, taking these factors into account, and must be explained to the patient before treatment starts. Specific guidelines in relation to retention are included in the management of each malocclusion type and appliance treatments (Section 11.4).

Final Presentation

Where two or more options exist with regard to treatment, these must be talked over thoroughly with the patient, parent and clinician so that an informed decision is arrived at steered by the patient's values, likes and dislikes. The 'pros' and 'cons' of each treatment option should be explained and the objectives of each stage of treatment clearly outlined in a form that is understandable to the patient and/or parent or guardian. Good colour photographs of any appliance to be used are very helpful. If anchorage reinforcement by headgear or temporary anchorage devices (TADs) is required, this must be explained. An outline of the likely appointment intervals and their length, together with an estimate of the overall duration of treatment and likely cost, is also necessary.

The commitment to maintenance of a high standard of oral hygiene, importance of regular dental attendance for routine dental care and level of compliance expected with treatment must be emphasised. The potential risks of treatment (Table 9.6) should be explained along with the benefits. When there is a risk with no treatment, this must also be highlighted.

Valid (voluntary and informed) consent individually adapted to each patient should then be obtained making certain there is an accurate grasp of all aspects mentioned above (details of treatment, risks and benefits, expected duration, commitment and cost). Written consent should be obtained acknowledging that this may require updating as treatment proceeds; the patient/parent/guardian should also be provided with a copy.

CREATING SPACE FOR DESIRED TOOTH MOVEMENT

Space Assessment

This entails evaluating the space required and space to be created during treatment; for the latter, the treatment aims

Table 9.6   Risks of Orthodontic Treatment.

RISKS	
Root resorption	0.5–1 mm loss of root length common, but large individual variation
	Suggested risk factors are force magnitude and method of application, length of treatment, appliance type (more with fixed than removable appliances), history of trauma, previous root resorption, blunt or pipette-shaped roots
	Current evidence indicates heavy forces and comprehensive treatment with fixed appliances increase incidence and severity; previous trauma and unusual root shape unlikely causes
Demineralisation/enamel damage	Greater risk with fixed than removable appliances; risk increases with poor oral hygiene and frequent intake of sugary foods/drinks
	Risk if occlusal contact with ceramic brackets and lack of care at debonding
Periodontal disease	Palatal gingival inflammation common with removable appliances if oral hygiene poor
	Marginal gingivitis common with fixed appliances; tends to resolve on appliance removal
	Occasionally 1 mm loss of attachment and 0.25–0.5 mm loss of alveolar bone adjacent to extraction sites
Pulpal/soft tissue damage	Loss of pulpal vitality, particularly if overactivation of appliance and previous history of trauma
	Abrasion/ulceration of mucosa more common with fixed than removable appliances
Relapse	More likely if teeth moved into unstable positions, retention regime inappropriate or not adhered to by the patient (see Section 11.4)
Iatrogenic	Greater risk with inexperienced operator (e.g. anchorage loss, inappropriate treatment mechanics)
Facial profile/ocular damage	Likely if poor diagnosis and treatment (see Limitations of Orthodontic Treatment and Profile Considerations under General Factors, Extractions)
	Headgear safety mechanisms not attached and patient carelessness with appliance (see Section 11.1, Headgear Safety)

need to be finalised. The following require space: relief of crowding; overbite reduction; overjet correction; centreline correction; contracting the arch width; adjusting incisor tip or torque. The mesiodistal width of the misaligned teeth compared to the space available in the arch allows the magnitude of crowding to be assessed and classified (see Section 9.3). Where the depth of the curve of Spee is 3 mm, 1 mm of space is estimated to be required for correction; more space will be required where the curve is deeper. Each mm of overjet reduction is reckoned to require 2 mm of space. Proclination of incisors will create space (2 mm gain for each mm). Space required for changes in incisor angulation or inclination is generally small.

Extractions

Extraction of teeth is required to provide space for either relief of crowding or to camouflage a class II or class III skeletal discrepancy. In general, to preserve symmetry, teeth are usually extracted from both sides of the same arch. The decision to extract teeth is governed by:

- general factors:
  - profile considerations
  - incisor relationship
  - appliance to be used
  - anchorage requirements.
- local factors:
  - the condition of the teeth
  - the site of crowding
  - the degree of crowding
  - the position of individual teeth.

General Factors
Profile considerations. Attempts to expand the arches anteroposteriorly to relieve crowding and improve facial aesthetics are unlikely to be inherently stable over the long term. Indeed, the extraction of premolars rather than second permanent molars may produce only 1–2 mm of retraction of the lips. Differences in lip thickness and growth pattern between individuals are likely to have greater bearing on the soft tissue profile than whether or not extractions are undertaken as part of treatment. However, where there is a marked class II skeletal discrepancy, retraction of the incisors is likely to produce a very unsatisfactory facial profile, and specialist advice should be sought.

Incisor relationships. In class I or class II, it is usual to extract at least as far forward in the upper arch as in the lower, but the opposite holds true in class III. Where the overbite is deep with a curve of Spee 5 mm or more, about 2 mm of space will be required for its reduction whereas 1.5 mm is likely to be required where the curve of Spee is 4 mm. Centreline discrepancies require greater space on one side of the arch than on the other to facilitate correction. To camouflage a moderate class II or class III skeletal problem, extraction of only upper first or lower first premolars, respectively, may be indicated.

Appliance to be employed. In crowded mouths, extraction of the same tooth from each quadrant encourages mesial drift and spontaneous space closure, but the choice of extraction is not so critical if fixed appliances are to be used for correction of the malocclusion.

Anchorage requirements. Bodily movement of teeth, particularly apical torque, is more demanding on anchorage than tipping movement, so space near to the site of the intended tooth movement is desirable. In addition, the anchorage balance (best thought of in terms of the combined root surface area posterior and anterior to the extraction site) is unfavourable for aligning crowded incisors the further posterior in the arch extractions are undertaken.

Local Factors

The condition of the teeth. Teeth with poor long-term prognosis should be considered for extraction even if treatment is made more difficult or prolonged as a result.

Site of crowding. Crowding in one part of the arch is more easily corrected if extractions are carried out in, or close to, that location. This is not true for the incisor areas: extraction of an incisor is not usually undertaken for relief of crowding because of the poor appearance that would result. First premolars, located midway between the front and back of the arches, often provide space for relief of crowding in both locations, whereas second permanent molars may be extracted for crowding confined to the posterior regions.

Degree of crowding. In the mixed dentition, mild crowding may resolve with the leeway space, but after this stage has passed, appliance therapy to either expand the arches or to move the buccal segments distally will be required to provide space. Where space shortage is of the order of 4 mm per quadrant, it may be dealt with in some instances without extractions, but extractions are more likely to be necessary for more severe crowding.

The position of individual teeth. Teeth that are grossly malpositioned and that would be difficult to align are often the choice for extraction. The position of the apex of the tooth must be considered as it is usually more difficult to move the apex than the crown.

Extraction of Teeth in the Buccal Segment

First premolars. These teeth are most commonly extracted for relief of moderate-to-severe crowding. Maximum spontaneous labial segment alignment is likely if the first premolars are extracted as the canines are erupting, provided they are mesially angulated, and is greatest in the first 6 months following extractions.

Second premolars. Extraction of these teeth is indicated in the following situations:

- Mild to moderate crowding, as the anchorage balance favours space closure by mesial movement of the molars; fixed appliances will be required for this.
- When the teeth are hypoplastic (usually as a result of extensive caries and pulpal pathology affecting the overlying second primary molar; Turner's hypoplasia), carious or absent.
- Where one or more second premolar is absent and crowding is mild to moderate, the second premolar may be extracted in the other quadrant(s), thereby balancing and/or compensating for the extractions; fixed appliances will be required to align the remaining teeth and close any residual spacing.
- One or more second premolar excluded from the arch either palatally or lingually following early loss of the second primary molar; the contact between the first permanent molar and the first premolar should be acceptable.

First permanent molars. See Section 10.1.

Second permanent molars. Extraction of lower second permanent molars may be considered for relief of slight premolar crowding or to compensate for upper second permanent molar extractions, being undertaken to facilitate distal movement of the buccal segments. First permanent molars must have a good prognosis. The best chance of providing space to disimpact a lower third molar successfully occurs when:

- it overlaps the distal of $\overline{7}$
- it makes $<30°$ angulation to the long axis of $\overline{7}$
- bifurcation is calcified.

Even when these criteria are met, the final position of $\underline{8}$ is unpredictable.

Third molars. Guidelines for removal are issued by The National Institute for Health and Care Excellence (NICE) and removal cannot be justified as a means of preventing or ameliorating late lower incisor crowding.

Extraction of Teeth in the Labial Segment

Lower incisors. Rarely, extraction of a lower incisor produces an acceptable solution for crowded incisors. Crowding of three lower incisors may occur due to a reduction in the lower intercanine width and a tendency for the labial segment to move lingually. Fitting six upper anterior teeth around five lower anteriors may lead to a reduction in the upper intercanine width and upper labial segment crowding. Therefore, extraction of a lower incisor is usually best considered only in the following situations:

- Poor prognosis due to caries, trauma or gingival recession.
- Severe crowding with one incisor excluded from the arch.
- Distally angulated canines with fanning of the lower incisors.
- Mild class III malocclusion in an adult with aligned buccal segments.
- Class I buccal and incisor relationships with severe lower incisor crowding; here subsequent changes in arch dimensions are likely to be minimal.
- Tooth-size discrepancy in the upper labial segment (i.e. small upper lateral incisors).

When extraction of a lower incisor is an option, it is wise to see what the final result is likely to be by carrying out a diagnostic set-up on a set of working casts. In each case, a lower fixed appliance is usually required to align and approximate the remaining teeth.

Upper incisors. A permanent central incisor is never a tooth of choice for extraction but may be considered if dilacerated or of poor prognosis due to trauma. Extraction of an upper lateral incisor is not recommended except in the following circumstances:

- $\underline{2}$ abnormally formed
- $\underline{2}$ on opposite side of the arch absent or abnormally formed
- $\underline{2}$ bodily excluded palatally with $\underline{1}$ and $\underline{3}$ in contact
- moderate crowding with $\underline{3}$ distally angulated.

The canine should be of good size, shape and colour to allow optimal dental aesthetics in the upper labial segment.

Canines

Lower canines. These should only be removed if the tooth is severely displaced or ectopic with good contact between first premolar and lateral incisor.

Upper canines. See Section 10.1.

Interproximal Reduction (IPR)

Using abrasive strips, discs or burs 0.25 mm of enamel can be removed from each proximal surface of the anterior teeth to give 2 mm of space. An extra 3–6 mm is possible per arch through enamel removal from the buccal segment teeth using fine tapered burs in a high-speed handpiece; the teeth should preferably be fairly well aligned with space created between them before this is carried out and fluoride applied after all enamel removal. IPR also flattens the contact points, re-shapes fan-shaped teeth and possibly reduces the chance of relapse.

Arch Expansion (Lateral or Anteroposterior)

Provided care is taken to limit lateral expansion to the confines of the supporting alveolar bone, lateral expansion in the upper arch may obviate the need for extractions (~0.5 mm per 1 mm of expansion). Expanding the lower intercanine distance should be avoided due to the propensity to relapse, but correction of a lingual crossbite in the premolar/molar areas by lower arch expansion is possible in some cases. For each mm of incisor proclination (anteroposterior arch expansion), ~2 mm of space is obtained in the arch.

Distal Movement of the Upper Molars

Space lost to unilateral mesial drift of the first permanent molar following early loss of a primary molar may be regained by use of a removable appliance with a screw and headgear support (Fig. 9.15). Bilateral distal movement of the upper first permanent molars by 2–3 mm is possible in well-motivated individuals and requires excellent co-operation with headgear wear or may be undertaken

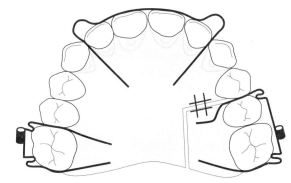

Fig. 9.15 An upper removable appliance (*URA*) with screw and headgear support to regain space lost to unilateral mesial drift. URA to move |56 distally. Screw section to |56; single Adams' clasp 6/ and double Adams' clasp |56 (both 0.7 mm SS wire); tubes for headgear soldered to clasp bridges; labial bow 2 1 | 1 2 (0.7 mm wire).

in conjunction with a fixed appliance attached to TADs. This may suffice to relieve a small amount of crowding or to reduce a small overjet but where space demands are greater, extractions in conjunction with distal molar movement will be necessary.

Combination of Means

In some circumstances, a combination of any or all of the methods listed may be appropriate to create space.

Self-Assessment: Questions

MULTIPLE CHOICE QUESTIONS (TRUE/FALSE)

1. The maxilla:
   a. Is derived from the second pharyngeal arch
   b. Completes growth in length before growth in width
   c. Grows partly by passive displacement of its articulation with the cranial base
   d. Is translated downwards and forwards by the condylar cartilage
   e. On average completes growth by 15 years in males
2. The mandible:
   a. Is derived from the first pharyngeal arch
   b. Ossifies medial to Meckel's cartilage
   c. Has a predictable pattern of growth in each individual
   d. On average follows the growth pattern of the maxilla
   e. Does not grow after age 18 years in males
3. Marked anterior mandibular growth rotation:
   a. Occurs when growth in posterior face height is less than in anterior face height
   b. Is more common than backward growth rotation
   c. Is often associated with a deep overbite
   d. Is associated with an increased maxillary/mandibular plane angle
   e. Is associated with a concave lower mandibular border
4. In the dental development of the 'average' child:
   a. Calcification of the primary incisors commences 6–8 months in utero
   b. Root calcification of the primary teeth completes 2–2.5 years after eruption
   c. Primary incisors erupt in contact and proclined
   d. Calcification of the first permanent molars commences at 8–10 months after birth
   e. The 'leeway space' is greater in the upper than in the lower arch
5. Space for the permanent upper incisors:
   a. Is obtained mostly by eruption palatal to their predecessors
   b. Is obtained by use of existing primary labial segments spacing
   c. Is obtained by intercanine width growth
   d. Is likely to be adequate where the primary incisors are crowded
   e. Is affected by the overbite
6. Expected maturational changes in the dentition include:
   a. A reduction in lower labial segment crowding
   b. An increase in upper labial segment crowding
   c. A reduction in lower intercanine width
   d. Increase in overjet
   e. An increase in interincisal angle
7. Clinical assessment of the anteroposterior dental base relationship:
   a. Is undertaken by viewing the patient from in front
   b. Should be undertaken with the teeth just out of occlusion
   c. Is best carried out with the patient supine
   d. Is reflected by the maxillary/mandibular planes angle
   e. Depends on the upper incisor angulation

8. A class II skeletal pattern:
   a. Is present when the mandible is protruded relative to the maxilla
   b. Can be assessed from the SNB angle
   c. Is usually associated with a retrognathic maxilla
   d. Can be assessed from the first permanent molar relationship
   e. Depends on the incisor relationship

9. The maxillary/mandibular planes angle (MMPA):
   a. Can be assessed clinically
   b. Reflects the anteroposterior skeletal pattern
   c. Indicates the vertical skeletal pattern
   d. Reflects posterior lower facial height and anterior lower facial height
   e. Is affected by lower incisor position

10. Class II division 2 malocclusion:
    a. Is defined by a half unit class II buccal segment relationship
    b. Exists when the lower incisor edges occlude anterior to the cingulum of the upper incisors
    c. Is characterised by retroclined upper central incisors
    d. Is usually associated with a minimal overjet
    e. May be associated with an increased overjet

11. A lateral cephalometric radiograph:
    a. Is taken with the head tilted up
    b. Is recorded with tube-to-midsagittal plane distance typically of about 15 cm
    c. Is an exact record of facial dimensions
    d. Is essential for orthodontic diagnosis
    e. May be useful in localising the position of an unerupted tooth

12. Cephalometrically:
    a. SNA (sella–nasion A point) angle describes the relationship of the mandible to the cranial base
    b. ANB angle is obtained by subtracting angle SNA from SNB (sella–nasion B point)
    c. Frankfort plane joins porion and nasion
    d. Mandibular plane joins gonion and menton
    e. Sella is the most anterior point on the cranial base

13. The ANB angle:
    a. Indicates the vertical relationships of the face
    b. Describes the anteroposterior skeletal pattern
    c. Tells about the relationship of the maxilla to the cranial base
    d. Is influenced by variation in the vertical position of nasion
    e. Is affected directly by the position of porion

EXTENDED MATCHING ITEMS QUESTIONS

Theme: Cephalometrics
For each of the clinical problems (a–e), select from the list below (1–25) the most appropriate cephalometric input to assist in your assessment (more than one may be correct). Each variable can be used once, more than once or not at all.

1. Nasion.
2. Porion.
3. Lower incisor angulation to mandibular plane.
4. Superimposition on Bjork's structures.
5. Orbitale.
6. ANB angle.
7. PNS.

8. Upper incisor angulation to maxillary plane.
9. MMPA.
10. Gonion.
11. ANS.
12. Interincisal angle.
13. Lower incisor tip to A–pogonion line.
14. Superimposition on S–N, holding at S.
15. Lower incisor tip.
16. Frankfort plane.
17. S–N line.
18. Maxillary plane.
19. No cephalometric assessment.
20. Prognosis tracing.
21. Mandibular plane.
22. Superimposition on anterior vault of the palate.
23. SNA angle.
24. SNB angle.
25. Menton.
   a. A 12-year-old girl presenting for treatment planning of her moderately severe class II division 2 malocclusion; you are asked to give priority to planning the lower labial segment position.
   b. An 18-year-old male patient on review for his worsening class III malocclusion, where an overall assessment is required of facial changes which have occurred in the 2 years since he was last seen (a cephalometric film is available from that time).
   c. A 14-year-old girl with a class II division 1 malocclusion seen for treatment planning, where it is necessary to evaluate upper incisor angulation and decide between tipping or bodily tooth movement for overjet correction.
   d. A 13-year-old male patient presenting for assessment of his class I malocclusion who indicates no desire to undertake orthodontic treatment.
   e. A 20-year-old female patient with an anterior open bite, class I skeletal and incisor relationships.

CASE HISTORY QUESTION

A 13-year-old female patient presents with a class I malocclusion with moderate upper and lower midarch crowding on a class I dental base with average FMPA. There is a history of recurrent oral ulceration.

1. What are the priorities in the management of this case?
2. Outline how you would go about orthodontic treatment planning for this patient.
3. What orthodontic treatment possibilities may exist?

PICTURE QUESTIONS

Picture 1

Examine the records in Fig. 9.16.

1. Classify the incisor relationship.
2. Classify the right and left molar relationships.
3. Classify the degree of crowding in the maxillary and mandibular arches (all permanent teeth are present).
4. What are the likely causes of this malocclusion?
5. What is the IOTN (DHC) score? (Additional information: no mandibular displacement associated with the crossbite; overjet 6 mm; lips competent.)

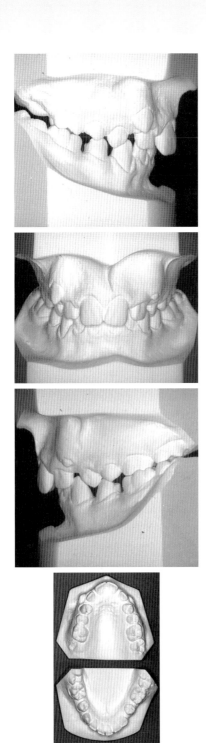

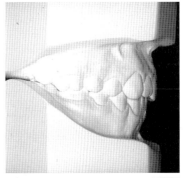

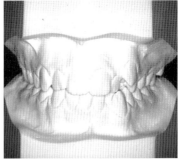

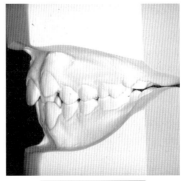

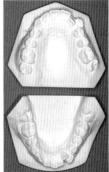

Fig. 9.16 Records for Picture question 1.

Fig. 9.17 Records for Picture question 2.

Picture 2

Examine the records in Fig. 9.17.

1. Classify the incisor relationship.
2. Classify the right and left molar relationships.
3. Assess the degree of crowding in the upper and lower arches.
4. What is the most likely cause of the upper arch crowding?
5. What is the IOTN (DHC) score? (Additional information: no mandibular displacement associated with | 2 or | 7 crossbites.)

DATA INTERPRETATION QUESTION

Given the following cephalometric values: SNA = 78°; SNB = 85°; SN to maxillary plane 7°; MMPA = 30°; 1 to maxillary plane = 130°; 1 to mandibular plane = 75°; answer the following questions, explaining your reasoning.

1. What is the anteroposterior skeletal pattern?
2. Classify the maxillary–mandibular planes angle. Explain your classification.
3. What feature of the malocclusion is expressed by the incisor angulation?

SHORT NOTE QUESTIONS

Write short notes on:

1. Angle's classification of malocclusion
2. The dental health component of the Index of Orthodontic Treatment Need (IOTN)
3. The aesthetic component of IOTN
4. Methods of creating space for relief of crowding other than by extraction.

VIVA QUESTIONS

1. What are the potential benefits/risks of orthodontic treatment? How would you assess the need for treatment?
2. Describe the occlusion of an average primary dentition in a child aged 5 years. What changes occur up to the age of 14 years leading to the establishment of a idealised permanent occlusion?
3. What factors should be considered when obtaining informed consent from a patient prior to orthodontic treatment?

SINGLE BEST ANSWER QUESTIONS

1. Postnatal maxillary growth is more akin to that of the following body tissue type:
   A. Cartilage
   B. Genital
   C. Lymphoid
   D. Neural
   E. Somatic
2. Anterior mandibular growth rotation is associated with:
   A. Concave lower mandibular border
   B. Increased Frankfort–mandibular plane angle
   C. Minimal overbite
   D. Pronounced antegonial notch
   E. Reduced lower facial height
3. Postnatal growth of the cranial vault is usually complete by:
   A. 7 years
   B. 10 years
   C. 12 years
   D. 15 years
   E. 18 years
4. The leeway space on each side of the lower arch is typically:
   A. 0.5 mm
   B. 1.5 mm
   C. 2.5 mm
   D. 3.5 mm
   E. 4.5 mm
5. The IOTN DHC Grade for an overjet of 9 mm is:
   A. 1a
   B. 2a
   C. 3a
   D. 4a
   E. 5a
6. The Zero-meridian line is a:
   A. Line perpendicular to the maxillary plane
   B. Measure of facial asymmetry
   C. Parallel to the occlusal plane
   D. Plane joining the condylar axes
   E. True vertical dropped from soft tissue nasion
7. The Zero-meridian line is used to assess the:
   A. Anteroposterior skeletal pattern
   B. Incisor inclinations to the lips
   C. Maxillary plane cant
   D. Tempero-mandibular joint axis
   E. Smile aesthetics
8. In an idealised smile the upper incisor edges:
   A. Are not visible
   B. Lie 1 mm below the upper lip
   C. Parallel the lower lip
   D. Touch the lower lip
   E. Are in line with the canine tips
9. Rotations are described by the tooth surface:
   A. Easiest to see from the line of the arch
   B. Furthest away from the line of the arch
   C. In the line of the arch
   D. Nearest to the line of the arch
   E. With the broadest tooth contact in the line of the arch
10. The Eastman standard cephalometric norm for the maxilla–mandibular planes angle is:
    A. 21° SD 1°
    B. 23° SD 2°
    C. 25° SD 3°
    D. 27° SD 4°
    E. 29° SD 5°
11. The mandibular plane joins the following cephalometric landmarks:
    A. ANS to PNS
    B. B point to pogonion
    C. Gonion to menton
    D. Porion to orbitale
    E. Sella to nasion
12. Orthodontic treatment has potential long-term benefits to dental health for:
    A. Completely lingually displaced erupted lower second premolar
    B. Increased complete non-traumatic overbite
    C. Mild crowded lower incisors
    D. Overjet of 10 mm with trauma risk
    E. Reverse overjet of 3 mm with no mandibular displacement
13. A reasonable estimate of the space required to reduce a 4-mm curve of Spee would be:
    A. 0.5 mm
    B. 1 mm
    C. 1.5 mm
    D. 2 mm
    E. 2.5 mm
14. Typically enamel removal by interproximal reduction from each proximal surface is:
    A. 0.1 mm
    B. 0.25 mm
    C. 0.5 mm
    D. 0.75 mm
    E. 1 mm

Self-Assessment: Answers

MULTIPLE CHOICE ANSWERS

1. a. False. Derived partially from first pharyngeal arch.
   b. False. Completes growth in width before growth in length.
   c. True.
   d. False. Condylar cartilage directs mandibular growth.
   e. False. In males, maxillary growth is complete, on average, by age 17 years; it is true in females.

2. a. True.
   b. False. It ossifies lateral to Meckel's cartilage.
   c. False. Pattern of growth is not predictable.
   d. False. Growth pattern is independent of maxillary growth pattern.
   e. False. Although, on average, mandibular growth will complete by 18–19 years in males, the mandible continues to grow, albeit at a considerably reduced rate, throughout the next three decades.

3. a. False. It occurs when growth in posterior facial height exceeds that in anterior facial height.
   b. True. A mild forward growth rotation is expected to produce a well-balanced facial appearance.
   c. True. The reduction in the anterior vertical facial proportions will promote overbite increase.
   d. False. Reduced maxillary/mandibular planes angle will result from marked anterior mandibular growth rotation, leading to increased overbite; see (c) above.
   e. False. It is associated with a convex lower mandibular border.

4. a. False. Typically at 3–4 months.
   b. False. Typically 1–1.5 years after eruption.
   c. False. Typically they are upright and spaced.
   d. False. Typically at birth.
   e. False. Greater in the lower than in the upper arch.

5. a. False. It is provided by their eruption in a more proclined angulation labial to the primary predecessors.
   b. True. This will help space requirements.
   c. True. Tends to be about 1–2 mm in primary dentition and 2–3 mm in mixed dentition.
   d. False. Crowding of the primary incisors is likely to provide insufficient space for the permanent incisors.
   e. False. Overbite will have no effect on potential space for the upper permanent incisors.

6. a. False. An increase in lower labial segment crowding is expected.
   b. False. An increase in lower labial segment crowding is expected.
   c. True. This will contribute to lower labial segment crowding.
   d. False. This is not a an expected finding.
   e. True. With uprighting of the lower incisors in response to facial growth changes, the tendency is for the interincisal angle to increase.

7. a. False. For anteroposterior assessment of the dental bases, the patient should be observed from the side.
   b. False. The teeth should be in maximum indigitation, ensuring that the mandible is not postured forward.
   c. False. The patient should be seated upright with the Frankfort plane horizontal.
   d. False. This assesses vertical dental base relationship cephalometrically and not clinical anteroposterior dental base relationship.
   e. False. Dental base relationship is not influenced by the upper incisor angulation.

8. a. False. This represents class III skeletal pattern; class II is present when the mandible is retruded relative to the maxilla.
   b. False. SNB angle tells about the relationship of the mandible to the cranial base; ANB angle tells the relationship of the mandible to the maxilla (i.e. the skeletal pattern).
   c. False. Class II is usually associated with a an as expected or prognathic maxilla.
   d. False. The anteroposterior skeletal pattern cannot be assessed by examination of the first permanent molar relationship, although Angle believed incorrectly that this was possible. It is possible for the first permanent molar relationship to be class II and the skeletal pattern to be also class II, but where early loss of primary teeth has occurred or if significant hypodontia is present, this will be altered.
   e. False. Incisor relationship does not influence the skeletal pattern. A class II skeletal pattern may be associated with a class II incisor relationship, but the latter does not have a direct bearing on the former.

9. a. False. The maxillary plane cannot be assessed clinically so this angle cannot be calculated. Frankfort–mandibular planes angle is assessed clinically.
   b. False. It reflects the vertical skeletal pattern. Anteroposterior skeletal pattern is reflected by the ANB angle.
   c. True. See (b) above.
   d. True. As it is an angular assessment of vertical skeletal pattern.
   e. False. It is not affected by lower incisor position but MMPA has an inverse relationship with lower incisor angulation. As MMPA increases, lower incisor angulation reduces and the converse is also True.

10. a. False. Class II division 2 is an incisor classification and is, therefore, not defined by the buccal segment relationship.
    b. False. This would be present in a class III incisor relationship. For class II malocclusion, the lower incisor edges lie posterior to the cingulum plateau of the upper incisors.
    c. True. This is a characteristic of this malocclusion type.
    d. True. This feature is also part of the British Standards Institute definition of this incisor relationship, although the overjet may also be increased.
    e. True. See (d) above.

11. a. False. The radiograph is taken with the Frankfort plane horizontal or the patient in natural head posture.
    b. False. The tube-to-midsagittal plane distance is usually standardised at the order of about 150 cm.
    c. False. Because of the magnification factor (which is in the range 8–12%), it is not an exact record of facial dimensions.

d. False. It is not essential for orthodontic diagnosis, although it may be of benefit in gaining an insight as to the cause of a malocclusion and in treatment planning.
e. True. It would not, however, be taken solely for this purpose.
12. a. False. It describes the maxillary relationship as 'A' point is on the maxilla.
b. False. The ANB angle is obtained by subtracting SNB from SNA.
c. False. It joins porion and orbitale.
d. True.
e. False. It is the midpoint of the sella turcica.
13. a. False. It indicates the anteroposterior skeletal pattern.
b. True. See (a) above.
c. False. This is reflected in the SNA angle.
d. True. This affects the angles SNA and SNB, and hence their difference ANB.
e. False. The position of porion does not affect the ANB angle.

EXTENDED MATCHING ITEMS ANSWERS

a. **3, 6, 9.** Lower incisor angulation should be assessed in conjunction with ANB and MMPA, observing any dento-alveolar compensation that has occurred for the antero-posterior and vertical skeletal discrepancies respectively. Lower incisor position to A–pogonion line (13) might also be assessed, but for treatment-planning purposes, priority should not be attributed to this parameter.
b. **14.** Superimposition of the two cephalometric tracings or digitisations on the S–N line holding at S will allow evaluation of facial changes.
c. **8, 20.** These will provide the information sought.
d. **19.** As the patient is not interested in pursuing orthodontic treatment, a cephalometric assessment is not indicated.
e. **9, 12.** The interincisal angle is directly related to the vertical relationship of the incisors, which may also be affected by MMPA.

CASE HISTORY ANSWERS

1. As with all orthodontic referrals, the patient's concern regarding appearance of her teeth as well as willingness to wear any likely appliances should be recorded. Medical history should be checked and a detailed history of the nature of the recurrent oral ulceration should be taken. The patient should be made aware that satisfactory wear of an orthodontic appliance may prove impossible depending on the nature and frequency of the recurrent oral ulceration. Thorough investigation of the ulcers should be undertaken, including referral to a consultant in oral medicine for blood tests if these are deemed necessary. If a systemic cause is identified, orthodontic treatment should be delayed until it is treated as the recurrent ulceration may resolve and allow comprehensive treatment with appliance therapy. If the ulceration is particularly severe, appliance therapy will need to be avoided.
2. Obtain all necessary records – study models recorded in centric occlusion and relevant radiographs (a lateral cephalometric film may be required if comprehensive treatment with upper/lower fixed appliances is likely). Decide on aims of treatment: aim for the ideal outcome but bear in mind the medical history; a plan that avoids the wearing of an orthodontic appliance would be optimal if the ulceration does not resolve. Plan the lower arch first: consider crowding (in this case moderate and midarch), canine inclination, overbite, centreline as well as anchorage requirements for all intended tooth movements. Then proceed to the upper arch and assess crowding, canine inclination, incisor angulation (anchorage requirements). Decide on the type of appliance required to effect tooth movements required and appropriate retention plan.
3. If the ulceration does not resolve, and appliance therapy is still warranted, consider fitting an upper removable appliance and monitor the oral reaction to wear before considering any likely extractions. If the ulceration resolves, upper removable appliance therapy alone or upper/lower fixed appliances may be justified, based on the assessment of the occlusal features.

PICTURE ANSWERS

Picture 1

1. Class II division 1.
2. Almost class II half unit on the right (mesiobuccal cusp of 6 occludes in a cusp-to-cusp relationship with 6); class I on the left.
3. Lower arch has mild crowding (note spacing); upper arch has moderate crowding (note spacing).
4. Possible causes are:
   - overjet, possibly mild class II skeletal discrepancy
   - lower arch crowding: early loss of primary molars: note tilting of 6s and distal drifting and rotation of 4s
   - upper arch crowding: inherent dento-alveolar disproportion most likely; early loss of primary teeth unlikely (observe the reasonably good alignment of the premolars).
5. 5i because of impaction of lower 5s.

Picture 2

1. Class I: the lower incisors occlude opposite the cingulum plateau of the upper central incisors.
2. Right is class I; left is half unit class II.
3. Lower arch has moderate crowding; upper arch has moderate crowding.
4. Inherent dento-alveolar disproportion.
5. 4d due to contact point displacement between |2 and |3.

DATA INTERPRETATION ANSWER

1. Class III. Subtracting SNB from SNA gives the ANB angle, a measure of the anteroposterior skeletal pattern. An ANB value of −5.5° after Eastman correction indicates a marked class III skeletal discrepancy.
2. This angle is average. The maxillary–mandibular planes angle may be classified as average ($27 \pm 4°$); high ($>31°$) or low ($<23°$).
3. The upper incisors are very proclined (average angulation $109 \pm 6°$) while the lower incisors are very retroclined (average angulation $93 \pm 6°$), indicating

dento-alveolar compensation for the class III skeletal discrepancy.

SHORT NOTE ANSWERS

1. Angle's classification is used nowadays to classify the anteroposterior molar relationship, although it was originally intended for classification of the anteroposterior dental arch relationship on the assumption that the first permanent molar erupted into a consistently reliable position in the face.
Three molar relationships exist:
Class I: mesiobuccal cusp of the upper first permanent molar occludes in the buccal groove of the lower first permanent molar.
Class II: mesiobuccal cusp of the upper first permanent molar occludes anterior to a class I relationship.
Class III: mesiobuccal cusp of the upper first permanent molar occludes posterior to a class I relationship.

2. This records occlusal features of a malocclusion using a MOCDO convention where M is missing teeth, O is overjet, C is crossbite, D is displacement of contact points and O is overbite. A specially designed ruler aids the process. A malocclusion is then ascribed to one of five categories of treatment need: Grades 1, 2, no/slight need; grade 3, borderline; grades 4, 5, great/very great need. Assessment by this means is objective, reliable and rapid.

3. This scores the need for treatment of a malocclusion based on the degree of aesthetic impairment of the anterior teeth. Assessment is made by viewing the anterior occlusion either clinically or from study models and comparing this with a set of 10 photographs of increasing aesthetic handicap. Treatment need is accorded as: grades 1–4, no/slight need; grades 5–7, borderline need; grades 8–10, definite need. The set of photographs does not include a full range of malocclusion types and assessment is subjective.

4. Space may be created by each of the following means:
a. Arch expansion: only indicated where a unilateral crossbite exists, especially if there is an associated displacement.
b. Distal movement of the buccal segments: may be undertaken in the lower arch if extraction of a lower second permanent molar is considered, but rarely adopted as an approach to relief of crowding. If undertaken, a fixed appliance is invariably required. In the upper arch, bilateral distal movement of the buccal segments using headgear may be undertaken to provide space for relief of mild upper arch crowding or correction of a small overjet. In these patients, the lower arch should be well aligned and the molar relationship no greater than half unit class II. Unilateral distal movement may be undertaken when space is required on one side of the arch only and may be undertaken using a screw section in a removable appliance, although provision for incorporation of headgear in the appliance is advisable. To remove the need for headgear use, a TAD may be used instead in combination with a fixed appliance to bring about the desired movement. Consider extraction of upper second permanent molar(s) to aid distal movement in the upper arch provided third molars are present and of good size and position.
c. Interdental stripping: only really a consideration in adults where a small amount of space is required for alignment. Usually confined to the lower labial segment. Involves the removal of ~0.25 mm from the mesial and distal surfaces of each tooth.
d. Any combination of above.

VIVA ANSWERS

1. The potential benefits of orthodontic treatment to the patient should outweigh the potential risks and side-effects.
The potential benefits of orthodontic treatment are quite limited. The relationship between dental caries and malocclusion is unproven. Periodontal health can be improved by orthodontic treatment of occlusal relationships traumatising the periodontal tissues, e.g. a traumatic overbite or incisor crossbite with mandibular displacement leading to mobility with/without gingival recession of a lower incisor. Where an impacted tooth is removed, the resorption risk to the associated teeth is reduced; the risk of incisor trauma may be reduced by overjet correction but the benefits of early intervention indicate no significant gains in this regard. Although TMD has been shown to be associated with crossbites, anterior open bite, class II due to mandibular retrusion and asymmetry, this is weak. Orthodontic treatment cannot be guaranteed to cure TMD. There are psychological benefits accruing from correction of increased overjet or anterior spacing which include improved self-concept and less negative experiences.
The potential risks are failure to achieve the aims of treatment; pulpal, gingival and mucosal damage; root resorption and loss of alveolar crestal height; and possibly instigation or exacerbation of temporomandibular joint dysfunction syndrome (see Section 9.4). With fixed appliances, the risk of decalcification is increased while there is a small but significant risk of facial or ocular damage from headgear.
The need for treatment may be assessed using the Index of Orthodontic Treatment Need (see Section 9.2). This has two components, but the dental health rather than the aesthetic component can only be assessed reliably.

2. In the average primary dentition at age 5 years, abcde have erupted in all quadrants. Although the 'ideal' features have been described as a generalised spaced dentition with specific space mesial to the upper and distal to the lower cs (anthropoid spaces), upright incisors with a relatively deep overbite and flush terminal planes, these rarely occur and great individual variation is encountered.
Where the overbite has been deep initially, it usually reduces by 5 years of age, and an edge-to-edge incisor relationship with attrition is common. From about age 6 years onwards, the permanent dentition starts to erupt, usually commencing with the eruption of the lower incisors or of the lower first permanent molars as growth posteriorly in the arch accommodates them. As the permanent incisors erupt lingual to their

predecessors, some incisor crowding is often seen, but this generally resolves with growth in the intercanine width.

Order and dates of eruption of permanent teeth are given in Tables 7.1 and 7.2 (Chapter 7, p. 194).

Space for the upper incisors is provided by the primary incisor spacing, intercanine growth (1–2 mm in the primary and .3 mm in the mixed dentition) and the more proclined inclination of the permanent incisors. Commonly, these teeth erupt spaced and distally inclined but the spacing reduces as the permanent canines erupt. These should be palpable in the buccal sulcus at age 10 years and are guided into position by the roots of the permanent lateral incisors.

Space for the premolars and permanent canines is provided by intercanine growth and the 'leeway space', typically 1–1.5 mm and 2–2.5 mm in the upper and lower arches, respectively. The greater space in the lower than in the upper arch also may allow the molar relationship to correct from a possible half a unit class II to a class I relationship.

By 14 years of age, the permanent occlusion should be all but complete apart from third molars, if present. The six features of a good ('ideal') permanent occlusion are given in Section 9.1.

3. All the points listed below should be gone through in a systematic order in a format that is understandable to the patient, with adequate time given to question any item that is not entirely clear.

   a. The diagnosis (problem list) should be outlined to the patient and/or parent together with the dental health component of IOTN. The significance of the latter should be explained.

   b. If there is more than one possible approach to treatment, the various options should be explained together with the 'pros' and 'cons' of each. If there are risks attached to undertaking no treatment, this must be explained also.

   c. Appliances to be used for treatment must be explained and examples demonstrated – colour photographs are a good means of doing this. If headgear is required,

this requires special consideration together with an explanation of the specific care required in its use. If a TAD is to be used, this should also be explained.

   d. Likely treatment intervals and an estimate of treatment length should be given.

   e. The compliance required from the patient during orthodontic treatment must also be emphasised: the need for maintenance of a high standard of oral hygiene; regular dental attendance for routine dental care; cooperation required with appliance wear, particularly if headgear or intraoral elastic wear is prescribed; and importance of attendance for appliance adjustment at the appointed times. The retention regimen and its importance should also be explained.

   f. Importance of risks of each treatment plan (i.e. root resorption, decalcification, alveolar bone loss, relapse potential) should be explained to the patient and parent/guardian, taking care not to dramatise sequelae, which are likely to be minor.

   g. An information sheet may be useful for the patient to take away to think over all the issues related to treatment prior to giving consent for treatment at a subsequent visit.

SINGLE BEST ANSWER QUESTION ANSWERS

Question 1: D
Question 2: E
Question 3: A.
Question 4: C.
Question 5: D.
Question 6: E
Question 7: A
Question 8: C
Question 9: B
Question 10: D
Question 11: C
Question 12: D
Question 13: C
Question 14: B

10 Orthodontics II: Management of Occlusal Problems

Overview

The management of malocclusion comprises a substantial part of orthodontic practice. It ranges from interception of developing occlusal problems through to comprehensive correction of established malocclusion in the adolescent or adult. It also encompasses the special requirements in orthodontic care of those with cleft lip and/or palate.

This chapter describes the management of the developing dentition and of all major anomalies of established malocclusion, including surgical correction. The occlusal problems particular to cleft lip and/or palate together with their management are also outlined.

10.1 Problem Solving in the Developing Dentition

LEARNING OBJECTIVES

You should:
- know the problems which are best dealt with in the developing dentition
- be able to classify supernumerary teeth
- know how to localise an unerupted tooth in the anterior maxilla
- understand the principles of management of an unerupted 1, ectopic 3 and first permanent molar with poor long-term prognosis.

Although most orthodontic treatment is undertaken when the permanent dentition is established, some aspects of the developing occlusion may be better dealt with in the mixed dentition. Such interception may eliminate the need for, or simplify, later treatment. Systematic and regular screening of the developing dentition is essential to this process.

ANOMALIES OF ERUPTION AND EXFOLIATION

Both eruption and exfoliation of primary and permanent teeth may be premature or delayed.

Natal Teeth

Natal teeth are usually lower incisors that are erupted at birth or appear soon after. Removal is indicated only if they interfere with suckling or if they are so mobile as to be at risk of inhalation.

Eruption of Teeth

Other than natal teeth, the following points should be borne in mind:

- There is greater variation in the eruption sequence of primary teeth between races than there is in eruption times.
- Poor diet and chronic ill-health in child populations may alter eruption sequence.
- Permanent teeth tend to erupt later in White European people compared to people of East and South East Asia, who in turn tend to have later eruption times than Black Central and Southern African people.
- Females tend to erupt their permanent teeth earlier than males, particularly second and third molars.

Factors causing premature exfoliation or delay in the eruption and exfoliation of primary or permanent teeth are given in Table 10.1.

To ensure that any deviation in the typical eruption sequence is detected early, clinical vigilance is required during the developing dentition, supported by radiographic investigations where necessary. Particular attention should be given to the permanent maxillary incisors and canines, as early recognition of an anomaly in their eruption improves the prognosis.

Table 10.1   Causes of Premature or Delayed Eruption of Primary or Permanent Teeth.

	Causes
Premature eruption	Familial tendency Primary dentition: high birthweight Permanent dentition: early-onset puberty, excess growth or thyroid hormone secretion
Delayed eruption	Primary dentition: very low birthweight, premature birth General causes: Down or Turner syndromes, severe nutritional deficiency, hypothyroidism/ hypopituitarism, cleidocranial dysplasia, hereditary gingival hyperplasia, cleft lip and palate Local causes: ectopic crypt position, supernumerary or odontome, developmental absence, retention of primary tooth, dilaceration, primary failure of eruption, crowding
Premature exfoliation	Commonly caries or trauma Rarely hereditary hypophosphatasia, developmental neutropenia, cyclic neutropenia, Chediak–Higashi syndrome, histiocytosis X
Delayed exfoliation	Developmental absence of permanent successor Ectopic position of permanent successor Trauma Severe periradicular infection of primary tooth

Hypodontia

The most common missing teeth are:

- third molars (25–35%)
- upper lateral incisors (2%)
- lower second premolars (3%)
- lower incisors (0.5%).

Hypodontia affects females more than males with a ratio of 3:2 and depending on the number of developmentally absent teeth, excluding third molars, may be classified as mild (1 or 2), moderate (3 – 6) or severe (greater than 6). The aetiology may be non-syndromic or syndromic, the former arising from a multifactorial interplay of environmental (systemic and local) and genetic (*MSX1*, *PAX9*, *AXIN2*) factors. Premolar and molar agenesis is related mostly to alterations in *MSX1* and *PAX9* respectively, whereas agenesis affecting several tooth types is linked to changes in *AXIN2*. With over a hundred syndromes associated with hypodontia, some of the more common are cleft lip and/or palate where almost 75% may be affected, Down syndrome, Ehlers–Danlos syndrome and ectodermal dysplasia. Additional dental features commonly found include microdontia, hypoplastic enamel, abnormal crown shape, infraoccluded primary molars and ectopic maxillary canines. Lower face height is also often reduced with an increase in overbite.

Absent Third Molars

Extraction of a second molar, either to facilitate distal movement of the upper buccal segments or to relieve posterior crowding, should not be considered in the absence of a third molar. These start to calcify any time between 8 and 14 years.

Absent Upper Lateral Incisors

Management options for the space created by absent upper lateral incisors are:

- space opening
- space maintenance
- space closure.

The final decision depends on:

- the patient's attitude to orthodontic treatment
- the anteroposterior and vertical skeletal relationships
- amount of exposure of the upper canines and incisors on smiling
- the colour, size, shape and inclination of the canine and incisor teeth
- whether the arches are spaced or crowded
- the buccal segment occlusion.

The possible plans are best assessed by carrying out a trial set-up of each on duplicate study models, followed by joint consultation with a restorative colleague.

SPACE OPENING. In uncrowded or mildly crowded arches, when the buccal segment occlusion is class I or, at most, half unit class II, or in class III where proclination of the incisors is likely to correct an anterior crossbite, space opening is best. In addition, in patients with low Frankfort-mandibular plane angle (FMPA) or where the maxillary canine is considerably darker than the incisors, it may be best to open rather than close the anterior spaces. A fixed appliance is required to localise space for the missing units, followed by at least 3–6 months of removable appliance retention ensuring that the space is maintained by placing wire spurs in contact with the adjoining teeth in addition to prosthetic tooth replacements. Where artificial teeth are added to a vacuum-formed retainer rather than to a Hawley retainer, the former must not be worn while eating or drinking. In selected cases, autotransplantation of lower premolars (extracted for relief of crowding) to the upper lateral incisor area may be possible but this may be difficult due to relative crown size differences. Rarely has a lower incisor been autotransplanted to an upper lateral incisor space but only if a satisfactory occlusal outcome is likely. More commonly, the missing units may be replaced on resin-retained bridgework, and occasionally by implants at a later date provided in the latter case that there is adequate width and height of alveolar bone along with root parallelism of the abutment teeth. If bridge work is planned, it is important to ensure that sufficient interocclusal clearance exists or has been created during appliance therapy for placement of the metal framework or for the pontic in the case of an implant. In the short term of 3–5 years, success rates of 85% and 95% have been reported with resin-bonded bridges and single-tooth implant-supported prostheses, respectively.

SPACE CLOSURE. In crowded mouths, early extraction of the primary canines should be carried out to encourage mesial drift of the posterior teeth, but a later phase of fixed appliance therapy is usually needed to align and approximate the upper anterior teeth, followed by bonded retention. Recontouring of the canines in addition to composite build-up of their mesio-incisal aspects is advisable before treatment starts to assist with definitive tooth positioning; final restorations are placed following appliance removal. Bleaching of the canines may also be required to enhance aesthetics. Overjet reduction by space closure may be more favourable than resorting to midarch extractions and space opening. Space closure is likely to be facilitated in patients with increased FMPA, crowding and where the buccal segment relationship is a full unit class II.

Absent Second Premolars

The primary second molar should preferably be retained where the arch is uncrowded or aligned. Prospects are good long term if they survive to 20 years of age. If the tooth starts to infraocclude, an occlusal onlay may be placed to maintain it in function. Removal of the lower second primary molar shortly after eruption of the lateral incisors will encourage spontaneous space closure in mildly crowded cases; in those with marked crowding, its extraction should be delayed until orthodontic treatment commences so that the resulting space may be used for arch alignment. Where it is necessary to extract the second primary molar and the resultant space is substantial, additional anchorage will need to be considered to move the lower molars forward without the lower labial segment being moved lingually. Alternatively acceptance of the space as it is out of sight and if not compromising occlusal function may be a possibility. In the upper arch, extraction of the second primary molar is best deferred until orthodontic treatment is about to start. Rarely, a lower second premolar develops late and necessitates an alteration in the original treatment plan.

Absent Lower Central Incisors

In the absence of permanent lower central incisors, root resorption and progressive incisal wear may lead to loss of the primary incisors in the late mixed dentition, although occasionally they can last longer. With one absent lower incisor, space closure is likely to increase the overjet and overbite, favourable where these are minimal and for correction of a class III incisor relationship; space opening is normally preferable in class II cases. Where both lower central incisors are absent, confining spacing to the lateral incisor areas is usually better due to the favourable characteristics afforded by the lower canines to support resin-retained bridgework.

Supernumerary Teeth

Teeth additional to the usual number are termed 'supernumerary'. Most common in the anterior maxilla (80%), they may occur between the central incisors (mesiodens) but often also develop distal to the last tooth in each dental series (lateral incisor, second premolar and third molar) as an exuberant growth of the dental lamina. The exact aetiology is not known but it seems genetic factors play a part. They are more common:

- in males than in females (relative reported frequency approximately 2:1 in White European populations)
- in the permanent than in the primary dentition (respective incidences around 2% and 1%)
- in children with cleft of the lip and alveolus, cleidocranial dysplasia and Gardner syndrome.

Those in the anterior maxilla can be categorised into three groups: conical, tuberculate and supplemental.

Conical Teeth

Conical teeth occur between the upper permanent central incisors; they are often singular but can sometimes occur in combination with others of similar form. They may have no effect if they are well above the apices of the incisors. If there is no risk of damage to adjacent teeth with tooth movement, they can be left in place and observed. Often, however, they may displace the adjacent teeth, perhaps creating a large diastema, or they may delay eruption. In these instances, removal is indicated. Occasionally, a conical supernumerary tooth erupts and can be extracted.

Tuberculate Teeth

Tuberculate teeth are the most common cause of an unerupted permanent maxillary central incisor. Suspicion should be raised if the lateral incisors erupt in advance of the centrals. In these cases, a radiograph of the premaxilla should be taken to allow early detection and localisation of any supernumerary, which should then be surgically removed. An attachment with gold chain should be bonded to the unerupted incisor to allow provision for orthodontic alignment if the tooth fails to erupt spontaneously within 12 months of surgery. In conjunction with surgery, space to accommodate the unerupted tooth must be maintained or opened by appliance therapy; the latter may entail extraction of the upper primary canines.

Supplemental Teeth

The supplemental tooth resembles the expected tooth in morphology and commonly produces crowding or displacement of adjacent teeth. Usually, the tooth, which is similar to the contralateral tooth, is better retained (provided it is not severely malpositioned) and the other incisor is extracted.

ANOMALIES OF DEVELOPMENT

First Permanent Molars With Poor Long-Term Prognosis

The first permanent molar is never the extraction of choice for orthodontic reasons but is invariably enforced because of poor prognosis resulting from caries and/or enamel hypoplasia. Molar incisor hypoplasia (MIH) has an unknown aetiology but is reckoned to be multifactorial with genetic and systemic (acute and chronic illnesses) factors thought to interact; it affects about one in seven children worldwide with no gender bias. It may lead to marked enamel breakdown, associated dental caries and dental sensitivity. Enamel demineralisation on the lingual aspect of lower first permanent molars or on the buccal aspect of upper first permanent molars should be treated seriously, as it is often a hallmark of a high caries rate and possible limited lifespan of these teeth. When a two-surface or deep occlusal restoration is indicated in one molar 2–3 years after eruption, careful assessment of the malocclusion and the condition of the other first permanent molars should be made. Timely removal may lead to considerable spontaneous correction of the malocclusion in certain patients but it does little for relief of incisor crowding or correction of an incisor relationship unless appliance therapy is instituted.

A 'cook book' approach to each patient with poor-quality first permanent molars is not possible but some guidelines are listed in Box 10.1.

Infraoccluded Primary Molars

Between 1% and 9% of children are likely to exhibit this anomaly but estimates regarding its incidence vary. A genetic tendency has been suggested with absent premolars, ectopic position of the first permanent molars and palatal canine displacement identified as associated factors. Infraocclusion results from ankylosis of the tooth while alveolar growth and eruption of the adjacent teeth continues. Provided the permanent successor is present, exfoliation will occur eventually, but removal is indicated in its absence and where the infraocclusion is marked, with the crown of the tooth just visible, or where root development of the unerupted premolar is almost complete.

Impaction of the Maxillary First Permanent Molar

Impaction of the maxillary first permanent molar occurs in 2–6% of children. It may correct spontaneously (unlikely after the upper lateral incisors erupt) or it may require disimpaction of the molar either by placing a brass wire separator between the adjacent teeth (in mild cases) or by appliance therapy (in more marked impaction). Extraction of the second primary molar is required if the impaction produces symptomatic resorption with pulpal involvement or to facilitate restoration of the first permanent molar. Crowding is exacerbated by the subsequent mesial drift of the first permanent molar, but this can be treated later.

Aberrant Position of Second Premolars

Occasionally, the second premolars appear in slightly unfavourable positions when viewed on a radiograph, but generally this is of no long-term consequence and their final position is usually satisfactory. A grossly ectopic second premolar is rare and may be observed or surgically removed.

Posterior Crossbite With Mandibular Displacement

Sometimes, a unilateral crossbite of the buccal segment teeth with mandibular displacement follows a prolonged finger- or thumb-sucking habit. In some children, grinding the primary canines can lead to correction and prevent perpetuation of the crossbite from the mixed to the permanent dentition; where this is not effective, arch expansion by using either a removable appliance and a midline screw or a quadhelix is required to reduce the chance of the crossbite being present in the permanent dentition. The latter treatment method is more efficient and cost-effective. Alternatively, correction may be deferred until the premolars erupt (Fig. 10.1).

TREATMENT OF ANOMALIES BY SERIAL EXTRACTIONS

In 1948, Kjellgren, a Swedish orthodontist, ascribed the term 'serial extractions' to the following three-stage procedure:

- Extraction of the primary canines at age 8.5–9.5 years to encourage alignment of the permanent incisors.
- Extraction of the first primary molars approximately 1 year later to encourage eruption of the first premolars.
- Extraction of the first premolars as the permanent canines are erupting.

The full extent of the original technique is never adopted in contemporary orthodontic practice, as three episodes of extractions are unpleasant for any child and may psychologically scar their attitude to subsequent dental treatment. In addition, simultaneous intervention at a time when the intercanine width is increasing makes gauging the extent

---

Box 10.1 Guidelines for Management of First Permanent Molars (FPM) With Poor Long-Term Prognosis.

- Institute preventive measures including oral hygiene motivation, dietary advice and fluoride therapy.
- Evaluate social circumstances, motivation for restorative and orthodontic treatment, level of dental awareness, general anaesthetic need, age and class of malocclusion.
- Ensure (radiographically) that all permanent teeth, particularly second premolars and third molars, are present and that all others are of good prognosis. Avoid extraction of an FPM in a quadrant with an absent tooth, or in uncrowded arches.
- Assess the need to balance or compensate for extraction of an FPM but balancing extraction of sound FPMs is seldom indicated. To avoid occlusal interference from overeruption of 7, consider extraction of the upper FPM when extraction of a lower FPM is required but the corollary does not apply.
- Timing of extraction of lower FPM is best when the bifurcations are calcifying (aged approximately 8.5–9.5 years) and moderate premolar crowding is present.
- Timing of extraction of upper FPM is less important because of the distal tilt and downward and forward eruption path of 7.
- Extraction of upper FPM is best delayed:
  - in Class III until the incisor crossbite is corrected
  - in Class II division 1 until 7s erupt
  - in severely crowded mouths until 7s erupt.
- Extraction of lower FPM may be deferred in Class III with marked incisor crowding until lower 7s erupt.
- Monitor eruption of second and third molars.

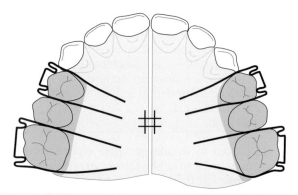

Fig. 10.1 Upper removable appliance to correct unilateral buccal segment crossbite with associated mandibular displacement. • Midline expansion screw; Adams' clasps 64|46 (0.7 mm SS wire); buccal capping.

of crowding problematic. The process was originally intended to remove the need for appliance therapy but, in practice, this is seldom the case. In children with class I malocclusion, however, aged 10–12 years, with moderate crowding, a full complement of teeth in favourable positions and no concern about the long-term prognosis of the first permanent molars, a reasonable outcome may be forthcoming from removal of the first premolars alone, without recourse to the earlier extraction of primary teeth. Planned extraction, however, of the primary canines is beneficial in the following instances:

- To allow labial movement of a permanent upper lateral incisor erupting palatal to the permanent upper central incisors and in potential crossbite.
- To create space in the upper labial segment for proclination of an instanding permanent lateral incisor or the eruption of a permanent incisor, where a supernumerary tooth has delayed its appearance.
- To promote alignment of a displaced permanent maxillary canine; this is particularly beneficial where the canine is displaced palatally.
- To facilitate lingual movement of a labially placed permanent lower incisor with reduced periodontal support or of the lower labial segment to aid anterior crossbite correction in class III malocclusion.

OTHER DEVELOPMENTAL PROBLEMS

Early Loss of Primary Teeth

Early loss of primary teeth is most commonly caused by caries but, occasionally, it results from premature exfoliation, often when there is severe crowding, or it may be planned (e.g. to encourage space closure by mesial drift of the buccal segments in children who are missing one or more permanent teeth). In all cases, consideration should be given to balancing (extraction of the same tooth on the opposite side of the arch) or to compensating (extraction of the equivalent opposing tooth) for an extraction, the respective justification being to avoid a shift of the midline or to ensure that the occlusion is not compromised. Premature loss of a primary tooth does not inevitably lead to premature eruption of the permanent successor.

The effects of early loss of a primary tooth depend on several factors including:

- the patient's age
- the degree of crowding
- the tooth extracted
- the arch from which it is removed
- the type of occlusion.

All of these influence the potential for crowding to be concentrated at the extraction site. In general, this potential is greatest in a young child with pre-existing crowding when a maxillary posterior tooth is removed with poor buccal segment intercuspation.

Incisors

Early loss of a primary incisor tends to have minimal effect as it usually exfoliates in the early mixed dentition. Premature loss of a primary incisor through trauma may, however, lead to dilaceration of the permanent successor.

Canines

Unilateral loss of a primary canine invariably leads to movement of the centreline and should be balanced to prevent this occurring.

First Molars

Occasionally, displacement of the centreline follows early extraction of a first primary molar, but the need for a balancing extraction is best assessed by checking the midlines at subsequent reviews.

Second Primary Molars

Where the second primary molar is extracted, the first permanent molar migrates mesially and may lead to considerable space loss if the extraction is carried out before the permanent molar erupts; hence, it is preferable to delay extraction until the first permanent molar has erupted. Provided the prognosis of the other second primary molars is favourable, in general, the need for a compensating or balancing extraction is unlikely but should be assessed on a case-by-case basis.

Space Maintenance for Early Tooth Loss

Space maintenance is indicated:

- when premature loss of a tooth promotes crowding in an otherwise acceptable occlusion
- in severely crowded mouths where all of the extraction space is required for alignment of the remaining teeth
- following traumatic loss of an upper permanent incisor.

A removable appliance will usually suffice in the upper arch but a lingual arch soldered to bands cemented to molar teeth is best in the lower. The impact on dental health and potential to strain co-operation with regard to further comprehensive treatment should be borne in mind.

Upper Median Diastema

Upper median diastema is a typical phase of dental development and reduces as the permanent maxillary canines erupt. It has a tendency to run in families or may be racial in origin or result from:

- a midline supernumerary tooth
- missing or small upper lateral incisors
- incisor proclination in class II division 1 malocclusion (Section 10.3) or due to a digit-sucking habit
- a more generalised spacing condition due to mismatch in tooth/arch size (Section 10.2).

A radiograph of the upper incisor area should be taken to exclude the presence of a supernumerary tooth in those with a large midline diastema. Rarely, a low-lying attachment of the labial frenum is a primary cause, as the attachment usually recedes as the incisors approximate. In a spaced arch, this does not occur, indicating that the frenum is associated with, but not causative of, the diastema.

Where the frenum is implicated in causing a diastema, blanching of the incisive papilla usually occurs when the lip is pulled upwards or outwards, with characteristic V-shaped notching of the alveolar bone between the two central incisors visible radiographically. The need for fraenectomy should be assessed after eruption of the permanent canines and is preferably undertaken during space closure as the scar tissue will aid approximation of the incisors. Treatment of the diastema in the early mixed dentition may be necessary if there is insufficient space for the lateral incisors and the diastema exceeds 3 mm but vigilance is needed to ensure that the lateral incisor roots are not moved into the path of the erupting canines. A fixed appliance is usually required to close an upper midline space, with bodily approximation of the incisors followed by palatal bonded retention.

Dilaceration

Dilaceration is a sudden angular alteration in the long axis of the crown or in the root of a tooth. Most commonly it results from intrusion of a primary incisor driving the crown of the permanent successor palatally, and it leads to enamel and dentine hypoplasia. On occasion, dilaceration is developmental in origin, more so in females and with a characteristic labial and superior coronal deflection of the tooth involved. Usually, a dilacerated incisor remains unerupted and when markedly affected requires surgical removal but, if the dilaceration is mild, surgical exposure and orthodontic alignment may be feasible when the root apex is destined not to perforate the cortical plate.

Traumatic Loss of an Upper Permanent Central Incisor

As the adjacent teeth tend to tilt towards the site of loss in the first days following trauma, the space must be maintained, ideally by immediate reimplantation of the tooth or by fitting a denture carrying a replacement tooth. Later, autotransplantation of preferably a single-rooted premolar (either upper second or a lower) with restorative modification or prosthetic replacement by adhesive or fixed bridgework or implant may be considered. This is generally preferable to space closure, as a lateral incisor rarely gives an optimum appearance in a central incisor position, even with coronal build-up and gingival recontouring. Involvement of oral surgery, paediatric dental and restorative colleagues is required for optimal treatment planning. Should autotransplantation be considered, provided that adequate space has been created and the donor site carefully prepared, this is best undertaken when two-thirds to three-quarters of the root is developed, ensuring an atraumatic technique and that the tooth is positioned at gingival level before splinting for 7 – 10 days. This procedure has good success with failure only reported in 10% – 15% of cases.

Incisors in Crossbite

Early correction of a crossbite involving a permanent incisor is essential to prevent displacing occlusal forces compromising the periodontal support of the lower anterior teeth and to allow the occlusion to develop around an undisplaced condylar position. Provided there is likely to be adequate overbite of 2–3 mm, an upper removable appliance with a double-cantilever spring to procline the instanding incisor and posterior capping to disengage the occlusion will usually suffice (see Section 10.5 and Fig. 10.2); a screw section clasping the teeth in crossbite

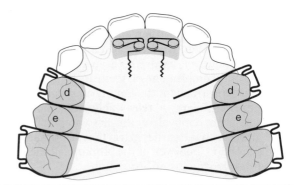

Fig. 10.2 Upper removable appliance to procline 1|1 in the early mixed dentition, assuming all primary teeth are in good condition. • Double-cantilever springs 1|1 (0.5 mm SS wire); Adams' clasps d|d (0.6 mm SS wire) and 6|6 (0.7 mm SS wire); posterior capping 2–3 mm in height to disengage the anterior occlusion.

will maintain appliance retention where two or more teeth need to be moved anteriorly. It may be necessary to remove the upper primary canines to facilitate crossbite correction on a permanent upper lateral incisor or the lower primary canines to allow alignment of a labially placed permanent lower incisor.

Habits

Depending on the positioning of a finger(s) or thumb, the frequency and intensity of a sucking habit may:

- procline the upper incisors
- retrocline the lower incisors
- increase the overjet, often asymmetrically
- reduce the overbite
- lead to a crossbite tendency of the buccal segments.

Gentle persuasion to discontinue the habit should be given and simple measures adopted to effect this. Fitting of a fixed habit breaker (palatal crib or palatal arch) may be considered if the child is eager to stop.

Increased Overjet

Where the overjet is greater than 3 mm, the risk of incisor trauma is more than doubled; trauma is more common in boys and the risk is greater with incompetent lips. An initial phase of functional appliance treatment to retract the incisors may be beneficial in these children or where the malocclusion is associated with bullying. A second phase with fixed appliances, however, is generally required to detail the occlusion with possibly premolar extractions for relief of crowding. As overall treatment time is increased and considerable demands placed on patient co-operation, the likely benefits of such early intervention must be deemed to outweigh potential disadvantages including the risk of upper incisor root resorption if these teeth are retracted into the eruption path of the upper canines.

Results of a North American clinical trial found that early skeletal effects produced by either functional or headgear therapy in the preadolescent period were not maintained long term. In addition, little or no differences existed following fixed appliance therapy in the permanent dentition between those who had been treated earlier or who had been observed until the permanent dentition erupted. Furthermore, a multicentre UK trial established that functional appliance treatment at 8–10 years of age did not result in a better skeletal or occlusal outcome. Consequently many clinicians now prefer to wait until the permanent dentition before starting treatment in these cases. Functional appliance treatment in the early mixed dentition, however, is indicated to reduce the risk of incisor trauma or where a child is being teased because of the malocclusion. The need for a custom-made mouthguard for sports should also be emphasised for all children with an increased overjet.

Ectopic Maxillary Canines

The maxillary canine is ectopic in approximately 2% of the population, with 15% of these buccal and 85% palatal to the arch. Development of the maxillary canine begins about 4–5 months after birth, the crown is complete around 6–7 years and eruption is typically at 11–12 years. From an initial position high in the maxilla, the tooth moves buccally downwards and forwards to be guided into its final position by the distal aspect of the lateral incisor root. For this reason, absence or diminution in the size of the lateral incisor increases the incidence of displacement (×2.4). There also appears to be a greater incidence of palatal canine displacement where the maxillary arch is spaced or in class II division 2 malocclusion; a polygenic multifactorial aetiology has been suggested for palatal displacement. With this, there is a familial and racial (more common in Europeans) tendency, greater prevalence in females than males and an increased bilateral occurrence than seems likely. In addition, there is an association with absent or small teeth, infraoccluded primary molars, impacted upper first permanent molars and other ectopic teeth. The long eruption path and in the case of more pronounced displacement, ectopic position of the tooth germ, are additional possible aetiological factors. Buccal displacement is more common in crowded arches. Where routine palpation of the buccal sulcus at 10–11 years fails to detect a canine prominence, the path of eruption is likely to deviate from the expected. In addition, considerable delay in the eruption of a canine compared with the opposite side of the arch points to canine displacement.

Transposition

Transposition occurs when the position of the canine is interchanged with that of an adjacent tooth. It has a prevalence of less than 1% and an aetiology involving genetic and environmental factors. In the upper arch, the maxillary canine and first premolar, or the lateral incisor and canine, are involved, although the former arrangement is more common. In the lower arch, the lateral incisor and canine teeth are solely affected.

Estimating the Maxillary Canine Position

CLINICAL ESTIMATE. Buccal and palatal palpation along with observation of the lateral incisor inclination give a hint to the canine position. When it is lying low and palatal or high and buccal, the lateral incisor is likely to be labially inclined.

RADIOGRAPHIC ESTIMATION. Although a dental panoramic tomogram is helpful in the initial assessment of the canine position, it underestimates its potential for alignment; the tooth is actually closer to the midline and at a more acute angle than it appears radiographically. Further radiographic views are needed to locate the position of the tooth. Most commonly an upper anterior occlusal view, preferably taken at 70 – 75°, or two periapical films taken with a tube shift are needed to allow localisation, using vertical or horizontal parallax respectively. The axial inclination, apex location and the vertical and mesiodistal position of the canine relative to the incisor roots should be assessed. The permanent incisors should be checked carefully to exclude resorption, and the root length of the primary canine noted. Resorption of incisors is more common in females than males and there is a 50% greater risk of its occurrence should the canine be at a greater than 25° angulation to the midline when viewed on a dental panoramic tomogram. If incisor resorption is detected, urgent treatment is indicated. Removal of the impacted canine may arrest the resorption but extraction of the incisor may be required in those with severe resorption. Cone-beam computed tomography (CBCT) can reveal the full extent of resorption.

Management of Canine Displacement

The management of buccal or palatal maxillary canine displacement including transposition is described in Table 10.2.

ANOMALIES OF SIZE AND FORM

Size

Teeth of a size that is greater or less than the norms for gender and for a given population are described as 'megadont' or 'microdont', respectively.

Megadontia has a prevalence of 1.1% in the permanent dentition, with maxillary central incisors most frequently affected, although lower second premolars are affected occasionally. The typical shape and absence of incisor notching distinguishes megadont maxillary incisors from 'double teeth'. Megadont teeth may be found unilaterally on the affected side in unilateral facial hyperplasia, but more generalised megadontia is associated with gigantism. A megadont upper incisor may produce crowding, an increased overjet or both. If the tooth is only slightly enlarged, removal of about 1 mm of enamel from each proximal surface and appliance therapy to close the resultant space may suffice. In gross enlargement, extraction of the affected tooth and placement of a pontic following any appliance treatment may be necessary.

Microdontia is frequently seen in association with hypodontia, in Down syndrome and in ectodermal dysplasia. The prevalence is 0.2–0.5% in the primary dentition and 2.5% in the permanent dentition, with diminutive upper lateral incisors accounting for 1–2% of the latter. Short roots are often found on these teeth, which may be a factor in the aetiology of palatally displaced canines. In crowded mouths, where the lateral incisor is peg-shaped on one side of the arch and of typical size on the opposite side, removal of both lateral incisors may be optimal to achieve symmetry

Table 10.2   Management of Maxillary Canine Displacement.[a]

	Treatment Options	Indications	Comments
Buccal displacement	Early removal of 4 before 3 erupts	Moderate crowding	May require removable or sectional fixed appliance to align 3 depending on axial inclination
	Exposure of 3	Delayed eruption of 3	Apically repositioned flap or replaced flap required at surgery Bond bracket or gold chain to 3 to facilitate alignment
	Removal of 3	Severe crowding with 2 and 4 in contact 3 severely displaced	May require fixed appliance to detail the occlusion or close any remaining space
Palatal displacement	Early removal of c[b]	Ectopic position of 3 detected at 10–13 years of age 3 overlaps up to half width of 2 3 crown below the apical third of 2 root 3 long axis to midsagittal plane ≤30° Ideally, crowding in arch no greater than mild	Extract contralateral c to prevent centerline shift; extraction of c may promote crowding Failure of 3 to erupt will leave space
	Exposure of 3	Well-disposed patient Good oral hygiene and dentition 3 overlaps less than half width of 1 and below the apical third of 2 root 3 root apex is not distal to 5 and 3 long axis ≤30° to midsagittal plane Spaced arch or possible to create space	Bond bracket or gold chain to 3 at surgery May commence alignment of 3 with removable appliance but fixed appliance usually required to align apex of 3 Prospects for alignment reduced and treatment time extended in adults
	Transplantation	Hopeless prognosis for alignment of 3 Adequate space in arch for 3 Intact removal of 3 possible Adequate buccal/palatal bone	Prognosis improved if root of 3 is two-thirds to three-quarters formed, minimal root handling at surgery, 3 not in occlusion with 6 weeks of sectional archwire splint Approximately 70% survival rate at 5 years
	Removal of 3	Hopeless prognosis for alignment of 3 Patient not keen for appliance therapy or evidence of incisor resorption or dentigerous cyst 2 and 4 in contact Good root length on c and aesthetics of c acceptable	Prosthetic replacement of c required when lost
	Retain 3	Occasionally in a young patient who is uncertain about treatment at present but may elect to proceed with alignment of 3 later	Periodic radiographic examination of incisors required to exclude resorption
Transposition	Accept	Transposition complete	
	Extraction of the most displaced tooth	If crowding present	
	Orthodontic	Sufficient space in the arch	Apical positions of the transposed teeth will determine whether alignment is carried out in the transposed positions or if these are corrected

[a]In each case, the patient's interest in orthodontic treatment, their level of dental awareness and general features of the malocclusion (including the degree of crowding or spacing and the condition of the primary canine (if present) and adjacent teeth) must be assessed before the final treatment plan can be devised.
[b]91% chance of normalisation of eruption path of 3 with extraction of c where 3 is mesially positioned and overlaps < half of root of 2; 64% chance of eruption of 3 if > half of 2 root overlapped. Recent evidence shows significant improvement in success rate of eruption of 3 with the use of RME and headgear (or headgear only) compared to untreated controls.

in the upper labial segment. If the diminutive lateral incisor is retained, orthodontic treatment should first create sufficient space to ensure that the tooth can be restored to ideal anatomical dimensions. This space is maintained for at least 3 months with metal spurs on a removable retainer prior to final restoration.

Form

Double Teeth

- Have a prevalence of 0.1–0.2% in the permanent dentition.
- Are equally common in males and females.
- Affect incisors more frequently than other tooth types.

Clinical appearance can vary from an incisal notch in a tooth of enlarged mesiodistal width to an anomaly resembling two separate crowns. Treatment is best delayed until the pulp has receded. Separation may be possible if there are two separate pulp chambers and root canals, but recontouring of the crown to resemble two separate teeth or reduction of its mesiodistal width may be possible where one pulp chamber exists.

The reported Prevalence in the primary dentition is 0.5–1.6% in White European populations and it affects teeth mostly in the mandibular labial segment. In the presence of hypodontia, double primary teeth are followed usually by absence of permanent teeth, but supernumerary teeth are more common in the permanent dentition if all of the primary teeth are present. Occasionally, eruption of the permanent successor is delayed if a double primary tooth exists, and its removal, possibly in conjunction with that of permanent supernumeraries, may be indicated to allow eruption of the permanent teeth.

Accessory Cusps and Evaginated Teeth

In the primary dentition, the maxillary molars are most commonly affected by additional cusps whereas the incisors, particularly the upper incisors, premolars and molars may be affected in the permanent dentition. An additional cusp on a maxillary incisor is termed a 'talon' cusp. As well as being unsightly, it may produce an occlusal interference or predispose to caries between the cusp and the palatal surface of the incisor. Treatment may be either by removal of the cusp and localised pulpotomy or by progressive grinding to encourage secondary dentine formation.

Evagination is characterised by a conical tuberculated prominence on the occlusal surface of a tooth and affects premolars most commonly. Treatment is as recommended for talon cusps.

10.2 Class I Malocclusion

LEARNING OBJECTIVES

You should:
- know the possible aetiological factors in class I malocclusion
- understand the principles of treatment planning.

Aetiology

Skeletal Factors
The skeletal pattern may be class I, class II or class III with the incisors compensating for any underlying skeletal discrepancy. An increase in lower anterior face height or a mild transverse skeletal discrepancy may also occur, creating an anterior open bite or buccal segment crossbite, respectively.

Soft Tissues Factors
Apart from bimaxillary proclination, where labial movement of the incisors may result from tongue pressure in the presence of unfavourable lip tone, the soft tissues are not prime aetiological factors.

Dental Factors
A tooth/dental arch size discrepancy leading to crowding or spacing is the principal cause of class I malocclusion. Other factors, however, such as early loss of primary teeth, large or small teeth, supernumerary or absent teeth, can also influence any inherent dento-alveolar disproportion.

Occlusal Features

There are several typical occlusal features:

- 'The lower incisor edges occlude with, or lie immediately below, the cingulum plateau of the upper central incisors' (British Standards Institute Classification). Not all of the incisors, however, may relate in this manner. Provided the overall anteroposterior labial segment relationship is class I, even where a crossbite exists on one or two upper incisors, the incisor relationship may be regarded as class I.
- The molar relationship is variable and depends on whether mesial drift has followed any previous extractions.
- Crowding is often concentrated in the upper canine and lower second premolar areas as these teeth often erupt last in each arch.
- Crowding may also displace one or more teeth into crossbite and create a premature contact on closure, with associated mandibular displacement and centreline shift.

TREATMENT

The need for treatment on dental health grounds is most commonly related to the presence of crowding or displacement of teeth; the latter may be caused by crowding, although ectopic developmental position, the presence of a supernumerary, retention of a primary tooth or, rarely, a pathological cause may be responsible. Treatment may be indicated also for spacing or for the management of vertical or transverse problems (see Sections 10.1 and 10.5).

Treatment Planning

The basic principles of treatment planning have already been outlined in Section 9.4.

Crowding
The possible measures to be considered in relation to the management of crowding have been presented in Sections 9.4 and 10.1. Some basic guidelines, however, regarding the management of crowding in class I malocclusion are as follows:

- Mild crowding, often present as the permanent incisors erupt, may resolve with some increase in intercanine width and use of leeway space. If present when the permanent dentition is established, it is best accepted.
- Moderate crowding is usually dealt with by first premolar extractions. Where this is undertaken in a growing patient, considerable spontaneous improvement in labiolingual alignment of the incisors and canines will ensue in the following 6 months provided the canines are mesially angulated and movement is not hindered by the occlusion. Thereafter, the potential for further spontaneous change is much less, and fixed appliances are usually required to correct residual occlusal discrepancies.
- Severe crowding often may be managed expediently by the removal of the most displaced teeth or, on occasion, by the extraction of more than one tooth per quadrant. Anchorage planning is most critical in this group and the placement of space maintainers prior to any proposed extractions is almost always necessary.
- Late lower labial segment crowding occurs commonly in late teens and gradually increases throughout the third and fourth decades, representing largely an adaptation to growth changes in the facial skeleton. Other factors have also been implicated (see Table 9.2, Chapter 9), but the evidence associating the mandibular third molar with late lower incisor crowding is weak. Mild crowding is best accepted and monitored.

■ Where the posterior occlusion is class I and the arches otherwise aligned with a mildly increased overbite, moderate-to-severe lower incisor crowding may be dealt with by extraction of one incisor (usually the most mal-positioned) followed by alignment and approximation of the remaining units using a sectional fixed appliance. A bonded lingual retainer is advisable to maintain the re-sult, but lingual movement of the lower labial segment may produce reciprocal palatal movement of the upper incisors and lead to their misalignment. This must be drawn to the patient's attention before treatment starts.

BIMAXILLARY PROCLINATION

Bimaxillary proclination (proclination of upper and lower incisors) is seen typically in Black people of Southern and Central Africa, and of African Caribbean heritage. It may also occur in White European populations in association with class I, class II division 1 or class III malocclusions. In class I, the overjet is increased because of the incisor inclina-tion. Treatment to retract the upper and lower labial seg-ments is generally unstable, as lingual movement of the lower incisors away from their zone of labiolingual balance tends to relapse post-treatment unless retained permanently. The prospect of stability may be improved where the lips have good muscle tone and become competent following incisor retroclination. Where the soft tissue factors are unfavourable (e.g. grossly incompetent lips), treatment is inadvisable.

SPACING

A spaced dentition is rare and is caused by a disproportion in the size of the teeth relative to the arch size or by absence of teeth. Where the spacing is mild, acceptance is usually best. Alternatively, consideration may be given to composite additions or porcelain veneers to increase the mesiodistal width of all the labial segment teeth. In more marked spac-ing, orthodontic treatment to concentrate the space at spe-cific sites prior to fitting of a prosthesis or implant place-ment may be necessary.

Space between the upper central incisors is more com-mon. Although this often exists in the early mixed denti-tion, it usually reduces considerably as the permanent maxillary canine erupts. Other factors that may cause an upper median diastema are given in Section 10.1. On aver-age, the mesiodistal width of the upper lateral incisor is 80% that of the central incisor. Where the lateral incisor is narrower, it should be enlarged by composite or porcelain additions to assist maintenance of diastema closure.

In patients with missing upper permanent lateral inci-sors, the resulting space may be opened, closed or accepted (Section 10.1).

10.3 Class II Malocclusion

LEARNING OBJECTIVES

You should:
- understand the possible aetiology of divisions 1 and 2 malocclusions
- appreciate those factors that require special consider-ation in treatment planning
- know the management options for class II malocclusion
- understand the difference between growth modification and camouflage treatment
- know the factors that promote post-treatment stability of class II malocclusion.

Class II malocclusions are divided into divisions 1 and 2.

DIVISION 1

Prevalence and Aetiology

Reported to occur in 15–20% of in white people, class II division 1 malocclusion may arise from the following factors.

Skeletal Relationships

Although the skeletal relationship is usually class II, class II division 1 malocclusion may exist on a class I or mild class III skeletal pattern. Where a class II skeletal pattern is pres-ent, mandibular deficiency is almost entirely the primary cause, although excessive maxillary growth or a combina-tion of the two may be factors in other instances. In con-trast, the developmental position or inclination of the teeth resulting from soft tissue or digit-sucking influences are to blame where the skeletal pattern is class I or mildly class III. The anterior vertical proportions of the face vary, and where these are greatly increased or reduced, treatment is likely to be difficult.

Lips, Tongue and Habits

The effects of the lips and tongue on the incisor position are determined principally by the skeletal pattern and thereaf-ter by the manner in which an anterior oral seal is achieved. Where the skeletal pattern is class II, an acceptable incisor relationship may be achieved by proclination of the lower incisors under the influence of the tongue. In general, how-ever, the greater the class II skeletal discrepancy, the more likely the lips are to be incompetent and to contribute to upper incisor proclination. Where lip incompetence exists along with a class II skeletal pattern and a reduced lower facial height, an anterior oral seal is likely to be produced by the lower lip lying under the upper incisors. This worsens the overjet by proclining the upper and retroclining the lower incisor teeth. In rare cases, the lower lip may be hy-peractive and contribute to a class II division 1 malocclu-sion by solely retroclining the lower incisors. Where the lower facial height is increased, an anterior oral seal is often produced largely by forward positioning of the tongue, thus tending to reduce the overbite further and compensate for the class II discrepancy by proclining the lower incisors.

In very rare instances, a primary atypical swallowing be-haviour will cause an overjet increase, but distinguishing this from an adaptive tongue thrust is difficult. The effect of a digit-sucking habit is to procline the upper incisors and retro-cline the lower incisors although the overjet increase may be asymmetric depending on the positioning of the digit.

Crowding

Labial displacement of the upper or lower incisors caused by crowding may respectively worsen or ameliorate an overjet.

Occlusal, Dental and Gingival Characteristics

As forward mandibular posturing to disguise the overjet increase is seen in some patients, it is important to ensure that the mandible is in centric relation before recording the occlusal features:

- 'The lower incisor edges lie posterior to the cingulum plateau of the upper incisors; there is an increase in overjet and the upper incisors are usually proclined' (British Standards Institute Classification).
- The upper incisors are often traumatised because of the increased overjet: the likelihood increasing more than two-fold when the overjet exceeds 3 mm compared to when it is less. In addition, the trauma risk is greater with incompetent lips and as the overjet increases.
- Drying of the gingivae labial to the upper incisors may occur with grossly incompetent lips, and this will aggravate an established gingivitis.
- The overbite varies depending on the skeletal pattern, the presence or absence of an adaptive tongue thrust on swallowing or the existence of a digit-sucking habit. It is commonly increased and complete, and sometimes traumatic, with the lower incisors impinging on the gingivae palatal to the upper incisors. It may also be incomplete or tend to an anterior open bite.
- Usually the molar relationship is class II, provided mesial drift following early loss of primary teeth has not occurred.

Treatment

There is little need for treatment where the overjet is mildly increased and the arches are aligned (overjet 3.5–6 mm with competent lips; dental health component of the Index of Orthodontic Treatment Need (IOTN) (Grade 2)). In such cases, the facial and dental appearance is usually acceptable and risks to dental health are minimal. Where the overjet increase is between 6 and 9 mm or greater than 9 mm, the need for treatment on dental health grounds is great or very great, respectively. The factors that must be considered regarding any potential treatment are discussed in Section 9.4.

Specific Factors in Treatment Planning

The skeletal pattern and profile, age and pattern of mandibular growth, soft tissue factors, space requirements and anchorage, stability and retention should be considered.

In general, the more the anteroposterior and vertical skeletal relationships deviate from the ideal, the more likely the profile is to be compromised and the more difficult treatment is likely to be. Where the nasolabial angle is obtuse or there is a marked 'gummy smile' or a short upper lip, treatment mechanics must ensure that overjet reduction does not worsen facial aesthetics. Non-extraction treatment may be preferable to address mild-to-moderate crowding and avoid potential compromise to facial profile from extraction-based treatment.

Whether a patient is growing depends on their age. The amount and pattern of mandibular growth can aid or detract from correction of a class II division 1 malocclusion in the growing patient. A forward mandibular growth pattern is favourable and is generally associated with a reduced lower facial height. A backward pattern of mandibular growth seen in individuals with increased lower facial height is unfavourable because the class II skeletal pattern is aggravated and the likelihood of lip competence post-treatment is reduced. In the non-growing patient, correction of both overbite and overjet of skeletal origin is difficult, and surgical correction may be required.

It is important to assess the likely impact of the lips and tongue in the aetiology of the malocclusion and, more importantly, whether a stable correction is possible by altering or correcting their influence. As a digit-sucking habit may affect the swallowing pattern and the incisor position, this should be ceased before treatment commences.

Space is required in the lower and upper arches for overbite reduction and overjet correction, respectively (the former always preceding the latter), in addition to that needed for possible relief of crowding (see Section 9.4). Anchorage must be planned, implemented and supervised appropriately. Where the lower arch is aligned, the buccal segment relationship typically half a unit class II and the overjet increase modest, space for overjet reduction may be obtained by moving the upper buccal segments distally using headgear or with the assistance of temporary anchorage devices (TADs). Fixed appliances produce the best outcomes, and where the crowding is more marked, removal of lower second and upper first premolars facilitates relief of crowding as well as correction of the incisor and buccal segment relationships. Further aspects regarding stability and retention are addressed later and in Section 11.4.

Treatment for an Underlying Class II Skeletal Relationship

Three possibilities exist.

GROWTH MODIFICATION. Growth modification is only possible in the growing child. Ideally the arches should be uncrowded. Treatment should be undertaken just before and/or during the pubertal growth spurt. Success depends on creating a differential in the rate of growth of the maxilla and mandible. Depending on the relative contribution of maxillary prognathism or mandibular retrusion to the skeletal class II malocclusion, an attempt may be made to restrain horizontal and/or vertical maxillary growth, stimulate mandibular growth or both. While headgear restrains maxillary growth with forces of up to 1000 g in total, a functional appliance accelerates mandibular growth; the final mandibular size, however, with functional appliance treatment is little if any greater than it would have been without treatment. Wear of either headgear or a functional appliance or both for 14–16 hours per day, in conjunction with favourable growth, is necessary for a successful outcome. The correction achieved by early treatment (before age 10 years) with a functional appliance or headgear has not been upheld long term; in addition, early treatment increases treatment duration, strains compliance and was not superior from a skeletal or occlusal perspective than when treatment was deferred to the late mixed dentition. Consequently, in current practice, early treatment is only considered in those cases with a risk of incisor trauma or with associated bullying/teasing.

When functional appliance treatment is planned, assessing standing height and secondary sexual characteristics assists in determining if a patient has begun the pubertal growth spurt. The stage of cervical vertebral maturation (CVM) viewed on a lateral cephalometric film has also been shown to be useful in the assessment of optimal treatment timing. Following overjet correction, often a second phase of treatment with fixed appliances and possibly extractions is necessary.

ORTHODONTIC CAMOUFLAGE. The skeletal discrepancy can be disguised by orthodontic tooth movement; this corrects the incisor relationship but the class II skeletal pattern remains. Invariably, treatment involves upper arch extractions, most commonly first premolars, and fixed appliance therapy to bodily retract the incisors. The effect of repositioning the teeth must not have a detrimental effect on the facial profile, otherwise 'camouflage' will have failed. Realistically this option is only acceptable where the class II skeletal pattern is no worse than moderate, the vertical facial proportions are good and the arches are reasonably well aligned so that the extraction spaces can be used for overjet reduction and not for relief of crowding. Where the lower incisors are retroclined by a habit, lip trap or deep overbite, it may be possible for them to be proclined by treatment and for this 'camouflage' to be stable.

ORTHOGNATHIC SURGERY. Where growth is complete and camouflage would not produce optimal facial and dental aesthetics, surgical correction of the malocclusion is best (see Section 10.6). In such an individual, an overjet >10 mm is the best indicator that successful correction by camouflage is unlikely. This is especially so if the mandibular incisors are proclined relative to a short and deficient mandible and/or the total face height is increased.

Retention and Post-Treatment Stability

The interincisal angle should be within average limits, the overjet completely reduced with the upper incisors in soft tissue balance (i.e. no tongue thrust) and the lower lip covering at least one-third of their labial surface. Where these criteria are met, the prospect of stability is good. Retention planning is discussed elsewhere (see Section 11.4).

DIVISION 2

Aetiology

Skeletal Relationships

The skeletal pattern in division 2 malocclusion is usually mildly class II, although it may be class I or mildly class III. A reduced lower anterior facial height is common with an associated anterior mandibular growth rotation, which tends to increase the overbite. A relatively wide maxillary base may lead to a lingual crossbite of the first premolars.

Soft Tissues

The high lower lip line (covering more than one-third of the upper incisor crowns) and resting pressure (about 2.5 times greater than that of the upper lip) are the most significant aetiological factors in retroclination of the upper incisors. The lower lip level depends largely on the lower anterior facial height; the more reduced the lower anterior facial height, the higher the lower lip line. Where the lower lip is also hyperactive, bimaxillary retroclination will result often associated with an anterior growth rotation and deep labiomental fold.

Dental Factors

The upper incisor cingulum is often reduced or absent, which may exacerbate the overbite. In addition, there is an increased likelihood of the teeth being smaller than average, as is the chance of a more acute crown/root angulation. Retroclination of the upper, and commonly of the lower, incisors also makes existing crowding worse.

Occlusal Features

The main occlusal features are the following:

- 'The upper central incisors are retroclined. The overjet is minimal but may be increased' (British Standards Institute Classification).
- The upper lateral incisors are often proclined and mesiolabially rotated but they may also be retroclined.
- Occasionally upper and lower incisors are retroclined, usually associated with a high lower lip line where the lip is hyperactive.
- The overbite may be traumatic: palatal to the upper incisors, labial to the lowers or, in severe cases, in both locations.
- Because of the discrepancy in arch widths and the class II skeletal relationship, a scissors bite is often present in the first premolar area as well as a class II molar relationship.

Treatment Planning

The following factors in particular must be considered: the profile and underlying skeletal discrepancy both anteroposteriorly and vertically, the growth potential and pattern of facial growth, the presence and degree of crowding, the lower lip level and masticatory muscle tone, the depth of overbite and inclination of the upper incisors.

Whether an associated class II skeletal pattern is to be camouflaged or corrected depends on the facial profile, preferred final upper lip support and incisor positions. The most appropriate means of overbite reduction is also determined by the underlying vertical skeletal pattern.

In a growing patient, correction of both a class II skeletal pattern and deep overbite is facilitated by favourable facial growth. Although a forward mandibular growth rotation aids correction of a class II skeletal discrepancy, it tends to increase the overbite.

Occasionally, a non-extraction approach may be adopted, usually in those with bimaxillary retroclination, to prevent the proposed risk of adverse profile change that may result from an extraction-based plan. There is, however, little difference in lip fullness with either approach. When the profile is particularly unfavourable in an adult, usually with a marked class II pattern and very reduced FMPA, a combined orthodontic/surgical approach will be required.

Lower arch extractions should only be considered where the crowding is marked. There is a risk of a deep overbite becoming traumatic as the lower incisors are allowed to drop lingually if extractions are undertaken in the presence of mild-to-moderate crowding. In addition, as the lower labial segment is constricted by the upper labial segment, some stable expansion of the lower intercanine width and proclination of the lower incisors may be feasible, thereby providing space for relief of mild-to-moderate crowding. Where extractions are necessary, a lower fixed appliance should be used to close residual spacing and prevent retroclination of the lower labial segment. In these cases, consideration should be given also to upper arch extractions and correction of the incisor relationship.

Where the lower lip level is at the gingival third of the upper incisor crowns or higher, correction of the incisor relationship may be difficult. Coincidentally increased tonicity of the masticatory muscles is linked to the reduced lower anterior facial height and may make overbite reduction problematic especially in adults.

Overbite reduction may be achieved by various means, including:

- molar eruption/extrusion
- upper and/or lower incisor intrusion
- lower incisor proclination
- upper incisor proclination followed by functional appliance treatment
- a combination of these methods
- surgery.

In a growing patient, use of a flat anterior bite plane on an upper removable appliance will retard lower incisor eruption while allowing the lower posterior teeth to erupt, thereby reducing the overbite. Facial growth then accommodates the increase in lower facial height. Extrusion of the upper molars by cervical headgear, or of lower molars using intraoral elastics attached to a fixed appliance, is only advisable in a growing patient as a means of overbite reduction. Attempts to intrude the incisors, for example by utility arches, are effective to a limited extent; however, the molars are also extruded somewhat. More apparent than real intrusion is likely.

Lower incisor proclination is not usually stable unless the lower incisors have been held in a retroclined position behind the cingulum of the upper incisors. Fitting an upper removable appliance with a flat anterior bite plane will allow spontaneous labial movement of the lower incisors to adopt a position of labiolingual balance. Careful planning by a specialist is required if active proclination of the lower incisors is considered.

A combined orthodontic/surgical approach is best in adults where the overbite is deep and the skeletal pattern is markedly class II.

Treatment

The depth of overbite and the inclination of the upper incisors determine the two approaches to treatment: either acceptance or correction of the incisor relationship.

ACCEPTANCE OF THE INCISOR RELATIONSHIP. Where the upper labial segment crowding and retroclination of the upper incisors are mild, and overbite onto tooth tissue, it is reasonable that no active treatment be undertaken. If treatment is provided, however, this is confined to relief of upper arch crowing and alignment of the upper labial segment alone.

CORRECTION OF THE INCISOR RELATIONSHIP. The interincisal angle and the overbite must be reduced for stable correction. Both are generally undertaken concurrent with that of management of any additional occlusal problems. The interincisal angle must be reduced to at least 135° (preferably less) to allow for an effective occlusal stop and may be corrected by various means.

ADJUSTMENT OF INCISOR ROOT TORQUE/LOWER LABIAL SEGMENT PROCLINATION. Usually fixed appliances are used to effect palatal root torque and reduce the overbite, sometimes by proclination of the lower incisors. Planning the final incisor positions requires considerable expertise, as proclination of the lower labial segment may stress the labial periodontium and create gingival recession, while the possible degree of palatal/labial root torque required is limited by the thickness of the alveolar processes. Anchorage demands are also increased because of the torquing movements.

Proclination of the labial segment or extractions will provide space for relief of mild-to-moderate or severe lower arch crowding, respectively, while in the upper arch, space to correct the incisor relationship may be created by moving the buccal segments distally (either by headgear or an alternative means) or by extractions. A non-extraction approach is preferred for correction of the incisor relationship and to enhance lip support. Where extractions are deemed necessary, to prevent lingual movement of the lower incisors, second premolars are favoured; upper first or second premolars may be chosen depending on the anchorage demands and space requirements.

PROCLINATION OF THE UPPER INCISORS AND GROWTH MODIFICATION. In a growing child with a mild-to-moderate class II skeletal pattern, with ideally a well-aligned lower arch, a functional appliance may be used to modify growth and correct the interincisal angle and overbite. To allow the mandible to be postured forward for the construction bite and to ensure favourable arch co-ordination posttreatment, the retroclined maxillary incisors must be proclined and the upper arch expanded prior to the functional appliance phase; the amount of upper arch expansion required, however, is often of a very modest nature due to the tendency for the maxillary arch form to be wider than that of the lower. If a twin-block functional appliance is used, this has a midline screw for upper arch expansion and springs may be incorporated in the upper appliance for incisor proclination (or their alignment may be undertaken simultaneously with a sectional fixed appliance), thereby avoiding the need for a preliminary separate phase of treatment. After functional treatment, detailing of the occlusion is usually completed by fixed appliances followed by retention.

ORTHOGNATHIC SURGERY. Where the facial profile is poor because of the marked skeletal discrepancy anteroposteriorly and/or vertically, and particularly in the adult with a deep traumatic overbite, a surgical approach in conjunction with orthodontics is best. A class II division 1 incisor relationship is created presurgically but the increased curve of Spee is maintained. A mandibular advancement osteotomy is then used to correct the overjet and facial profile; afterwards the lower buccal segment teeth are extruded to level the arch and close the lateral open bites followed by retention.

Post-Treatment Stability

Two features of class II division 2 malocclusion are particularly prone to relapse:

- The alignment of the upper lateral incisors, especially where these were rotated pretreatment.
- The overbite reduction.

Bonded palatal retention long-term is advisable to maintain rotational correction, ensuring that this is supervised appropriately.

Proclination of the lower incisors so their long axes lie on or 2 mm ahead of the mid-upper incisor root (centroid) has been proposed to aid stability of the corrected overbite. An increase in lower anterior facial height and inferior movement of the lower lip away from the upper labial segment also aids correction of the interincisal angle but is dependent on favourable vertical facial growth. Even where these features are evident, the closing pattern of mandibular growth tends to increase the overbite into adulthood. Following overbite correction, an upper removable retainer incorporating a flat anterior bite plane is recommended to be worn at night long term.

10.4 Class III Malocclusion

LEARNING OBJECTIVES

You should:
- understand the possible aetiology of class III malocclusion
- account for specific factors in treatment planning
- know the treatment possibilities.

AETIOLOGY

Skeletal Pattern

The skeletal pattern is most usually class III although it may be class I with the class III malocclusion due to incisor position or inclination. Mandibular, maxillary and cranial base factors often make a combined contribution to the underlying class III skeletal relationship. Characteristically, relative to class I occlusion, with class III malocclusion the mandible is longer, the glenoid fossa positioned more forward, the maxilla shorter and/or retrognathic in addition to a shorter anterior cranial base. The vertical relationship of the skeletal bases varies from increased to average or reduced and is generally reflected in the depth of overbite, which may alter depending on the pattern of facial growth. Where this is vertical rather than horizontal, an anterior open bite is likely.

Commonly, a transverse discrepancy exists in the dental base relationship because of the narrow maxillary and wider mandibular bases, although this is often worsened by the class III skeletal pattern.

Soft Tissues

The soft tissues contribute little to the aetiology of the malocclusion. Instead, where the lips are competent, the lips and tongue induce retroclination of the lower and proclination of the upper incisors (dento-alveolar compensation); as a result, the incisor relationship masks the true severity of the skeletal pattern. Where the lower anterior facial height is increased, however, the lips are frequently incompetent, with an adaptive tongue thrust on swallowing which may procline the lower incisors.

Dental Factors

Crowding is more common and more severe in the upper than in the lower arch, often resulting from the difference in length and width of the arches: the upper frequently is short and narrow compared with a longer and wider lower arch.

Occlusal Features

- 'The lower incisor edges lie anterior to the cingulum plateau of the upper incisors, the overjet is reduced or reversed' (British Standards Institute Classification).
- The overbite may be increased, average or reduced. Where the vertical facial proportions are increased, there is often an anterior open bite.
- Frequently, the upper incisors are proclined and the lower incisors retroclined, compensating for the underlying class III skeletal pattern.
- Upper arch crowding is common, often because of a short and narrow dental base, while the lower arch is more commonly aligned or spaced.
- Crossbites of the labial and/or buccal segments are common, resulting from the underlying class III skeletal discrepancy as well as from differences in the length and width of the arches. Crossbites may be associated with a mandibular displacement (see Section 9.3), particularly where a unilateral buccal segment crossbite exists. In the case of an anterior crossbite, the possibility of displacement should be assessed by checking if the patient can bite with the upper and lower central incisal edges contacting. Lower incisor mobility and occasionally gingival recession may be associated with the anterior crossbite.

TREATMENT

Treatment Planning

Account must be taken of the following factors.

The Degree of Anteroposterior and Vertical Skeletal Discrepancy

The degree of anteroposterior and vertical skeletal discrepancy is the most important factor in planning treatment and assessing the prognosis. As it is usually directly reflected in the facial and dental appearance, it will also influence the complexity of treatment undertaken through the patient's perception of these features.

The Potential Direction and Extent of Future Facial Growth

The general trend for downward and forward mandibular growth to surpass that of the maxilla is unfavourable for class III correction. Relevant family history, the age and gender of the patient, together with assessment of the vertical facial proportions, may help in making a 'guesstimate' as to the likely changes with growth. A reduced or average anterior facial height is often associated with a closing mandibular growth rotation, and a horizontal pattern of mandibular growth worsening the reverse overjet. With an increased vertical facial height, there is a tendency for a backward mandibular rotation to increase the likelihood of anterior open bite.

The Incisor Inclinations

The incisor inclinations indicate the degree of dento-alveolar compensation; if this is already marked (proposed thresholds are 120° and 80° for upper and lower incisors, respectively), further compensation by orthodontic means is unlikely to be stable or to produce an aesthetic result.

The Amount of Overbite

It is essential that there is an adequate overbite post-treatment to improve the prospects of stable overjet correction. Where the overbite is average or increased pretreatment, stability is more likely than where the overbite is reduced. Proclination of the upper incisors reduces the overbite while retroclination of the lower incisors increases it. Both movements may be necessary in some cases.

The Ability to Achieve an Edge-to-Edge Incisor Relationship

If it is not possible to achieve an edge-to-edge incisor relationship, correction of the incisor relationship by simple means is unlikely.

The Degree of Upper and Lower Arch Crowding

The following should be borne in mind. Upper arch extractions should be delayed until a reverse overjet and/or buccal crossbites have been corrected. This may provide space for relief of mild-to-moderate upper arch crowding. Where *extractions are undertaken in the upper arch only*, the reverse overjet may worsen with palatal movement of the upper labial segment. Where *mid upper arch extractions are necessary*, extraction of lower first premolars is usually advisable to allow correction of the incisor relationship.

Treatment

No treatment is an option when the skeletal pattern is mildly class III and/or the incisor relationship is acceptable, with minimal crowding and no mandibular displacement.

Treatment in Class I or Mild Class III Skeletal Pattern

Where the lower anterior facial height is increased, the overbite is usually minimal and the incisor relationship should be accepted. Treatment should focus on aligning the arches, with possible extractions. Upper arch expansion for crossbite correction will create space for relief of crowding. When this is indicated, fixed appliance mechanics must be used to minimise unfavourable dropping of the palatal cusps of the premolars and molars, as this will reduce the overbite further.

Provided the lower anterior facial height is average or reduced, with an average or increased overbite and upright upper incisors, proclination of the upper labial segment may be undertaken. This is often best carried out in the early mixed dentition before the permanent canines move labial to the lateral incisor roots, thereby increasing the risk of root resorption if their proclination is attempted. In such cases, treatment is best deferred until the canines have been retracted, removing the obstruction to crossbite correction of the lateral incisors. An upper removable appliance, incorporating a screw or Z-springs and posterior capping, may be used to correct the anterior crossbite (see Fig. 10.2), but a fixed appliance may be indicated depending on the presence of other occlusal features.

The need for upper arch extractions should be reassessed after the incisor relationship has been corrected, as some additional space for relief of crowding will be forthcoming from anteroposterior expansion. Movement of the upper buccal segments distally is not a favoured option as restraint of maxillary growth is likely. Often, extraction of the lower primary canines in the early mixed dentition, or of first premolars in a crowded lower arch in the permanent dentition, is advantageous in allowing the lower labial segment to drop lingually and increase the overbite.

Treatment in Mild-to-Moderate Class III Skeletal Pattern

Where the overbite is average or increased, two options exist: growth modification and orthodontic camouflage.

GROWTH MODIFICATION. In general, attempts to modify growth in class III malocclusion are disappointing, largely because the inherent tendency for growth is unfavourable. Where the underlying skeletal problem is mild, however, caused by either maxillary deficiency or mandibular excess, an effort may be made in the early mixed dentition to augment forward maxillary growth or 'restrain' mandibular growth. Maxillary protraction facemask treatment applies tension to the posterior and superior maxillary sutures, typically via a bonded or banded rapid maxillary expansion splint, and is ideal where maxillary retrognathia exists in combination with average or reduced vertical facial proportions, and upright, or slightly proclined, upper incisors.

Treatment must be started in the early mixed dentition, definitely before 10 years of age and preferably younger, to maximise the chances for successful forward movement. Forces of ~350–450 g per side are applied for 12–14 hours per day with a slight downward direction (~30°) from the maxillary splint to the facemask frame. The need for simultaneous rapid palatal expansion is disputed. The overall skeletal correction is brought about by moving the maxilla down and forward which rotates the mandible down and back. Additionally, the mandibular teeth are displaced backward and the maxillary teeth forward. There is often rebound of mandibular growth when treatment is discontinued and surgical correction may be required after adolescence. Results of a recent randomised controlled trial indicate maxillary protraction treatment in children under 10 years to be successful in 70% of cases (i.e. a positive overjet was achieved). There was, however, no discernible psychosocial improvement. In late adolescence, 68% of cases retained a positive overjet; surgical correction, however, was felt to be needed in twice the number of controls compared to the treated group (two-thirds versus one-third, respectively). To maximise the skeletal changes, it is now possible to use mini-plates in the infrazygomatic crest of the maxillary buttress and between the lower canine and lateral incisors with class III intermaxillary elastic traction. Results so far are promising but long-term follow-up is required.

Compressive forces applied to the condylar area via a chin cup have never been very successful, but if the force is aimed below the condyle, redirection rather than restraint of mandibular growth occurs. In essence, a downward and backward mandibular rotation is effected which increases the lower anterior facial height and reduces chin prominence. Lingual tipping of the lower incisors helps to correct the incisor relationship.

A functional appliance, particularly a Frankel III, may also be used for correction of mandibular prognathism, although only limited posterior mandibular posturing is possible. Mandibular growth is not restrained and the effects are similar to chin cup therapy where the force is directed below the condyle. For both chin cup and functional appliance therapy, the skeletal pattern should ideally be mildly class III with reduced vertical facial proportions, and the ability should exist to achieve an edge-to-edge incisor relationship with upright or proclined lower incisors. In all class III situations where growth modification is attempted, there is a need for prolonged follow-up during and after adolescence in order to monitor mandibular growth.

ORTHODONTIC CAMOUFLAGE. Orthodontic camouflage may be considered where the overbite is mildly reduced. Treatment aims to correct the incisor relationship by retroclination of the lower labial segment and/or proclination of the upper labial segment. Lower arch extractions may be necessary in conjunction with class III intermaxillary traction to upper and lower fixed appliances. Expansion of the upper arch will tend to compromise the overbite (as the palatal cusps tend to drop down) unless undertaken with rectangular wire incorporating additional torque to upright the premolars and molars. Extrusion of the upper molars ought to be avoided as this will also reduce the overbite. Lower arch extractions must only be undertaken where the likelihood of achieving successful overjet correction is favourable. Should the result relapse with further mandibular growth, surgical correction may be required. Any decompensation will need to be undone as part of presurgical orthodontics, which will result in opening up of the extraction spaces.

Treatment in Severe Class III Skeletal Pattern

ORTHOGNATHIC SURGERY. Where the skeletal discrepancy is more marked in the anteroposterior (often with an associated lateral discrepancy), and/or vertical dimension and therefore not amenable to satisfactory correction by orthodontic camouflage, the arches may be aligned and the incisor relationship accepted or correction may be brought about by orthognathic surgery. ANB <4° and lower incisor inclination <80° to the mandibular plane have been suggested as indicators for surgery rather than camouflage. The former is preceded by fixed appliance therapy to decompensate the arches. The nature of the surgical procedures (see Section 10.6) is specific to the underlying skeletal problems but often involves a combination of maxillary advancement and/or posterior impaction with mandibular set back, and possibly a reduction genioplasty, to attain the optimal profile change.

10.5 Open Bite and Crossbite

LEARNING OBJECTIVES

You should:
- be aware of the aetiology of open bite and crossbite
- appreciate treatment possibilities and limitations of open bite management
- be able to classify crossbite
- know how to manage anterior crossbite correction and buccal crossbite correction of a premolar or molar with an upper removable appliance.

OPEN BITE

An open bite may exist anteriorly or posteriorly in the arch.

Anterior Open Bite

The incisors do not overlap vertically when the posterior teeth are in occlusion.

Aetiology

SKELETAL PATTERN. An increase in lower facial height and high FMPA leads to an increase in the distance between the upper and lower incisors. Where it is not possible for the incisors to erupt sufficiently to compensate for this, an incomplete or anterior open bite results. This is worsened by the downward and backward pattern of mandibular growth, which contributes to the likely additional class II skeletal pattern.

SOFT TISSUES. Rarely an open bite is caused by the action of the tongue. The forward positioning of the tongue to achieve an anterior oral seal is usually adaptive in those with increased vertical skeletal proportions, as there is a greater tendency for the lips to be incompetent. In addition to the latter skeletal and soft tissue features, the overall poor facial and labial muscle tone with disharmonious tongue/lip activity may account for open bite in muscular dystrophy and cerebral palsy. An adaptive swallowing pattern is also often observed in children with an open bite caused by a digit-sucking habit. Where a tongue thrust is endogenous/primary (which is rare), there is often a lisp and some proclination of upper and lower incisors.

HABITS AND OPEN MOUTH BREATHING. A persistent digit-sucking habit inhibits eruption of the incisors, often producing an asymmetric anterior open bite. Occasionally, a posterior crossbite is produced through unopposed action of the cheek muscles as the tongue is lowered by the presence of the digit during sucking. Research shows that, in the main, open mouth breathing, due to nasal obstruction or habit and which may lead to altered head posture and increased lower facial height, does not have a major role in the aetiology of anterior open bite.

LOCALISED FAILURE OF ALVEOLAR DEVELOPMENT AND TRAUMA. A localised failure of alveolar development may occur in those with clefts of the lip and palate, but it can also occur where no cause is readily discernible.

Traumatic intrusion or avulsion of an incisor(s) as well as ankylosis following reimplantation may also create an open bite (see Chapter 8, Section 8.1).

Treatment

With the exception of an anterior open bite caused by a habit, treatment is complex and is best managed by a specialist. Where the open bite is due to intrusion trauma, potential exists for re-eruption until apical closure completes but orthodontic alignment or repositioning surgically may be necessary. For such cases and where ankylosis ensues following trauma, liaison with paediatric dental, restorative and oral surgical colleagues is required for optimal treatment planning.

MONITOR AND/OR ACCEPT. The open bite may be monitored/accepted if it is mild or where the prospect of stability is poor because of adverse skeletal and/or soft tissue factors, notably grossly incompetent lips and/or the suspicion of a primary tongue thrust.

ORTHODONTIC AND SURGICAL MANAGEMENT. The aim is to increase or at least maintain the overbite. Extrusion of molars, which may occur through use of a flat anterior bite plane on an upper removable appliance or cervical-pull headgear, must be avoided. Expansion of the upper arch, which is likely to extrude the palatal cusps and 'prop open' the bite, should also be avoided.

Assuming that there are no adverse growth or soft tissue factors, growth modification may be possible using high-pull headgear to the upper molars in mild open bite, or by attaching high-pull headgear to a removable or functional appliance with buccal capping where a class II skeletal pattern and a more marked anterior open bite exists. Where an anterior open bite is associated with a 'gummy smile', high-pull headgear to a full-coverage maxillary splint is indicated. As extrusion of the incisors to close an anterior open bite is unstable, the aim in all cases is to attempt to maintain the vertical position of the maxilla while preventing eruption of the upper posterior teeth. Attempts to intrude the maxilla and modify growth require excellent patient co-operation, with a minimum of 14–16 hours per day wear of the headgear and any other appliance. Following correction of the anterior open bite, fixed appliances are often required, sometimes in conjunction with extractions, to detail the occlusion.

For camouflage treatment, use of multiple loops in the archwires configured to tip the molars distally (Kim mechanics), in conjunction with vertical anterior elastics, closes the open bite as the vertical posterior facial height decreases. Use of 'rocking horse' archwires can also accomplish similar results. Maximal molar intrusion without buccal tipping can be obtained by placing TADs (screws or plates) palatally and buccally. Maintenance of the skeletal anchorage to the retainers for at least the first year is advised to combat relapse. Occasionally, camouflage by incisor retraction following relief of crowding can be stable if the lips become competent post-treatment. The contention that extraction of molars may aid overbite increase is unproven.

Where the anterior open bite is severe, a combined orthodontic/surgical approach is best when growth is complete. Treatment aims to impact the maxilla, more posteriorly than anteriorly, allowing the mandible to auto-rotate to close the open bite; additional mandibular advancement surgery may be required to correct an underlying skeletal class II problem.

TREATMENT OF OPEN BITE CAUSED BY HABITS. Weak evidence suggests that positive or negative reinforcement, a fixed habit breaker or both are effective at improving cessation of a digit-sucking habit. Gentle discouragement in the early mixed dentition is often a good starting point although it could take several years for the overbite to be regained.

Posterior Open Bite

Posterior open bite exists where there is no contact between the buccal segment teeth when the remainder of the dentition is in occlusion.

It is rare and the exact aetiology often incompletely understood. Causes include unilateral condylar hyperplasia. Here removal of the condyle is required if growth is excessively active. It is also caused, rarely, when the molar teeth fail to erupt despite apparent bone resorption in advance of the teeth (primary failure of eruption which solely influences

molars), or eruption is arrested at a certain occlusal level while adjacent teeth maintain contact with the opposing teeth; the former has a genetic link. In some instances in both case types, extraction of the molar is often the only treatment option. A lateral open bite is occasionally seen in the buccal segments with infraocclusion of primary molars (see Section 10.1) resulting from ankylosis. Lateral tongue spread has been given as a possible cause in some other cases but it is likely that additional factors are involved. Transient lateral open bites usually occur bilaterally during twin-block therapy but resolve as the buccal blocks are trimmed and the posterior teeth erupt into occlusion.

CROSSBITE

A crossbite is a buccolingual malrelationship of the upper and lower teeth. It can be anterior or posterior, unilateral or bilateral and may be associated with a mandibular displacement on closing such that an occlusal contact deflects the mandible laterally or anteriorly to allow maximum interdigitation. With a lateral displacement, there is often a centreline shift. By convention, the lower teeth are described relative to the upper so where the lower teeth occlude buccal to the opposing teeth, a buccal crossbite exists. Conversely, where the lower teeth occlude lingual to the palatal cusps of the upper teeth, a lingual (scissors) crossbite exists.

Aetiology

Skeletal Factors

A mismatch in the widths of the dental arches or an anteroposterior skeletal discrepancy may produce a crossbite of a complete arch segment – a lingual crossbite commonly found in class II – whereas a buccal and/or anterior crossbite is often associated with a class III malocclusion. A lingual or buccal crossbite may be unilateral or bilateral.

Growth restriction of the maxilla following cleft repair or of the mandible secondary to condylar trauma may lead also to buccal segment crossbite.

Soft Tissue Factors

With a digit-sucking habit, the tongue position is lowered and contraction of the cheeks during sucking is unopposed. This displaces the upper posterior teeth palatally and often creates a crossbite.

Crowding

Where the arch is inherently crowded, the upper lateral incisor may be displaced palatally and the upper second or third molar pushed into a scissors bite.

Local Causes

Retention of a primary tooth or a supernumerary tooth may produce a crossbite while early loss of a primary second molar in a crowded arch could lead to the successor erupting in crossbite.

Treatment

It is important to realise that where a crossbite is associated with a mandibular displacement, there is a functional indication for its correction, as displacing occlusal contacts may predispose to temporomandibular joint problems in susceptible individuals and a unilateral crossbite to possibly asymmetric mandibular growth. In addition, a traumatic displacing anterior occlusion may deflect a lower incisor labially and compromise periodontal support.

Treatment of Anterior Crossbite

Where one or two incisors are in crossbite, there is usually a mandibular displacement, and correction early in the mixed dentition is advisable provided adequate overbite exists to maintain correction. Space must be present in the arch (or can be created by extraction) to allow alignment of the tooth. If the tooth inclination is amenable to tipping, an upper removable appliance with buccal capping to free the occlusion and a Z-spring for proclination may be used (see Fig. 10.2). Anterior retention must be good to resist the displacing force caused by the action of the spring. Alternatively, an appliance with a screw section, clasping the teeth to be moved, overcomes this problem. Where insufficient overbite is likely to exist post-treatment, or the incisor is bodily displaced, treatment is better carried out with a fixed appliance in the permanent dentition which also affords the option of reciprocal lingual movement of the opposing lower incisor(s) if required. Treatment of anterior crossbite involving two or more incisors is considered in Section 10.4.

Treatment of Unilateral Buccal Crossbite

An upper removable appliance incorporating a T-spring or screw section may often be considered for correcting a crossbite on a premolar or molar, respectively (Figs 10.3 and 10.4). However, where reciprocal movement of opposing teeth is needed, fixed attachments should be placed and cross-elastics used to achieve the desired movement. Where a single tooth is mildly displaced from the arch, relief of crowding may be necessary to aid crossbite correction. In those with more marked tooth displacement, extraction rather than orthodontic alignment may be a better option.

Where a unilateral buccal segment crossbite is associated with a mandibular displacement, this usually results from a mild mismatch in widths of the dental bases, sometimes as a result of narrowing of the upper arch caused by digit-sucking. Upper arch expansion using a removable appliance with

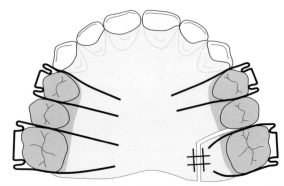

Fig. 10.4 Correction of a crossbite on a molar – upper removable appliance to move |6 buccally. • Screw section to move |6 buccally; Adams' clasps 64|64 (0.7 mm SS wire); buccal capping.

midline expansion screw and buccal capping to disengage the occlusion, or a quadhelix appliance, may be used for correction provided the teeth are not tilted buccally already. The quadhelix consists of a 1-mm stainless steel wire with four coils; it is attached to bands cemented to a molar tooth on each side of the arch. Alternatively, a preformed appliance may be slotted into welded attachments on the palatal aspect of the molar bands. Differential slow arch expansion anteriorly and/or posteriorly may be achieved following customary activation of half a tooth width per side. Slight overcorrection is advised to compensate for the relapse tendency. Although treatment with an upper removable appliance or quadhelix produced similar results, treatment with a quadhelix has been shown to be more cost-effective. With a full arch fixed appliance, crossbite correction, albeit by tipping of the crowns buccally, may also be achieved via an auxiliary expansion (E) arch. This is a straight length of 018 in or 020 in stainless steel wire placed in the headgear tubes of the molar bands and ligated to the base archwire in the upper midline.

Treatment of Bilateral Buccal Crossbite

A bilateral buccal crossbite is seldom associated with functional problems. Generally, as its existence indicates an underlying symmetrical transverse skeletal discrepancy, it is best accepted unless correction is planned as part of overall treatment, when rapid expansion of the midpalatal suture should be attempted only by a specialist. This is achieved by turning a midline screw (Hyrax) connected to bands cemented on first premolar and molar teeth, twice daily for 2 weeks. Expansion of the suture must be carried out no later than in early teenage years. Overcorrection is advisable as it appears that only half of the expansion achieved is maintained. Surgically assisted rapid palatal expansion (SARPE) (see Section 10.6) may be considered in the adult.

Treatment of Lingual Crossbite

Crowding may displace a single tooth into lingual crossbite. Once the crowding is relieved, the crossbite may be corrected, provided the occlusion is disengaged. Where a complete unilateral lingual crossbite is associated with a mandibular displacement, lower arch expansion and upper arch contraction with either removable or fixed appliances can produce a stable result provided a good buccal intercuspation is

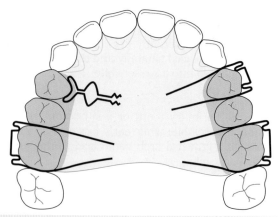

Fig. 10.3 Correction of crossbite on a premolar – upper removable appliance to move 4| buccally. • T-spring 4| (0.5 mm SS wire); Adams' clasps 6|46 (0.7 mm SS wire); buccal capping relieved over 4|.

achieved. Surgical correction may be indicated to correct a complete bilateral lingual crossbite or unilateral lingual crossbite with no displacement.

10.6 Adult and Surgical–Orthodontic Treatment

LEARNING OBJECTIVES

You should:
- be aware of special considerations in undertaking orthodontic treatment in adults
- know the indications for surgical–orthodontic treatment
- understand how surgical–orthodontic treatment is planned and executed
- be aware of common orthognathic surgical procedures.

ADULT ORTHODONTICS

Orthodontic treatment in adults is the most rapidly expanding area of contemporary orthodontic practice. The increased focus on facial and dental appearance allied with improved awareness of the potential of orthodontic tooth movement to improve dental aesthetics and greater social acceptability of appliances account for this.

Special Consideration in Adults

There are a number of factors that are specific for orthodontic procedures in adults:

- Adults are generally highly motivated orthodontic patients, able to specify their concerns, but they tend to have higher expectations of the final result than younger patients.
- The dentition may be compromised because of periodontal disease, tooth loss or extensive restorative treatment. Careful pretreatment assessment is required and all systemic and dental disease must be controlled before orthodontic treatment starts. Occasionally existing bridgework may need to be removed to allow tooth movement to proceed. Often, input from a variety of other disciplines (restorative, periodontal, prosthodontic and surgical) is necessary to achieve the best result, and integrated treatment planning must be co-ordinated in a logical sequence.
- There is also a greater likelihood of systemic illness impacting on the treatment plan in adults.
- Due to the absence of growth, skeletal discrepancies (other than mild) are best dealt with by orthodontics in combination with surgery rather than by camouflage.
- Where camouflage is considered and so long as an optimal smile is still possible, overbite reduction by intrusion of the incisors rather than by extrusion of the molars is necessary. The resultant increase in anterior facial height with the latter is unstable without compensatory facial growth.
- Anchorage planning is often more demanding than in the younger patient because of previous tooth loss and the possibility of reduced bony support of the remaining teeth. Headgear is not a realistic treatment option and alternatives such as palatal arches or temporary anchorage devices must be considered.

- Because of the reduced cell population and often reduced vascularity of the alveolar bone, the initial response to orthodontic forces is slow; once tooth movement starts, however, it tends to progress as efficiently as in adolescents. Nonetheless, the bone remodelling process necessary for tooth movement is slower in those taking oral bisphosphonates for osteoporosis (see Section 9.3).
- Some pain is common for 3–4 days following appliance adjustment, and light forces should be applied initially in all cases and throughout treatment where periodontal support is compromised.
- To improve the appearance of the appliance, aesthetic brackets (plastic or ceramic) and wires (Teflon or rhodium coated) or lingual appliances are options. In selected cases, treatment by a series of clear vacuum-formed thermoplastic aligners may be considered. Made of aluminium oxide, ceramic brackets offer better aesthetics than plastic alternatives composed of polycarbonate, polyurethane or polyoxymethylene. Special care, however, is required at debond due to their high bond strength and possibility of enamel fracture. Ceramic brackets should not be bonded in occlusion with the opposing teeth due to the risk of enamel wear; tie wing fracture is also common.
- Bands should be avoided in those with periodontal breakdown; fully bonded appliances should be used instead and indeed are generally preferable in adults due to longer clinical crowns.
- Irrespective of whether the dentition is periodontally compromised which leads to the gingival margins shifting apically, interproximal reduction is frequently required near the end of treatment to eliminate unsightly 'black triangle' spaces between the gingival margins and the contact points.
- Following diagnosis by a sleep physician, adults with obstructive sleep apnoea (OSA) may be treated by mandibular advancement splints which resemble functional appliances used for class II correction.

Adjunctive or Comprehensive Orthodontic Treatment in the Adult

Adjunctive Treatment

Adjunctive treatment involves carrying out tooth movement to correct one aspect of the occlusion to improve dental health or function, although the final occlusal result may not be necessarily ideal for class I. Treatment duration is usually about 6 months and typically is integrated with periodontal or advanced restorative procedures. Uprighting of teeth that have tilted into an extraction space or redistribution of space prior to bridgework, extrusion of teeth with a subgingival fracture margin to allow placement of a coronal restoration on sound root surface, intrusion of teeth that have over-erupted to allow restoration of the opposing space and anterior alignment to facilitate the best appearance of restorative work are examples of some adjunctive treatments.

Comprehensive Treatment

The aim of comprehensive treatment is to achieve the optimal aesthetic and functional occlusal result. Where the skeletal discrepancy is mild, camouflage by dento-alveolar movement is possible using fixed appliances. The principles of treatment planning and treatment follow similar lines to those adopted for class I, class II division 1 and division 2 and class III malocclusions (see Sections 10.2–10.4) but with due consideration of the smile margins, overbite reduction must be achieved by intrusion of incisors rather than by extrusion of molars. In those with a more marked skeletal discrepancy, a combined orthodontic and surgical approach is required to ensure that the best facial and occlusal results are achieved (see later).

Where significant periodontal breakdown has occurred, comprehensive treatment may still be possible provided disease is controlled and a regular maintenance scheme operates throughout orthodontic treatment. Because of the reduced periodontal ligament area, forces should be as light as possible, and anchorage planning is critical. Fixed appliances using a sectional arch approach are often indicated as is interproximal reduction for 'black triangle' spaces. Permanent retention with a bonded retainer is usual with the requirement for related patient maintenance of optimal oral hygiene.

SURGICAL–ORTHODONTIC TREATMENT

Surgical–orthodontic treatment involves correction of dentofacial deformity through a combined surgical and orthodontic approach. In contemporary practice, surgery to correct a jaw deformity (orthognathic surgery) is rarely undertaken independent of concurrent orthodontic treatment, as otherwise the final result is likely to be compromised.

Timing of Treatment

Treatment is usually deferred until growth is essentially completed, which is generally in late teens in males and slightly earlier in females. This delay is most important where growth is excessive, particularly in class III cases, as it safeguards against relapse brought about by further growth. Where the temporomandibular joint is ankylosed or the dentofacial deformity is causing severe psychological distress, earlier intervention may be considered.

Indications

Surgical–orthodontic treatment is indicated where the dentofacial problem cannot be dealt with satisfactorily by orthodontics alone. This includes moderate-to-severe anteroposterior, vertical and lateral skeletal discrepancies, severe dento-alveolar problems as well as craniofacial anomalies, including cleft lip and palate. Patients most likely to benefit from treatment may be recognised by the Index of Orthognathic Functional Treatment Need (IOFTN; see Section 9.1).

Planning Surgical–Orthodontic Treatment

A team approach is required, involving the orthodontist and oral and maxillofacial surgeons. Input from a plastic surgeon, restorative specialist, speech therapist and clinical psychologist may be required.

The patient's complaint and what is expected from treatment must be ascertained. Complaints may relate to dental and/or facial appearance, masticatory (including temporomandibular joint) function, speech or a combination of these. Where the primary concern relates to speech or temporomandibular problems, advice from a speech therapist or restorative specialist respectively is prudent. In such cases, although surgical–orthodontic treatment may improve matters somewhat, complete resolution is unlikely.

Occasionally, a patient may be overly concerned about some relatively minor skeletal or dental anomaly, which is blamed for lack of success in some aspect of life with resultant unrealistic expectations of treatment. In these instances, there is often a deep-rooted psychological problem and referral to a clinical psychologist or psychiatrist is indicated.

A detailed medical and dental history together with a thorough examination must then be performed, including an analysis of facial form in full face and profile. The height and width proportions of the face including, among others, the alar base width, nasolabial angle, upper incisor exposure at rest and when smiling, relation of the upper dental midline to the other facial midlines and the location of any cranial, maxillary, nasal, mandibular or chin deformities should be noted. Comparisons may be made to data that exists ensuring that consideration is given to race, gender and age. Temporomandibular joint signs or symptoms and any speech problems must be documented. Dental and periodontal health, the degree of upper and lower arch crowding and any dento-alveolar compensation should be recorded.

Facial and dental photographs, panoramic and lateral cephalometric films and dental casts should be obtained. A posteroanterior cephalometric film is indicated if facial asymmetry is apparent. Where available, CBCT and three-dimensional (3D) facial images may be taken for more detailed evaluation.

Record Analysis and Planning

The patient's cephalometric film should be digitised and assessment carried out using specific analyses of how the cranium and cranial base, nasomaxillary complex, mandible and respective dentitions relate to each other. Comparisons may be made to appropriately matched norms for ethnicity, gender and age to indicate sites of discrepancy and dentofacial disharmony. Bolton templates, while useful for preliminary assessment, are North American composites for males and females. Formerly, planning involved enlargement of the photographic negative profile to match 1:1 with the cephalometric film and then 'cutting and pasting' to simulate the desired surgical changes.

Newer techniques allow superimposition of the patient's soft tissue profile, from a digital photograph, on the cephalometric tracing; then, the image is adjusted in line with proposed orthodontic/surgical moves. The patient may view the predicted impact on the soft tissue profile of various 'simulated' treatment options, the risks and benefits of which should be explained to facilitate decision making. It must be emphasised that these 'predictions' are not an assurance of the likely outcome. 3D planning combining CT scans, 3D facial images with incorporation of digital models is now being used more frequently.

Surgical movement may also be simulated on a duplicate set of dental casts. Where a maxillary procedure is planned, the casts should be mounted on a semi-adjustable articulator.

The impact of presurgical decompensation, which usually worsens facial appearance, must also be understood. It may, on occasion, be helpful for a prospective patient to have an opportunity to discuss the process with another individual where a successful outcome has been achieved. In addition, provision of information leaflets and direction to respected Internet resources are valuable to ensure the patient has a complete perception of treatment and assist with informed decision making.

Orthodontic Management

Presurgical Orthodontics and at Surgery

All dental and periodontal disease must be managed before treatment can get underway. Presurgical orthodontics allows the jaws to be positioned in their desired location without interference from tooth positions. This phase of treatment takes about 1 year but may be slightly longer where there is severe crowding or protrusion. It aims to align and co-ordinate the arches or arch segments as well as to establish the vertical and anteroposterior position of the incisors. Usually, this involves placing the incisors at an average inclination to their respective bases, decompensating for any existing dento-alveolar compensation (nature's attempt to camouflage a skeletal discrepancy). The full extent of the skeletal problem is thus revealed so maximum surgical correction can then be achieved. Intermaxillary traction for class III or II cases is often used to aid decompensation. Depending on the degree of crowding and space requirements, extractions may be necessary to allow the tooth movements required. Consideration should also be given to the removal of impacted third molars at this stage.

In some cases, it is not possible or advisable to decompensate fully for the incisor position because of anatomical constraints (e.g. a narrow symphysis or thin labial gingival tissue in a class III malocclusion). Marked gingival recession is likely in the latter if the lower incisors are proclined.

Space must be created interdentally to allow access for surgical cuts when a segmental procedure is planned. Some tooth movements (e.g. levelling of a curve of Spee in patients with a short face) are managed in a more expeditious manner postsurgically while other movements (e.g. correction of a bilateral skeletal crossbite of the upper arch) can be managed simultaneously with Le Fort I correction for other skeletal problems at the time of surgery. Where there is an obvious height discrepancy between the posterior and anterior maxillary arch segments in cases of anterior open bite, in the interest of stability it is more appropriate to align these separately avoiding upper incisor extrusion.

When presurgical orthodontics is completed, photographic images, radiographs (including a lateral cephalometric film) and impressions should be taken. Arch co-ordination, and the other desired tooth movements, should be checked on a set of work casts. Adjustment to tooth position(s) may be necessary and, in some cases, the surgical plan may require slight amendment. Rigid rectangular stabilising archwires with ball hooks, to allow for intermaxillary fixation, should be placed. An interocclusal acrylic wafer, made from casts positioned to simulate the desired occlusal result, is required to ensure accuracy of the postsurgical result. If maxillary or bimaxillary surgery is planned, a face-bow recording is necessary to allow the casts to be positioned on a semi-adjustable articulator. At surgery, the interocclusal wafer is used to locate the jaws or jaw segments accurately; in the maxilla, the bone segments may then be fixed

semirigidly in position by mini-plates while in the mandible, these may be used with or without screws.

In certain cases, surgery may be undertaken before the orthodontic phase. This may shorten the treatment time and reduce soft tissue interference in some tooth movements once the skeletal relationships are rectified.

Surgical Procedures

Surgery may be carried out on the maxilla, mandible or on both jaws depending on the nature and severity of the skeletal problem.

Maxilla

LE FORT I OSTEOTOMY. The Le Fort I osteotomy is the most common maxillary orthognathic procedure. Access is usually provided by an incision in the buccal sulcus from left to right first molar areas. The maxilla is sectioned above the apices of the teeth so that it can be 'downfractured' from its anterior wall, tuberosities, lateral nasal walls and nasal septum but remains pedicled on the palate. With additional bone removal or placement of a bone graft, superior or inferior movement respectively is then possible; anterior movement is also possible but posterior repositioning is not realistic.

LE FORT II OSTEOTOMY. With the Le Fort II procedure, the incisions pass through the bridge of the nose and lower border of the orbit, allowing the correction of marked maxillary retrognathism and nasal retrusion.

LE FORT III OSTEOTOMY. Via a bicoronal flap, the whole midface including the zygomas is separated from the cranium. This is most frequently employed in correction of rare craniofacial anomalies (e.g. Crouzon's syndrome where the coronal and orbital sutures fuse early, leading to cessation of forward maxillary growth).

SEGMENTAL PROCEDURES. Rarely used nowadays, the Wassmund osteotomy involves separating the premaxilla by vertical cuts distal to the canines; the cuts are then extended horizontally across the palate. It may be used for overjet correction in the presence of premaxillary prominence or correction of a 'gummy smile'. Lack of interdental space for surgical cuts and damage to the adjacent teeth as well as compromised segmental blood supply are potential problems.

SURGICALLY ASSISTED RAPID PALATAL EXPANSION. Following the cuts for a Le Fort I osteotomy but eliminating the down-fracture, this procedure in conjunction with rapid maxillary expansion allows correction of severe maxillary constriction.

Mandible

SAGITTAL SPLIT OSTEOTOMY. A sagittal split osteotomy is the most frequently undertaken mandibular procedure. The inner and outer parts of the ramus are split through a cut made horizontally above the lingula and obliquely across the retromolar area. These cuts are extended vertically through the buccal cortical plate to the inferior aspect of the mandible. The tooth-bearing part can then be moved forwards or backwards or rotated slightly, but inferior alveolar nerve damage is a common complication.

VERTICAL SUBSIGMOID OSTEOTOMY. The mandible is sectioned via an extra- or intraoral incision by a vertical cut through the sigmoid notch, passing behind the lingula, to the mandibular angle. This procedure is used for correction of mandibular prognathism. With an extraoral approach, there is a residual scar.

BODY OSTEOTOMY. Surgical cuts are made in the mandibular body, ideally where a space exists anterior to the second premolars. This operation is valuable in those with marked mandibular prognathism but is seldom undertaken.

GENIOPLASTY. Using a horizontal sliding osteotomy and muscle pedicle, with/without bone removal or bone grafting, the chin can be repositioned in a variety of locations, often producing dramatic profile changes. In some cases, it may be used alone as a masking procedure.

Bimaxillary Procedures

Correction of the skeletal problems in many individuals involves surgery to both the maxilla and mandible to produce optimal dentofacial harmony.

Distraction Osteogenesis

Based on manipulation of a healing bone, this technique stretches an osteotomised site by an extra- or intraoral distractor in advance of calcification, which induces the generation of new bone formation and investing soft tissue. Where large distances of movement are required and/or deficient jaws increased in size at an early age, this technique has its greatest applications. The maxilla or mandible can be moved forward with distraction but as the force vector is difficult to control, it lacks the precision of standard orthognathic procedures in terms of placement of the jaws or teeth in pre-planned positions. Patients with craniofacial syndromes, for example moderately severe hemifacial microsomia with a rudimentary ramus on the affected side or those with severe maxillary deficiency as found in Apert's or Crouzon's syndrome, are prime candidates for distraction. The mandibular symphysis may also be widened by this procedure.

Adjunctive Facial Procedures

To improve the soft tissue contours beyond those attainable by orthognathic surgery, several adjunctive facial procedures can be employed. These include chin augmentation, rhinoplasty, implants for facial soft tissue contours, liposuction and platysma lift procedures. Injection of collagen or Botox (Allergan Inc., Irvine, California, USA) tends to produce a temporary aesthetic improvement.

Postsurgical Orthodontics and Follow-Up

Lasting usually between 3 and 9 months, this phase starts within weeks of surgery by typically placing light round stainless steel archwires and light elastic traction to aid occlusal settling, followed by further detailing to ensure that good interdigitation is achieved. This is followed by a retention regimen that generally follows a standard fixed appliance therapy. Surgical follow-up should be for a minimum of 2 years.

Stability and Relapse

In general, stability is enhanced and relapse minimised when:

- surgical and orthodontic plans are correct and realistic, well-integrated and executed competently
- surgical movement is modest – no greater than 5–6 mm vertically or anteroposteriorly in the maxilla or 8 mm in the mandible; does not place the soft tissues under tension and the condyles are not distracted at surgery

- aberrant soft tissue factors are absent (e.g. tongue thrust or previous surgical scarring, as may occur in repaired cleft palate) and lips are competent
- teeth have been placed in soft tissue balance and not extruded presurgically
- patient is compliant with all aspects of treatment, particularly postsurgical wear of elastic traction
- fixation is adequate.

The most stable procedures are maxillary impaction and mandibular advancement while inferior positioning of the maxilla and mandibular setback are least stable.

10.7 Cleft Lip and Palate

LEARNING OBJECTIVES

You should:
- know the likely aetiological factors in orofacial clefting
- be aware of the common clinical features
- understand how care is managed and the role of the general dental practitioner.

Management of patients with cleft lip and palate is best undertaken in specialist centres. The general practitioner should, however, understand the timing and sequence of treatment for these patients and the importance of providing a high standard of preventive and routine dental care.

Aetiology

Whether a cleft occurs in isolation or as part of a syndrome, both genetic and environmental factors interact in its aetiology. A distinct family history exists in 40% of those with cleft lip (with or without palate involvement) and in 20% of those with cleft palate only. Environmental factors such as folic acid deficiency, nicotine, anticonvulsant drug therapy, aspirin and cortisone may act synergistically in a susceptible, genetically predisposed individual to promote clefting. Clefting of the lip and primary palate follows from failure of fusion of the medial nasal, lateral nasal and maxillary processes at around the sixth week of intrauterine life. Clefts of the secondary palate follow failure of fusion of the palatal shelves from 8 to 10 weeks. Elevation of the palatal shelves from a vertical to a horizontal position occurs later in females than males, allowing for more lateral facial growth, which possibly contributes to the greater prevalence of isolated cleft palate in females.

Classification

Several classification systems exist, but the cleft is easiest described as involving the primary (lip and alveolus to the incisive foramen) and/or secondary palate (hard palate from incisive foramen back and soft palate) as being unilateral or bilateral, complete or incomplete (Fig. 10.5). A submucous cleft may not be detected for some time as the overlying mucosa is unaffected, but it is usually noticed when speech development is poor.

Prevalence

Clefts of the lip and/or palate occur in 65% of all craniofacial deformities. In the White European population, the

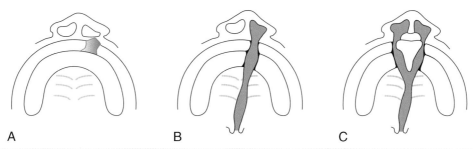

Fig. 10.5 Classification of cleft lip and palate. • (A) Left incomplete cleft of primary palate. (B) Left unilateral complete cleft of primary and secondary palate. (C) Bilateral complete cleft of primary and secondary palate.

reported prevalence is about 1 in 700 live births for cleft lip and palate, and 1 in 2000 live births for isolated cleft of the secondary palate, although the prevalence is on the rise in the former group. Cleft lip and palate more frequently affects males and is more common on the left than on the right side, while females are more often affected by cleft palate alone. The latter may also be associated with syndromes such as Pierre Robin, Treacher Collins and Down syndrome.

Common Clinical Features

Skeletal Features

- Both the maxilla and mandible tend to be retrognathic (particularly with cleft palate only) relative to non-cleft individuals; the maxillary position is partly attributable to growth restriction postsurgically.
- Upper facial height tends to be reduced but the lower facial height tends to be increased, with an excess freeway space.
- Class III skeletal relationship often results from the retrusion of maxilla and mandible but is aggravated by mandibular overclosure to allow posterior tooth contact.

Dental and Occlusal Features

On the side of the cleft, the following anomalies often exist:

- The lateral incisor is absent, of atypical size and/or shape, hypoplastic or appears as two conical teeth on the medial and lateral side of the cleft.
- A supernumerary or supplemental tooth may be present on either side of the cleft.
- The central incisor is often rotated and tilted towards the cleft and may be hypoplastic, particularly in bilateral clefts.

Elsewhere in the mouth, tooth size tends to be smaller and eruption delayed, with a greater prevalence of hypodontia and supernumerary teeth, enamel hypoplasia and aberrant tooth shape than in unaffected individuals. The delay in eruption worsens as the extent of the cleft increases.

A class III incisor relationship is common with a crossbite of one or both buccal segments and occasionally a lateral open bite.

Growth

Postsurgical scarring in those with cleft lip and palate restricts anteroposterior, vertical and transverse growth of the midface. These changes do not seem to occur to any significant extent in unrepaired clefts. About 40% of those with clefts have evident maxillary retrusion.

Hearing and Speech

Where the cleft involves the posterior palate, the action of tensor palati on the eustachian tube is impaired, often leading to hearing difficulties. This, in addition to palatal fistulae and adverse palatopharyngeal function, means that speech is often affected (hypernasal). Regular assessment of hearing and speech is essential before and during school years.

Anomalies of Other Body Tissues

Prevalence of cardiac and digital anomalies varies worldwide but is most common in those with clefts of the secondary palate only.

Care Management

Care management is best co-ordinated in a specialised centre by a team usually comprising an orthodontist, speech therapist, dedicated nurse, health visitor, psychologist and plastic, ear–nose–throat and maxillofacial surgeons. General dental care must be monitored regularly by a caring and interested general dental practitioner.

Neonatal Period

Maternal support, with discussion of the potential of what current treatment offers, should be provided by designated individual(s) from the cleft team. Emphasis should also be placed on the importance of a high standard of dental care for later treatment. The mother must be instructed in feeding using special bottles and teats (e.g. Rosti bottle and Gummi teat). A specialised health visitor should be available for provision of ongoing advice and support. This may be augmented by contact with a member of the Cleft Lip and Palate Association (CLAPA).

Repositioning the displaced cleft segments by removable acrylic appliances to idealise their relationship and facilitate surgical repair (presurgical orthopaedics, PSO) is not universally adopted. Modifying the appliance, however, by extending the acrylic into the nostril on the cleft side in an effort to mould the nose (naso-alveolar moulding) has seen a resurgence in the practice of PSO, particularly in North America, but the long-term value of this approach is as yet unproven.

Lip closure, by Millard, Delaire or straight-line techniques, is usually undertaken at around 3 months with the aim to accurately reposition anatomically the alar base and upper labial musculature. In bilateral clefts, both sides are now mostly repaired together but doing each side separately is still practised in some centres. Due to its negative impact on future growth, primary bone grafting is not advocated to restore alveolar integrity. Repair of the hard and soft palate aims respectively to separate the nasal and oral cavities as well as assist comprehensible speech by restoring velopharngyeal function and closure. Usually this is carried out between 6 and 9 months, commonly by means of a two-layered procedure (vomer flap for the nasal layer and muco-periosteal flaps minimising bone exposure for the oral layer). Delaying until at least 5 years, as practised in some European centres, is inadvisable due to the detrimental effects on speech development.

Primary Dentition

Preventive advice including dietary counselling and possibly provision of fluoride supplements is essential. Speech should be assessed formally at about 18 months and speech and hearing assessed regularly. Speech therapy can be instituted as necessary. Pharyngoplasty to address velopharnyngeal incompetence and/or lip revision may be required around 4 – 5 years of age, usually prior to starting school.

Mixed/Permanent Dentition

In preparation for alveolar bone grafting at 9–10 years of age, upper incisor(s) alignment and arch expansion is usually undertaken to facilitate access. Extraction of any primary teeth in the upper arch, if required, should take place at least 3 weeks prior to surgery to allow healing. Bone is harvested from the iliac crest or the chin, placed in the cleft site and the wound closed with keratinised flaps. An alternative of bone substitution is bone morphogenetic protein but this is currently expensive and not so widely available. Alveolar bone grafting, in addition to allowing eruption of the permanent canine and space closure, supports the alar base and helps to close oronasal fistulae; in bilateral cases, it also stabilises the premaxilla.

Once the permanent canine has erupted (~10–15% require exposure), further treatment usually involves centreline correction and space closure by mesial movement of the buccal segment teeth so that the canine replaces a missing or diminutive lateral incisor. The treatment plan should be finalised with input from a restorative colleague. Crowding should be relieved in the non-cleft quadrant if necessary and in the lower arch if orthodontic correction of the malocclusion is likely. Otherwise, lower arch extractions should be delayed until surgical correction of the malocclusion is planned.

Where gross midface retrusion is present in late teenage years, a Le Fort I or II surgical advancement is likely (required in about 25% of cases treated to a standardised protocol), with possible mandibular setback and/or genioplasty depending on the severity of the skeletal problem. Presurgical orthodontics proceeds along conventional lines (see Section 10.6). Rhinoplasty may be required as a later procedure to optimise the facial profile.

Retention

Because of scar tissue in the cleft area, treatment where maxillary arch expansion has been undertaken has a high relapse potential, so long-term retention is necessary in these cases.

Self-Assessment: Questions

MULTIPLE CHOICE QUESTIONS (TRUE/FALSE)

1. Hypodontia:
   a. Affects the upper permanent lateral incisors in 20% of cases
   b. Affects lower second premolars more than upper second premolars
   c. Is more common in males than females
   d. Has not a familial link
   e. Of third molars can be determined definitively by 8 years of age
2. Supernumerary teeth:
   a. Occur in about 10% of the population
   b. Are more common in females than males
   c. May occur in the lower incisor area
   d. May cause spacing of 1/1
   e. May have no effect on the dentition or occlusion
3. Removal of a 6 deemed of poor prognosis in a class I (incisors and molars) malocclusion with generalised moderate premolar crowding where all other teeth are sound:
   a. Is advisable when the bifurcation of the 8 is calcifying, to maximise the potential for spontaneous correction of malocclusion in that quadrant
   b. Should be compensated
   c. Should be balanced
   d. Is likely to lead to overjet increase
   e. Is likely to lead to 3-mm overbite increase

4. Extraction of cs may be indicated:
   a. To allow spontaneous correction of potential crossbite on erupting 2s
   b. To allow space to be created for an unerupted upper central incisor whose eruption has been inhibited by the presence of a supernumerary
   c. To allow the lower incisors to drop lingually in a developing class III malocclusion
   d. To encourage improvement in the position of a displaced 3
   e. Along with bs in early mixed dentition to encourage space closure in children in whom 2s are absent
5. Extraction of a lower right first primary molar:
   a. Is described as balanced when extraction of the upper left first primary molar is requested also
   b. Is described as compensated when extraction of the lower left first primary molar is requested also
   c. Should be compensated to prevent a centreline shift
   d. Should be balanced to prevent overbite reduction
   e. Should be requested if the crown of the tooth is submerged level with the gingival margin
6. A persistent thumb-sucking habit may produce:
   a. An increased overbite
   b. An asymmetric increase in overjet
   c. A buccal segment crossbite
   d. An adaptive tongue thrust
   e. Upper incisor root resorption

7. Buccal displacement of 3/ may be contributed to by:
   a. Crowding in the arch
   b. Retention of c/
   c. An increased overbite
   d. Early loss of lower primary molars
   e. Absent 2/
8. Bimaxillary proclination:
   a. Represents inclination of the upper/lower incisors less than the mean for White European populations
   b. Is common with cleft lip and palate
   c. Results when lip pressure is higher than tongue pressure
   d. May exist with incisor relationship class I
   e. Has a high chance of stability when corrected
9. Factors that may aggravate an already increased overjet include:
   a. A persistent thumb-sucking habit
   b. Upper arch crowding
   c. A bilateral buccal segment crossbite
   d. An anterior mandibular growth rotation
   e. Proclination of the lower incisors
10. Prognosis for stable correction of a 10-mm overjet in a 12-year-old female patient with average overbite is enhanced when:
    a. The underlying anteroposterior skeletal pattern is class I
    b. There is a backward pattern of mandibular growth
    c. The lower lip lies under the upper incisors post-treatment
    d. A thumb-sucking habit persists
    e. A buccal segment crossbite is present pretreatment
11. A functional appliance for correction of a class II division 1 malocclusion:
    a. Works by maintaining the mandible in its rest position
    b. Is least effective during active growth
    c. Is ideal for treating irregularities in tooth alignment
    d. Requires 14–16 hours per day wear to be effective
    e. Requires post-treatment retention until growth has ceased
12. Deep overbite in class II division 2 malocclusion is associated with:
    a. A reduced interincisal angle
    b. A high lower lip line
    c. Average cingulum thickness on the upper incisors
    d. A forward pattern of mandibular growth
    e. Early loss of a mandibular primary first molar
13. Relative to class I malocclusion, cephalometric features of class III malocclusion may include:
    a. A short maxillary length
    b. A more posterior position of the glenoid fossa
    c. A reduced mandibular length
    d. A more protrusive position of the maxilla
    e. Retroclined lower incisors
14. An anterior open bite may be caused by:
    a. A low Frankfort-mandibular planes angle
    b. An endogenous tongue thrust
    c. A cleft of the lip and alveolus
    d. A digit-sucking habit
    e. A horizontal pattern of facial growth
15. A buccal crossbite on 5/ may result from:
    a. Early loss of e/
    b. Submergence of ē/

c. A repaired cleft palate
   d. A prolonged thumb-sucking habit
   e. A class III malocclusion
16. In a 30-year-old adult male patient:
    a. Overbite reduction is generally easier than in an adolescent
    b. Molar extrusion is the approach of choice for overbite reduction orthodontically
    c. Lighter forces are desirable for tooth movement if the dentition is periodontally compromised
    d. Anchorage demands may be less if teeth have been lost
    e. Significant skeletal discrepancies may be addressed by growth modification
17. Factors associated with dental and/or skeletal relapse following mandibular advancement osteotomy include:
    a. Mandibular advancement greater than 8 mm
    b. Condylar distraction during surgery
    c. Adequate fixation
    d. Poor co-operation with wear of intermaxillary elastics
    e. Tongue thrust
18. Common dental anomalies in a 10-year-old child with a left unilateral cleft of lip and palate include:
    a. Enamel hypoplasia of /1
    b. Delayed eruption of the permanent dentition
    c. Absent /2
    d. A lingual crossbite of the buccal segments
    e. Anterior crossbite
19. Alveolar bone grafting in patients with cleft lip and palate:
    a. Is best undertaken before age 8 years
    b. Improves alar base support
    c. Provides bone through which 6 can usually erupt
    d. Stabilises a mobile premaxilla in a bilateral cleft
    e. Should be undertaken simultaneously with any extractions on the cleft side

EXTENDED MATCHING ITEMS QUESTIONS

Theme: Occlusal management
For each of the clinical problems (a–e), select from the list below (1–13) the most appropriate course of action (more than one may be correct). Each item can be used once, more than once or not at all.

1. Removal of lower second primary molars after eruption of the permanent lateral incisors.
2. Early removal of the associated upper primary canine.
3. Retention of a lower second primary molar.
4. Observe but take no specific action.
5. Removal of supernumerary.
6. Carry out a balancing extraction.
7. Extraction of the same tooth type in contralateral quadrants.
8. Autotransplant a lower premolar.
9. Prescribe a radiograph to check if a supernumerary tooth is present.
10. Upper permanent incisor proclination with an upper removable appliance.
11. Fit an upper removable appliance space maintainer.

12. Extraction of the upper left second primary molar.
13. Prescribe a dental panoramic tomogram and an upper anterior occlusal radiograph.
    a. A 9-year-old boy with class I incisor and molar relationships who has large carious lesions in the upper left and lower right first permanent molars (all permanent teeth are developing on a dental panoramic tomogram).
    b. A 10-year-old girl with a class II division 2 malocclusion where the upper right permanent canine is not palpable buccally; subsequent radiographic assessment reveals the tooth to overlap less than half the width of the upper right permanent lateral incisor and to be located at the mid-third of its root; the long axis of the unerupted right maxillary canine is <30° to the midsagittal plane.
    c. An 18-year-old girl with a class III malocclusion and generalised mild crowding who is not keen to proceed with fixed appliance orthodontic treatment; a single conical supernumerary is identified radiographically well above the apices of the upper incisors.
    d. A 9-year-old boy with the upper permanent incisors fully erupted and a median diastema of 4 mm.
    e. An 8.5-year-old girl presents with caries on the medial aspect of the upper left first permanent molar which is impacted into the upper left second primary molar producing resorption of half the width of its distobuccal root resulting in pain.

CASE HISTORY QUESTIONS

Case History 1

An 8-year-old girl presents with her mother, who is very concerned about her daughter's large (5 mm) upper median diastema.

1. What are the causes of an upper median diastema in an 8-year-old?
2. What are the management options?

Case History 2

A 10-year-old child presents with an anterior open bite.

1. What are the possible causes of the open bite?
2. What treatment options may be considered?

Case History 3

A 7-year-old boy presents with 1/1 in crossbite but otherwise has features of a class I malocclusion.

1. What is the possible aetiology of the crossbite?
2. When is early treatment advisable?
3. What factors must be considered regarding treatment possibilities?
4. List the desirable features in the design of an upper removable appliance to correct the incisor relationship.

PICTURE QUESTIONS

Picture 1

Fig. 10.6 is a radiograph.

1. What features are visible?

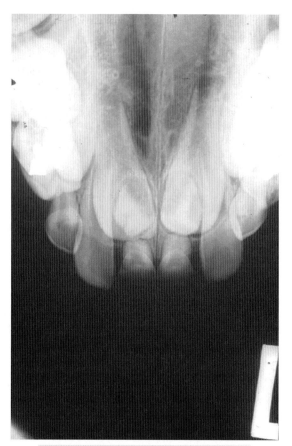

Fig. 10.6 Upper anterior occlusal radiograph.

2. What other common factors or conditions may produce a similar effect?
3. How would you manage the case?

Picture 2

Fig. 10.7 shows the anterior occlusion of a 13-year-old female.

1. What anomaly is visible?
2. What is its likely aetiology?
3. What are the management options?
4. What factors would dictate your decision regarding treatment?

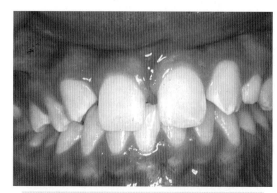

Fig. 10.7 Anterior occlusion of a 13-year-old female.

Picture 3

Fig. 10.8 shows an intraoral view of an 8-year-old girl.

1. What occlusal anomaly is visible?
2. What clinical assessment would you wish to perform and why?
3. What is the possible aetiology?
4. What are the treatment options?

Picture 4

Fig. 10.9 is a dental panoramic tomogram.

1. What anomaly is visible?
2. What factors may account for this?
3. How would you aid localisation?
4. What interceptive method may have helped to avoid this problem developing?
5. What factors determine whether orthodontic alignment is possible?

Picture 5

Fig. 10.10 is a lower intraoral occlusal view in a 19-year-old male patient.

1. What anomaly is present?
2. How may this arise?
3. What advice would you give?
4. What management possibilities exist?

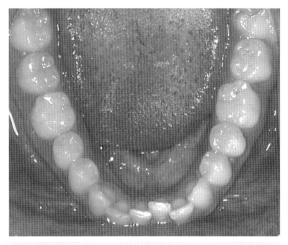

Fig. 10.10 Lower intraoral occlusal view in a 19-year-old male.

Picture 6

Fig. 10.11 shows the frontal view of a 22-year-old female who presented for orthodontic treatment with an obvious facial anomaly, which she reported to be gradually worsening.

1. What obvious facial anomaly is present?
2. What investigation is shown in Fig. 10.12? What does this show?
3. What occlusal features would you expect?
4. How would you manage the patient?

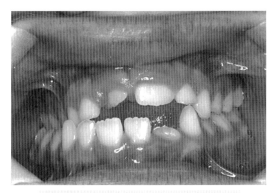

Fig. 10.8 Intraoral view in an 8-year-old girl.

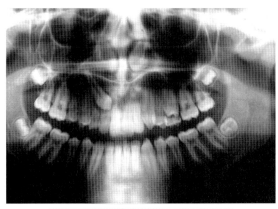

Fig. 10.9 Dental panoramic tomogram.

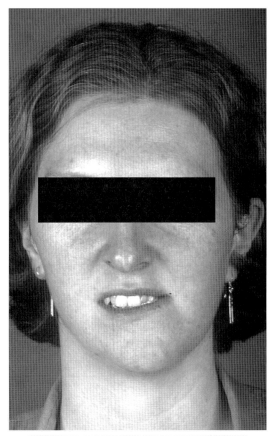

Fig. 10.11 Frontal view of a 22-year-old female.

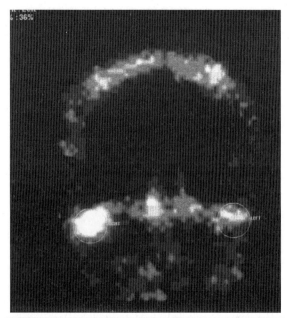

Fig. 10.12 An image from a bone scan with technetium-99m.

Picture 7

The intraoral views (Fig. 10.13) are of a 2-day-old infant with a cleft.

1. Classify the cleft and outline the anatomical aetiology.
2. What would be the initial management (first weeks)?
3. When would surgical intervention usually be considered?
4. What would be your management during the primary dentition?

SHORT NOTE QUESTIONS

Write short notes on:

1. infraoccluded primary molars
2. impacted 6s
3. serial extractions
4. transposition
5. space maintenance
6. methods of overbite correction
7. growth modification for class II correction
8. camouflage therapy for class II correction
9. bilateral buccal crossbite
10. differences in orthodontic treatment in adults compared with adolescents
11. maxillary osteotomies
12. aetiology of clefting.

VIVA QUESTION

1. What are the possible effects of early loss of primary teeth on the permanent dentition? What factors determine the severity of these effects and how may the impact of any undesirable effect be minimised?

SINGLE BEST ANSWER QUESTIONS

1. The term 'compensating' extraction refers to extraction of:
   A. Another tooth in the opposing quadrant
   B. Another tooth on the opposite side of the arch
   C. Same tooth in the diagonally opposite quadrant
   D. Same tooth in the opposing quadrant
   E. Same tooth on the opposite side of the arch
2. In the mixed dentition, planned extraction of both upper primary canines is advisable where:
   A. An upper second premolar is impacted
   B. Bilateral buccal crossbite exists of the upper arch
   C. Large upper median diastema is present
   D. Unilateral permanent maxillary canine is ectopic palatally
   E. Upper permanent incisors are very mildly crowded
3. The reported prevalence of children affected by molar incisor hypoplasia is:
   A. One in five
   B. One in four
   C. One in seven
   D. One in six
   E. One in seven
4. Exposure and alignment of a palatally displaced maxillary canine is unlikely to be successful if the crown position mesio-distally relative to adjacent teeth is:
   A. Across the distal half of the lateral incisor
   B. Beyond the midline of the central incisor
   C. Crosses into the mesial half of the lateral incisor
   D. Lies between the lateral incisor and the first premolar
   E. Over the distal half of the central incisor

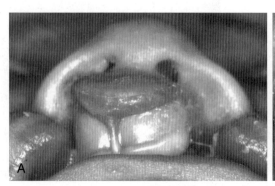
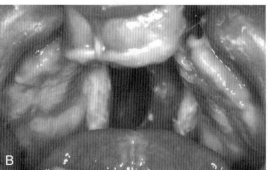

Fig. 10.13 Intraoral views of a 2-day-old infant with a cleft.

5. Correction of a unilateral buccal segment crossbite with mandibular displacement in the mixed dentition is best undertaken by a:
   A. Functional appliance
   B. Midline expansion screw in an upper removable appliance
   C. Occlusal grinding of the primary canines
   D. Quadhelix appliance
   E. Rapid maxillary expansion

6. Early functional appliance treatment for class II division 1 malocclusion:
   A. Is likely to increase patient co-operation for further treatment
   B. Leads to a superior skeletal change compared to later treatment
   C. May be considered to reduce the risk of upper incisor trauma
   D. Produces better final occlusal results
   E. Shortens the overall length of treatment

7. The best radiographic technique for detecting suspected resorption of a maxillary lateral incisor by a maxillary canine is:
   A. CBCT
   B. Dental panoramic tomogram
   C. Lateral cephalogram
   D. Maxillary anterior occlusal
   E. Periapical film

8. The reported percentage of cases in the mixed dentition where protraction facemask therapy is effective for class III correction is:
   A. 20
   B. 30
   C. 50
   D. 70
   E. 90

9. A class II division 2 malocclusion commonly exhibits which occlusal feature:
   A. Buccal crossbite of the first molars
   B. Class III molar relationship
   C. Lingual crossbite of first premolars
   D. Proclined upper incisors
   E. Reduced overbite

10. The most stable orthognathic procedure is:
    A. Advancement genioplasty
    B. Lower labial segment setdown
    C. Mandibular setback
    D. Maxillary impaction
    E. Surgically assisted maxillary expansion

11. The most aesthetic orthodontic appliance for adult treatment is:
    A. Ceramic labial brackets
    B. Clear aligners
    C. Lingual appliances
    D. Stainless steel labial brackets
    E. Plastic labial brackets

12. In a child with compete unilateral cleft of lip and palate, surgery to close the hard and soft palate should be undertaken at:
    A. 4 weeks
    B. 2 months
    C. 6–9 months
    D. 1 year
    E. 12–18 months

Self-Assessment: Answers

MULTIPLE CHOICE ANSWERS

1. a. False. Affects upper lateral incisors in 2% of cases.
   b. True. Affects lower second premolars (3%) more so than upper second premolars (less than 2%).
   c. False. Hypodontia and microdontia are more common in females than males.
   d. False. Hypodontia has a strong tendency to run in families.
   e. False. Third molars start to calcify any time between 8 and 14 years so one must wait until age 14 years before making a definite diagnosis of hypodontia of third molars.

2. a. False. Occur in about 2% of the population in the permanent dentition (~1% in primary dentition).
   b. False. More common in males.
   c. True. Typically as a supplemental lower incisor.
   d. True. Typically by a conical mesiodens.
   e. True. For example, a conical mesiodens high above the apices of 1/1.

3. a. False. Timing of removal is best when the bifurcation of /7 is calcifying (aged ~8.5–9.5 years) and not when bifurcation of /8 is calcifying.
   b. True. In a class I malocclusion with a class I molar relationship, a compensating extraction (i.e. removal of /6) is advisable to prevent the 'plunger cusp' effect of overeruption of /6 into the lower extraction site.
   c. False. There is no need to balance for the extraction with removal of 6 | as all other teeth are sound; however, an extraction from the lower right quadrant will be necessary to relieve the moderate premolar crowding.
   d. False. Removal of one lower first permanent molar is not likely to lead to an overjet increase.
   e. False. There is likely to be no overbite increase.

4. a. True. Timely removal of cs may allow this to occur.
   b. True. Extraction of cs will provide space to allow for 2s to be moved distally with appliance therapy, thereby creating space for alignment of an unerupted upper permanent incisor.
   c. False. Extraction of s will have no effect on the position of lower incisors.
   d. True. Displaced 3 may align spontaneously with timely extraction of c (usually about age 10 years) provided position of 3 and space conditions in the arch are favourable.
   e. True. As this will favour mesial drift particularly where there is inherent crowding.

5. a. False. A balancing extraction would involve extraction of a lower left primary molar.

b. False. A compensating extraction would involve removal of the upper right first primary molar.

c. False. Extraction should be balanced to prevent centreline shift.

d. False. Balancing extraction will not prevent overbite reduction.

e. True. Early removal is advisable to prevent adjacent teeth tilting into its space and making removal more difficult.

6. a. False. An open bite is characteristic.

b. True. The upper incisors are proclined and lower incisors retroclined, often in an asymmetric manner through positioning of the thumb.

c. True. The action of the cheek musculature is unopposed in sucking because the tongue is displaced out of the palatal vault by the insertion of the thumb.

d. True. Because of the anterior open bite, this is necessary to achieve an anterior oral seal for swallowing.

e. False. No evidence to support this.

7. a. True. Buccal displacement is likely in a crowded arch as 3s are the last teeth to erupt in the buccal segments with exception of second and third molars and therefore may be displaced buccally if the arch is intrinsically crowded.

b. True. This will deflect the eruption path of 3/.

c. False. This will have no effect on position of 3/.

d. False. Early loss of primary molars in the lower arch will not affect crowding in the upper arch.

e. False. This will not produce buccal displacement of 3/.

8. a. False. Inclination of upper/lower incisors is more proclined than the mean value for White European populations.

b. False. Bimaxillary retroclination is more common with cleft lip and palate.

c. False. Typically lip pressure is less than tongue pressure.

d. True. Overjet may be slightly increased because of the incisor inclination, although the incisor relationship may be class I.

e. False. Stability is generally poor and at best guarded as any retroclination of upper/lower incisors is prone to relapse owing to encroachment on tongue space.

9. a. True. This will procline upper incisors and retrocline lower incisors, worsening the overjet.

b. True. If the upper arch is inherently crowded, the upper incisors may be displaced labially making the overjet worse.

c. False. This will have no effect.

d. False. This will tend to reduce the overjet; a backward mandibular growth rotation will tend to make the overjet worse.

e. False. This will tend to mask an increased overjet.

10. a. True. The greater the class II skeletal pattern, the more difficult stable correction is likely to be.

b. False. A backward pattern of mandibular growth will tend to worsen the prognosis.

c. False. Coverage of one-third to one-half of the labial surface of the upper incisors by the lower lip confers a better prognosis.

d. False. This will promote overjet increase.

e. False. This will not affect the prognosis for overjet correction.

11. a. False. The mandible is held in a forward postured position.

b. False. The appliance is most effective during the growth spurt.

c. False. Typically the appliance has no components to treat irregularities in tooth position; these are best dealt with by other appliance systems, particularly fixed appliances.

d. True. Full-time wear is generally not required but at least 14–16 hours' wear per day is required to give the best chance of success.

e. True. Wear of the appliance on a night-only basis until the late teens is advisable to minimise overjet relapse.

12. a. False. A high interincisal angle would produce a deep overbite.

b. True. This will retrocline upper incisors.

c. False. Maxillary incisor cingulae tend to be poorly developed.

d. True. This will tend to increase overbite.

e. False. No evidence to support this.

13. a. True. This leads to maxillary retrusion.

b. False. The condylar head is in a more anterior position, producing mandibular prognathism.

c. False. Increased mandibular length leads to mandibular protrusion.

d. False. More retruded position of the maxilla leads to maxillary retrusion.

e. True. Because of dento-alveolar compensation for the skeletal pattern.

14. a. False. A low angle would tend to produce a deep overbite and a high angle an anterior open bite.

b. True. This will procline upper and lower incisors and reduce the overbite.

c. True. As this would inhibit vertical alveolar growth.

d. True. As upper incisors are proclined, and eruption of lower incisors is inhibited.

e. False. A vertical pattern of facial growth would lead to anterior open bite.

15. a. True. As this will allow 6/ to migrate forward in a crowded arch displacing 5/ palatally.

b. False. This will not produce a buccal crossbite but perhaps allow overeruption of 5/.

c. True. As transverse maxillary growth is likely to be restricted.

d. True. See 6 (c) above.

e. True. As a wider part of the lower arch opposes a relatively narrower part of the upper arch.

16. a. False. As successful overbite reduction depends on favourable growth and growth can be regarded as ceased in the adult, treatment is generally more difficult than in the adolescent.

b. False. Incisor intrusion rather than molar extrusion is the preferred approach for overbite reduction. Molar extrusion will increase the vertical posterior facial height and is likely to relapse.

c. True. As the pressure (force per unit area) on the periodontium will be greater for a given force in a periodontally compromised dentition, forces need to be lighter than where there has been no loss of periodontal support.

d. False. Anchorage demands are likely to be greater where teeth have been lost as there are fewer teeth to incorporate in the anchor unit.

e. False. Although small increments in growth occur in adulthood, for the purpose of any orthodontic treatment, adults can be regarded as non-growing. Growth modification is, therefore, not a viable treatment option.

17. a. True. Movement greater than 8 mm is likely to place the soft tissues under tension and tend to induce relapse.

b. True. Distraction of the condyles will lead to relapse when they return to the condylar fossae.

c. False. This is likely to promote stability.

d. True. Non-compliance with elastic wear is likely to lead to relapse in the occlusal result.

e. True. Tongue thrust would tend to lead to relapse of the incisor occlusion, particularly an overjet increase and an incomplete overbite.

18. a. True. As the enamel organ in the site of the cleft is affected.

b. True.

c. True. Teeth are often absent in the line of a cleft as all tissues (dental as well) are affected.

d. False. A buccal crossbite is common following post-surgical restriction in transverse growth of the maxilla.

e. True. Collapse and inward rotation of the cleft segment commonly leads to anterior crossbite.

19. a. False. If grafting is undertaken before 8 years, it may interfere with transverse anterior maxillary growth.

b. True. The added bone improves alar base support.

c. False. It provides bone through which 3 usually (not 6) may erupt.

d. True. A bony bridge will reduce mobility of the premaxilla.

e. False. Extractions should be undertaken at least 3 weeks prior to bone grafting to allow keratinised mucosa to heal.

EXTENDED MATCHING ITEMS ANSWERS

a. 7. In view of the patient's age, occlusal features and radiographic findings, this treatment is likely to lead to a satisfactory buccal occlusion when the second permanent molars erupt.

b. 2, 6. Removal of the upper right primary canine is required to encourage alignment of the upper right permanent canine; removal of the upper left primary canine is required also to prevent an upper centreline shift.

c. 4. The supernumerary may be observed and no arrangements made for its surgical removal as no orthodontic tooth movement is planned and it is well away from the upper incisor apices.

d. 9. In view of the magnitude of the diastema, it would be wise to check radiographically regarding the presence of a supernumerary tooth. If present, a surgical opinion should be requested.

e. 12. This is required in view of the symptomatic resorption and the need to restore the first permanent molar.

CASE HISTORY ANSWERS

Case History 1

1. An upper median diastema occurs routinely as a developmental stage of dental development (formerly referred to as the 'ugly duckling' stage), which tends to reduce as the permanent maxillary canines erupt. It can also be caused by:
   - missing or small upper lateral incisors
   - generalised spacing in the upper arch
   - proclination of the upper incisors in a class II division 1 malocclusion or digit-sucking
   - supernumerary tooth, i.e. mesiodens
   - low-lying frenal attachment may be associated with a midline space; blanching of the incisive papilla when the frenum is put under tension and a characteristic 'V'-shaped notch radiographically in the alveolar bone between the incisors implicate involvement of the frenum.

2. There are a number of treatment options:
   - If a supernumerary tooth is interfering with approximation of the incisors, removal is indicated ensuring no damage to the adjacent teeth. Otherwise wait until 3s erupt before considering treatment.
   - Where the lateral incisors are absent, space opening or space closure are options. If the latter is the preferred option, consider early extraction of primary teeth to encourage mesial drift of the buccal segments. Fixed appliances are usually required later to complete alignment and space closure, followed by recontouring of the cusp tips of 3/3 and composite additions to their mesial aspects (or veneers) followed by bonded retention to 31/13.
   - If space opening is deemed a better option, wait until 3/3 erupt and then create space for 2/2, followed by their replacement initially on a partial denture/removable retainer and at a later stage by either resin-retained bridgework or implants.
   - In class II division 1, or crowded maxillary arches where 3 is upright/distally inclined and of favourable colour and form, space closure is generally preferable to space opening. Conversely where a class III incisor relationship or spacing exists, space opening is usually the option of choice.
   - If spacing is generalised and mild, advise the patient to accept it or consider composite additions or veneers to close the anterior spaces when older. Where the spacing is more marked in those with severe hypodontia, orthodontic treatment is usually required to reposition the teeth and localise space prior to prosthetic or implant replacement.
   - Correction of a class II division 1 malocclusion should eliminate the midline diastema; early treatment with a functional appliance may be indicated. If the space is caused by digit-sucking, the patient should be advised to stop. In some instances, fitting an upper removable appliance to act as a reminder may be useful.
   - If a frenal involvement is suspected, fraenectomy prior to completion of space closure will be advantageous, the scar tissue encouraging incisor approximation.

Case History 2

1. There are a number of possible causes:
   - Skeletal: an increased FMPA and anterior lower facial height.
   - Soft tissues: an endogenous tongue thrust (often difficult to distinguish from an adaptive tongue thrust), although lisping and proclination of both upper and lower incisors are thought to be characteristic.
   - Digit-sucking habit: this arrests eruption of the incisors.
   - Cleft of the lip and primary palate: this may produce a local failure of development of the alveolus.

2. If the open bite is caused by digit-sucking, gently persuade the child to stop. Otherwise wait until the permanent dentition is fully established. Ensure that the habit is stopped before considering correction of an overjet, otherwise relapse is likely, although occasionally the habit may stop if appliance therapy is instituted. If it is not caused by digit-sucking, monitor, and where growth is likely to be favourable with no adverse soft tissue factors, consider growth modification with a maxillary intrusion splint and high-pull headgear or with a functional appliance incorporating high-pull headgear (depending on whether there is an underlying class II skeletal problem). Accept the open bite if it is mild or if the soft tissue factors are adverse (endogenous tongue thrust or grossly incompetent lips). Crowding may, however, be relieved and the arches aligned accepting the vertical discrepancy. Orthodontic correction may be possible in a limited number of children, particularly where the arches are crowded with bimaxillary proclination and the lips are likely to become competent post-treatment. Orthognathic surgery is required in severe anterior open bite and is best carried out when growth is complete.

Case History 3

1. Retention of a/a may deflect the path of eruption of the permanent successors into crossbite. A mild class III skeletal pattern may also produce an incisor crossbite, even though the malocclusion is otherwise class I. In those with repaired cleft lip and palate, scar tissue contraction may restrain maxillary growth, producing an incisor crossbite.

2. Early treatment is advisable if the crossbite is associated with a mandibular displacement on closure, as this may predispose to temporomandibular joint dysfunction syndrome. In addition, displacing occlusal contacts may push the mandibular incisors labially and compromise periodontal health.

3. The factors to be considered include the following:
   - The inclination of the upper incisors: this will determine if tipping or bodily movement will be necessary.
   - The inclination of the lower incisors: lingual movement of the lower incisors in addition to labial movement of the upper incisors may be needed.
   - The amount of overbite likely: a positive overbite is necessary for stability.
   - The amount of space available for 1/1 proclination.

4. Desirable features include:
   - activation: individual Z-springs may be used to procline each of the incisors (or one double-cantilever spring to procline both) but activation may displace

the base plate away from the palate; use of a screw section clasping the teeth to be moved will overcome this problem
   - retention: typically Adams' clasps on 6/6 (if a screw section is used to procline the incisors, these may be clasped also)
   - anchorage: from all teeth other than 1/1, and the palate contacted via the base plate
   - base plate: posterior capping is necessary to disengage the anterior teeth by about 2 mm, thereby facilitating crossbite correction.

PICTURE ANSWERS

Picture 1

1. Unerupted 1/1 owing to the presence of two supernumerary teeth with retained a/a.
2. Delayed eruption of 1/1 may also occur through ectopic position of the tooth germs, dilaceration, delayed exfoliation of a/a, crowding or cleft lip and palate.
3. Remove the supernumerary teeth and bond gold chain to the unerupted 1/1; maintain/create space to accommodate the unerupted 1/1 (some operators may choose to swap the order of these steps). This will involve fitting an upper removable appliance with palatal finger springs to move 2/2 distally. It may be necessary to extract cs also. If 1/1 do not erupt spontaneously, then traction can be applied to the gold chain to extrude them into alignment.

Picture 2

1. Absent 2/2.
2. Strong genetic link and is more common in females than males. The 2s may also be absent in cleft lip and palate owing to absence of the tooth-forming tissues in the line of the cleft.
3. Management options include: accept, open spaces for prosthetic replacement (possibly by implants) of missing units, close spaces orthodontically, restorative build-up of the teeth on either side of the space with either composite or veneers.
4. Consider what the patient wishes, level of oral hygiene, dental status, interest and likely co-operation with orthodontic treatment/complex restorative treatment. Space closure is best considered where the upper arch is crowded, FMPA is increased, an overjet exists, size/shape/colour of 3s will give satisfactory aesthetics beside 1s and the buccal segment relationship is a full unit class II. Space opening is best considered where there is no crowding/spacing in the arch, FMPA is average or reduced, morphology of 3s will not give good aesthetic result when approximated to 1s, buccal segment relationship is class I/half unit class II and/or there is a class III incisor relationship where proclination of incisors will correct an anterior crossbite.

Picture 3

1. A crossbite of the right buccal segments.
2. It would be essential to determine if there is a mandibular displacement associated with the crossbite. This may be assessed by asking the child to touch the back of the hard palate with the tongue and to maintain this while

gently closing the mouth. It is wise to correct a crossbite with an associated mandibular displacement sooner rather than later to allow the remaining occlusal development to occur in an undisplaced position.

3. This may result from a thumb-sucking habit (although in this case none of the other features associated with such a habit are visible); the anterior open bite is due to partial eruption of the permanent incisors rather than to a digit-sucking habit). It may also be skeletal resulting from a mismatch in the width of the upper and lower dental arches. Condylar hypoplasia and hemimandibular hypertrophy are rarer causes.

4. If a mandibular displacement is present due to initial contact on the primary canines, these may be ground in an initial attempt to remove the displacement and correct the crossbite. Other management strategies are expansion of the upper arch either by a midline screw incorporated in an upper removable appliance with buccal capping to disengage the occlusion or by a quadhelix appliance. If no displacement is present, the crossbite may be accepted unless correction as part of more comprehensive treatment is considered at a later stage. Should hemimandibular hypertrophy or asymmetric mandibular deficiency be the cause, then careful planning with a maxillofacial surgeon is required so that intervention is timed appropriately. For hemimandibular hypertrophy, either condylar or ramus surgery should be considered depending on the outcome of a technetium-99m bone scan. For asymmetric mandibular deficiency with some condylar translation on the affected side, a custom-designed 'hybrid' functional appliance may be used to address the vertical and anteroposterior deficiency aspects of the asymmetry. Where little or no translation of the condyle exists, early surgical intervention is indicated followed by hybrid functional therapy to release ankylosis and guide subsequent growth.

Picture 4

1. Ectopic position of 3/.
2. The following factors have been implicated in the aetiology of maxillary canine impaction:
   - Recent evidence suggests a strong genetic influence.
   - 3 has the longest path of eruption of any tooth in the dental arches and has therefore a greater likelihood of becoming displaced.
   - Absent or short-rooted 2. 3 is guided into position by the root of 2, and where 2 is absent or has a short root, there is a two-fold increase in the incidence of palatal displacement of 3.
   - A higher incidence of palatal canine ectopia has been identified also in class II division 2 malocclusion, where small teeth in well-developed arches have been noted.
   - Absence of crowding: palatal impaction of 3 is more likely in a spaced rather than a crowded arch.
3. Clinical palpation of the buccal sulcus and palatal mucosa should have been undertaken before any radiographic investigation. A dental panoramic tomogram will give an indication as to the position of 3: if the image is enlarged relative to 3 on the opposite side of the arch, the tooth is likely to be palatal in 80% of cases. However, two views are required to localise the position of 3; the

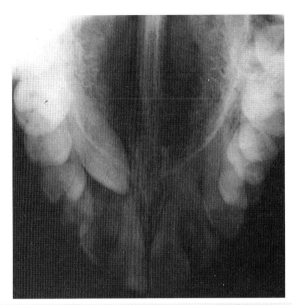

Fig. 10.14 Localisation of 3/ position, upper anterior occlusal view.

panoramic view may be supplemented with an upper anterior occlusal view (Fig. 10.14) or by two periapical films. Parallax is then employed to locate the tooth: if the tooth moves in the same direction as the tube shift, it is palatal; if it remains stationary, it is in the line of the arch; if it moves in the opposite direction to the tube shift, it is buccal.

4. Removal of c/ at age 10 may have helped to encourage improvement in the position of 3/. The extraction of c/ would require a balancing extraction of /c to prevent centreline deviation.
5. Exposure and orthodontic alignment of 3/ depend on the following:
   - General factors: motivated patient with a well-maintained mouth.
   - Local factors: adequate space for 3/, or likely from extractions.
   - 3/ below apical third of incisor roots, overlapping less than half the mesiodistal width of 1, less than 30° to the midsagittal plane and the apex not distal to 5.

Picture 5

1. Late lower labial segment crowding.
2. This is an expected development with aging. This has a multifactorial aetiology including uprighting of the lower labial segment (possibly owing to increased tissue tone in the lips with maturation and in response to mandibular growth rotation), tendency for intercanine width to reduce in late teens, mesial drift and anterior component of force. Third molar presence/eruption has been implicated in its aetiology but is only weakly associated. One possibility is that as 8 erupts, it pushes the incisors forward; alternatively 8 blocks dispersion of forces created by mandibular growth whereby the mandibular dentition moves distally relative to the mandibular body.
3. Explain that it is a common maturational change in the occlusion. Study models should be taken to act as a baseline record from which to monitor any further change.

The patient may be seen again if the crowding worsens considerably.

4. Management option initially is to accept and monitor. If crowding worsens, consider interdental stripping in moderate cases or extraction of a lower incisor in severely crowded mouths and alignment with a fixed appliance followed by bonded retention.

Picture 6

1. Marked facial asymmetry with chin point displaced about 1 cm to the left.

2. An image (anterior Towne's view with the mouth open) from a bone scan with technetium-99m. It shows a 'hot spot' in the right condylar area and the difference in isotope uptake between the right and left sides.

3. One would expect a buccal crossbite of the left buccal segments with the lower centerline displaced to the left.

4. Management. If the referring practitioner or the patient has previous dental casts, the magnitude of any occlusal change in the intervening period can be assessed. Similarly the degree of facial change can be assessed from previous facial photographs. As the condyle is still actively growing, producing hemimandibular hypertrophy, this will require a high 'condylar shave'. When the condition has stabilised, orthodontic treatment – in combination with orthognathic surgery – will be required to ensure a satisfactory facial appearance and occlusion.

Picture 7

1. Complete bilateral cleft of lip and palate. Failure of fusion of the medial and lateral nasal process on each side with the corresponding maxillary process produces the bilateral cleft lip (probably at about 6 weeks of intrauterine life). Failure of fusion of the palatal shelves, which form the secondary palate at about 8 weeks of life, leads to the cleft palate.

2. Initial management. The weeks following the birth of a child with a cleft are very difficult for the parents, who invariably feel somewhat shocked and disappointed. Great sensitivity on the part of the nursing staff and support from family and other members of the cleft team are required. Instruction in bottle feeding with the aid of special teats is necessary and introduction to a support group, such as the Cleft Lip and Palate Association, who can provide counselling, is invaluable. The likely future management should also be explained by a member of the cleft team and a contact person identified who can provide advice as required. In some centres, feeding plates are made and presurgical orthopaedics commenced with the intention of reducing the size of the cleft to make surgical closure easier. The benefits of this intervention are disputed and it is not so widely practised nowadays.

3. Usually lip closure is undertaken at about 3 months of age. With a bilateral cleft, one side may be repaired at a time. Palatal repair is usual at about 9–12 months.

4. During the primary dentition, the following are advisable:
   - Regular care by the general dental practitioner and prescription of fluoride supplements if required.
   - Speech assessment at about 18 months and speech therapy as required; regular monitoring of speech

and hearing should be carried out during childhood.
   - Lip revision, closure of palatal fistulae and possible pharyngoplasty may be undertaken at about 4–5 years of age if required.

SHORT NOTE ANSWERS

1. Infraoccluded primary molars occur in about 1–9% of children although estimates vary. They arise most probably because of ankylosis of the primary molar while alveolar bone growth and development of the adjacent teeth continues. Exfoliation will occur eventually if the permanent successor is present and not in an ectopic position. Removal, however, is indicated where the submergence is marked, with the crown of the tooth just visible or where root development of the unerupted premolar is almost complete.

2. This occurs in 2–6% of children but its prevalence is ~25% in cleft lip and palate. A number of factors have been implicated in its aetiology, including a more mesial eruption path of 6, a larger mean size of primary first and second molars and a retruded maxilla. Impaction may be reversible and self-correct, although this is uncommon after 8 years. In mild cases, placement of a brass wire separator for a few months may allow disimpaction, but appliance therapy to move 6 distally may be required in more marked cases. Removal of e may be required if symptomatic resorption has occurred or to allow restoration of 6. Extraction of e will aggravate existing crowding by facilitating mesial drift of 6 but can be managed at a later stage.

3. This was advocated by Kjellgren in 1948 as an interceptive procedure in a developing malocclusion to eliminate the need for any further intervention later. It involves removal of cs at age 8.5–9.5 years to encourage relief of incisor crowding; removal of ds at about 1 year later to encourage 4s to erupt; removal of 4s as 3s are erupting. A class I malocclusion with generalised moderate crowding is required for this to have the best chance of success, but even where these features are present there is no guarantee that appliance therapy will not be required later. For this reason and because three episodes of dental extractions, often requiring three episodes of general anaesthesia, are required, the full extent of serial extractions is not practised nowadays. Rather, extraction of cs alone may be considered in some circumstances: removal of cs to allow the position of ectopic 3s to improve in the early mixed dentition; to allow a 2, which is likely to erupt in crossbite, to move labially; to create space for crossbite correction on 2 or for alignment of 1 following removal of a supernumerary which has impeded its eruption. Removal of D s may be considered to facilitate lingual movement of a lower incisor that is being displaced labially by a crossbite relationship with the upper incisor teeth, or of the whole lower labial segment lingually in a class III malocclusion.

4. Transposition is a positional interchange of two adjacent teeth (particularly of their roots) or the development of a tooth in a position occupied typically by an adjacent tooth. It is an uncommon dental anomaly (0.1–0.2% prevalence). It affects 3,4 and 2,3 most commonly. Management involves acceptance of the transposition if it is complete, extraction of the most displaced

tooth if crowding is present or orthodontic alignment where sufficient space exists in the arch. The apical positions of the transposed teeth will determine whether alignment is carried out with the teeth in their transposed positions or if these can be corrected.

5. Space maintenance is indicated:
   - typically in the late mixed dentition where there is likely to be no crowding in an arch, if mesial drift can be withheld and the leeway space used to provide space for arch alignment
   - where there is moderate/severe crowding in an arch such that there will be just sufficient space for the remaining teeth following removal of a unit/units. In the upper arch, it involves fitting either a removal appliance or palatal arch, whereas a lingual arch is best in the lower arch.

6. An increased overbite may be reduced by several means. In a growing child, a flat anterior bite plane on a removable appliance restrains eruption of the lower incisors while allowing the lower molars to overerupt, thereby reducing the overbite. Lower incisor capping on a functional appliance will effect overbite reduction by similar means. Extrusion of the upper molars by cervical headgear to upper molar bands in a growing patient will also reduce overbite. In the child patient, facial growth then compensates for the increase in vertical facial height. Where the overbite increases through overeruption of the upper labial segment, often with an associated 'gummy' smile, intrusion of the upper incisors with either high-pull headgear to a full-coverage maxillary splint or by a fixed appliance is indicated. In the adult, overbite reduction must be by incisor intrusion with a fixed appliance rather than by molar extrusion as there is unlikely to be any favourable vertical facial growth. In adults where the overbite is greatly increased, overbite reduction by orthognathic surgery will be required. Presurgical orthodontics does not involve overbite reduction. Rather, where class II correction is undertaken by mandibular advancement, overbite is reduced postsurgically by extrusion of the buccal segment teeth into occlusion to close the lateral open bites. In some patients, segmental osteotomies to 'set down' the lower labial segment and/or impact the upper labial segment may be indicated.

7. Growth modification is indicated in moderate-to-severe class II malocclusion in the mixed dentition when the child is growing. Treatment should commence just prior to the pubertal growth spurt so that maximum advantage is taken of the growth potential. Depending on the contribution of maxillary prognathism or mandibular retrusion to the aetiology of the malocclusion, treatment attempts to restrain maxillary vertical and forward growth and/or encourage mandibular growth. In doing so, the growth expression of the maxilla and/or mandible is altered but the amount of growth of both is unaffected. This is carried out by either a functional appliance or headgear (1000 g required to restrain maxillary growth), or by a combination of the two. At least 14 hours per day wear is required of any appliance trying to modify growth. After occlusal correction, the appliance should be worn until growth is reduced to adult levels in late teens or until a second phase of treatment commences, possibly with extractions and fixed appliances.

8. Where growth modification is no longer a viable treatment option, the skeletal discrepancy can be disguised by tooth movement so that the incisor relationship is corrected, but the class II skeletal discrepancy remains. The skeletal pattern should be no worse than moderate and the vertical facial proportions good. Upper arch extractions are required (usually first premolars) to provide space for overjet correction by bodily retraction of the incisors. Importantly, the profile must not be worsened by this tooth movement, otherwise camouflage will have failed. The arches should be reasonably well aligned so that the extraction spaces are used for overjet reduction and not for relief of crowding. Proclination of the lower labial segment, in selected cases, may also camouflage for a class II problem.

9. Bilateral buccal crossbite exists where the lower buccal segment teeth occlude buccal to the opposing upper teeth. It indicates underlying symmetrical transverse skeletal discrepancy. It is common in class III malocclusions, often resulting from the anteroposterior skeletal discrepancy. It may also result from growth restriction laterally in a patient with repaired cleft palate. Rarely is there a functional problem associated, so it may be accepted unless being corrected as part of comprehensive treatment in a cleft patient. Where correction is considered, it may be undertaken by rapid maxillary expansion: turning a midline screw connected to bands cemented to premolar and molar teeth, twice daily for 2 weeks. This must be undertaken before early teens and overcorrection is advisable.

10. Adults are usually very specific about their complaint and have high expectations of treatment. The dentition may be compromised by periodontal disease or it may be heavily restored with perhaps apical pathology or retained roots. All dental disease must be controlled before orthodontic treatment can be considered. Anchorage may be a problem because of loss of bony support and previous tooth loss. Headgear is not realistic to reinforce anchorage, and alternatives such as palatal arches or bone anchorage devices may be needed. The appearance of the appliance may be improved by the use of aesthetic brackets, vacuum-formed clear aligners or lingual orthodontics. Initial response to tooth-moving forces is generally slower, but subsequent progress is as efficient as in the adolescent. Lighter forces should be used in the periodontally compromised dentition. Retention is often for longer as periodontal and alveolar bone remodelling takes longer. Permanent retention is essential in the periodontally compromised dentition. The absence of growth has two implications: overbite reduction should be by incisor intrusion rather than by molar extrusion and skeletal discrepancies other than mild are best dealt with by orthognathic surgery.

11. The type of maxillary osteotomy undertaken depends on the nature and severity of the skeletal problem. Maxillary osteotomies are classified according to the fracture lines described by Le Fort or they may be segmental. Le Fort I is the most common osteotomy and allows the maxilla to be repositioned superiorly, inferiorly or anteriorly. Posterior movement is not realistic. The maxilla is disarticulated from its anterior wall, tuberosities, lateral nasal wall and nasal septum but

pedicled on the palate to retain its blood supply. Le Fort II osteotomy is used for correction of marked maxillary retrognathia and nasal retrusion. Le Fort III osteotomy is employed for correcting rare craniofacial anomalies including Crouzon's syndrome. The Wassmund osteotomy separates the premaxilla with cuts distal to the canines, which are then extended horizontally across the palate. Although previously popular for overjet correction where premaxillary prominence exists, it is used rarely nowadays. Lack of interdental space and damage to adjacent teeth from the interdental cuts are potential problems.

12. Genetic and environmental factors interact to produce clefting. Positive family history exists in 40% of cleft lip (with or without palate) and in 20% of cleft palate only. Environmental factors (e.g. folic acid deficiency, maternal infections, anticonvulsant drug therapy, aspirin and cortisone) may act in a genetically susceptible individual to promote clefting. A cleft of the lip and primary palate results from failure of fusion of the medial nasal, lateral nasal and maxillary processes at around the sixth week of intrauterine life. Failure of the palatal shelves to fuse at about 8–10 weeks leads to cleft palate. As palatal shelf elevation is later in females, it may promote cleft palate as there is greater potential for more lateral facial growth.

VIVA ANSWER

1. Early loss of primary teeth may have no effect (e.g. early loss of a primary incisor rarely has an effect on the permanent dentition) or it may cause:
   - dilaceration of the root of the permanent successor or hypoplasia of its crown if the loss results from trauma
   - mesial drift: leading to worsening of inherent crowding, which may displace the permanent successor into crossbite and create a premature contact with associated mandibular displacement, or to tooth impaction or complete exclusion of a tooth
   - centreline shift if the loss is asymmetric
   - temporary relief of labial segment crowding.

   The following factors determine the effects:
   - Which tooth is lost: loss of a or b rarely has any detrimental effect, although dilaceration of the permanent incisor root or hypoplasia of the crown may

follow trauma; loss of c or d tends to improve labial segment crowding, often temporarily; unilateral loss of c or d will result in a centreline shift; loss of e facilitates mesial drift of the first permanent molar, which may lead to impaction of the second premolar but has minimal effect on the centreline. Age at which the tooth is lost: in general, the earlier a tooth is lost, the greater the impact on the occlusion.
   - The arch from which it is lost: as there is a greater tendency to mesial drift in the upper arch, the effects of early loss are generally more marked in the upper than in the lower arch.
   - The occlusion: provided good interdigitation exists of the teeth on either side of the extraction site, minimal mesial drift is likely where a tooth is lost early from one arch.
   - Other losses: the potential for space loss is enhanced where a tooth is lost from the opposing arch also.
   - The presence/absence of underlying crowding: where the arches are spaced, there is little untoward effect, but where crowding is inherent or likely, this is exacerbated by early loss.

   Undesirable sequelae may be minimised by:
   - retaining a primary molar where possible by root treatment and placement of a stainless steel crown; this necessitates a co-operative child with a high level of dental motivation and very supportive parents
   - considering the need to balance or compensate if an extraction is deemed necessary
   - space maintenance (see Short note question 5 earlier).

SINGLE BEST ANSWER QUESTION ANSWERS

1. D
2. D
3. C
4. B
5. D
6. C
7. A
8. D.
9. C
10. D
11. C
12. C

11 Orthodontics III: Appliances and Tooth Movement

Overview

Central to the success of any orthodontic treatment is selection of the appropriate appliance and competence in its handling. It is, therefore, necessary to be aware of the scope and limitations of each appliance system and the care required with its use.

In this chapter, removable, fixed, and functional appliances are discussed. Anchorage management is also considered. Histological aspects of tooth movement are addressed, and the factors that must be considered in planning retention are presented.

11.1 Removable Appliances

LEARNING OBJECTIVES

You should:
* know the indications for removable appliance therapy
* know how to design, fit and adjust an upper removable appliance
* understand what is meant by anchorage
* be aware of those factors that influence anchorage loss
* realise the potential hazards and safety requirements with headgear.

Aside from clear vacuum-formed thermoplastic appliances that may be used in the upper and lower arches, removable appliances consisting primarily of wire and acrylic components are used almost exclusively in the upper arch. Lower appliances of the latter components are poorly tolerated because of encroachment on tongue space and the difficulty in achieving satisfactory retention due to the lingual tilt of the molars; they are, however, usually used for the sole purpose of retention post-treatment. Clear thermoplastic appliances may also be used in either arch as retainers; they are also capable of minor tooth alignment and have gained acceptance by adults for this purpose. Although functional appliances are also composed of wire and acrylic, they have a different mode of action and are dealt with in Section 11.3.

INDICATIONS FOR REMOVABLE APPLIANCE THERAPY

In the contemporary management of malocclusion, the role of 'traditional' removable appliances composed of wire and acrylic is much more restrictive than it has been formerly; a greater awareness of their limitations and the widespread use of fixed appliances account mainly for this. Removable appliances, however, may be considered in the following situations:

* Where tilting movement of teeth is desirable and acceptable.
* To maintain space in the mixed or early permanent dentition.
* To help to transmit forces to groups of teeth, e.g. for arch expansion or distal movement of buccal segments (possibly with intrusion); extraoral traction may be applied quite easily to the appliance to produce the latter movements.
* To free the buccal occlusion and facilitate crossbite correction or other tooth movement.
* To produce overbite reduction.
* As an adjunct to fixed appliance treatment.
* As a retainer following removable or fixed appliance treatment.

DESIGNING A REMOVABLE APPLIANCE

Some important points should be remembered in relation to appliance design for those that involve acrylic and wire components:

* Always design the appliance with the patient in the dental chair; this helps to avoid design errors.
* Keep the design as simple as possible: aim to carry out a few tooth movements with each appliance.
* Use the acronym ARAB to help to design the appliance in a logical sequence, ensuring nothing is overlooked: A, activation; R, retention; A, anchorage and B, base plate.

Active Components

Springs. The force (F) delivered by a spring is expressed by the formula $F \propto dr^4/l^3$, where d is the deflection of the spring when activated, r is the radius of the wire and l is the length of the spring. Radius and wire length, therefore, have most effect on wire stiffness.

Screws. Where the teeth needed for retention of the appliance are those to be moved, a screw rather than springs may be useful. Screws, however, are more expensive than springs and make the appliance bulky. The sections of the base plate are moved apart by 0.25 mm with each quarter-turn activation.

Elastics. Intraoral elastics designed for orthodontic purposes may be used to apply elastic traction; the size and force of elastic chosen is determined by the root surface area [RSA] of the tooth to be moved and the distance the elastic is stretched.

Retention Component

The retention component maintains the appliance in the mouth, and it is generally advisable to have the clasps located to optimise retention. The following components are commonly used.

Adams' clasp. Retention is achieved by the arrowheads, which engage about 1 mm of the mesial and distal undercuts on the tooth. This clasp is the most common means of gaining posterior retention. For molars, 0.7 mm wire is used, but 0.6 mm wire is advisable for premolars and primary molars. The clasp is easily modified to incorporate two teeth for retention, hooks for elastic traction or soldered tubes for extraoral anchorage. To move the arrowhead towards the tooth and to engage more gingivally, adjustment should be made in the middle of the flyover; otherwise, close to the arrowhead is all that may be necessary.

Southend clasp. This 0.7 mm clasp is recommended anteriorly with the U-loop engaging the undercut between the incisors. Pushing the loop towards the base plate is the only adjustment usually required.

Long labial bow. This bow is constructed from 0.7 mm (0.8 mm if designed with reverse loops) wire and is useful in preventing buccal drifting of teeth during mesial or distal movement. Alternatively, it may be fitted to the teeth as a retainer.

Adjustment depends on the design, but for a U-looped bow, it is usual to squeeze the legs of the U-loop, followed by an upward adjustment anteriorly to restore its optimal vertical position.

Anchorage

Anchorage is the resistance to the force of reaction generated by the active components and is best thought of in terms of the available space for the intended tooth movement. The anchorage demands should be assessed before treatment commences and may be classified as:

- *low*: where the space from an extraction will provide excess space to achieve the desired result. Revision of the treatment plan would seem advisable, or methods used to encourage space closure
- *moderate*: where some residual extraction space is likely to remain following the intended tooth movement, but this should be kept under surveillance during the treatment period
- *high*: where all the space from an extraction is needed to align the remaining teeth or reduce an overjet; anchorage must be reinforced from the start of treatment

- *very high*: the extraction space will not allow successful achievement of the desired tooth movement and either additional extractions or distal movement of the buccal segments is required to gain further space. The treatment aims may need amendment.

Patients for whom anchorage demands are high or very high are best treated by a specialist.

The anchorage demands are influenced by the following:

- How many teeth are being moved and the intended final tooth positions: greater demand is placed on anchorage when several teeth, rather than one tooth, are being moved and when the intended final tooth position requires teeth to be moved large distances.
- The force applied: tipping movement (~30–60 g) places less demand on anchorage than bodily movement (~100–150 g; see Section 11.2).
- The RSA: teeth with larger RSA or a block of teeth with a large RSA will resist anchorage loss more than those with a smaller RSA.
- Mesial drift tendency: this is greater in the upper than in the lower arch.
- Frankfort mandibular planes angle (FMPA): space loss has been proposed to be easier with increased than with reduced FMPA, which may be related to the different musculature associated with each facial form.
- Occlusal interdigitation: where this is good, mesial drift is less likely.

Intraoral reinforcement of anchorage with an upper removable appliance may be:

- intramaxillary, using teeth in the same arch by incorporating the maximum number of teeth in the anchor unit.
- by palatal coverage of the base plate.

Extraoral Reinforcement of Anchorage

Headgear may be used to pull upward and backward on a facebow attached to an upper removable appliance, against the cranial vault. Forces of 200–250 g for 10–12 hours/day are needed. If distal molar movement is required, extraoral traction is necessary with forces of 400–500 g for 14–16 hours or more per day.

Safety with Headgear

Safety is a priority because of the potential hazards to the eyes and face. Two safety mechanisms must be fitted to each headgear assembly, preferably a facebow with locking device and a safety release spring mechanism attached to the headcap. Verbal and written instructions must be issued to the patient and parent or guardian emphasising that:

- the headgear is only to be assembled and removed in the way demonstrated by the orthodontist
- no horseplay is permissible when the headgear is attached
- if the headgear ever comes out at night, discontinue wear and contact the orthodontist as soon as possible
- if it ever damages the face or eyes, contact the local hospital immediately; discontinue wear and contact the orthodontist.

Base Plate

The base plate connects the other components of the appliance and may be passive or active.

Anterior bite plane. An anterior bite plane is required when overbite reduction is necessary or when removal of an occlusal interference is required to allow tooth movement. Three essential elements must be addressed:

- The bite plane should be flat: if inclined, it may procline or retrocline the lower incisors.
- It must have sufficient extension posteriorly to contact the lower incisors; to ensure this, a measurement of the overjet ($+3$ mm) should be forwarded to the laboratory at the time of appliance fabrication.
- It should separate the molar teeth by about 2 mm; it will be necessary, in most cases, to add cold-cure acrylic to the flat anterior bite plane during treatment to continue overbite reduction.

Posterior bite planes. Posterior bite planes are required to remove occlusal interferences and facilitate tooth movement when overbite reduction is unnecessary. This is commonly the case when correcting a unilateral buccal crossbite with mandibular displacement or an incisor crossbite. The acrylic coverage should be just sufficient to disengage the occlusion but must be adjusted to give even contact of the posterior teeth. The bite planes should be removed when the malocclusion is corrected, and the appliance should then be worn as a retainer while the posterior occlusion settles.

COMMON TOOTH MOVEMENTS REQUIRED

Table 11.1 summarises some common desired tooth movements and the active components to achieve these. Box 11.1 describes the steps involved in fitting a removable appliance.

MANAGING PROBLEMS DURING TREATMENT

Problems that arise commonly during treatment are listed in Table 11.2 together with the most likely causes and necessary treatment.

CLEAR ALIGNER THERAPY

This form of treatment involves creating a series of aligners (clear vacuum-formed thermoplastic appliances). Scanned dental casts or impressions are used to create digital models, which are then related using the bite registration. Alternatively, the teeth and bite registration may be scanned and transferred to the manufacturer. Following the clinicians prescription, the technician moves the teeth small amounts

(0.25 mm for incisors and canines; 0.33 mm for premolars and molars), incorporating any adjunctive treatments (interproximal reduction, placement of attachments and inter-arch elastics) until all treatment objectives have been achieved. The full series of movements should be reviewed using a three-dimensional (3D) visualisation software and any changes made before finalising the plan for the manufacturer to produce the sequence of aligners. Although there are differences between aligner systems with regard to types of tooth movement possible, these appliances perform well, particularly in adults, where tipping movements are required for relief of mild-to-moderate crowding. This treatment is combined with interproximal stripping and/or expansion. Clear aligners have also achieved success with lower incisor extraction for severe crowding, closure of mild-to-moderate spacing, posterior dental expansion and where intrusion of one or two teeth is required. With choice of an apt sophisticated aligner system in conjunction with attachments to allow suitable force application and an experienced operator, it is possible to extend their use to more complex cases, such as alignment of very ectopic teeth, molar uprighting, molar translation, closure of anterior open bite and extraction space closure.

The initial aligner is fitted active to be worn a minimum of 22 hours/day and is likely to produce discomfort that may require relief with mild analgesics. The patient must be told how to assess change in tooth position so timely progress can be made to the next aligner in the sequence. Depending on the tooth movements required, attachments may need to be added during treatment. The clinician should review treatment progress regularly by comparing the anticipated with the actual movement. On completion of treatment, retainers must be fitted (see Section 11.4).

11.2 Fixed Appliances

LEARNING OBJECTIVES

You should:
- be aware of the components of a fixed appliance
- know the indications for a fixed appliance
- be aware of how management of fixed and removable appliances differ
- be aware of different fixed appliance types.

A fixed appliance is attached to the teeth.

Table 11.1 Common Tooth Movements and Related Active Components.

Tooth Movement Required	Component and Wire Diameter	Activation
Upper arch expansion	Two or more teeth: screw	Instruct the patient to turn screw once or twice per week
Distal movement of upper first permanent molar (FPM)	0.6 mm palatal finger springs to retract banded FPMs	1–2 mm activation of springs, with headgear worn 12–16 hours/day with a force 200–250 g per side Must fit with two safety mechanisms (e.g. 'Ni Tom' facebow and 'Snap-away' headcap)
Proclination of incisor(s)	Z-spring 0.5 mm Double cantilever springs 0.6/0.7 mm Screw appliance	Pull the spring 1–2 mm away from the base plate at ~45° angle to direction of wanted movement As for Z-spring Instruct patient to turn screw one or two turns per week

Box 11.1   Fitting a Removable Appliance.

1. Check that the working model and appliance are those of the patient, and that the appliance has been well made to your design.
2. Check the fitting surface for roughness and any sharp edges of wire tags. These should be smoothed off with an acrylic bur or green stone, respectively.
3. Try the appliance in the patient's mouth. If any teeth have been lost or extracted since the impression was taken, some adjustment is likely to be required to get the appliance to fit well.
4. Adjust the posterior, and then the anterior retention until satisfactory.
5. Trim any anterior or posterior bite plane to the correct height.
6. If extractions are required to provide space for the tooth movements required, leave all springs passive for the first 2 weeks until the patient has adapted to wearing the appliance. Otherwise, gentle activation of the springs may be undertaken.
7. Show the patient in a mirror how to insert and remove the appliance, stressing that it is important not to damage any springs. Let the patient practise this several times under your supervision.
8. Instruct the patient and parent or guardian in wear and care of the appliance, emphasising the following:
   - full-time wear, including mealtimes, is essential; it will take a few days to get used to eating with the appliance in, but you must persevere
   - sticky and hard foods, particularly toffees and chewing gum, must not be eaten. Fizzy drinks are also to be avoided
   - the appliance must be taken out after meals for cleaning and for contact sports (when it should be stored in the strong plastic container provided)
   - speech is likely to be affected for the first week but will recover thereafter
   - mild localised discomfort is to be expected if the appliance is gently activated on one or two teeth. An analgesic, usually that taken for headache, may be taken for relief as required
   - if the appliance cannot be worn as instructed or breaks or discomfort other than mild ensues, the clinic must be contacted immediately. A list of written instructions

should be issued and a note to this effect made in the patient's file.
9. Explain that any extractions will be requested once there is evidence of full-time wear.
10. Make a review appointment for 4 weeks if the appliance is active, otherwise for 2–3 weeks to review wear and request any extractions necessary.

Subsequent Visits

1. Check that the appliance is being worn full time; if so:
   - speech should be clear with no lisp
   - the patient should be able to remove and insert the appliance unaided by a mirror
   - the base plate should have lost its shine
   - if there is an anterior or posterior bite plane on the appliance, there should be occlusal markings from the opposing teeth
   - mild gingival erythema and a slight mark across the posterior extent of the appliance on the palate should also be present.
2. If full-time wear is not apparent, the patient should be questioned as to why and informed that treatment will be terminated unless total compliance is forthcoming.
3. Check oral hygiene.
4. Check for anchorage loss by recording the buccal segment relationship and the overjet. If headgear is being worn, ask if there have been any problems. These must be documented, and if none are apparent, this should be noted. Check for evidence of headgear wear and for how long it is worn by assessing the time sheet. Check the headgear safety mechanisms.
5. Assess the intended tooth movement; record the changes in the patient's case records.
6. Adjust the retention of the appliance if necessary.
7. Check the base plate so that there is no impediment to the intended tooth movement, and/or that its height is satisfactory for overbite reduction or to prevent occlusal interference.
8. Adjust the active component(s) if necessary.
9. Indicate in the patient's records the action plan for the next visit.

COMPONENTS

The appliance is composed of three elements: the attachments (brackets/bonded molar tubes/bands), the archwires and the accessories.

Brackets, Bonded Molar Tubes and Bands

It is becoming increasingly popular to bond all teeth, including molars. Bonding of brackets or molar tubes, which mainly have a mesh base, is primarily undertaken using composite resin following acid-etching of the enamel, although self-etching primers (SEPs, which combine etchant and primer to avoid the need to wash the etchant away) may also be used. Resin-modified glass ionomer cements, which release and uptake fluoride in an attempt to prevent enamel demineralisation, are an alternative. These newer systems, however, are not as popular as the two-stage etch and prime system. Adhesive precoated brackets are also available; these are claimed to reduce excess composite or to absorb it internally, save on clean-up time and give a more consistent bond.

The bonded brackets and molar tubes allow the teeth to be directed by the active components comprising the archwire and/or accessories. Brackets may be made from stainless steel, titanium, polycarbonate, ceramic or a combination of polycarbonate/ceramic. Molar tubes are made from stainless steel or titanium. Ceramic brackets are more aesthetic than metal but have disadvantages. They are hard and brittle so may wear the opposing teeth, increase friction with the archwire and can cause enamel fracture at debond due to the strong bond to the adhesive (common with the early-marketed types). The problems with friction and enamel fracture have now been overcome by a polycarbonate base on a ceramic-faced bracket with a metal insert in the bracket slot.

Despite the trend to use bonded tubes instead of bands on molars, bands are particularly indicated for the upper molars especially if headgear, a palatal arch or rapid maxillary expansion is being used. Other indications include teeth with short clinical crowns, as placement of bonded attachments is difficult, and teeth with repeated bond failure or those that are heavily restored. Bands are usually cemented using a glass ionomer cement. Separation of the teeth, commonly with elastomeric rings, is required for up to 1 week to facilitate band placement and guarantee best fit.

Table 11.2 Problems During Treatment.

Problem	Cause	Management
Base plate fracture	Existing crack Base plate too thin	Check co-operation; caution the patient if necessary If small fracture, cold-cure acrylic repair; if large fracture, consider remake with heat-cured acrylic
	Damage by patient out of the mouth	
	Clicking habit	Discourage habit
	Eating sticky/hard foods	Reinstruct the patient regarding avoidance of inappropriate foods
Wire fracture	Work hardened from repeated bends or occlusal loading Damaged while trimming base plate	If arrowhead fracture on Adams' clasp, use solder; otherwise replace component; ensure component is not loaded by the occlusion
	Clicking habit	Discourage habit
	Eating sticky/hard foods	Dissuade from eating inappropriate foods
Rapid deterioration in retention	Clicking habit	Discourage
Palatal hyperplasia	Failure to trim base plate to allow tooth movement	Ensure base plate trimmed appropriately
	Poor oral hygiene	Oral hygiene instruction, but if marked, additional four times a day application of antifungal agent (e.g. Nystatin) to the fitting surface
Slow progress	Lack of full-time wear	Caution the patient and encourage to wear the appliance full time
	Active component not adjusted as instructed or spring overactivated/passive/distorted	Reinstruct or adjust/reposition spring correctly
	Incorrect positioning of springs by patient	Reinstruct in appliance insertion and removal
	Acrylic, wire or the opposing occlusion preventing movement	Remove acrylic/adjust wire/increase height of any bite plane
	Retained root fragment/ankyloses	Consider removal of root fragment; if tooth ankylosed, reassess and consider other treatment options
Lack of overbite reduction	Appliance not worn at meals	Caution and reinforce importance of full-time wear
Marked tipping of tooth	Incorrect spring positioning	Relocate spring to just above gingival margin
	Excess force	Reduce force
Anchorage loss	Appliance not being worn full time	Reinforce importance of full-time wear
	Anchorage demands exceed those required	Reassess anchorage need carefully; consider revised treatment plan, appliance design, anchorage reinforcement

Archwires

Archwires may be round or rectangular.

With its easy formability, good stiffness and reasonable cost, stainless steel is the most popular archwire material; however, nickel–titanium, cobalt–chromium and beta–titanium – all with greater flexibility than stainless steel – may also be used at different stages of treatment. Nickel–titanium has two unique properties – shape memory and superelasticity – that relate to phase transitions between the martensitic and austenitic alloy forms. Even with a large deflection, a relatively constant low force is applied, making these archwires an excellent choice for initial alignment. They are, however, more expensive than stainless steel archwires, which because of the properties given above are especially suitable later in treatment.

Cobalt–chromium alloy (Elgiloy) may be shaped while in a soft state, and then hardened by heat treatment and may be used for a quadhelix or a utility arch for incisor intrusion. Titanium molybdenum (TMA) has excellent strength and springiness, mid-way between nickel–titanium and stainless steel, making it ideal for intermediate and finishing stages of treatment.

Accessories

Elastics, elastomeric modules/chain/thread, wire ligatures. Latex elastics produced for orthodontic purposes may be used for intra- or intermaxillary traction. A range of sizes is available. Elastomeric modules are used to maintain an archwire in an edgewise bracket slot (see later), while elastomeric chain or thread may be used to move teeth along an archwire, or for derotation. Stainless steel wire ligatures continue to be used particularly when maximum contact is desired between the wire and the bracket slot or to maintain space closure.

Springs. Uprighting or rotation of teeth may be carried out by auxiliary springs, while space opening or closure may be undertaken by coil springs.

INDICATIONS FOR FIXED APPLIANCES

Indications include:

- bodily movement of incisors to correct mild-to-moderate skeletal discrepancies
- overbite reduction by incisor intrusion
- correction of rotations
- alignment of grossly misplaced teeth, particularly those requiring extrusion
- closure of spaces
- multiple movements required in either one or both arches.

Tooth Movement

As with a removable appliance, a fixed appliance may also tip teeth but has the additional possibilities of producing bodily movement (crown and root apex move in the same direction), uprighting, torqueing, rotation, intrusion and extrusion of teeth. Torquing is a complex movement involving apical bucco-lingual movement in addition to no or negligible crown movement in the equivalent direction.

ANCHORAGE CONTROL

Because the palate is not covered by a base plate, anchorage control is more critical with a fixed than with a removable appliance. In addition, bodily rather than tipping movement places greater strain on anchorage.

Anchorage may be reinforced by:

- increasing the anchorage unit by bonding more teeth and ligating them together.
- preventing forward tipping of the molars by anchor bends in the archwire (placed between premolar and molar at 30° to the occlusal plane).
- placing torque in the archwire ensuring that the anchor teeth can only move bodily, thereby increasing resistance to unwanted movement; a twist is placed in the plane of the wire so that on insertion in a rectangular bracket slot, it exerts a bucco-lingual force on the root apex.
- palatal and/or lingual arches: these link molar teeth across the arch, which increases RSA of the anchor unit to resist mesial drift and molar tipping.
- intermaxillary traction (see Section 11.1): as well as reinforcing anchorage, the incisor relationship may be corrected, the direction of the elastic traction depending on the malocclusion: class II traction pulls backward on the upper labial segment and forward on the lower buccal segment; class III traction pulls forward on the upper molars and backward on the lower labial segment.
- placement of a Temporary Anchorage Device (TAD); may be an implant, mini-plate attached with screws to maxillary or mandibular basal bone or a mini-screw (usually 6–12 mm long and 1.2–2 mm wide) in the alveolus. Mini-screws are the most popular and as not osseointegrated, they do not provide absolute anchorage.
- extraoral means, including reverse headgear (see Sections 10.4 and 11.1).

APPLIANCE TYPES

Preadjusted Appliances

The preadjusted edgewise appliance uses an individual bracket with a rectangular slot for each tooth to give it 'average' tip, torque and bucco-lingual position and to allow the placement of flat archwires; some individual adjustment bends, however, are often required to the wire to compensate for these 'average' values. 0.018 and 0.022 systems (which describes the bracket slot height in inches) exist and bracket prescriptions by Andrews, Roth and MBT are available. Round flexible wires are used for initial alignment, and rectangular wires are required for precise apical control. Clinical time is saved and good occlusal results are achieved consistently with these appliances.

Tip-Edge appliance. This system was developed from the Begg appliance to overcome some of its deficiencies and uses brackets with rectangular slots. The Begg appliance uses a bracket with a vertical slot and round wires exclusively held in place loosely with brass pins. Tipping movement is facilitated, but auxiliaries are necessary for rotational and apical movement. With the Tip-Edge appliance, although round wire is used for most of the treatment as with the Begg technique, the facility exists to place rectangular wire in the final stages, affording greater control of tooth positions without the need for additional springs, which the latter required.

Lingual appliance. Brackets are bonded, usually indirectly, to the lingual or palatal surfaces of the teeth. With the Incognito system, brackets are fully customised to be low profile and are supplemented with individualised archwires fabricated by a robot. More expensive than conventional labial appliances, chairside time is also increased due to difficulty with adjustment. In addition, there is interference with speech and tongue irritation.

Self-ligating appliances. These remove the need for elastomeric or stainless steel wire ligation of the archwire to the bracket. Available systems include Damon, Speed and SmartClip. Because the archwire is not pressed firmly against the base of the bracket, as is the case with use of an elastomeric module or wire ligature, friction is reduced. Claims that the need for extractions is reduced, and that overall treatment time is significantly shorter than with conventional preadjusted edgewise appliances have not been upheld, although there is some evidence of reduced chairside time.

Fully Customised Appliances

Aside from fully customised lingual appliances, similar labial appliances (Insignia) have been developed but are costly. These have not been shown to shorten treatment time or to improve treatment quality compared to non-customised self-ligating designs.

Appliance Management

An excellent standard of oral hygiene is essential prior to and during fixed appliance treatment. All patients must be instructed specifically in relation to diet and optimal oral hygiene practices following placement of the appliance to minimise the risk of enamel demineralisation. Mucosal ulceration is common in the early stages of treatment, and it is wise to give the patient some soft ribbon wax to place over any components that are causing minor trauma. Adjustment visits are usually at intervals of 4–10 weeks. Repairing fixed appliances occupies more chairside time than does removable appliances. Some discomfort is to be expected for a few days following adjustment and is usually overcome by mild analgesics.

11.3 Functional Appliances

You should:
- have an appreciation of how functional appliances work
- know the indications for functional appliance therapy
- be familiar with the practical management of a patient with a functional appliance
- be aware of differences between functional appliance types
- know the skeletal and dental effects of functional appliance therapy.

Functional appliances correct malocclusion by using, removing or modifying the forces generated by the orofacial musculature, tooth eruption and dentofacial growth.

MECHANISM OF ACTION

How functional appliances work is not completely understood. They are not efficient at managing malaligned teeth or addressing asymmetry between upper and lower arches. Instead, they operate by applying (through stretching) or eliminating forces that are generated via the facial and masticatory musculature and by harnessing those that occur through natural growth processes. They are, therefore, only effective in growing children, preferably just prior to their pubertal growth spurt.

The specific force system set up by any appliance will depend on its particular design. Essentially, forces are developed by posturing the mandible – either downward and forward in class II or downward and backward in class III. This applies intermaxillary traction between the arches, as can be produced by elastics with fixed appliances. As the scope for posturing the mandible backward is far less than for posturing it forward, functional appliances are more successful in, and are indicated almost exclusively for, class II malocclusion. For this reason, the possible mechanisms of action will only be considered for class II malocclusion. In these cases, the result is a forward tipping of the lower incisors and the entire mandibular dentition, with acceleration of mandibular growth, as well as a backward tipping of the upper incisors and restraint of maxillary growth. Overall mandibular growth is modified – the total amount is unaffected, but the expression of growth is altered.

INDICATIONS

Where used for correction of class II malocclusion, the following should ideally be present:

- Patient should be actively growing, preferably just prepubertal.
- Mild-to-moderate skeletal class II owing to mandibular retrusion.
- Average or reduced FMPA.
- Uncrowded arches.
- Lower incisors upright or slightly retroclined; proclined lower incisors usually contraindicates functional appliance therapy.

In most cases, a further phase of fixed appliances is required to detail the occlusion. In moderate class II malocclusion with crowding, this may involve extractions also (see Section 10.1). In more severe cases, the prospect of successful correction of the malocclusion by functional appliance therapy alone is limited; if this is undertaken, the likely need for subsequent extractions and fixed appliances or even combined surgical–orthodontic treatment should be explained.

PRACTICAL MANAGEMENT OF PATIENTS WITH A FUNCTIONAL APPLIANCE

Box 11.2 outlines the general steps involved in using a functional appliance. The orthodontist must be confident about the ability of the appliance to work and relay this enthusiastically to both the patient and parent as compliance with wear is critical to success.

Types of Functional Appliance

The following account describes some standard functional appliances. Current thinking, however, regarding design is to 'pick and mix' the components that are necessary for the specific correction of a particular malocclusion. Such a 'components approach' to design requires considerable insight into the working of these appliances, which necessitates specialist knowledge and expertise. Functional appliances may be removable or fixed, tooth borne or tissue borne.

Twin-Block Appliance
The Twin-block appliance consists of upper and lower appliances incorporating buccal blocks, with interfacing inclined planes at 70° that posture the mandible forward on closure. Although a labial bow was incorporated in the upper appliance with the original design, this has now been shown not to be necessary (Fig. 11.1). Full-time wear is facilitated by the two-part design. Where the mandible needs to be postured further forward during treatment to reactivate, acrylic may be added to the inclined bite planes. When the overjet is corrected, trimming of the upper buccal blocks or a modified retainer with a steep anterior inclined plane is required to close the lateral open bites that develop, especially evident where the overbite is deep to start with. Variants for treatment of class II division 2 and class III malocclusions also exist.

Herbst Appliance
This fixed-functional appliance consists of splints cemented to the upper and lower buccal segment teeth connected by a rigid arm to posture the mandible forward. Although costly and subject to breakages, speaking and eating are reported to be easier than with the Twin-block.

Bionator
A labial bow is extended back to hold the cheeks out of contact with the buccal segment teeth and allow arch expansion, while a thick palatal loop takes the place of acrylic. Full-time wear is advisable except for meals.

Medium Opening Activator
Particularly useful where deep overbite correction is required, this appliance has molar clasping, a palatal base

Box 11.2   Management Technique for a Patient With a Functional Appliance.

1. Ensure that the patient is keen for treatment and is growing.
2. A lateral cephalometric film, in addition to the usual diagnostic records, is essential before treatment starts. Staging of skeletal maturity may be assessed from the cervical vertebrae with specific changes in shape of C3 and C4 coinciding with peak mandibular growth.
3. In some patients, a preliminary phase of arch expansion and/ or alignment is necessary before proceeding to functional appliance treatment. The upper incisors will need to be proclined and aligned in class II division 2 malocclusion to allow forward posturing of the mandible to obtain the construction bite; the appliance used for the first stage of treatment may then be worn as a retainer at all times when the functional appliance is out of the mouth. (Alternatively, if a Twin-block appliance is used, the design can be modified to incorporate these movements simultaneously with anteroposterior correction of the buccal segments.)
4. Obtain well-extended upper and lower impressions and a construction bite, the specifics of which depend on the functional appliance chosen. Generally, the construction bite is taken with the mandible postured forward, ideally to an edge-to-edge incisor relationship and in the case of a Twin-block appliance open 2–3 mm (some operators recommend 5–6 mm). Where the overjet is markedly increased, it may be necessary for patient comfort to reduce the initial advancement by 25% of the maximal possible, and then to reactivate the appliance as treatment progresses.
5. Record the patient's standing height at the appointment when the appliance is fitted. Recording height over several visits will give an indication of the rate of growth. Greatest growth in the maxilla and mandible corresponds with a period of maximum increase in height.
6. The Herbst and other fixed class II correctors can be worn full time. For other appliances, the number of hours of prescribed wear is appliance-dependent, but a minimum is likely to be evenings and bedtime. While prescribed wear of the Twin-block appliance has usually been full time, apart from sports and appliance hygiene after meals, it appears from the results of a recent clinical trial that prescribed wear for a minimum of probably 8–12 hours/day may suffice. Although a time sheet could be used to record the number of hours of wear and should be brought along for inspection at each review visit, this is subject to overestimation. Compliance with prescribed wear is better assessed with microsensors (TheraMon) embedded in the acrylic, but this incurs an additional cost and makes the appliance bulkier. Granting that patients appear not to comply with prescribed full-time or part-time wear of the Twin-block appliance, the latter has proved as effective at overjet reduction as the former.
7. Warn the patient that minor discomfort is common initially, particularly muscular and temporomandibular joint tenderness, but this usually subsides after 1–2 weeks. Mild analgesics may be taken as required. If an area of mucosal ulceration develops, the patient must return for appliance adjustment.
8. Review 1–2 weeks after appliance fitting to check appliance wear, to make any necessary adjustments and, most importantly, to assess and encourage compliance. Then recall at intervals of 6–8 weeks.
9. Measure the overjet and check the buccal segment relationships at each recall visit, ensuring that the patient's mandible is retruded maximally – otherwise, a false indication of any progress will arise. Check the time sheet or microsensor (TheraMon) data at each visit and encourage if progress is good; about 1 mm of overjet reduction per month is usual in co-operative, growing individuals. If the appliance is not being worn as instructed, careful counselling, highlighting that this form of treatment is only effective for a finite time while the patient is growing, may improve co-operation.
10. Depending on the initial construction bite, at 4–6 months in treatment, reactivation of the appliance (or a new appliance) may be necessary, with further posturing of the mandible to achieve the desired incisor relationship.
11. If there is no discernible progress in 6 months, stop treatment and reassess.
12. Slight overcorrection of the occlusion is advisable, and then the appliance should be worn as a retainer at nights until growth reduces to adult levels or until a second phase of treatment (possibly with extractions and fixed appliances) gets underway. It may be necessary to make a new appliance for this purpose. In the case of treatment with a Twin-block appliance, in order to facilitate closure of the lateral open bites that are created, acrylic may be trimmed away from the occlusal surfaces of the upper block or an upper retainer with a steep anterior inclined bite plane may be fitted.

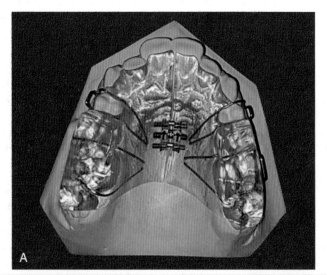
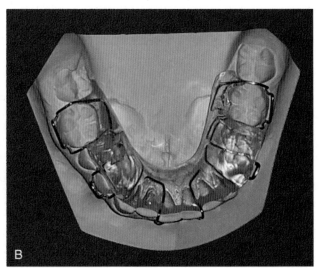

Fig. 11.1 The Twin-block appliance. (A) Upper occlusal view. (B) Lower occlusal view. The design is modified from the original developed by Clark. (Reprinted with permission from Millett D, Day P, *Clinical Problem Solving in Orthodontics and Paediatric Dentistry*. 3rd ed. © 2017 Elsevier Ltd. All rights reserved. ISBN: 9780702058363.)

plate, acrylic extensions lingual to the lower incisors and no buccal capping; acrylic struts link the upper to the lower, and the lower buccal segment teeth have scope to erupt. Full-time wear with the usual exceptions is possible.

Frankel Appliance

Originally termed a 'function regulator', this may have particular use in the management of atypical soft tissue pattern, for example, hyperactive mentalis muscle. The only soft tissue–borne functional appliance, buccal shields hold the cheeks away from the teeth and stretch the mucoperiosteum at the sulcus depth, intending to expand the arches and widen the alveolar processes. There are three types: FR 1 for class I and class II division 1 malocclusions; FR 2 for class II division 2 malocclusion and FR 3 for class III malocclusion. Wear is built up over the first weeks until full time, apart from sports and while eating. Frankel appliances are complex in design, expensive to make and repair and easy to damage and distort. They can, however, be reactivated by sectioning the buccal shields and repositioning them forward.

Headgear Addition to Functional Appliances

In cases where maximal anteroposterior and vertical maxillary restraint is desirable, usually in association with considerable upper incisor and gingival display, occipital-pull headgear may be added to tubes incorporated in the acrylic or soldered to the clasp bridges. Forces of about 500 g should be used for 14–16 hours/day, and the usual headgear safety precautions and instructions should be followed (see Section 11.1). If the FMPA is increased, molar capping is essential to promote a closing rotation of the mandible and prevent molar eruption, thereby facilitating an increase in overbite. The addition of high-pull headgear to the appliance will facilitate this process.

Effects of Functional Appliances

For class II malocclusion with deep overbite, these are:

Dentoalveolar

- Retroclination of the upper incisors and proclination of the lower incisors are usual, although the latter is not found consistently and is best minimised by placing acrylic capping on the lower anterior teeth.
- Inhibition of lower incisor eruption and promotion of eruption of the posterior teeth lead to levelling of the curve of Spee. This process is facilitated by lower incisor capping on the appliance.
- Guidance of eruption of the lower posterior teeth in an upward and forward direction while preventing eruption and forward movement of the upper posterior teeth encourages correction of a class II buccal relationship.
- Arch expansion is intended through the buccal shields of the Frankel appliance, the buccal wire of the Bionator or by adjustment of the midline screw of the Twin-block.

Skeletal

- Enhancement of mandibular growth is brought about by movement of the mandibular condyle out of the fossa, promoting growth of the condylar cartilage and forward migration of the glenoid fossa. This effect is very variable.
- Restraint of forward maxillary growth.

- An increase in lower facial height is mediated by the alterations in the eruption of the posterior teeth, as described above.

The skeletal effects (1–2 mm mostly) only account for a small portion of the treatment effects even when efforts are made to limit the amount of tooth movement. Treatment is successful in about 70–80% of cases. Treatment process or outcome was no better with incremental (2 mm advancement initially and 2 mm at 6-week intervals) than with maximum bite advancement (edge-to-edge) during Twin-block treatment. Again with the Twin-block appliance, treatment undertaken in the early mixed dentition before 10 years of age has been shown to be no more effective than treatment undertaken in the late mixed dentition in terms of overjet reduction, skeletal change, occlusal improvement or extraction need. Furthermore, early treatment increases the overall treatment duration and taxes co-operation. Despite this, as self-esteem is improved temporarily and the trauma risk to the incisors reduced by maximally 40%, early treatment is indicated if a child is being teased or bullied because of dentofacial appearance (see Sections 9.4 and 10.1) or where the incisors are deemed to be at serious risk of trauma.

The limited indications, use and effects of functional appliances in class III malocclusion are dealt with in Section 10.4.

11.4 Orthodontic Tooth Movement and Retention

LEARNING OBJECTIVES

You should:
- know the histological response in areas of pressure and tension with orthodontic tooth movement, and how tipping differs from bodily movement
- be able to give the range of force required for each type of tooth movement
- know the undesirable sequelae of orthodontic forces
- understand the rationale for retention and factors to be considered in planning retention.

ORTHODONTIC TOOTH MOVEMENT

The biological response to a sustained force is determined mainly by the force magnitude and duration, which generate zones of pressure and tension within the periodontal ligament, their extent and location depending on the intended movement. It is the cells of the periodontal ligament which detect, instigate and coordinate the process of bone remodelling and tooth movement.

Pressure Zones

The cellular response relates to whether a light or heavy force is applied. With a light sustained force, movement occurs within a few seconds as periodontal ligament fluid is squeezed out and the vascular supply is compressed, setting off a complex biochemical response. Osteoclastic invasion occurs within 2 days and frontal resorption follows.

When a heavy sustained force is applied, the periodontal ligament is compressed to such a degree that the blood flow is cut off completely, producing an area of sterile necrosis (hyalinisation). Small zones of hyalinisation are inevitable even with light forces, but the area of hyalinisation is extended with forces of greater magnitude. Osteoclastic differentiation is impossible within the necrotic periodontal ligament space but, after several days, osteoclasts appear adjacent to and within the adjacent cancellous spaces. From there, they invade the bone adjacent to the hyalinised area, and tooth movement eventually occurs by undermining resorption, albeit delayed by 10–14 days.

Tension Zones

Following initial application of a light force, the blood vessels vasodilate and the periodontal ligament fibres are stretched. In response to escalation in extracellular kinase signalling which stimulates release of a transcription factor (RUNX-2), fibroblast and osteoblast proliferation occurs. The stretched fibres become embedded in osteoid, which later mineralises. The typical periodontal ligament width is eventually regained by simultaneous collagen fibre remodelling.

With heavy forces, rupture of blood vessels and severing of the periodontal ligament fibres are likely, but these are restored with the remodelling processes.

Mechanisms of Tooth Movement

Although the histological response to an applied orthodontic force has been investigated extensively, the mechanism by which a mechanical stimulus effects a cellular response is complex and at present unclarified. It is likely that vascular changes in the periodontal ligament in areas of pressure and tension, electrical signals generated in response to flexing of alveolar bone following force application, cytokine (bone morphogenetic proteins (BMPs); interleukin-1 (IL-1)) and prostaglandins (such as PGE-2) interact in the process.

Types of Tooth Movement, Force Magnitude and Duration

Although it was previously thought that tipping of a single-rooted tooth (Fig. 11.2) occurred about a point almost midway along the root, rotation now appears to take place near the apical third within an elliptically shaped area. Half of the periodontal ligament is stressed, with maximum pressure created at the alveolar crest in the direction of movement and at the diagonally opposite apical area. For bodily movement and rotation, a force couple must be applied, loading uniformly the whole of the periodontal ligament in the direction of translation so both crown and root move in the same direction by equal amounts (Fig. 11.3). With extrusion, all of the periodontal ligament is tensed, but when a tooth is intruded, the force is concentrated at the apex. An element of tipping is unavoidable with extrusion, intrusion and rotation.

For tooth movement to occur optimally, the force per unit area within the periodontal ligament should ideally not occlude the vascular supply, yet be sufficient to induce a cellular response. A force should, therefore, be as light as possible for the movement intended, taking into account the root surface area over which it is spread. Optimal force ranges for various tooth movements are:

- tipping: 50–75 g
- extrusion: 50–100 g

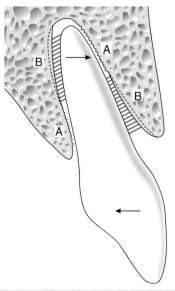

Fig. 11.2 The effect of tipping movement. A = area of periodontal ligament compression/alveolar bone resorption; B = area of periodontal ligament tension/alveolar bone deposition.

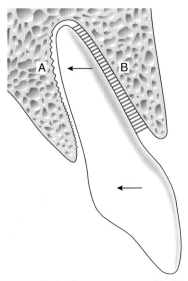

Fig. 11.3 The effect of bodily movement. A = area of periodontal ligament compression/alveolar bone resorption; B = area of periodontal ligament tension/alveolar bone deposition.

- bodily movement: 100–150 g
- rotation: 35–60 g
- uprighting: 75–125 g
- intrusion: 15–25 g.

Although tooth movement can occur in response to heavy forces, these should not be applied continuously; intermittent application may be clinically acceptable. Not only must a force be of sufficient magnitude to effect the movement desired, but it must also be sustained for sufficient time. For successful movement, a force must be applied for about 6 out of 24 hours, and continuous application of light forces is optimal. This is favoured, because control of tooth movement and anchorage is facilitated, while the risks of pulpal and radicular damage are minimised. Excessive mobility is avoided and movement is more efficient with less discomfort. Movement of the order of 1 mm in a 4-week period is regarded as optimal, with faster progress recorded in children than in adults. This is largely a consequence of the greater cellularity of the periodontal ligament, more cancellous alveolar bone and faster tissue turnover in a growing patient, which ensure a more rapid response to an applied force.

Accelerated Tooth Movement

Various non-surgical and surgical means, which kindle bone resorption/deposition or reduce the bony resistance to tooth movement, respectively, have and are currently being explored as means of promoting bone remodelling and a faster rate of orthodontic tooth movement. Intraoral devices which apply supplementary vibrational forces for around 20 minutes/day have been assessed mostly as a non-surgical option, although pulsed electromagnetic waves and localised laser radiation of low energy have also been tested. Surgical adjuncts explored are primarily corticotomy/piezocision and micro-osteoperforation. Good quality evidence has not found supplementary vibrational forces to speed up tooth movement and further high-quality evidence is required regarding non-surgical methodologies.

Furthermore, pharmacological means of stimulating tooth movement, some with local application, are being considered but require further investigation.

Undesirable Sequelae of Orthodontic Force

Pulpal Damage

A mild pulpitis following initial force application is common, but has no effect long term. Where the apical blood vessels are severed by the use of heavy continuous force or by injudicious root movement through the alveolar plate, pulp death is likely, although this is usually associated with previous trauma.

Root Resorption

Areas of cementum resorbed during tooth movement are usually repaired. Some permanent loss of root length is found, however, on nearly all teeth following bodily movement over long distances. The maxillary incisors, then the mandibular incisors and first permanent molars, are primarily affected. Fortunately, in most instances, loss of 0.5–1.0 mm of root length is of no long-term significance. Suggested risk factors include: root resorption before treatment, a history of previous trauma, roots that are pipette-shaped, blunt or demonstrate a marked apical curvature, use of excessive forces and apical contact with cortical bone. Genetic risk factors are also involved. Comprehensive orthodontic treatment increases the severity and incidence, and that heavy forces produce most root resorption.

Loss of Alveolar Bone Height

With fixed appliance treatment, 0.5–1 mm loss of crestal alveolar height is common, with the greatest loss occurring at extraction sites. In the presence of good oral hygiene, this appears of little concern.

Pain and Mobility

Even with appropriate force magnitude, ischaemic areas develop in the periodontal ligament after activation of an orthodontic appliance, leading to mild discomfort and pressure sensitivity. These usually last for 2–4 days and return when the appliance is reactivated. Some increase in mobility is common, as the periodontal ligament space widens and the fibres reorganise in response to the applied force. With heavy orthodontic forces, however, the likelihood of almost immediate onset of pain and marked mobility is increased, as the periodontal ligament is crushed and further undermining resorption occurs.

Retention

Following tooth movement, a period of retention is usually required to hold the teeth passively, preventing them returning to their pre-treatment position while the periodontal fibres and alveolar bone adapt to their new locations. As part of informed consent, the retention phase should be planned and discussed fully with the patient before treatment starts. The following factors are likely to destabilise the final result.

Forces From the Supporting Tissues

Reorganisation of the principal periodontal ligament fibres and supporting alveolar bone occurs within 4–6 months, but at least 7–8 months is required for the supracrestal fibres to reorganise because of the slow turnover of the free gingival fibres. Rotational correction is, therefore, liable to relapse, but this tendency may be reduced by surgical sectioning (pericision) of the supracrestal fibres. Overcorrection of the rotation early in treatment may help to minimise relapse; however, irrespective of strategy, bonded retention is required to guarantee alignment.

Where periodontal support is compromised, indefinite retention will be necessary following orthodontic treatment. When the maxillary labial frenum is suspected in the aetiology of a diastema (see Section 10.1), a fraenectomy is recommended. This is best undertaken during space closure so incisor approximation is aided by scar formation, although indefinite retention is required.

Soft Tissues

Following appliance therapy, the teeth should be in a position of soft tissue balance. The original mandibular archform should remain unchanged, as markedly altering the angulation of the lower incisors will promote relapse. Limited proclination of the lower labial segment may be stable, however, where the lower incisors have been retroclined by a digit-sucking habit, a lower lip trap or by retroclined upper incisors. In addition, some retroclination of the lower incisors may be stable in class III correction where the upper incisors have been proclined and, as a result, the labiolingual position of the incisors is, in effect, interchanged.

In class II division 1, a pre-treatment assessment of the degree of lip incompetence and mechanism of achieving an anterior oral seal should be made, followed by an estimate of the likely post-treatment coverage of the upper incisors by the lower lip. One-third to one-half of the labial surface of the upper incisors should be covered to give the best chance of stable overjet correction.

Occlusal Factors

A good buccal segment interdigitation, although unproven, and an interincisal angulation of about 135° promote stability. In addition, following incisor proclination, a positive overbite is necessary to prevent relapse.

Facial Growth

Continuing growth in the original pattern that contributed to the malocclusion is particularly likely to occur post-treatment in class III, open bite and deep bite cases. Some overcorrection of these incisor relationships is recommended, and retention should be continued until growth is complete. To prevent facial growth impacting the development of late lower incisor crowding, permanent retention to the lower labial segment is now widely advocated.

Retention Strategies

There are no specific rules as to the most appropriate retention strategy for each patient; this must be devised on an individual basis. As it is impossible to predict which cases will and which will not stay relatively stable, indefinite retention is advisable in all cases or until the patient decides to cease retainer wear themselves. In advance of treatment, the clinician must notify the patient of the post-treatment need for retention, select the most suitable retainer type, provide information on the manner by which any associated risks may be reduced and plan for their long-term upkeep. The patient must wear and maintain the retainers as instructed as well as take responsibility for having them inspected on a regular basis for as long as they are worn.

Selection of a Retention Regime

This requires consideration of the following:

Patient factors: starting malocclusion and growth pattern, oral health, demands, likes, potential compliance
Occlusal factors: final occlusion and prospects of stability
Retainer factors: ease of care
Need for adjunctive procedures: pericision or interproximal reduction

Retainers

These may be removable or fixed.

Removable. Aside from a positioner, which is constructed to teeth ideally repositioned on a working cast and is therefore active when fitted initially to encourage occlusal settling but subsequently worn as a retainer, these appliances are devoid of active components. The two most common removable retainers are the Hawley retainer and the clear plastic retainer; the latter looks better, is cheaper and easier to make, has less impact on speech and fractures less easily. The Hawley and clear plastic retainer are equally effective at maintaining upper arch alignment, but the latter is superior in the lower arch. Night-only wear of either retainer is sufficient.

The Hawley retainer may be modified to incorporate an acrylated labial bow (useful following alignment of rotated teeth), an anterior bite plane for maintenance of overbite correction or an acrylic prosthetic tooth with metal stops either side of a potential pontic space.

Carbonated beverages must not be consumed with the either removable retainer in place, but especially with the clear plastic retainer, as there is a serious rick of demineralisation of the tooth surfaces in prolonged contact with any residual drinking solution. Furthermore, the clear plastic retainer should not be run under hot water, as it will distort the fit. Neither should it be cleaned with toothpaste, as this damages the surface; special cleaning solution should be used instead. As retention is by engagement in the undercut below the contact points, where the gingivae are inflamed, an alternative design may be better to ensure a good fit.

Fixed. Fixed bonded retainers are particularly indicated where initially teeth are markedly rotated or severely displaced, the dentition exhibits generalised spacing, a median diastema, root resorption or is periodontally compromised. Following treatment of cleft of lip and palate, where treatment has considerably adjusted the intercanine width or moved the lower incisors appreciably in a lingual or labial direction or where lip competence is not present after correction of an increased overjet, fixed retention is also advisable.

Bonded passively to the inner surface of each of the labial segment teeth, stainless steel multistranded wire is most frequently used with 0.0195 inch recommended. The retainer may be bonded directly or indirectly using light-cured composite following acid-etching of the enamel. Alternatively, the retainer may be attached to the canine teeth only. This, however, runs the risk of the incisors misaligning, but access for oral hygiene is enabled. Other types of retainer include single strand rectangular titanium, CAD/CAM nickle titanium (Memotain), flexible chain (stainless steel or gold) or fibre-reinforced polymer bonded to each tooth. Regular review is required to confirm periodontal and dental health are maintained and to ensure the retainer is intact with no induced unwanted tooth movement, although this is rare.

Fixed retainers make compliance with wear easier for the patient as they are in situ, whereas removable retainers rely entirely on patient compliance for wear but facilitate oral hygiene.

Adjunctive Procedures

By severing the supracrestal fibres above the alveolar bone, pericision reduces rotational relapse by 30%, is more successful in the maxilla than in the mandible and has no long-term periodontal consequences. Interproximal reduction removes 0.25 mm of enamel from each proximal surface. It is useful where teeth need to be reshaped to flatten the contact area which is thought to promote stability.

Self-Assessment: Questions

MULTIPLE CHOICE QUESTIONS (TRUE/FALSE)

1. A removable appliance:
   a. Is indicated for bodily tooth movement
   b. Is particularly effective as a lower arch space maintainer in the mixed dentition
   c. May act as a retainer following active tooth movement
   d. Provides less anchorage than a fixed appliance
   e. Is indicated for correction of premolar rotations
2. When designing an upper removable appliance:
   a. It is not recommended to do so with the patient in the dental chair
   b. It is advisable to incorporate as many active components as possible
   c. Using the acronym ARAB is helpful
   d. The overjet measurement minus 2 mm gives an accurate indication of the required extent of a flat anterior bite plane
   e. It is advisable to specify the wire dimensions of the appliance components
3. A flat anterior bite plane:
   a. Is indicated for lower incisor proclination
   b. Is an aid to correction of anterior open bite
   c. Should contact at least two lower incisors
   d. Should separate the molar teeth by 5 mm
   e. Should allow the lower incisors to occlude posterior to it
4. Retention of an upper removable appliance may be improved by:
   a. A T-spring
   b. An Adams' clasp
   c. A Southend clasp
   d. Palatal finger springs
   e. Minimal extension of the base plate
5. The following removable appliance components are usually made from 0.6 mm stainless steel wire:
   a. A Z-spring to procline 1
   b. A coffin spring
   c. An Adams' clasp on d
   d. A T-spring
   e. A Southend clasp
6. The force exerted by a typical 0.5-mm palatal finger spring to retract a maxillary canine is:
   a. Directly proportional to the length of the wire
   b. Inversely proportional to the wire diameter
   c. Inversely proportional to the deflection of the spring at activation
   d. Directly proportional to the thickness of acrylic covering the terminal end of the spring in the base plate
   e. Inversely proportional to the number of retention components on the appliance
7. A fixed appliance is indicated for:
   a. Correction of rotations
   b. Space closure
   c. Bodily retraction of upper incisors for overjet reduction
   d. Alignment of grossly misplaced teeth
   e. Overbite reduction by incisor intrusion

8. Active components on a fixed appliance may be:
   a. The molar bands
   b. The archwire
   c. Elastomeric chain
   d. The base plate
   e. A Nance palatal arch
9. The following are types of functional appliance:
   a. Begg
   b. Frankel
   c. Tip-edge
   d. Bionator
   e. Edgewise
10. The Twin-block appliance for class II correction:
    a. Cannot be worn while eating
    b. Has buccal shields to allow arch expansion
    c. Has six subtypes
    d. Is usually constructed using a wax registration with the patient opened 2 mm in the first permanent molar region
    e. May have headgear added to the lower appliance
11. There is a greater likelihood of anchorage loss:
    a. When light forces are used to move teeth
    b. On average, in the upper than in the lower arch
    c. When few teeth are being moved in an intact arch
    d. When the buccal interdigitation is good
    e. In the upper arch with a full arch fixed appliance than with a removable appliance
12. Anchorage may be reinforced with an upper removable appliance by:
    a. Extending the base plate maximally
    b. Using intermaxillary traction
    c. Addition of headgear
    d. Using a close-fitting labial bow
    e. By minimising the number of clasped teeth
13. Application of excessive force for tooth movement:
    a. Leads to loss of pulp vitality
    b. Hastens tooth movement
    c. Conserves anchorage
    d. Is likely to evoke a pain response
    e. Has no effect on root length

EXTENDED MATCHING ITEMS QUESTIONS

Theme: Appliance components and appliance types
For each of the patients (a–e) that you might be asked to assess, select from the list below (1–16) the most appropriate appliance components to incorporate in an appliance or a specific appliance type (more than one may be correct) for correction of the occlusal problem(s) given. Each item can be used once, more than once or not at all.

1. Adams' clasps 6/6.
2. Adams' clasps d/d.
3. Southend clasp 1/1.
4. Flat anterior bite plane.
5. Posterior capping.
6. Z-spring(s).
7. T-spring.
8. Screw sectional.

9. Roberts' retractor.
10. Labial bow from 3/ to /3.
11. Lingual arch.
12. Extraoral traction.
13. Twin-block appliance.
14. Frankel III appliance.
15. Bionator appliance.
16. Herbst appliance.
   a. An 8-year-old boy with both permanent upper central incisors in crossbite; there is an anterior mandibular displacement on closure on 1/1 and a 5-mm overbite on these incisors. 6edc21 are present in each quadrant.
   b. A 13-year-old girl who has completed upper fixed appliance treatment for her class I malocclusion; there were no incisor rotations pre-treatment; 7 to 1 are erupted in each quadrant.
   c. A 12-year-old boy with an uncrowded class II division 1 malocclusion on a class II skeletal base with average FMPA.
   d. An 11-year-old girl scheduled for fixed appliance therapy where slightly more space than that provided by extraction of upper first premolars will be required for upper arch alignment.
   e. A 12.5-year-old boy where all the extraction space from lower second primary molar extractions (both lower second premolars are absent) will be needed for relief of crowding and fixed appliance alignment of the remaining teeth.

CASE HISTORY QUESTIONS

Case History 1

A 14-year-old male patient presents complaining of slow progress of upper removable appliance therapy to retract 3/3 following extraction of 4/4. Treatment commenced 8 months ago, and the canine teeth are still not in a class I relationship. On examination, 3/3 only appeared to have moved 3 mm in the past 8 months.

1. What are the possible reasons for slow treatment progress?
2. What investigations would you undertake?
3. How would you manage treatment from now on?

Case History 2

A 16-year-old female patient presents complaining of increase in the prominence in her upper incisor teeth following Twin-block functional appliance therapy, which was concluded 14 months previously.

1. What may account for the overjet increase?
2. How may it have been prevented?
3. What management options are there?

PICTURE QUESTIONS

Picture 1

Fig. 11.4 shows a patient wearing an upper removable appliance.

1. What is the active component?
2. What is it used for?
3. What are its wire dimensions?
4. What problems may arise with its use?

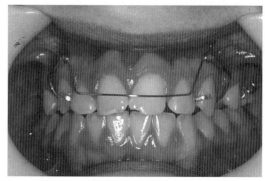

Fig. 11.4 A patient wearing an upper removable appliance.

Picture 2

Fig. 11.5 shows an appliance.

1. Specify the appliance type.
2. What are the indications for its use?
3. How does it work?
4. What factors determine whether the occlusal correction achieved will be stable long term?

Picture 3

Fig. 11.6 shows components of an orthodontic appliance.

1. List the components shown.
2. What functions are served by the two components shown in the upper and lower middle section of the figure?
3. When would you use this appliance?
4. What instructions would you issue with it?

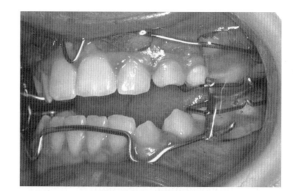

Fig. 11.5 An appliance.

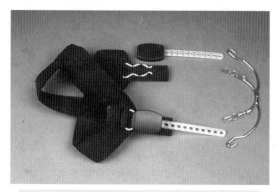

Fig. 11.6 Components of an orthodontic appliance.

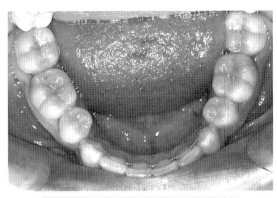

Fig. 11.7 Occlusal view of the lower arch.

Picture 4

Fig. 11.7 is an occlusal view of the lower arch.

1. What is visible lingual to the lower anterior teeth?
2. What is its purpose?
3. When would you consider its use?
4. What alternative approaches are there to treatment?

SHORT NOTE QUESTIONS

Write short notes on:

1. Adams' clasp
2. disadvantages of removable appliances
3. orthodontic screws
4. preadjusted edgewise fixed appliances
5. optimal force range for tipping, bodily movement, rotation, intrusion
6. intermaxillary traction
7. the histological effects that occur with a tipping movement to retract a maxillary canine
8. retention procedures to minimise/prevent rotational relapse.

VIVA QUESTIONS

1. What instructions would you give a patient who was issued with an upper removable appliance to procline/1?
2. How would you know if a passive removable appliance you had issued 4 weeks previously was being worn full time?
3. a. Classify functional appliances.
   b. Outline your management of a class II division 1 malocclusion to be treated by a functional appliance.
   c. Explain the mode of action and effects of a functional appliance in such a case.
4. Define what is meant by the term 'anchorage'. Classify anchorage and describe how anchorage can be preserved and monitored during removable appliance therapy. What special measures may need to be taken with anchorage reinforcement?

SINGLE BEST ANSWER QUESTIONS

1. The optimal wire size for a Z-spring to procline an upper permanent incisor in crossbite is:
   A. 0.4 mm
   B. 0.5 mm
   C. 0.6 mm
   D. 0.7 mm
   E. 0.8 mm
2. To be effective, the daily wear in hours of an aligner should be:
   A. 6
   B. 10
   C. 14
   D. 20
   E. 22
3. Fixed appliances, in comparison with removable appliances:
   A. Lessen the risk of enamel demineralisation
   B. Occupy less chairside time
   C. Place greater demand on anchorage
   D. Produce less discomfort after adjustment visits
   E. Rarely lead to mucosal ulceration after placement
4. Nickle–titanium is a favoured wire choice for initial alignment because of its:
   A. Ability to exert heavy forces
   B. Cost
   C. Ease of permanent deformation
   D. Shape memory
   E. Stiffness
5. A tissue-borne functional appliance is the:
   A. Bionator
   B. Frankel
   C. Herbst
   D. Medium opening activator
   E. Twin-block appliance
6. The Twin-block appliance for correction of a class II division 1 malocclusion typically incorporates:
   A. A palatal wire to the upper incisors
   B. An upper midline expansion screw
   C. Buccal shields
   D. Lower incisor capping
   E. No molar capping
7. Treatment undertaken with a Twin-block before age 10 years, compared to that undertaken during adolescence:
   A. Enhances the occlusal outcome
   B. Gives superior skeletal change
   C. Lessens the need for extractions
   D. Produces more stable overjet reduction
   E. Reduces the risk of incisal trauma
8. Skeletal effects produced by a functional appliance amount to about:
   A. 1–2 mm
   B. 2–3 mm
   C. 3–4 mm
   D. 4–5 mm
   E. Greater than 5 mm
9. The optimal force range for intrusion is:
   A. 15–25 g
   B. 50–75 g
   C. 50–100 g
   D. 75–125 g
   E. 100–150 g
10. Greatest root resorption is likely with:
   A. Apical root curvature
   B. Heavy forces
   C. Light class II elastics
   D. Pipette-shaped roots
   E. Short treatment

11. The need for retention after orthodontic treatment should be discussed first with the patient:
    A. As part of informed consent
    B. As treatment starts
    C. At end of treatment
    D. Mid-way through treatment
    E. Near end of treatment

12. After orthodontic treatment, reorganisation of the principal periodontal ligament fibres and alveolar bone occurs mostly at:
    A. 1–2 months
    B. 2–3 months
    C. 4–6 months
    D. 6–9 months
    E. 8–12 months

Self-Assessment: Answers

MULTIPLE CHOICE ANSWERS

1. a. False. It is only capable of a tipping tooth movement, not bodily tooth movement.
   b. False. Removable appliances are generally poorly tolerated in the lower arch, as they encroach on tongue space. In addition, retention is not as good as in the upper arch because of the lingual tilt of the lower molars, which makes clasping difficult.
   c. True. It is indicated most commonly for retention following active tooth movement.
   d. False. A removable appliance provides greater anchorage than a fixed appliance owing to palatal coverage by the base plate.
   e. False. Rotational correction is best carried out by a fixed rather than a removable appliance.
2. a. False. The appliance should be designed with the patient in the dental chair to avoid errors.
   b. False. The number of active components should be kept to a minimum.
   c. True. ARAB stands for activation, retention, anchorage, base plate; this sequence is useful when designing a removable appliance.
   d. False. The overjet plus 3 mm should be forwarded to the laboratory at the time of fabrication to ensure accurate extension of the flat anterior bite plane.
   e. True. This reduces the likelihood of error in wire selection particularly for components that may be fabricated in one of two wire diameters, e.g. a buccal canine retractor may be made as 0.5 mm sleeved or in 0.7 mm wire.
3. a. False. A flat anterior bite plane is indicated for overbite reduction.
   b. False. See (a) above. An anterior bite plane would worsen an anterior open bite.
   c. True. This will distribute the occlusal load. Contact on one incisor may lead to periodontal trauma and mobility.
   d. False. Molar separation of about 3 mm is sufficient initially. Addition of cold-cure acrylic to the bite plane can be made, as required, to reduce the overbite further.
   e. False. It should be constructed so that the lower incisors occlude on the anterior bite plane. If the lower incisors occlude posterior to the flat anterior bite plane, overbite reduction will not ensue.
4. a. False. This is an active component and hence will not improve retention.
   b. True. This is a retentive component.
   c. True. This is a retentive component.

d. False. These are active components.
e. False. Maximal extension of the base plate would improve retention; minimal extension would not aid retention.
5. a. False. This is usually made from 0.5 mm wire.
   b. False. This is usually made from 1.25 mm wire.
   c. True. This is usually made from 0.6 mm wire; clasps on 6s may be made in 0.7 or 0.8 mm wire.
   d. False. This is usually made in 0.5 mm wire.
   e. False. This is usually made in 0.7 mm wire.
6. a. False. Inversely proportional to wire length to the power of three.
   b. False. Directly proportional to the radius to the power of four.
   c. False. Directly proportional.
   d. False. Not relevant.
   e. False. Not relevant.
7. a. True.
   b. True.
   c. True. Bodily movement is necessary in all cases (a–e).
   d. True.
   e. True.
8. a. False. On their own, these are not active components but become active through the interaction of the archwire with the slot in the molar attachments.
   b. True. The archwire may be active or passive.
   c. True. This is used for space closure or to aid correction of rotations.
   d. False. Fixed appliances do not have a base plate; this is a component of a removable appliance.
   e. False. This is used to support anchorage.
9. a. False. This is a type of fixed appliance.
   b. True.
   c. False. This is a type of fixed appliance.
   d. True.
   e. False. This is a type of fixed appliance.
10. a. False. It is issued to be worn full time, and the patient is instructed to wear it while eating.
    b. False. These are incorporated in the Frankel appliance.
    c. False. There are two principal subtypes.
    d. False. The bite should be open 4–5 mm in the first permanent molar region.
    e. False. Headgear may be added to the upper appliance, not the lower appliance; sometimes elastic traction may be added from the lower appliance to a facebow attached to the upper appliance.

11. a. False. Lighter forces are less likely to produce anchorage loss.
    b. True. As there is a greater tendency to mesial drift.
    c. False. There will be less total force than when a larger number of teeth are being moved.
    d. False. As this will resist mesial drift.
    e. True. A fixed appliance does not have a base plate, so resistance to unwanted movement is less; a few teeth will only be moved by tipping movements with a removable appliance, both factors tending to reduce the likelihood of anchorage loss.
12. a. True. As this will spread the reaction force over a greater area.
    b. False. This is not appropriate with an upper removable appliance, as it will tend to dislodge the appliance.
    c. True. As it will prevent or minimise mesial drift.
    d. True. This will prevent the overjet increasing in response to any forward reaction force from the active components.
    e. False. This will tend to make the appliance loose and encourage mesial drift of the posterior teeth if the fit then becomes poor.
13. a. True. As apical blood flow is compromised.
    b. False. As extensive hyalinisation of the periodontal ligament takes place, followed by undermining resorption, tooth movement is likely to be slowed.
    c. False. Anchorage is likely to be lost as the reaction force to the active force may be sufficient to make the anchor teeth move.
    d. True. Likelihood of pain is greater as extensive areas of the periodontal ligament will be compressed.
    e. False. Likelihood of root resorption is increased.

EXTENDED MATCHING ITEMS ANSWERS

a. 1, 2, 5, 6. An upper removable appliance incorporating these components is required to correct the anterior crossbite.
b. 1, 10. An upper removable retainer (Hawley design from the components chosen) is necessary.
c. 13 or 16. Either appliance should produce all desired occlusal changes if compliance is optimal.
d. 12. In a compliant patient, through distal movement of the upper buccal segments, this should provide the small increments of additional space needed for upper arch alignment.
e. 11. Anchorage reinforcement via this means is required to ensure sufficient space for the requisite tooth movements.

CASE HISTORY ANSWERS

Case History 1

1. Possible reasons for slow progress include the patient not wearing the appliance full time, not placing the springs in the correct position, underactivation/overactivation or distortion of the springs, movement impeded by acrylic/wire/opposing occlusion/retained root of 4.
2. Ask the patient about the length of time the appliance is worn on a daily basis. Check that the springs are positioned correctly and are not overactivated, underactivated,

or distorted. Check if acrylic/wire/opposing occlusion is impeding tooth movement. Enquire from the patient if there was any mention from the practitioner who carried out the extraction as to whether any root fragment was retained. Radiograph the extraction sites of 4/4 to ensure that there is no root remnant of the extracted units if any doubt exists and to check if the bone density and periodontal architecture as expected.
3. If the appliance has not been worn as instructed, discuss this with the patient and warn him that if full-time wear is not forthcoming, treatment will be terminated. Reinstruct the patient in correct positioning of the springs if this is the problem. Check the activation is correct; if the springs are distorted, it may be possible to improve this. However, in some instances, it may be necessary to construct a new appliance. Remove acrylic if it is preventing tooth movement; if a wire component is preventing movement, it can be removed if possible, or it may be necessary to remake the appliance with a slightly different design to allow movement to proceed. Acrylic addition to the bite plane or to posterior capping may be required if the occlusion with the opposing arch is impeding movement. If a retained root is identified on radiograph, arrangements should be made for its removal, and tooth movement then recommenced after a period of healing.

Case History 2

1. Overjet increase following conclusion of functional appliance therapy represents relapse. This may result from insufficient wear of the appliance as a retainer following correction of the malocclusion. Ideally, it should be worn until growth is almost complete, in the late teens. A poorly interdigitating occlusion, persistent thumb-/finger-sucking habit, lip trap or tongue thrust may also account for overjet relapse, as may a posterior mandibular growth rotation.
2. Prevention could involve the following:
   - Checking that the final occlusion was well interdigitating and ensuring that there was slight overcorrection.
   - Reducing wear of the appliance to night-time only, and then maintaining wear at that level until late teens. Alternatively, an upper removable appliance with steeply inclined anterior bite plane may be constructed and worn for a similar duration.
   - Ensuring that digit-/thumb-sucking habits had ceased before commencing treatment.
   - If the lower lip coverage of the upper incisors was not at least one-third to one-half of the upper incisor crowns at completion of overjet reduction, the patient should have been informed that retention may be lengthy and perhaps require the placement of a bonded retainer at a later stage. A tongue thrust should also have been checked for and, if present (it may be adaptive if the lips are incompetent), retention carefully monitored. A pre-treatment cephalometric radiograph would have given an indication of the growth pattern, and if this is likely to be more backward and vertical than forward and horizontal, then prolonged retention is likely to be required as the former is likely to be less favourable for overjet stability.

3. Management options are as follows. As a 16-year-old female patient will be beyond her pubertal growth spurt, recommending functional appliance therapy is not a realistic option. If the overjet relapse is only minimal (of the order of a few millimetres), with the patient's consent, it could be monitored by recording the occlusion on study casts and reassessing it in 6 months when further treatment could be embarked on should there be evidence of further relapse. Further treatment options are orthodontic camouflage with, most likely, extraction of the upper first premolars and upper/lower fixed appliance therapy. Alternatively, if the relapse is significant and the underlying skeletal pattern/facial profile unlikely to benefit from camouflage treatment, orthognathic correction when growth is complete is the only other satisfactory solution.

PICTURE ANSWERS

Picture 1

1. A Roberts retractor.
2. It is used for overjet reduction.
3. Its wire dimensions are 0.5 mm wire sleeved in 0.5 mm internal diameter stainless steel tubing.
4. If the coils are positioned too high in the buccal sulcus, ulceration is likely. Also where the acrylic is not relieved sufficiently behind the upper incisors, the gingivae will become heaped up between the base plate and the palatal surfaces of the upper incisors during overjet reduction.

Picture 2

1. Frankel III appliance.
2. Indications are a growing child in the early mixed dentition (preferably 7–8 years), with a mild Class III skeletal discrepancy and reduced FMPA who is able to achieve an edge-to-edge incisor relationship. Dentoalveolar compensation should be minimal, or ideally lower incisors proclined and upper incisors upright.
3. The appliance is constructed to a wax registration recorded with the mandible postured open slightly and backwards as much as possible. The wire labial to the lower incisors is fabricated to a groove cut into the teeth on the work casts so it is active at insertion. A wire palatal to the upper incisors pushes them labially. The buccal shields allow upper arch expansion and maintain lower arch width. Other components aid retention of the appliance.
4. Stable correction of the class III incisor relationship is enhanced by achieving adequate overbite and by favourable mandibular growth.

Picture 3

1. Headcap, safety release spring mechanism (in two parts) and a facebow with locking device.
2. The spring mechanism connects the headcap to the facebow and controls the amount of force applied.
3. Headgear is used either to reinforce anchorage or for extraoral traction. For anchorage, wear of the appliance for 10–12 hours/day with 200–250 g force is required; for extraoral traction, the appliance should be worn for at least 14 out of 24 hours and force

magnitude is 400–500 g. Forces over 500 g with even longer wear prior to and during the pubertal growth spurt are necessary to restrain maxillary downward and forward growth.
4. Headgear must be fitted with two safety mechanisms and safety instructions issued. The following instructions are necessary: wear the appliance as instructed; it must never be worn without the safety mechanisms attached. Do not adjust the force yourself at any time. The headgear should not be worn during sports or other activity. If it ever becomes detached from the appliance, discontinue wear and return to the orthodontist. If the headgear ever becomes detached and rubs your face or eyes, go immediately to your doctor or hospital; cease appliance wear and report to your orthodontist.

Picture 4

1. A bonded canine to canine lower retainer.
2. It is used to maintain alignment of the lower labial segment following orthodontic movement.
3. As the lower labial segment will tend to crowd with time in all cases irrespective of the original malocclusion and the type of orthodontic treatment undertaken, it is now advocated by many that some form of permanent retention be used, particularly following fixed appliance therapy, to prevent relapse. This may involve placing a bonded retainer as seen here. Bonded retention is particularly indicated where rotations are present, where the lower labial segment has been proclined intentionally and in periodontally involved dentitions.
4. A lower removable (Hawley) retainer may be issued instead, but these are not good at maintaining rotational correction and may not be well tolerated. An alternative is a clear vacuum-formed retainer with full occlusal coverage, which has been shown to be more effective than a Hawley retainer at maintaining lower arch alignment.

SHORT NOTE ANSWERS

1. An Adams' clasp is used to provide retention for a removable appliance. Designed for this purpose to engage the mesiobuccal and distobuccal undercuts on a first permanent molar, it may be used also to provide retention on primary molars or premolars. It is usually made from 0.7 mm hard drawn stainless steel wire, but 0.6 mm wire is used for primary molars and premolars. Tubes may be soldered for extraoral anchorage or the clasp may be modified to incorporate hooks for elastics. Adjustment mid-flyover or closer to the arrowhead leads to respective down and inward or inward only movement of the clasp toward the tooth.
2. Disadvantages of removable appliances include: appliance is removable and can be taken out of the mouth by the patient; lower appliances are not well tolerated; speech is affected; limited to tipping movements only and not efficient where multiple tooth movements are required; intermaxillary traction cannot be used and good technical support is required.
3. A screw may be used as the active component rather than a spring where several teeth need to be moved or

where these also are required for retention of the appliance. There are two types: a Landin screw, which has a piston-like action and is used for movement of a single incisor tooth, and a Glenross screw, which has two interlocking pieces and is generally used to move several teeth. The disadvantages of screws are that they make the appliance bulky as well as being more expensive and less versatile in action than a spring. Activation is dependent on the patient remembering to adjust the screw as instructed – each turn producing about 0.25 mm of movement.

4. This appliance uses individual attachments with a rectangular slot for each tooth with 'average' tip, torque and 'in-out'. Brackets are available in a range of prescriptions including Andrews, Roth and MBT. Flat archwires may be placed. Clinical time is saved and a high standard of occlusal finish is achieved more consistently with these techniques than with non-preadjusted ('standard') edgewise techniques.

5. For tipping movement, forces in the range 35–60 g are appropriate; for bodily movement, 70–120 g; for rotation 35–60 g; for intrusion 10–20 g.

6. Intermaxillary traction is a means of producing tooth movement in one arch using teeth in the opposing arch as anchorage. It is the means of tooth movement employed by functional appliances but may be applied also with fixed appliances. It is not practical to employ intermaxillary traction with removable appliances, as it will dislodge the appliance. With fixed appliances, intermaxillary traction takes the form of either Class II or Class III traction with application of inter-arch elastics; the force necessary is decided by selecting elastics of appropriate size and weight. For class II traction, the elastics are stretched from the posterior aspect of the lower arch (usually the hook attached to the buccal molar tube or band) to an attachment on the anterior aspect of the upper arch, commonly to either a hook on the canine bracket or a soldered hook on the archwire. For class III traction, the elastics run from posteriorly in the upper arch (usually first permanent molar area) to anteriorly (canine area) in the lower arch. Class II elastics may be used to reduce an overjet while simultaneously closing buccal segment spacing in the lower arch. Both types of traction may extrude molar teeth and increase the vertical facial proportions, which would be undesirable in individuals where this is already increased. Proclination of lower incisors is a possible side effect of Class II traction and may be best avoided depending on the objectives of treatment.

7. A tipping force applied to a maxillary canine will induce areas of pressure and tension within the periodontal ligament space: pressure at the alveolar crest margin distally and at the apical area diagonally opposite; tension at the other sites. In the pressure areas, the blood vessels are compressed and osteoclasts invade within 4–5 days, leading to frontal alveolar bone resorption. In the tension sites, the blood vessels are dilated and the periodontal ligament fibres are stretched, with osteoblast invasion leading to osteoid deposition along the fibre bundles in the direction of tooth movement. Eventually, this is mineralised. All of the socket is remodelled in response to the tooth movement.

8. Once the rotation has been corrected, percision to sever the free gingival fibres may be undertaken to reduce the amount of relapse. Prolonged retention, often with a bonded retainer, is also necessary to prevent relapse.

VIVA ANSWERS

1. a. The appliance should be worn full time with the exception of after meals (when it should be removed for cleaning) and also for contact sports. Please place it in the hard plastic container provided when it is removed for contact sports.
   b. The main difficulties you will experience are likely to be in the first week, particularly during eating and speaking, but these should resolve after that.
   c. You may experience mild discomfort related to /1 for a few days. Take a mild analgesic, if necessary.
   d. You should not eat sticky or hard foods; avoid consuming fizzy drinks.
   e. The appliance should be removed after meals for cleaning, when you should also brush your teeth.
   f. If there are any problems with appliance wear, or if the appliance breaks, return immediately.

2. a. The patient's speech should be clear.
   b. The patient should be able to insert and remove the appliance unaided by a mirror.
   c. The base plate should have lost its shine, and there may be bite marks on a bite plane if this is part of the appliance.
   d. There is likely to be mild gingival erythema in relation to the base plate adaptation to the gingival margins and across the palate.
   e. The appliance will have lost some of its retention through being inserted and removed.

3. a. Classification could be tooth-borne passive (e.g. Andresen), tooth-borne active (e.g. Bionator), tissue borne (e.g. Frankel appliance).
   b. Obtain full diagnostic records, including a lateral cephalometric film. Take well-extended upper and lower impressions. With the patient sitting upright, instruct them in posturing the mandible to the desired position. Place a roll of softened wax over the upper teeth and gently instruct the patient to close into the rehearsed postured position – the exact extent of the forward posturing and mandibular opening will depend on the appliance chosen. Chill the wax registration, and check it in the mouth, ensuring that the centrelines are not displaced if they were already coincident. When the working casts have been constructed, mount them on an articulator using the construction bite to allow appliance fabrication. Wear of any appliance should be generally increased slowly over the first few weeks until it is being worn for at least 14 out of 24 hours. This is with the exception of the Twin-block appliance, which should be worn full time from the start. A time chart should be issued for recording wear. It is wise to see the patient 2 weeks after fitting the appliance to discuss any problems and to encourage co-operation with wear. Thereafter, an interval of 6–8 weeks between review appointments is usual. At each visit, with the appliance removed and the mandible fully retruded, the

overjet and buccal segment relationship should be recorded; the appliance adjusted for comfort and to facilitate eruption of permanent teeth, if necessary; the standing height checked; and the time chart checked and encouragement given regarding wear. Overcorrection is advisable. The appliance should be worn as a retainer until growth is ceased unless a further phase of treatment is planned with fixed appliances, and possible extractions to detail the occlusion.

c. The mode of action of a functional appliance is incompletely understood, but its primary function is to posture the mandible downwards and forwards, displacing the condyles out of the glenoid fossae. This stretches the orofacial musculature and generates a force vector that tends to procline the lower incisors, while the reaction force is transmitted backwards through the appliance to the upper teeth and maxilla. The effects, therefore, are to procline the lower incisors (which in most cases is undesirable, and can be resisted by capping of the incisal edges), and to retrocline the upper incisors. Condylar growth is stimulated and the glenoid fossae may be positioned more anteriorly, while downward and forward maxillary growth is restrained. Overbite reduction occurs by restraining eruption of the lower incisors while the posterior teeth are allowed to erupt.

4. Anchorage is the resistance to the force of reaction generated by the active components. It may be classified as intra- or extraoral anchorage. Intraoral anchorage can be simple, where movement of one tooth is pitted against that of several others for which movement is not desired, or reciprocal, where movement of one group of teeth is used as anchorage for movement of another group of teeth in the opposite direction; for example, closure of a median diastema or upper arch expansion. Extraoral anchorage is anchorage obtained by wearing headgear.

Anchorage may be preserved by:
- moving a few teeth at a time
- control of the force magnitude to 0.3–0.5 N for tipping
- maximum base plate extension
- clasping additional teeth to increase resistance to movement
- preventing the incisors from tipping labially by placing a close-fitting labial bow
- fitting headgear.

Anchorage may be monitored by:
- careful measurement of the space required for the intended tooth movement at each visit
- measurement of the overjet in class II division 1 and/or the buccal segment relationship is useful. If extraoral anchorage is fitted, two safety mechanisms must be added to the headgear: a locking device on the facebow (Ni Tom) and a safety release headcap with spring mechanism. Specific instructions regarding wear (10–12 hours), placement and removal, as well as warnings regarding possible facial and eye injuries, must be given together with a contact number should any problems arise. Patient and parent must understand these.

SINGLE BEST ANSWER QUESTION ANSWERS

1. B
2. E
3. C
4. D
5. B
6. B
7. E
8. A
9. A
10. B
11. A
12. C

12 Professionalism, Law and Ethics

Overview

Professionalism is a multi-faceted and complex phenomenon. As members of a healing profession, dental surgeons are expected not only to obey the law of the land but also to abide by ethical principles in their professional and personal life. Ethics are moral principles or rules of conduct expected in the professional and personal conduct of someone practising a profession. To assist dental surgeons in ethical matters, national regulatory bodies regularly issue requirement and guidance documents. In the United Kingdom, an example of this is the standards and guidance produced by the General Dental Council (GDC). In 2013, the GDC published *Standards for the Dental Team*, which sets out standards of conduct, performance and ethics for dental professionals in the United Kingdom. The GDC has also produced a wide range of guidance documents on specific topics, such as *The professional duty of candour, Guidance on child protection and vulnerable adults* and *Guidance on using social media*. All GDC advice documents are available online (www.gdc-uk.org). Dental professionals have a duty to understand and abide by the requirements of the country in which they work.

The authors of this chapter are based in the United Kingdom, and it is recognised that many aspects mentioned are UK specific; however, other countries will have in place organisations, structures and systems that have similar functions and comparable policies. The other item to highlight is the continuous development and updating of some of the areas discussed in this chapter. Regulatory aspects are often not static, and it is important to be aware of this and understand the sources that can be accessed in order to keep in touch with such updates. Keeping up-to-date and being aware of current developments is just one of the facets of being 'a professional'.

(Note: For an explanation of the acronyms used here, please refer to the Acronyms section at the end of the chapter.)

12.1 Principles

In addition to the GDC, the Federation Dentaire International (FDI) World Dental Federation at its 1997 General Assembly approved a statement on 'International Principles of Ethics for the Dental Profession', which is still available on the FDI website, together with further guidance, and they have also produced an ethics manual (www.fdiworldental.org). As previously mentioned, in terms of UK dentistry, the GDC has published *Standards for the Dental Team*, which sets out standards of conduct, performance and ethics for dental professionals. *Standards for the Dental Team* was implemented on 30 September 2013 and replaced *Standards for Dental Professionals*, which had been in effect from 2005 to 2013. When *Standards for the Dental Team* was introduced, the booklet was sent to the registered address of all GDC registrants, it is now available to download and print on the GDC website. The content of this document is applicable to all dental professional registrant groups. One of the requirements for those managing a dental team is that they must display information so that it can be seen by patients. This information includes both the nine principles in *Standards for the Dental Team* and the fact that dental professionals are registered by the GDC.

The nine principles in *Standards for the Dental Team*, which GDC registered dental professionals must observe at all times are:

- Put patients' interests first.
- Communicate effectively with patients.
- Obtain valid consent.
- Maintain and protect patients' information.
- Have a clear and effective complaints procedure.
- Work with colleagues in a way that is in patients' best interests.
- Maintain, develop and work within your professional knowledge and skills.
- Raise concerns if patients are at risk.

■ Make sure your personal behaviour maintains patients' confidence in you and the dental profession.

The principles are not listed in order of priority and have equal importance. The format of the document presents principles, standards, guidance and also includes what patients expect. The principles listed in *Standards for the Dental Team* are supplemented by further guidance documents found on the GDC website; these must also be followed. There are also scenarios and case studies based around this content on the GDC website.

(Note: The GDC is reviewing *Standards for the Dental Team*. If new documentation is developed, it will be available on the GDC website [www.gdc-uk.org].)

12.2 The General Dental Council

LEARNING OBJECTIVES

You should:
- understand the roles and functions of the GDC
- be aware of its membership.

The first attempt to control the practice of dentistry in the United Kingdom was the Dentists Act of 1878, which created the first official Dentists Register. Only a registered person was able to use the title 'Dentist' or 'Dental Practitioner'. In the late 19th and early 20th centuries, there were two ways to become a dentist: either by serving an apprenticeship as a dental technician followed by being apprenticed to a dentist, or by studying at a university or college and obtaining either a degree or a diploma in dentistry.

The 1921 Dentists Act prohibited the practice of dentistry by unregistered persons. It set up the Dental Board of UK, which was administered by the General Medical Council (GMC). After that date, only persons with a degree or diploma in dentistry from a recognised university or college could apply to join the register. However, anyone who had completed apprenticeship dental training, and was over 21 years of age when the register was formed, was admitted to that register.

The Dental Board of UK was dissolved by the Dentists Act of 1956 and it established the independent GDC to take over the role of governing the dental profession. This Act also permitted the use of the additional title of 'Dental Surgeon' and permitted the introduction of registered ancillary dental workers. All previous laws relating to the practice of dentistry were consolidated into one Act by the Dentists Act 1957.

The Dentists Act 1983 altered the composition of the GDC by increasing the number of elected dentists to 18 and Privy Council nominated lay members to six. However, the 17 nominated dental members from the universities and colleges giving dental degrees and diplomas plus the four UK Chief Dental Officers still made up over 40% of the membership. This Act also strengthened the disciplinary procedures undertaken by the Professional Conduct Committee (PCC) and introduced a Health Committee to deal with dentists who had health rather than disciplinary problems. The Dentists Act 1984 consolidated the 1957 and 1983 Acts into a single piece of legislation.

In 2005, the Dentists Act 1984 was amended by the Dentists Act 1984 (Amendment) Order 2005 (a Section 60 Order).

This Order updated several aspects of the Act to allow for changes the GDC wished to make. The most important provision of this Order is that it allows for future amendments to the Dentists Act 1984 to be made as 'Orders in Council' by the Privy Council. This method of making any amendments that may prove necessary in the future is much simpler and involves very little legislative time. The 2005 Order also allowed for the registration of dental care professionals (DCPs).

Another important part of this Order made it compulsory for dentists to have 'adequate and appropriate insurance' to remain on the Dentists Register. This insurance must indemnify the dentist by providing sufficient insurance cover for liabilities that may be incurred in carrying out work as a dentist.

As the Health and Social Care (Quality and Safety) Act 2015 required all health and social care professions and organisations '*to secure that the services provided cause no avoidable harm*', further amendment of the Dentists Act 1984 was needed. This meant that the over-arching objective of the GDC is to protect the public.

Pursuant to this, as stated on the GDC website, the objectives and purpose of the Council are:

■ to protect, promote and maintain the health, safety and well-being of the public
■ to promote and maintain confidence in the dental profession
■ to promote and maintain proper professional standards and conduct for members of these professions.

The GDC regulates Dentists and Dental Care Professionals in the United Kingdom. The following groups are registered with the GDC:

■ Dentists
■ Clinical Dental Technicians
■ Dental Hygienists
■ Dental Nurses
■ Dental Technicians
■ Dental Therapists
■ Orthodontic Therapists

The GDC website has a search function which permits searching of the Dentist, DCP and specialist lists. It allows the public to check: a dental professional's registration; the status of a registration, for example, if there are any conditions on that registration; the type of registration held. This includes whether a dentist is registered as a Temporary Registrant, or if dentists or DCPs are registered as Visiting Practitioners. Information was reported on the GDC website that in November 2019, there were approximately 42,000 dentists and 70,000 DCPs registered with the GDC.

The GDC protects the public by means of its statutory responsibilities for dental education, registration, professional conduct and health.

The membership of the GDC, and how the membership is appointed, has changed over time. The Council has become smaller and, since 2009, no longer has a majority of dentists in its membership. To illustrate the evolution of the Council, in 2003, the GDC was reconstituted, and comprised of:

■ six lay people appointed by the Queen on the recommendation of her Privy Council
■ 15 dentists elected by dentists on the Dental Register

- four elected from the professions complementary to dentistry (PCDs) elected by registered PCDs (note: in September 2005, in line with new legislation, the GDC agreed to use the term 'Dental Care Professionals' instead of PCDs)
- four associate members, who have no voting rights; these are the four Chief Dental Officers for England, Scotland, Wales and Northern Ireland.

In 2009, in line with government plans for health care regulation, the membership of the GDC and the way that membership was appointed changed. The new GDC was smaller, comprising:

- eight dentists
- four DCPs
- 12 lay people.

This meant that from 2009, the GDC no longer had a majority of dentists in its membership. Following national advertisements, all members of the GDC are now appointed by the government's Appointments Commission within the parameters set down by the GDC. The purpose of this change was to remove any perception by the public that professional members of the GDC, and of other health care regulatory bodies, are representing those who elected them, rather than being purely responsible for the effective regulation of that profession.

In 2013, a new Council convened. The Council is now formed of 12 members: six appointed registrant and six appointed lay members.

REGISTRATION WITH THE GDC

In the United Kingdom, only dental surgeons registered with the GDC are entitled to practise dentistry. Graduates and licentiates in dentistry of universities and Royal Surgical Colleges of the United Kingdom may be registered on completion of the appropriate application and payment of the prescribed registration fee. The universities and royal colleges in the United Kingdom provide the GDC with lists of their dental graduates or licentiates. Registration has to be renewed annually as long as a dentist wishes to practise in the United Kingdom. The annual renewal process includes three actions: making an Indemnity Declaration; payment of the Annual Retention Fee (ARF); making a Continuing Professional Development (CPD) statement.

Prior to the U.K. withdrawal from the European Union (Brexit) holders of an appropriate European Dental Diploma who were nationals of member states of the European Union (EU) were also entitled to register, as were Icelandic and Norwegian graduates, since Norway and Iceland are members of the European Economic Association (EEA), as are dentists who qualified in Switzerland. Any European dentist applying for registration required documentary evidence of:

- identity
- academic attainment
- a knowledge of the English language which, in the interest of themselves and their patients, is necessary for the provision of dental services
- good standing
- good health.

Disqualification from practice in any EU/EEA member state is most likely to bar a dentist from registering with the GDC.

Up to 2001, dentists holding a primary dental diploma from certain overseas universities that the GDC had visited to check educational standards could also be fully registered with the GDC and are still able to continue to be registered. These universities are in Commonwealth or former Commonwealth countries where dental education is similar to that in the United Kingdom. No other qualifications were automatically accepted by the GDC for full registration and therefore the right of undertaking independent dental practice in the United Kingdom.

There are several ways by which dentists with qualifications that do not fit into the above categories can register with the GDC.

Temporary Registration

Temporary registration is available to allow such dentists to teach, do research work or obtain postgraduate instruction in certain approved hospital, dental school or other approved institution posts for a limited period. Temporary registration only lasts for the period of a particular post or employment and may be renewed by application up to a maximum of 5 years.

Dentists with temporary registration can only practise dentistry under the supervision of a named, fully registered dentist of consultant status in the United Kingdom.

International Qualifying Examination

The International Qualifying Examination (IQE) replaced the Statutory Examination in 2001. At the same time, the GDC ceased to recognise the primary dental diplomas from certain universities overseas. From 2001, all dental surgeons who do not have a primary dental qualification gained through a dental school or Royal Surgical College in the United Kingdom, the EU or the EEA had to sit the IQE. The IQE closed to new applicants in 2007.

Overseas Registration Examination

In 2007, the Overseas Registration Examination (ORE) became the new statutory examination to permit overseas dental graduates to apply for admission to the Dentist's Register, it replaced the IQE.

Additionally, since October 2011, before applying to sit the ORE, prospective candidates need to demonstrate that their dental course and qualification is comparable to EU training and assessment requirements. A statement to this effect has to be obtained from the UK National Recognition Information Centre (UK NARIC). This organisation has been set up by the UK government to check comparability of all professional qualifications. Other EU countries have set up similar organisations. A NARIC Statement of Comparability has to be submitted with the application to sit the ORE. Prospective candidates must also demonstrate that their clinical experience satisfies the requirements set (a set number of hours is required of personal treatment of patients in the dental chair) and English language requirements are met.

The ORE is comprised of two parts:

Part 1 consists of two, 3-hour written papers, comprising short answers, which are undertaken on a computer, to test the candidates' application of knowledge in clinical practice:
Paper A: this covers clinically applied dental science and clinically applied human disease.

Paper B: this covers aspects of clinical dentistry, including law and ethics and health and safety.

Part 2: the purpose of this part is to test candidates' ability to demonstrate clinical skills safely and consists of four elements:

1. three practical exercises on a dental manikin in 3 hours
2. an Objective Structured Clinical Examination (OSCE)
3. a diagnosis and treatment planning exercise
4. an examination in medical emergencies, including cardiopulmonary resuscitation using a manikin.

Up to four attempts each are allowed for Part 1 and Part 2 of the ORE. Also, Part 2 has to be passed within 5 years of the first attempt at Part 1 of this examination.

Additionally, to register with the GDC, candidates will need, as part of the application process, to provide evidence of good standing.

To be able to work in National Health Service (NHS) primary care dental services, those who have passed the ORE have been expected to show equivalence to dental foundation training (DFT).

There are various local rules and legislation governing dentists moving to a new country. It is beyond the scope of this book to cover all eventualities, and the reader is recommended to engage with border and immigration services and the professional regulator to determine the requirements, e.g. in the United Kingdom, the GDC and the UK Visas and Immigration.

Licence in Dental Surgery

The Licence in Dental Surgery (LDS) examination is open to applications from qualified dentists and is awarded by the Royal College of Surgeons of England (RCS Eng). Again, there are criteria which must be satisfied when applying to sit this examination. Successful candidates are eligible to apply for GDC registration.

The LDS is comprised of two parts:

Part 1 consists of two, 3-hour written papers comprising short answers, to test the candidates' application of knowledge in clinical practice:

Paper A: this covers clinically applied human disease and clinically applied dental science.

Paper B: this covers elements of clinical dentistry, including health and safety, law and ethics.

Part 2: the purpose of this part is to test candidates' ability to practise clinical skills safely and consists of three elements:

1. an Objective Structured Clinical Examination
2. an operative test on a dental manikin
3. an unseen case examination including diagnosis, treatment planning and clinical reasoning.

Up to four attempts each are allowed for Part 1 and Part 2 of the LDS. Also, Part 2 has to be passed within 5 years of the first attempt at Part 1 of this examination.

Continuing Professional Development

CPD includes professional development through learning, training or other activities, which maintain and further develop an individual's practice or intended practice. It is the duty of all dental professionals to keep their knowledge and skills up-to-date. It is also a requirement for all dentists and DCPs in order to remain registered with the GDC. The GDC made CPD compulsory for dentists on 1 January 2002; since then, there have been different schemes and requirements, and these have included the need for concise and appropriate educational aims and objectives, in addition to a quality control mechanism. Compulsory CPD for DCPs was introduced in 2008.

The 5-year CPD cycle was phased in over a period of 3 years depending on the date of first registration with the GDC:

- First registered between 1990 and 2001, 5-year cycle started on 1 January 2002.
- First registered between 1980 and 1989, 1 January 2003.
- First registered before 1979, 1 January 2004.

These first 5-year cycles therefore ended on 31 December in 2006, 2007 and 2008, respectively.

Dentists whose first registration date is on or after 1 January 2002 commence their 5-year cycle on 1 January of the year following their first registration. Also, dentists applying to rejoin the register will have to show that they have met CPD requirements prior to being readmitted to the Dentists Register.

The current legislation governing CPD requirements for Dentists and Dental Care Professionals is the General Dental Council (Continuing Professional Development) (Dentists and Dental Care Professionals) Rules Order of Council 2017, which came into force on 1 January 2018. The enhanced Continuing Professional Development (eCPD) scheme started in January 2018 for dentists and August 2018 for DCPs. The scheme has a number of features and includes:

- A requirement for a Personal Development Plan (PDP).
- A minimum number of verifiable hours of eCPD for each registrant group (these should be evenly spread over a 5-year cycle).
- A requirement to declare the number of hours completed in an annual declaration to the GDC.
- A requirement to plan CPD activities according to the field of practice of the individual dental professional.
- The GDC has set development outcomes, and CPD should also be aligned to these. Full descriptors of the development outcomes can be found on the GDC website, but briefly these include:
  A. Communication with patients and the dental team. This includes aspects of obtaining consent, managing complaints and raising concerns
  B. Patient management, management of the dental team and management of self-leadership as appropriate
  C. Maintenance and development of knowledge and skill;
  D. Maintenance of skills, behaviours and attitudes which put patients' interests first and maintain patient confidence.

The GDC website also holds a list of highly recommended topics for CPD, for which they recommend certain levels of engagement (number of hours) based on field of practice:

- Medical emergencies;
- Disinfection and decontamination; and
- Radiography and radiation protection.

They also recommend CPD in the following areas:

- Legal and ethical issues;
- Complaints handling;
- Oral cancer: early detection;
- Safeguarding children and young people; and
- Safeguarding vulnerable adults.

The 2018 Enhanced CPD scheme requires dentists to complete a minimum of 100 hours of verifiable CPD per 5-year cycle and to ensure hours are spread evenly over the cycle, at least 10 hours must have been completed during any 2-year time period.

For DCPs under the 2018 Enhanced CPD scheme, completion of a minimum of 50 hours of verifiable CPD is required for dental nurses and dental technicians during the 5-year cycle. A minimum of 75 hours verifiable CPD per cycle is required for dental therapists, dental hygienists, orthodontic therapists and clinical dental technicians. Again, at least 10 hours must be completed during any 2-year period.

A written record of CPD must be kept by each registrant, together with documentary evidence (e.g. certificates from the CPD provider). Details of what CPD records must include are available on the GDC website.

A CPD declaration is made annually by each registrant. The 'annual CPD statement' includes: the number of hours of CPD which have been completed; a declaration that a CPD record has been kept; a declaration that a PDP is in place; a declaration that the CPD is relevant to the current or intended field or practice, and that the statement is full and accurate.

Periodic checks are carried out by the GDC, and they can randomly select registrants to check CPD records.

The previous GDC CPD scheme ran from 2008 to 2017 and included a combination of both verifiable and non-verifiable requirements. Transitional arrangements exist until 2022 for certain registrants, depending on where they are in the 5-year cycle.

Personal Development Planning

A PDP provides an opportunity to identify areas for further development, record development objectives and encourage life-long learning. It also aids development of a strategy to achieve the goals set.

Following a learning or development activity, the participant should take time to consider what they have learnt, whether their learning objective from their PDP has been met and how they may benefit from their learning, and possibly how others may benefit (e.g. the team they work with).

Personal development plans are not static and may need to be revised following reflection, or if learning needs alter or if the individual's field of practice changes.

GDC requirements are for a PDP that must include the CPD which is planned during the registrant's 5-year cycle (this must be relevant to field of practice).

Reflective Practice

Reflection is important in development, and reflective practice aims to allow individual practitioners to assess their professional experiences, recognise positives and where improvements could be made. Identification of opportunities to improve may guide personal development planning and learning. Reflection may be individual, but multi-disciplinary and team reflection can be important for development and improved practice.

In June 2019, a joint statement of support on the benefits of becoming a reflective practitioner was made by the Chief Executives of the United Kingdom's statutory regulators of health and care professionals. This included the General Dental Council. Whilst approaches of reflective practice from each regulator may vary, this statement demonstrates the importance and value placed on reflection in learning and development.

Professional Standards Authority

The government originally set up the Council for the Regulation of Healthcare Professionals (CHRP) in April 2003, and it consisted of 10 lay members and nine members nominated by health care professions regulators, including a GDC nominee. In the Health and Social Care Act (2008), the name of the council was changed to the *Council for the Regulation of Healthcare Excellence (CHRE)*. The Council for Healthcare Regulatory Excellence (CHRE) was renamed under the Health and Social Care Act 2012 and became the Professional Standards Authority (PSA).

The PSA is independent and accountable to the UK parliament. It oversees nine regulators who 'register' health and care professionals; one of these is the General Dental Council. The PSA encourages co-operation and greater consistency in the work of health care regulators and promotes good practice. One of the PSA's powers is to review decisions of a health care regulator about practitioners' 'fitness to practise' and appeal to the appropriate court of law against a decision where it considers that such a decision has been over-lenient.

The PSA board consists of eight members; none of whom are health or care professionals. The board set the strategic directions and are responsible for determining overall policies. The PSA has adopted the approach of *right touch regulation*, which includes ensuring understanding of a situation and proportionate regulation. Further information about the Professional Standards Authority and *right touch regulation* is available on their website (www.professionalstandards.org.uk).

12.3 Titles and Descriptions

You should:
- understand what dental specialties are available
- know the scope and limitations of the tasks that Dental Care Professionals undertake.

DENTISTS

Registration with the GDC allows the use of the titles Dentist, Dental Practitioner or Dental Surgeon. Also, since November 1995, the GDC has accepted the use of the courtesy title Doctor, provided that it is not used in a way to suggest that the user is anything other than a dentist. The services offered must be clear and must not imply that the user is a medical doctor.

Before 1998, no other title was permitted, but the GDC is now empowered to set up and maintain specialist lists of practitioners who can show they have received sufficient postgraduate training to be considered specialists in a particular field. Practitioners on these lists are permitted to use the appropriate titles (e.g. 'Specialist in Endodontics').

Entry to the lists is determined by European and GDC regulations. There are two methods of entry to these specialist lists:

1. At the end of the appropriate time in a recognised training post, the appropriate postgraduate diploma and an assessment by the Specialist Advisory Committee for the specialty.
2. By virtue of current specialist practice and previous training. Consideration of equivalents is known as *mediated entry*. There was also a pathway open for 2 years following the establishment of each individual specialist list, this was referred to as *transitional arrangements*.

There are currently 13 specialist lists. These are:

Dental and Maxillofacial Radiology
Dental Public Health
Endodontics
Oral and Maxillofacial Pathology
Restorative Dentistry
Oral Medicine
Oral Microbiology
Oral Surgery
Orthodontics
Paediatric Dentistry
Periodontics
Prosthodontics
Special Care Dentistry

The specialty of restorative dentistry involves training in endodontics, periodontics and prosthodontics; it therefore involves a longer training period than that required for specialisation in only one of the other three recognised restorative specialties.

In 2019, the GDC began quality assuring specialty training and education programmes in the United Kingdom. Specialty curricula are developed by the Special Advisory Committees (SACs) for a given specialty, for example, the Specialist Advisory Committee for Special Care Dentistry. Curricula are then approved by the GDC. There is a reference guide for postgraduate training in the United Kingdom, *The Dental Gold Guide*, which is produced by the UK Committee of Postgraduate Dental Deans and Directors (COPDENDs). The *Dental Gold Guide* sets out a framework for the operational management of postgraduate specialty training. In addition to outlining roles and responsibilities of the organisations involved in specialty training, the guide outlines stages in undertaking a training programme and how trainees progress through a programme. The guide can be downloaded from the COPDEND website (www.copdend.org). For medical postgraduate training in the United Kingdom, the *Gold Guide* is the reference guide, and this is produced by the Conference of Postgraduate Medical Deans of the United Kingdom (COPMeD). This guide, which is

regularly updated, is available on the COPMeD website (www.copmed.org.uk).

The GDC is currently reviewing aspects of specialty listing and training; this includes specialty curricula and assessments and the mediated entry process to specialist lists. Mediated entry and equivalents of specialty training are currently under a comprehensive review. There is considerable flux around entry to the specialist lists in the United Kingdom, and a number of stakeholders are currently involved, including the GDC, the SACs and Health Education England (HEE).

Since the GDC originally established specialist lists, the specialties included have altered. The original 13 specialist lists established by the GDC were:

SPECIALTY	END OF TRANSITIONAL ENTRY PERIOD
Dental and maxillofacial radiology	31 May 2002
Dental public health	15 April 2000
Endodontics	31 May 2000
Oral medicine	30 June 2001
Oral microbiology	31 May 2002
Oral pathology	31 May 2002
Oral surgery	15 April 2000
Orthodontics	30 June 2000
Paediatric dentistry	30 June 2000
Periodontics	31 May 2000
Prosthodontics	31 May 2000
Restorative dentistry	15 April 2000
Surgical dentistry	31 May 2000

Surgical dentistry was confined to dento-alveolar surgery, whereas oral surgery encompassed surgery to surrounding structures and the treatment of maxillofacial injuries. At the December 2005 meeting, the GDC decided to merge the surgical dentistry list into the oral surgery list. Current surgical dentistry trainees and future trainees were then expected to train to the oral surgery core competences. Those previously admitted to the surgical dentistry list were reminded that the professional duty is to practise only within the limits of their competence. This change brought the United Kingdom in line with the situation in the EU and in many other countries. This merger took place in April 2007.

In 2008, the GDC added another specialty, 'Special Care Dentistry', again with a 2-year transitional period for those already competent in that specialty.

Maxillofacial surgery is considered to be a medical specialty by the EU, and maxillofacial surgeons are registered with the GMC.

DENTAL CARE PROFESSIONALS (FORMERLY PROFESSIONS COMPLEMENTARY TO DENTISTRY)

Since 1956, the GDC has been responsible for maintaining a register of dental hygienists and dental therapists. The 2005 amendments to the Dentists Act of 1984 allowed for the registration of other groups of dental care workers. In

2005, the title *Professions Complementary to Dentistry* was changed to *Dental Care Professionals*. Several new classes of DCPs were eligible for registration, and 'grand parenting' arrangements were agreed for dental nurses and dental technicians, but only for the first 2 years of this register.

The GDC Dental Care Professionals' Register opened in July 2006 and is separate from the Dentists Register. Registration for dental nurses and dental technicians became compulsory in July 2008. Also, it became illegal for a non-registered person to use any of the recognised DCP titles as they are protected by law. For two of the new classes of DCPs, clinical dental technicians and orthodontic therapists, registration has been compulsory since this register opened.

The GDC *Scope of Practice* document can be found on the GDC website and describes the skills and abilities each DCP registrant group should have. The GDC makes it clear that registrants should ensure they have the necessary skills, are appropriately trained, competent and indemnified for the patient care they deliver. The *Scope of Practice* document also includes the additional skills a registrant may develop if they have attended appropriate additional training and in some cases undertaken appropriate assessment. The following descriptors of dental care professionals are based on the GDC's *Scope of Practice* document; the reader is recommended to refer to the GDC documentation to appreciate the full scope of practice of each registrant group.

Dental Hygienists

This group of dental professionals help patients to maintain their oral health by promoting good oral health practice. They also work by preventing and treating periodontal disease. Among a range of other skills, *dental hygienists* use indices to screen and monitor periodontal disease, undertake supragingival and subgingival scaling and root surface debridement and also apply certain prophylactic materials to the surface of teeth. They provide advice on preventive oral care and smoking cessation. Hygienists who qualified prior to 1992 and who administer local anaesthetic infiltration analgesia must have attended a course and received a certificate in administration of local infiltration analgesia, or hold the Diploma of Dental Therapy.

Dental Therapists

Among a range of other skills in the scope of the dental hygienist, dental therapists undertake direct restorations on primary and secondary teeth, can carry out pulpotomies on primary teeth and extract primary teeth. Before 2002, dental therapists were only allowed to work in the community dental service or in the hospital service, but now they also work in general dental practice.

Dental Nurses

Dental nurses provide clinical and other support to registrants and patients. This includes, amongst other roles, preparation of the clinical environment, chairside support to other registrants during treatment and monitoring, support and reassurance to patients. Following appropriate additional instruction, *additional skills* dental nurses could develop include further skills in oral health promotion and oral health education. Additional skills carried out on prescription from, or under direction of, another registrant could include taking radiographs, removing sutures after the wound has been checked by a dentist or taking impressions to the prescription of a dentist.

Orthodontic Therapists

Orthodontic therapists are permitted to carry out certain parts of orthodontic treatment under prescription from a dentist. Their roles can include taking impressions, inserting removable orthodontic appliances, fitting orthodontic headgear, separators and orthodontic bands, placement of direct bonded orthodontic attachments and the ligation and removal of archwires previously fitted by a dentist and the removal of orthodontic bands and excess cement.

Dental Technicians

This group of dental professionals make dental devices to the prescription of a dentist or clinical dental technician. They are also able to repair dentures direct to members of the public. In addition to the construction of appliances, they can take tooth shades of patients for the construction of prostheses.

Clinical Dental Technicians

This registered group of dental professionals, who are also qualified dental technicians, provide complete dentures direct to patients, and other dental devices on prescription from a dentist. Clinical dental technicians can refer patients to a dentist if they are concerned about a patient's oral health, or if they need a treatment plan. Patients who have implants or natural teeth must be seen by a dentist before a clinical dental technician can do any treatment.

Maxillofacial prosthetists and technologists were originally included in the GDC's list of PCDs, but as much of their work is non-dental, the Institute of Maxillofacial Prosthetists and Technologists, on the recommendation of the Department of Health, has elected to be registered with the Health Professions Council rather than the GDC.

Direct Access

In the United Kingdom, since 2013, the GDC has allowed certain DCP's to provide a range of services directly to the general public without the need for a referral or a prescription from a registered dentist.

Before undertaking direct access, registered DCPs must:

- be appropriately trained, competent and indemnified for any tasks they undertake
- continue to work within their scope of practice regardless of this change in status
- follow the GDC's *Standards for the Dental Team*
- DCPs do not have to offer direct access and should not be made to offer it.

Dental Hygienists and Dental Therapists can carry out their full scope of practice without prescription or having to see a dentist first if they are confident that they have the skills and competences required. They are not permitted to directly undertake tooth whitening or botulism toxin treatment and are not able to prescribe local anaesthesia. Those who were trained and registered prior to 2002 may require 'top-up' training.

Dental Nurses can participate in preventative programmes without the patient(s) having to see a dentist first.

Orthodontic Therapists can carry out Index of Orthodontic Treatment Need (IOTN) screening, but the majority of their work remains under the prescription of a dentist.

Clinical Dental Technicians can continue to provide and maintain full dentures for patients. Other work must have a prescription from a dentist.

Dental Technicians, apart from denture repairs, continue to carry out work only on the prescription of a dentist.

12.4 Requirements for the Practice of Dentistry

LEARNING OBJECTIVES

You should:
- understand how the GDC carries out its regulatory tasks and how disciplinary matters are dealt with
- understand the educational and indemnity requirements of being a member of a profession.

REGULATION BY THE GENERAL DENTAL COUNCIL

It is the GDC's duty to maintain the Dentists Register and the Dental Care Professionals Register. The Registrar and Chief Executive of the GDC is responsible for ensuring the accuracy of these registers. The Registrar must remove the name of any dentist or DCP who fails to satisfy requirements for ongoing registration. A name can only be restored to the register by formal application and the payment of a restoration fee in addition to the annual retention fee. Evidence of CPD may also be required, depending on how long someone has been off the register. Further information may also be required depending on circumstances; this may include a Certificate of Current Professional Status (CCPS) and/or demonstration of English language knowledge. There are mechanisms to appeal erasure from the list; these depend on the reason for removal. Further information is available on the GDC website.

Education

The Dentists Act (1984) gives the GDC the responsibility to supervise all stages of dental education, postgraduate as well as undergraduate. The GDC quality assures new and existing programmes which lead to registration. The GDC determines minimum standards and sends an inspection panel to dental schools and other training establishments to check on standards of teaching and of examination of students. It has the power to recommend that the recognition of a dental qualification by the GDC is withdrawn should the council consider that the training or examination no longer secures sufficient knowledge and skill to practise dentistry.

The 2005 Amendment Order requires the GDC to determine the appropriate standard of proficiency required and to specify the content and standard of education and training required for the registration of DCPs.

The GDC document *Preparing for Practice: Dental Team Learning Outcomes for Registration* (2015 revised edition) presents the learning outcomes which an individual must be able to demonstrate at the end of a period of training for each of the professions registered by the GDC.

The outcomes are presented by profession (dentist, dental therapist, dental hygienist, dental nurse, orthodontic therapist, clinical dental technician and dental technician) in a domain structure, with varying content and numbers of outcomes for each group. The four domains included are:

- clinical
- communication
- professionalism
- management and leadership.

Quality assurance processes for education and training programmes leading to registration with the GDC are outlined in the GDC *Quality Assurance Guidance for Education Providers* document. A further document, *Standards for Education*, outlines the standards required by providers of UK dental GDC accredited training programmes. *Standards for Education* highlights three areas of requirements: patient protection; quality evaluation and review of the programme; and student assessment.

Education providers of qualifications that lead to registration as a dentist with the GDC must hold dental authority status; this is a legal status granted by the Privy Council. *Standards for Education* forms the basis of the quality assurance processes and monitoring/inspection of programmes leading to registration. If the required level is achieved, programmes that lead to registration as a dentist are found 'sufficient' and programmes leading to DCP registration are 'approved' (the terminology is dictated by the Dentists Act 1984).

A number of resources are available for students on the GDC website. These are aimed at supporting understanding and how standards may be applied in specific situations. An example of this is the resources on student professionalism, which include guidance and case studies.

As discussed in the previous section, in 2019, the GDC became responsible for quality assurance of specialty education. The *Standards for Specialty Education* document contains the standards and requirements for programme and examination providers. Requirements are presented under the areas of: patient protection (programme providers only); quality evaluation and review of the programme and specialty trainee assessment. Specialty curricula are currently under review and new curricula are expected to be implemented in 2022.

Conduct

The GDC also has a duty to remove from the Dentists Register or the Dental Care Professionals Register any member who is shown to have behaved in a manner unsuitable for continued registration. The GDC has regularly issued written advice on the standards required by the professions it regulates; further information is available on the GDC website.

At all times, the dentist's and dental care professional's conduct must be of the high standard that the public and the profession expect. The dentist's first priority is a responsibility to patients. If a dentist's conduct falls below this high standard, the GDC has the power to suspend or remove the dentist's name from the register. Conviction for a criminal offence or serious professional misconduct can be grounds for refusal of admission, erasure or suspension from the register. Conduct or behaviour prior to qualification is also considered by the GDC; therefore, this power also applies to students. Any dentist or DCP who is found guilty of serious professional misconduct in another country may not be entitled to register with the GDC.

Serious professional misconduct by a dentist cannot be precisely defined. However, it is considered to be conduct by a dentist that falls short of the standards of conduct expected among dentists, and that this should be a serious omission/commission. Specifically, the GDC has to decide upon a dentist's *Fitness to Practise* (FtP) if a concern is raised. In the case of DCPs, the GDC uses the more general term of 'misconduct' for matters that may be investigated and be subject to disciplinary action. Also, any criminal conviction in the United Kingdom of a person on a GDC register is automatically forwarded to the council by the police, who may also inform the GDC of formal cautions and other matters of concern. *Standards for the Dental Team* also requires registrants to report any criminal proceedings or regulatory findings made against them, anywhere in the world, directly to the GDC.

When Concerns Are Raised

In addition to criminal convictions, a patient, a member of the public, another dentist or a DCP may raise a concern to the GDC. If serious concerns are raised about a dental professional's ability, health or behaviour to the GDC, they can look into these if there is a suggestion these could lead to significant harm to patients, the general public or colleagues and/or undermine public confidence in the profession.

The GDC has a responsibility to investigate when concerns are raised regarding possible impaired fitness to practise of a registrant.

Until 2004, disciplinary hearings were conducted by various committees made up of GDC members. The GDC started discussing major reforms in 2000 to update its functions and membership to make the organisation fit and appropriate for the 21st century. One of the reforms was to set up an independent Fitness to Practise Panel made up of people who are not members of the council. A pool from which the membership of the disciplinary committees would be formed thus allowed the council to concentrate on strategy, such as setting standards, and also ensuring that there was no risk of compromising the integrity and impartiality of conduct hearings. This pool consists of dental professionals (dentists and dental care professionals) and lay members.

Panel members are initially appointed for 5 years and have been given appropriate training for their task. As has always been the case, appropriate legal advice is always available for all conduct hearings.

Fitness to Practise Investigations

Outlined below are stages and committees which can be involved if concerns are raised to the GDC. The details have the potential to change over time, and these processes are related to the United Kingdom; however, they are likely to be mirrored by regulators/organisations around the world. For location-specific information and specific detail, the reader should access information directly from the relevant regulator.

Initial Assessment of Concern or Received Information

When concerns are raised to the GDC, they undergo an initial assessment by the Initial Assessment Decision Group (IADG); this consideration uses the Initial Assessment Test (IAT). The group considers whether, in principle, the concern would be a fitness to practise issue if it were proven true and also the risk involved which informs the urgency of any investigation. If a more urgent process is indicated, this is the Interim Orders Committee (IOC).

There are specific circumstances when IADG may refer low-level concerns which do not give rise to a fitness to practise concern, to the NHS. There are categories within which concerns referred to the NHS must fit.

Investigating Committee

The Investigating Committee (IC) considers if allegations should be referred to a Practice Committee for a full inquiry. Meetings of this committee, which is made up of trained members drawn from an independently appointed pool, are held in private. This committee can:

- close the case should no further action be needed
- adjourn the case for further information
- issue a letter of advice
- issue a letter of warning to the registrant, which, if appropriate, may be published on the GDC's website, or
- refer the case to a Practice Committee for a full inquiry and, if necessary, refer the case immediately to the Interim Orders Committee to consider if action is required before a full inquiry by a practice committee.

The remaining committees are drawn from the FtP Panel.

The Interim Orders Committee

At any stage in the investigation, a case may be referred to this committee. This committee has the power when necessary to protect the public, the public interest or the registrant themselves pending the outcome of the case. It does not investigate allegations or conduct a fact-finding exercise. If necessary, this committee can:

- suspend a registrant for up to 18 months, with 6-monthly reviews
- impose conditions on a registrant for up to 18 months, with 6-monthly reviews
- decide that no order is necessary.

The Practice Committees

There are three Practice Committees whose role is to determine whether a registrant's fitness to practise is impaired and, if so, what action has to be taken to protect patients. Also, these committees have the direct power to impose interim suspension, or conditions limiting the field of practice, if it is considered that immediate action to protect the public is needed pending the final outcome of a particular case. If one of these committees considers it appropriate, it can refer a case directly to another practice committee.

These committees are:

THE PROFESSIONAL CONDUCT COMMITTEE. This committee investigates cases involving conduct issues. It has the power to:

- conclude a case without further action if it is considered that fitness to practise is not impaired
- issue a reprimand
- impose conditions on the registrant for up to 3 years, for example, prohibiting a registrant from working in a particular field of practice, to take immediate effect if required
- suspend a registrant for up to 12 months, with or without a review. Again, with immediate effect if required
- erase a registrant from the register, which recently became for a compulsory minimum of 5 years.
- refer the case back to case examiners, the Investigating Committee or to the Interim Orders Committee or one of the other practice committees.

After July 2006, any new case reported to the GDC that is assessed by the Professional Conduct Committee is no longer judged as being guilty or not guilty of *serious professional misconduct* but whether or not their *fitness to practise is impaired*. Also under these rules, the committee can sanction a *suspension with review*, which gives the committee the power to recall the suspended registrant before the end of the period of suspension to check whether or not the suspended person is fit to be returned to the register.

THE PROFESSIONAL PERFORMANCE COMMITTEE (PPC). This committee deals with cases where it appears that a registrant's performance may be deficient, and that deficiency would mean an impairment to fitness to practise.

This committee can impose conditions or suspend registration in the same way as the Professional Conduct Committee.

THE HEALTH COMMITTEE. The Investigating Committee refers cases to this committee where it appears that fitness to practise is due to a health condition. This committee can impose the same sanctions as the other practice committees, including referral back to case examiners, the Investigating Committee or other practice committees. It cannot, however, erase a dentist from the register if it determines that fitness to practise is impaired solely as a result of adverse physical or mental health.

The GDC, on their website, have learning points from the *fitness to practise* process, including the types of issues represented. Examples include the types of clinical treatment concerns, conduct concerns and consent concerns which have led to cases being opened for further investigation.

Advertising

Guidance on advertising has been issued by the GDC, which took effect from 30 September 2013. This incorporates important recommendations in the Code of Ethics for Dentists in the EU. The GDC clearly states that whenever the name of a registrant appears on any form of advertising, it remains the responsibility of that individual dental professional to ensure the accuracy of their personal information appearing.

It states specifically that:

- the registrant must ensure information is current and accurate
- his or her GDC registration number is included

- if mentioned on a website as providing dental care as a dental professional, his or her professional qualification(s) and the country where it was obtained is stated
- clear language that patients will understand is used
- all claims made are backed up with facts
- ambiguous statements are avoided
- no statements of claims are made that could create an unjustified expectation of achievable results
- only dentists on a GDC specialist list can refer to themselves as a 'specialist in ...'
- dentists not on a specialist list should not use specialist titles such as Endodontist, Orthodontist, etc.
- dentists who limit their practice completely or mainly to a particular form of treatment should use terms such as 'practice limited to...'; 'experienced in...' or 'special interest in...'.

All information and publicity regarding dental services should meet the following criteria:

- Be legal, decent, honest and truthful.
- State whether the practice is NHS, mixed or wholly private.
- Information should be balanced, factual and in a language that patients understand to help them make informed choices about their treatment.
- Products should only be recommended if they are the best way to meet patients' needs.

Websites

In addition to the above, websites should include:

- the name and geographic address of the dental practice/service
- full contact details of the practice/service, including telephone number and email address
- the GDC's full contact details or a link to the GDC website
- details of the practice's complaints procedure, and details of who patients may contact if they are not satisfied with the response from the practice
- the date when the website was last updated.

Websites should be regularly updated to accurately reflect the current personnel and the services offered. No comparative information comparing the skills or the qualifications of one dental professional with another should ever be displayed. Listing memberships of professional associations and societies, or honorary degrees, can be misleading and imply additional skills. It would be sensible for registrants to consider this information and how it may mislead patients or be criticised as misleading patients, and ensure current guidance is followed.

OTHER REQUIREMENTS FOR THE PRACTICE OF DENTISTRY

Following qualification, a dental surgeon is immediately eligible for full registration with the GDC. Before commencing the practice of dentistry, however, there are several requirements or recommendations that should be carried out in addition to registering with the GDC.

Professional Indemnity

Dentists have always been advised to have professional indemnity (insurance) cover in the unfortunate occurrence that they are sued for damages or their actions are investigated by a statutory body. However, since November 2015, the GDC has made proof of sufficient indemnity cover a requirement of being on the Register. This was in further clarification of the Amendment Order 2005 (of the Dentists Act 1984), which made adequate and appropriate insurance (professional indemnity) compulsory for retention on the Dentists or the Dental Care Professionals Registers.

Until 2019, there were three organisations in the United Kingdom that provide indemnity for dentists and doctors. These are mutual organisations, which mean that the organisation belongs to the members and all profits made by these organisations have to go to the benefit of the members (unlike a limited company where owners or shareholders reap the benefit of any profits). These organisations are:

- the Dental Defence Union (a subsidiary of the Medical Defence Union)
- Dental Protection (a subsidiary of the Medical Protection Society)
- the Medical and Dental Defence Union of Scotland.

These non-profit making (mutual) organisations provide members with indemnity against any legal action brought by patients; advice and assistance on medicolegal matters; legal representation at courts, tribunals or professional committee hearings on disciplinary matters and general advice on professional conduct.

Hospital trusts and health authorities as employers of salaried practitioners have corporate indemnity should a patient sue the organisation or individual employees. However, this cover does not include representation of a practitioner at tribunals or disciplinary hearings of any sort. Therefore, it is advisable to belong to one of the professional protection organisations; these organisations offer lower rates of subscription for those practitioners who have indemnity from their employers.

In 2019, the British Dental Association set up its own indemnity scheme restricted to British Dental Association (BDA) members who practice in the United Kingdom (excluding those practising in the Isle of Man or the Channel Islands). This is a hybrid scheme, where advice, assistance and case management is provided by an expert team of senior BDA members, whilst legal representation and financial indemnity is provided by a major UK insurance company.

The indemnity cover with all the above organisations is 'occurrence based,' which means that the policy has to be active when an unfortunate incident or treatment occurred. This is important as patients have the automatic right to claim in court for up to 3 years after they were aware of any damage or negligence from treatment. Also, in extenuating circumstances, the courts may extend this 3-year limit.

Professional indemnity is also available on the commercial market, but this normally has a maximum limit of indemnity and only provides cover within the time of the insurance contract (i.e. a 'claims made' contract, so that it may be necessary to continue to have the insurance for several years after retirement!). Therefore it is important to carefully check the contract of your insurance to ensure continuing cover. This is an important factor, which is recognised and covered by the professional protection organisations, as there may be a delay of several years

between an incident occurring and a patient bringing an action for damages, and is referred to as 'Incurred But Not Reported' (IBNR). Also, it is unlikely that advice on medicolegal matters, legal representation at tribunals or professional committee hearings on disciplinary matters, or general advice on professional conduct would be available with commercial insurance cover.

Whoever you choose to obtain professional indemnity from, the premium that will be charged will depend on the scope of your practice.

The First Steps

For many years, there was nothing to prevent a dental surgeon on qualification and initial registration from setting up in single-handed private practice, but the benefit of a period of a supervised practice cannot be overemphasised. The majority of UK dental graduates undertake a year of Dental Foundation Training (DFT) in general practice on qualifying. Foundation training, previously known as Vocational Training (VT), is under the supervision of Regional Postgraduate Dental Deans and provides a very good introduction to the practice and business of dentistry. Successful completion of Dental Foundation Training allows entry to the NHS Performers List in England and Wales and Health Boards in Scotland and Northern Ireland.

Recruitment to Dental Foundation Training in England, Wales and Northern Ireland is by a national recruitment process, and recruitment to Scottish schemes is currently managed separately. National recruitment involves competitive assessment, and at the time of writing included online Situational Judgement Testing (SJT) and face-to-face assessment stations. *The Dental Foundation Training Curriculum*, which includes a competency framework and detail of assessment, can be found on the COPDEND website (www.copdend.org).

Continuing Education

There are several important aspects to postgraduate training and education.

Further information and detail of postgraduate and specialty training can be found on the specialty training section of the NHS Health Education England website (www.hee.nhs.uk), on the postgraduate training section of the COPDEND website (www.copdend.org) and the dental faculty sections of the Royal Surgical Colleges.

Dental Core Training (DCT)

This is a recognised, standalone period of training with a number of exit points. It occurs after DFT and prior to entry to specialty training. There are DCT 1, 2 and 3 posts, each with competitive entry. Trainees will have clinical and educational supervisors, the level of skills and attributes develops through the training years. Further information about DCT recruitment and the curriculum can be found on the COPDEND website.

Specialist Training

There is a national recruitment and benchmarking process for places on specialty training programmes. The benchmarking process ensures that individuals who gain entry to specialty training have demonstrated an appropriate level of knowledge, clinical skills and experience. On successful completion of the appropriate period of higher professional training and obtaining any required postgraduate qualifications, a certificate of completion of specialist training (CCST) will be issued, and that dentist will then be eligible to apply to join a specialist list held by the GDC.

General Dental Practice

There is no formalised postgraduate equivalent training in general dental practice, but general practitioners can undertake further study to sit for various diplomas awarded by the Royal Surgical Colleges.

The Royal Surgical Colleges are associated with numerous opportunities for postgraduate development. An example of recognition of additional training is through the award of Fellowships and Memberships of the various Colleges. In addition to examinations and assessments, the Colleges offer learning through events and courses and support in personal development.

Continuing Professional Education

It is essential that dental surgeons, or members of any other profession, continue to update their knowledge and expertise throughout the whole of their professional practising life. Learning more about dentistry should continue until at least retirement to provide the best for one's patients.

As detailed previously, continuing professional education/development is now a prerequisite to remaining registered with the GDC.

Professional Organisations and Societies

It is not compulsory to join any organisation or society connected with dentistry, but all dentists practising in the United Kingdom are recommended to join the BDA. The BDA is the official negotiating body with the government on matters concerning general dental practice and the community dental service. It also contracts with the British Medical Association to negotiate on behalf of the hospital dental service and clinical academic staff.

Advice on all aspects of dental practice is available to members from the BDA, and it has a large library available to members. The BDA publishes many advice booklets, which are regularly updated, as well as giving individual advice on request. The *British Dental Journal* is published on behalf of the BDA and contains scientific papers and useful review articles. Also in the BDJ Portfolio of publications is the *BDJ In Practice*, published monthly, which updates members on developments and issues affecting dental practices including legal and ethical matters pertaining to all aspects of dentistry. As it is a registered trade union, the BDA can assist members who have problems relating to their employment.

There are also many specialist dental societies, and it is worthwhile joining those related to any special interest. Dental surgeons undergoing higher professional training are strongly recommended to join the appropriate specialist society or societies pertaining to their specialty.

Ability and Experience

Ability and experience are essential matters of self-regulation throughout one's professional life, not just at the beginning. Prior to undertaking any particular item of treatment for a patient, a dental surgeon must be certain that (s)he has both the ability and the experience to complete the treatment successfully in the patient's best interest, as well as having the necessary equipment and materials available to complete the task.

Referrals

If a dental surgeon does not feel competent to complete a particular treatment for their patient, or if the patient requests a second opinion, then that patient should be referred to a colleague or specialist. Referrals can be made by multiple routes of communication including paper-based or electronic means, but in cases of acute emergency or life-threatening conditions, telephone referral can be acceptable.

All correspondence of referral should contain:

- the patient's full contact details and appropriate demographic information
- the reason for the referral
- whether the patient is referred for:
  - an opinion only
  - a special investigation only, e.g. advanced imaging
  - treatment of a specific condition
  - complete and continuing treatment.
- the patient's medical history
- details of any relevant treatment already carried out
- whether the patient has requested NHS or private treatment.

There are specific criteria for referrals for general anaesthesia and sedation, which are described later in this chapter.

It would be considered best practice for the person receiving the referral to focus treatment and advice to that requested by the referrer. It could be considered negligent to not offer comment on observations made during a consultation. It would be expected that the person receiving the referral should inform the referring practitioner of their decision, observations made and any proposed treatment, by written correspondence. In the case of a referral for an investigation, rather than treatment, a comprehensive report of that investigation would be expected to be sent to the referring dentist.

On completion, a letter of information should be sent to the referrer, with a copy to any other party relevant to the patient's care (e.g. the patient's general medical practitioner), and offered to the patient.

12.5 Records and Documentation

LEARNING OBJECTIVES

You should:
- realise the importance of neat contemporaneous records detailing all aspects of patient care
- have a clear understanding of informed consent prior to undertaking any treatment
- be aware of the importance of a chaperone.

RECORDS

The patient's records do not just consist of clinical notes but also include radiographs, referral letters and replies, study models, occlusal recordings, photographs, dental laboratory cards and investigation results. Consent forms, copies of treatment plans and cost estimates should also be retained with patients' records. If patients are receiving treatment under NHS regulations, NHS documentation should also be retained. Appointment books and day sheets may be useful should any query arise concerning the timing and extent of a particular patient's treatment; consequently, their retention can be extremely helpful. Telephone messages and any other memoranda concerning patients should be stored with their records. Finally, all records should be stored in a safe and secure place where they are easily retrievable when next required. Paper records must be kept in a locked container (e.g. a filing cabinet); electronic records must be protected using appropriate electronic security measures. Access to data must be restricted to personnel who have a legitimate reason for that access.

When records are eventually disposed of, they must be destroyed under confidential conditions.

Data Protection

Failure to comply with data protection has been a criminal offence since the Data Protection Act (1998). The holding and processing of personal data was made more stringent by the General Data Protection Regulation (GDPR) that was approved by the Parliament in 2017 and came into effect in May 2018. Personal data is any information relating to an identified or identifiable person and includes:

- names
- addresses and telephone numbers
- dates of birth
- name of general medical practitioner
- hospital record numbers.

There are also special (sensitive) categories of personal data, such as:

- health details
- ethnicity
- sexual orientation
- religion
- political views.

With the exception of non-profit making organisations, all organisations have to register with the Information Commissioners Office (ICO). All (including non-profit making organisations) have to appoint a Data Controller who will probably be the head of the organisation and a Data Protection Officer (DPO) who is responsible for the control of all data processing activity; one person can undertake both of these roles in small organisations. The DPO has to decide who in the organisation can process or have access to personal data (a data processor). All data processors have to formally agree to abide by their legal obligations under GDPR in their contracts of employment, or their independent involvement in the organisation if they are self-employed. To ensure compliance with these regulations, it is advisable that all staff are made aware of their obligations under these regulations. The ICO must be given the contact details of the DPO.

All patients have to formally consent to the retention of their personal data by the organisation, be informed of the limitations governing the use of that data and given a Privacy Notice informing them what the data will be used for.

The Privacy Notice should also be available on the premises and the organisation's website; it should include:

- the Data Controller's identity
- the Data Protection Officer's contact details
- the purpose of the data processing
- the legal basis for data processing
- categories of personal data processed
- potential recipients of personal data
- details of retention periods of data
- a list of data subjects rights, including the right to complain to the ICO if they have any concerns about the handling of their data.

Retention of Records

Records should be retained in accordance with the current legislative requirements.

The UK Department of Health, via *NHS Digital*, publishes a Records Management Code of Practice for Health and Social Care. This was last updated in 2016. This document contains detailed retention schedules. Timescales for retention of records are dependent on a number of criteria – full details of this Code of Practice and detailed retention schedules are available on the *NHS Digital* website (https://digital.nhs.uk).

It cannot be overstated that records should be:

- accurate
- complete
- comprehensive
- contemporaneous
- legible
- retrievable
- retained in accordance with the current legislative requirements.

Medical History

It should never be forgotten that medical history is an essential part of dental or medical records. Medical history should always be taken at the initial visit of a patient and rechecked and updated at every subsequent appointment.

Confidentiality and Disclosure

All health care records are confidential between the patient and those involved in their care and should not be disclosed to a third party without the patient's permission. There are occasionally circumstances when a Court Order may be produced which would compel disclosure. As the rules governing disclosure vary according to the circumstances, the advice of the dentist's defence/protection organisation should be sought on this matter. It is essential that all staff employed by a dentist are aware of patient confidentiality and do not break any confidences. Any breach of confidentiality by a member of staff is the responsibility of the dentist both legally as an employer and ethically as a member of a caring profession.

CONSENT AND RELATED MATTERS

No treatment can be carried out on a patient without that patient's or their legal guardian's valid informed consent for that specific treatment to be undertaken. Undertaking treatment without consent is an assault on the patient. Consent can be implied, verbal or written.

Implied Consent

Examples of implied consent:

- If a patient has previously been presented with a treatment plan and arranges further appointments for this treatment plan to be carried out, implied consent can be assumed.
- If a patient requests local anaesthetic for fillings and opens his/her mouth to allow local anaesthetic to be administered.

Verbal Consent

For example, a dentist may say:

- 'Would you like a local anaesthetic for me to put the filling in your tooth?'
- 'I am going to give you local anaesthetic for this filling/extraction'.
- 'I think that the most urgent treatment you need is a filling in this tooth'.

The patient either verbally agreeing to the above or opening his/her mouth to allow the dentist to proceed would be valid consent, providing the dentist is confident that the patient understands what is going to happen. If there is any doubt regarding the patient's capacity to understand the treatment fully, no treatment should be undertaken.

Implied or verbal consent is frequently sufficient for treatment without any form of anaesthetic or when treatment is undertaken with local analgesia, as the patient can request that the treatment is stopped at any time, and they may wish to withdraw consent.

Written Consent

Written consent must be obtained if the patient is having treatment under sedation or general anaesthesia when they are not fully conscious of the treatment being carried out and are, therefore, in no position to ask for the treatment to be stopped should they wish to withdraw consent. Written consent is also advisable for any complicated and/or expensive treatment even when this is carried out without any form of anaesthetic or with local analgesia.

Written consent is advisable when carrying out a procedure that carries one or more specific risks. For example, prior to the removal of an impacted lower wisdom tooth, a patient should be warned of the possibility of swelling, trismus and the risk of trauma to the inferior dental nerve, which would lead to labial anaesthesia/paraesthesia, or trauma to the lingual nerve, which would cause similar problems with the tongue. The use of the mnemonic STALL (swelling, trismus, anaesthesia of lingual or labial nerves) may ensure that appropriate warnings are given. These warnings should be entered in the patient's record. It is essential that written consent should contain details of the procedure, the type of anaesthetic or analgesic that will be used and any complications that may occur during treatment. Without being patronising, consent should be worded in a language that the particular patient understands, avoiding the use of jargon and abbreviations to describe a particular clinical procedure.

As part of the consent procedure, the clinician should advise the patient of all treatment options, as well as any risks of not having the suggested treatment. Also, if appropriate, the patient should be informed of the current national guidelines relating to the treatment of the condition. When discussing risks, it is essential to have knowledge of the patient's circumstances; for instance, the likelihood of nerve damage resulting from the removal of impacted wisdom teeth will need to be quantified as it could affect the livelihood of, for instance, a lecturer, singer or musician.

For treatment carried out under sedation of general anaesthesia, it is advisable to undertake the consent process at an initial consultation, and to confirm the consent when the patient attends for the actual treatment. Particularly under these circumstances, except in an emergency, consenting just as treatment is about to commence is not advisable.

Additionally, after the patient has been made aware of all choices including alternatives and any risks, this does not diminish the duty of care that the operator has to act carefully and skilfully when carrying out a procedure, as obtaining consent is no defence for inadequate treatment or a poor technique.

Because of the nature of dentistry in the United Kingdom at the present time, it is essential that the patient is aware of whether they are consenting to treatment under the NHS or by private contract before treatment commences.

Special Cases

Age of the Patient

The minimum age for valid consent is considered to be 16 years; however, if a practitioner is satisfied that someone of less than 16 years of age fully understands the treatment to which they are consenting, their consent may be valid. Particularly in the case of sedation or general anaesthesia, the consent of a parent or guardian or someone over 18 years should be obtained as well as from the patient themselves for those between 16 and 18 years of age.

Adults Lacking Capacity

These patients may be unable to give informed consent, it is recommended you review local legislation that will govern these circumstances. In the UK, this is covered by the Mental Capacity Act.

According to the Mental Capacity Act of 2005, a person is unable to make their own decision if they cannot do one or more of the following four things:

- understand information given to them
- retain that information long enough to be able to make the decision
- weigh up the information available to make the decision
- communicate their decision – this could be by talking, using sign language or even simple muscle movements such as blinking an eye or squeezing a hand.

For any major treatment, it is normal practice for the agreement of two practitioners of consultant status to be obtained prior to treatment. Alternatively, as a result of the 2019 Amendment to the Mental Capacity Act, a trained Independent Mental Capacity Advocate (IMCA) can be appointed to look after the patient's best interests.

Patients With Specific Ethnic Customs or Beliefs

Practitioners should always be sympathetic to specific patient beliefs and requests (e.g. the avoidance of blood transfusions to Jehovah's Witnesses, the avoidance of materials derived from any animals for vegetarians and from certain animals for religious or cultural reasons). It should also be remembered that certain cultures object to women receiving treatment from male practitioners.

Life-Saving Procedures

Occasionally, it may be necessary to carry out a life-saving procedure on an unconscious person. Under these circumstances, informed consent is normally unobtainable, but any treatment under these circumstances should be limited to that which is life-saving. Non-life-saving treatment should be delayed until consent is obtained.

CHAPERONES

It is always advisable to have a chaperone present for all patient contact even if active treatment is not involved. The presence of a third person can be useful in confirming consent and may be required to avoid any allegation of impropriety. When carrying out treatment, the dentist should normally be assisted by a dental nurse, who can also act as a chaperone. It should be remembered that whether attending a patient in the dental surgery or on a domiciliary visit, another member of the dental team or another person should be present at all times. It would be considered good practice to take into account who would be appropriate as a chaperone in individual situations; this may, for example, include gender or cultural considerations.

12.6 General Anaesthesia and Sedation

LEARNING OBJECTIVES

You should:
- know who can administer general anaesthesia and sedation to your patients
- understand the role of the dental operator under these circumstances.

When patients are receiving treatment under general anaesthesia or sedation, it is essential that written informed consent is obtained prior to the procedure being undertaken. Whenever possible, this consent should be obtained at a consultation and treatment planning appointment, as signing the consent form when the patient arrives for this treatment and immediately before the anaesthetic and sedation is administered could be considered as signing under duress.

Any patient who is to receive treatment under general anaesthesia or sedation must be accompanied by a friend or relative who can take responsibility for the patient's care following treatment. The presence of this accompanying person, and confirmation of their availability for the time required for the patient to recover sufficiently to not need support, must be established prior to administering any general anaesthesia or sedation.

Prior to November 1998, dental surgeons who had received the appropriate training were allowed to administer general anaesthesia to patients. The ethical guidance on general anaesthesia from the GDC clarified the roles and responsibilities of those involved in carrying out dental treatment under general anaesthesia, and it specifically precludes dentists from administering general anaesthesia.

GENERAL ANAESTHESIA

The Referring Dentist

Any dental surgeon who refers a patient for treatment under general anaesthesia must:
- take a full medical history
- explain to the patient the risks involved
- offer alternative methods of pain control
- obtain consent.

When sending a patient for treatment under general anaesthesia, the dentist's referral letter should contain full justification for the use of general anaesthesia and proper records must be kept by the referring dentist.

The Dentist Treating a Patient Under General Anaesthesia

The dentist treating a patient under general anaesthesia must:
- repeat the history taking
- repeat the explanations concerning risk and the alternative methods of treatment and pain control
- obtain the patient's or the parent's written consent
- give written pre- and postoperative instructions
- keep careful records.

Treatment Under General Anaesthesia

For treatment of a patient under general anaesthesia, it is essential that:
- the dentist/surgeon has an appropriately trained dental/general nurse available for assistance
- the anaesthetic is administered by an anaesthetist on the GMC's Specialist Register; if a trainee anaesthetist/non-consultant career-grade anaesthetist gives the anaesthetic, that doctor must be working under a named consultant anaesthetist
- the anaesthetist is supported by someone experienced in monitoring the patient's condition and able to assist the anaesthetist in an emergency
- the anaesthetist and the dental surgeon have an agreed written protocol for the provision of advanced life support, including agreed arrangements for the immediate transfer of a patient to a critical care facility
- recovery and discharge is the responsibility of the anaesthetist, and recovery nurses must be properly trained and responsible to the anaesthetist
- all personnel involved in anaesthetics train together.

The GDC makes it clear that it is the responsibility of the treating dentist to ensure that these protocols for general anaesthesia are adhered to.

SEDATION

Conscious sedation is defined as a technique in which the use of a drug or drugs depresses the central nervous system, thus enabling treatment to be carried out, but during which communication with the patient can be maintained. The modification of the patient's state of mind should be such that the patient will respond to command throughout the period of sedation. Techniques used should carry a margin of safety wide enough to render unintended loss of consciousness unlikely.

A suitably experienced and trained dental surgeon can administer sedative drugs as well as operating on the patient, providing at least one other appropriately trained person is present throughout the procedure. This other person must be capable of monitoring the clinical condition of the patient and of assisting the dental surgeon in the event of an emergency. An appropriately trained dental or general nurse can fulfil this duty; ideally, this person should be present in addition to the dental nurse providing close support for the dental treatment.

The GDC recommends that normally a single drug should be used for intravenous sedation; if more than one sedative drug is utilised, the provision of advanced life support must be immediately available. Whatever sedation techniques are used, contemporary appropriate standards of patient monitoring should be adopted during conscious sedation. As intravenous sedation is unpredictable in children, it is recommended that this technique is used only under very special circumstances.

Before undertaking treatment under sedation, a dental surgeon must:

- carefully assess the patient, including a full medical and dental history
- explain the sedation technique proposed
- advise on appropriate alternative methods of pain and anxiety control
- provide clear and comprehensive pre- and postoperative instructions in writing
- obtain written informed consent for the sedation and treatment proposed
- ensure that proper equipment for the administration of the sedation technique is available
- ensure that the facilities are adequate
- adopt contemporary standards of monitoring the patient
- ensure that appropriate drugs for resuscitation of the patient are readily available
- ensure that the dentist and staff are trained in the sedation procedure being used and resuscitation techniques. It is essential that all those involved in the provision of sedation and/or the supervision of recovery of sedated patients should train together as a team to deal with any emergencies, and that this training should include frequent practice of resuscitation routines in a simulated emergency
- ensure that patients recovering from sedation will be appropriately supervised, protected and monitored in adequate recovery facilities.

Monitoring of patients should be undertaken either by the sedationist or by an appropriately trained person responsible to the sedationist. When the sedationist considers the patient is sufficiently recovered to leave the premises, they must be accompanied by a responsible adult. Where nitrous oxide/oxygen sedation alone has been used for an adult patient, a dental surgeon may exercise discretion as to whether that patient is fit enough to be discharged unaccompanied.

CHAPERONES

During treatment under general anaesthesia or sedation and in the recovery room following general anaesthesia or sedation, the presence of a third person is mandatory. It is advisable that either the dentist or another person present is of the same sex as the patient, or is a relative of the patient.

12.7 Complaints Procedure and Negligence

LEARNING OBJECTIVES

You should:
- understand how the health complaints procedure works in the United Kingdom so that you are able to deal with any complaints expeditiously
- understand the meaning of negligence
- be aware of how best to avoid an accusation of negligence.

All health care organisations must have a complaints procedure; this applies to all branches of dentistry, including general dental practice. There has to be designated person/persons in each health care organisation to accept complaints, acknowledge the receipt of all complaints and keep the complainant informed of how the complaint is progressing. Complaints should be answered within a reasonable time of the complaint being made. Mediation between the parties, rather than confrontation, is encouraged to allow the resolution of any grievance the patient may have. As part of the GDC's information, standards and guidance, there are principles published for complaints handling best practice and a publication entitled *Handling Feedback and Complaints in the Dental Practice*. This is available to download from the GDC website along with other useful resources.

Adaptation and flexibility are important when handling complaints, and whilst there is no one correct way to approach their management, there are a number of key areas to consider. These include ensuring complaints are recognised, a thorough investigation ensuring all of the facts are gathered, establishing what is needed to resolve dissatisfaction and an appropriate response. It is also important to consider what learning that can be taken forward following complaints for future personal/practice development and risk management. This may include review of aspects which led to the complaint and processes and protocols which are currently in place.

Further advice, face-to-face training and web-based resources are available from a variety of organisations to gain further understanding of key areas of how you should approach the management of a complaint. These include dental indemnity providers.

'MIXING'

Mixing is the term used for providing some treatment under the NHS for a patient and other treatment for the same patient privately. It is a situation fraught with difficulties and is best avoided if at all possible. It is advisable that any course of treatment be undertaken entirely under NHS regulations or entirely under a private contract. If this is not possible, it is important that:

- it is not implied to the patient that NHS treatment is inferior to private treatment
- the patient fully understands which items are being carried out under NHS regulations and which privately and consents to this, preferably in writing
- the NHS-funded treatment is completed prior to undertaking items of treatment that will be charged privately.

When dealing with complaints, as previously mentioned, every provider of health care is obliged to set up a system for dealing with complaints from patients. Since 2009, a complainant can complain directly to the primary care organisation responsible for the service or directly to the service provider. In secondary care, the complaint should be made to the hospital or other institution providing the care. Each part of the United Kingdom (England, Scotland, Wales, Northern Ireland) has slightly different protocols for this, which can be found on the appropriate websites. For England, it is *the Local Authority Social Services and National Health Service Complaints [England] Regulations 2009.*

Every effort should be made to deal with complaints as quickly as possible, as the longer a feeling of dissatisfaction or aggravation continues, the more entrenched the parties become, which makes the problem more difficult to solve.

In addition to a complaints procedure, organisations may wish to have processes in place to actively seek and encourage comments and suggestions from patients.

It is hoped that the vast majority of complaints will be dealt with locally. If a patient makes a complaint in person, the designated person should endeavour to discuss the nature of the problem at the time the complaint is made. Any discussion should take place in a private office to protect patient confidentiality and give an atmosphere conducive to resolution of the complaint. The term 'Complaints Manager' is probably best avoided, but the person designated to deal with complaints (the *responsible person*) should inform the complainant of their name and status in the practice or organisation.

Organisations have a responsibility to develop an effective complaints procedure. These will vary dependent on local circumstances and must be compliant with their legal and contractual obligations. The contracting agreement will contain specific details of what the complaints process should contain and the timelines within which this should be actioned. Practitioners should ensure their patients are aware of the local complaints policy. Some complaints processes include scope for a local resolution meeting.

Parliamentary and Health Service Ombudsman

This body makes final decisions on complaints which have not been resolved by the NHS in England and UK government departments and other UK public organisations. Any patient still dissatisfied after the NHS complaints procedure has been completed may ask the Parliamentary and Health Service Ombudsman to investigate the case. This ombudsman is completely independent of both the NHS and the government and can investigate complaints about NHS services and how the complaints procedure is working. The Ombudsman is not obliged to investigate every complaint and will not generally consider any case that has not first been through the NHS complaints procedure, nor any case that is being dealt with by the courts.

GDC Complaints Service

The 2005 Amendment Order to the Dentists Act of 1984 allowed the GDC to set up a complaints scheme for private patients. This is known as the *Dental Complaints Service* and was launched in 2006. This service is funded by the GDC. They will look into complaints raised with them within 12 months of the treatment happening or within 12 months of the patient becoming aware they have something to complain about. Again, patients are recommended to attempt local resolution in the first instance. If local resolution is not successful, a complaints officer discusses the matter further with the patient and the practice to attempt resolution. This service has also set up complaints panels consisting of two lay people and one dental professional who have been given appropriate training. If the patient remains dissatisfied and the complaints officer is unable to resolve the complaint, the service will convene a complaints panel if it believes this is appropriate. The panel will listen to both parties, independently and impartially in a non-legalistic way. After the panel has considered the complaint, it is able to endorse any appropriate agreement reached between the dental professional and the patient, or if an agreement cannot be reached, recommend one or more of the following:

- That no further action should be taken.
- That the dental professional reviews their future practice.
- An apology to the patient.
- An offer of a refund of part or all of the fees.
- A contribution towards remedial treatment up to the amount of fees paid.

Further information is available on the dental complaints service website (https://dcs.gdc-uk.org).

NEGLIGENCE

In the treatment of patients, the following may be considered negligent:

- Failure to exercise reasonable skill and care.
- Omitting to do something that a reasonable person would do, considering what normally regulates the conduct of human affairs.
- Doing something that a prudent reasonable person would not do.

Every dentist is expected to exercise reasonable skill and care in every treatment she/he carries out by virtue of their dental qualification (i.e. a similar degree of skill and care as exercised by the majority of colleagues). A general practitioner would be compared with other general practitioners, and a specialist with other specialists in the same field. Also, no dentist should undertake treatment for which he/she is not trained and competent to undertake; consequently, failure to refer to a specialist when appropriate could be considered negligent.

A practitioner is expected to exercise reasonable skill and care whether a patient is being treated privately, under the NHS, as an act of friendship or even as a 'good Samaritan act' in an emergency.

To recover compensation for negligence, it is necessary to prove:

- that the practitioner owed a duty of care to the patient at the time
- that there was a breach of that duty
- that damage or suffering occurred as a result of the action of the practitioner.

This means that if the patient suffered no harm or damage as a result of the practitioner's action, there is nothing for the patient to be compensated for, so no compensation will be paid.

A dentist cannot guarantee that all treatments provided will be uneventful or free from accident even if there is no lack of care and skill. To prove negligence, the patient (plaintiff) has to prove that harm has been caused as a result of lack of care and/or lack of reasonable skill that the practitioner (defendant) had a duty to apply. Unless the plaintiff can satisfy the court of this, the claim will fail.

If a very obvious mistake or damage has occurred to a patient, the patient's legal adviser will make a plea of *res ipsa loquitur*. This legal term basically means 'the thing speaks for itself'. Carrying out treatment on the wrong tooth or treating the wrong patient could be considered as examples.

Contributory Negligence

If something occurs or is made worse by an action or failure by the patient, the defendant can plea contributory negligence, which may reduce or negate any damages that are awarded. An example of this would be failure on the part of the patient to follow pre- or postoperative instructions or grabbing the dentist's arm when he was using a sharp instrument or a dental handpiece.

Unsuitable Treatment

Dentists should always resist being talked into undertaking treatment by a patient that is unsuitable or of very poor prognosis (e.g. advanced restorative treatment on teeth with gross periodontal disease). Carrying out treatment that is very likely to fail or cause severe problems is as much negligent as any other professional act a dentist performs.

Vicarious Liability

As an employer, a dentist can be held responsible for any acts or omissions of his/her staff. This applies to all grades of staff, whether or not that member of staff was or was not acting in accordance to instructions. At the same time, however, the employee is responsible for his/her own acts. Therefore, a claim for negligence could be brought against the employer, employee or (as is more commonly the case) against both. In the case of partnership agreements, each partner is individually and jointly liable for the actions of other partners. Therefore, it is essential that all partnership agreements include the provision to provide indemnity for the partnership as a whole.

The Bolam Principle Test

The Bolam principle has been used as the benchmark in the assessment of professional negligence. In 1957, Judge McNair in the High Court directed the jury in the case of *Bolam* v. *Friern Hospital Management Committee* that 'a doctor is not guilty of negligence if he has acted in accordance with the practice accepted as proper by a reasonable body of medical men skilled in that particular art'. This means that, if there is more than one respectable body of professional opinion concerning diagnosis or treatment, there is no negligence should a practitioner choose one protocol in preference to another.

The Bolam principle was re-examined in 1997 in an appeal to the House of Lords (*Bolitho* v. *City and Hackney Health Authority*). This particular case involved an omission to carry out a procedure on a patient that several experts supported but others did not. Their Lordships opined that the use of the adjectives 'responsible, reasonable or respectable' concerning a body of opinion may not be sufficient, but that experts' views should include scientific evidence on the comparative risks and benefits to decide whether or not an act or omission is defensible. With the advent of clinical governance and evidence-based medicine leading to clinical guidelines, the Bolitho judgement replaced the Bolam principle as the benchmark for negligence.

Where there is more than one accepted medical/dental opinion in a particular case, it is the clinician's decision which is most appropriate. It is not a decision for the court to make, as there is seldom any one answer exclusive of all others to the problems of professional judgement. Even if a court prefers one body of opinion to another, that is no basis for a conclusion of negligence (*Maynard* v. *West Midland Regional Health Authority*, 1984).

Further guidance arose following the case of *Montgomery* v. *Lanarkshire Health Board* (2015) in which the UK Supreme Court opined that as it was not recorded that the patient had not been informed of a risk that a reasonable patient may wish to take into account before deciding whether or not to proceed with a particular treatment option, the clinician was negligent. This reinforced the decision made by the High Court in 1985 (*Sidaway* v. *Board of Governors of Bethlem Royal Hospital*) concerning risks of treatment. The conclusions from these cases confirm that the patient must be informed of any material risks as well as the benefits of treatment, as it is the patient who will have to live with any complications that occur. The process of obtaining consent must be patient centred, rather than the former paternalistic approach of the clinician as the one who 'Knows Best'.

Time Limits

Claims for negligence normally have to be made within one of the following time limits:

- Within 3 years of the plaintiff becoming aware of having suffered damage.
- Within 6 years of the incident occurring.
- Within 6 years of reaching the age of majority (18 years) in the case of alleged negligence occurring in a minor.

At the Court's discretion, claims can be brought outside these limits if the plaintiff can persuade the Court that there is a good reason for ignoring them.

In 1999, two important legal changes have occurred affecting all claims for compensation, not just medical and dental claims: legal aid/contingency fees and the Woolf report.

Legal Aid/Contingency Fees

The government has introduced further limits to the payment of legal aid so that fewer plaintiffs will be eligible to receive legal aid. By way of compensation for this restriction of legal aid, solicitors are now able to work on a contingency fee basis. Contingency fees, which have been accepted in the United States for many years, involve the lawyer only receiving a fee if the client's claim is successful. It has the advantage that if the plaintiff/client does not have sufficient capital available to pay legal fees, these will not be charged should the case be unsuccessful. This gives an additional impetus to the lawyer to make certain of success. Disadvantages may include lawyers charging higher fees, which may be fixed or a percentage of the total compensation obtained, and a reluctance of lawyers to take on any cases except those with an almost certain chance of success. Even with this system, there may be some cost to the claimant, as solicitors may be unwilling to fund such fixed costs as specialist medical reports necessary to support a claim – unless, that is, they can find dental/medical experts who are also willing to work on a contingency fee basis.

The Woolf Report

In July 1996, Lord Woolf published his report to the Lord Chancellor on proposed reforms of the Civil Justice System for England and Wales. These recommendations came into effect on 26 April 1999 and affect the legal profession more than the dental and medical professions in that a very strict timetable is laid down for each stage of the procedure. These rules are detailed in the Civil Procedure Rules published in January 1999. The over-riding objective of these rules is to enable the courts to deal with cases justly. This includes the following:

- Ensuring that the parties are on an equal footing.
- Saving expense.
- Dealing with the case in ways that are proportionate to:
  - the amount of money involved
  - the importance of the case
  - the complexity of the issues
  - the financial position of each party.
- Ensuring that the case is dealt with expeditiously and fairly.

- Allotting to a case an appropriate share of the court's resources, while taking into account the need to allot resources to other cases.
- Requiring the parties involved to help the court in the furtherance of the above objectives.
- Restricting expert evidence to that which is reasonably required to resolve the proceedings; this means that, whenever possible, a single joint expert is appointed to act on behalf of the court, rather than the plaintiff/claimant or the defendant. This can occur either by agreement with the parties involved or, if necessary, an expert can be appointed by the court.
- The plaintiff/patient will in future be called the claimant. Claims will be divided into three types:
  - *Small claims track*: this is for claims of compensation of up to or equal to £5,000 in most cases but is limited up to £1,000 in personal injury.
  - *Fast track*: this is for claims of up to £15,000; complicated claims of under or equal to £15,000 may not be considered suitable for the fast-track system; dental/medical negligence claims may often come into this category and have to be dealt with under the multi-track system.
  - *Multitrack*: this is for cases which are complicated or where claims are in excess of £15,000.

On occasions, potential claims may start as a complaint. In this case, dealing with the complaint fairly and expeditiously with a clear explanation, as recommended earlier, may mean that a claim does not arise. However, should the patient be dissatisfied, she/he may consult a solicitor for advice regarding whether or not a claim for damages should be made. The solicitor may request a copy of the patient's health records from the health care provider (HCP), and these should be disclosed within 40 days. If this time limit is not kept, the patient's solicitor can apply to the court for an order for pre-action disclosure, and the HCP will be responsible for any costs involved in this. Should the patient or their legal adviser decide there are grounds for a claim, a detailed letter of claim should be sent to the HCP. This letter should contain:

- a clear summary of the facts of the case
- the main allegations of negligence
- the injuries incurred, present condition and future prognosis
- any financial losses and damage
- reference to any relevant documents.

The HCP then has 3 months to respond to this letter of claim before court proceedings are issued. During this period, either side may negotiate or offer to settle the claim. Either side may support its position with an appropriate dental/medical report. Should this not lead to the resolution of the matter, there are strict protocols and timetables that have to be observed, or the defaulting party may be liable to any additional costs of the other side.

Fast-Track Timetable

It is intended that any fast-track cases will come to trial within 30 weeks of the court issuing a Notice of Allocation following the submission of a claim. In fast-track cases, the trial is expected to last a maximum of 1 day. The timetable following the date of the Notice of Allocation is:

- 4 weeks for the disclosure of documents by both parties
- 10 weeks for the exchange of witness statements between the parties
- 14 weeks for the exchange of expert reports between the parties
- 20 weeks for sending a list of questions to the court and the other party for clarification
- 22 weeks for response to questions from the other side or the court (note: each side is limited to one request for clarification and cannot delay matters by asking further questions at a later date)
- 30 weeks for the court hearing, unless the case has been previously resolved.

Under the Civil Procedure Rules (2009), there is an appendix setting out the fast-track standard directions, which it is expected that the parties will use to ensure that the timetable is adhered to.

Multitrack Timetable

It is expected that the majority of clinical negligence claims will be dealt with by the multitrack system even if they are below or equal to £15,000 in value. This is because they are regarded as too complex for the fast track. The multitrack timetable is not as tight as the fast track, but the court will have far greater control of cases than previously. Once a case has been allocated, a case management conference will be called. At the case management conference:

- both parties and/or their legal representatives will be expected to be present
- a substantial amount of information will be expected from all parties, including details of witnesses to be called and experts whose evidence will be heard; this means that parties must have their case in order at a very early stage, and this may facilitate settlement in some cases
- the timetable for the case will be set, which will be closely controlled by the court, who will not allow delay
- trial dates will be fixed at, or soon after, the case management conference, and these dates will be immovable.

To ensure that the case is dealt with expeditiously, the courts have power to impose sanctions should, for example, either party fail to comply with the pre-action protocol. These sanctions include costs, penalties and the disallowing of evidence.

To further speed resolution of a case, the court may suggest mediation, and it is expected that courts will build up a list of mediators suitable for different categories of claims. In addition, the trial judge will hold a pretrial review of the case. Normally, additional evidence or reports cannot be submitted following the case management conference without the permission of the court and the other parties.

These changes basically mean that the court will control the timetable and scrutinise the progress of the case. The court will now act without prompting by one of the parties, which means that the lawyers will no longer be able to determine the timetable of the case.

12.8 Laws and Regulations

LEARNING OBJECTIVES

You should:
- realise the extent that the law of the land governs you as a dentist, an employer and an employee
- be aware of the need to seek professional advice whenever it is appropriate
- understand agreements and contracts of employment as they affect dental practice.

A dentist may be an employer and/or an employee, both of which involve a myriad of legislation. The Dentists Act of 1984, which has had several minor amendments over the years, makes the practice of dentistry illegal other than by registered practitioners and enrolled auxiliaries. It is this Act that gives the GDC the powers that have already been discussed.

A summary of other important legislation is listed below; as it is so extensive and complicated, appropriate professional advice should always be sought. This list should be used only as a guide to those situations or occasions when further details should be sought and/or appropriate professional advice obtained. Ignorance of the law is not acceptable for defence or mitigation.

EMPLOYMENT

All employees should have a written contract of employment.

There is a nationally agreed contract for the employment of foundation dentists, and the BDA offers specimen contracts for various types of employee and working agreements to its members on request.

Termination

There is specific legislation regarding the termination of employment, redundancy and unfair dismissal. Legal advice should be sought on this matter.

Discrimination

This now comes under the aegis of the Equality and Human Rights Commission in the United Kingdom, which was established under the Equality Act 2006. Under this legislation, there are nine *protected grounds* against discrimination both within the workplace and in general:

- age
- disability
- sex
- race
- religion or belief
- pregnancy and maternity
- marriage and civil partnership
- sexual orientation
- gender reassignment.

Employers' Liabilities

These include the safety of employees, customers and the general public, as well as the collection of income tax and National Insurance contributions.

Premises and Working Environment

Legislation involving factories, offices and other workplaces prescribes standards of cleanliness, levels of occupation, the provision of appropriate protective clothing for employees and the provision of sanitary facilities of any workplace. Specific legislation concerning, for instance, eye protection, air compressors, autoclaves and the safety of all electrical appliances are among those applicable to dental practice.

Health and Safety at Work Legislation

This states that every employer has a general duty to ensure the health, safety and welfare at work of all employees. There are many general and specific regulations under this umbrella. Every employer has to:

- provide and maintain safety equipment and systems of work
- ensure safe handling and storage of any potentially harmful substances
- maintain entrances and exits in a safe condition
- provide a working environment for employees that is no risk to their health
- provide instruction, training and supervision necessary to ensure health and safety.

The Health and Safety Executive has the duty to enforce legal requirements and provide advisory services. Its inspectors have the power to enter premises and carry out investigations.

If an inspector notes a risk to health and safety, she/he can issue a Prohibition Notice preventing the continuance of that risk activity until remedial action as specified has been taken. In the case of a less severe risk, an Improvement Notice may be issued, which requires action within a specified time to remove that risk. Failure to comply with either of these notices within a specific time can lead to prosecution of the offender (employer).

Under the health and safety umbrella, there are several specific regulations that are particularly important to dentistry:

Ionising Radiations Regulations

The Ionising Radiation Regulations (IRRs) are concerned with the safety and maintenance of X-ray equipment, quality assurance and the health and safety of employees and the general public.

The protection of patients is covered by the Ionising Radiations (Medical Exposure) Regulations (2000) (IRMERs). IRMERs came into force on 13 May 2000 and are mainly concerned with the protection of patients and specify the responsibilities of those ordering and taking radiographs. They are to ensure that only necessary examinations are undertaken and that the dose of radiation that the patient receives is kept to a minimum.

As there is no doubt that dental radiography is included in medical exposures, these regulations have to be fully covered in all undergraduate dental courses in the United Kingdom. Additionally, all dentists and ancillary staff involved in ordering and/or taking radiographs for patients must undertake a formal radiation protection course of at least 5 hours of verifiable CPD covering these regulations every 5 years.

The IRRs and IRMERs were updated in 2017, and the new IRMERs came into force in February 2018. Since then, all organisations that use ionising radiation have to be registered with the UK Health & Safety Executive and appoint a Radiation Protection Adviser (RPA). Also, these regulations lowered the maximum permissible doses to certain organs of the body.

Each organisation using ionising radiation has to have a Legal Person to ensure that this legislation is abided by and that good working practices are implemented. In dental practice, the Legal Person is usually the practice owner.

In dentistry the Legal Person must:

- ensure that there are written protocols for all radiation procedures
- keep training records of all staff undertaking X-ray examinations
- make up referral criteria for all X-ray examinations
- ensure there are written protocols for each radiographic examination and all X-ray equipment
- publish Diagnostic Reference Levels (DRLs) for each category of X-ray examination
- have procedures for investigating and managing any overexposures to ionising radiation
- keep an inventory of all X-ray equipment
- register the X-ray equipment with the Health & Safety Executive (HSE)
- appoint an appropriately qualified member of staff as the Radiation Protection Supervisor (RPS) whose duty is to ensure the implementation of 'Local Rules' for X-ray usage
- ensure that staff dosage is as low as reasonably practicable (ALARP)
- appoint an RPA to examine and test X-ray equipment, undertake risk assessments, quality assurance and training. This needs to be undertaken at least every 5 years and when any new X-ray equipment is installed.
- appoint a Medical Physics Expert (MPE) to advise on patient dosage, X-ray examination techniques and radiation protection.

It is worth noting that a suitably qualified medical physicist can act as both RPA and MPE.

Any incident involving an excessive dose of radiation must be reported to the RPA/MPE, who will decide if the incident needs to be reported to the relevant statutory body.

There are three categories of staff involved in X-ray examinations; however, in dental practice, they are often the same person.

Referrer: the person who refers the patient for the X-ray examination and ensures that the referral is in line with reference criteria.

IRMER Practitioner: who must justify the need for an X-ray examination, ensuring that the benefit to the patient outweighs the detriment of that X-ray exposure.

Operator: is the person who carries out the investigation on the patient, and is responsible for identifying that it is the correct patient, taking and processing the image, evaluating that the exposure is appropriate and is responsible for quality assurance of the equipment.

There are two terms that have specific meanings in regard to the use of ionising radiation in diagnosis.

Justification: this is an estimation of the benefit to the patient and includes:

- ensuring that the patient will benefit from the X-ray examination and that the benefit will outweigh the risk
- checking that the X-ray examination has not already been undertaken in the recent past
- ensuring that there is no suitable diagnostic alternative to the exposure.

Optimisation: the operator must ensure that:

- The dose is as low as reasonable practicable.
- The technique is in line with protocols.
- They have sufficient skill to carry out the procedure.
- The exposure is within diagnostic reference levels.
- There is a clinical evaluation of the image(s) and ensure that those findings are recorded in the patient's records.

Control of Substances Hazardous to Health Regulations 2002 (COSHH)

Within these regulations are occupational exposure limits and maximum exposure limits. In dental practice, for example, substances such as glutaraldehyde, mercury, methylacrylate, phenol and trichloracetic acid are common and could cause hazard if mishandled. The employer has the duty to make a risk assessment on all hazardous substances and to reduce any identifiable risk as much as possible.

The Control of Mercury (enforcement) Regulations 2017

Since July 2018, dental amalgam must not be used for dental treatment in:

- primary dentition
- children under 15 years of age
- pregnant or breastfeeding women.

Amalgam may be used when deemed strictly necessary by the dental practitioner based on the specific medical or dental needs of the patient. If advising the use of dental amalgam in any of the above groups, discussion with the patient or their legal guardian is required and consent is essential.

Reporting of Injuries, Diseases and Dangerous Occurrences Regulations (2013)

Any serious injuries, accident, work-related diseases or dangerous incidents that could potentially cause harm arising out of or in connection with work affecting the employer, an employee or a member of the public on the premises must be reported to the Health & Safety Executive.

Freedom of Information Act (2000 or 2002 in Scotland)

Dentists who provide NHS treatment are considered to be a 'public authority' and are therefore covered by this legislation. This Act allows patients to examine any records held by the practice and allows the primary care organisation and individuals to request information such as NHS contract value and Unit of Dental Activity (in NHS dental treatment) (UDA) targets. Dentists are also able to request information held by the primary care organisation.

Care Quality Commission

This body is the independent regulator of health and adult social care in England; it is an executive non-departmental public body sponsored by the Department of Health and Social Care of the United Kingdom. It was established in 2009; its purpose is the regulation of organisations and the premises where health and social care is undertaken. The Care Quality Commission (CQC) set out fundamental standards of care which encompass quality and safety. They also monitor, inspect and regulate services to ensure these standards are met. Their findings are published and publicly accessible. The CQC has had a rolling programme of inspecting dental practices since 2015. These inspections are judged in five key areas—is the practice:

- safe
- effective
- caring
- responsive
- well-led.

The CQC remit covers all health and social care organisations, not just dentistry. Its fundamental standards are to insure that there is:

- person-centred care
- dignity and respect
- need for consent
- safe care and treatment
- safeguarding service users from abuse and improper treatment
- meeting nutritional and hydration needs
- suitable premises and equipment
- receiving and acting on complaints
- good governance
- staffing
- fit-and-proper persons employed.

There is a Primary Care Dental Services Provider Handbook available from CQC covering details of what is expected to demonstrate that a practice is well-led and compliant.

At the time of writing, the information taken from the CQC website shows that the CQC currently registers and regulates:

- hospitals
- dental practices
- ambulance services
- care homes
- children's services
- healthcare clinics
- services based in the community
- GP and doctor services
- hospices
- mental health services
- services in secure settings
- home care services.

Further information about the Care Quality Commission is available on their website (www.cqc.org.uk).

Disclosure and Barring Service (DBS)

The Disclosure and Barring Service is an executive non-departmental public body sponsored by the Home Office of the United Kingdom. Previously, this facility was provided by the Independent Safeguarding Authority and later by the Criminal Records Bureau. Any individual working with vulnerable groups, for example, treating or caring for children or vulnerable adults, has to undergo checks by this organisation. They will check whether the applicant has any criminal record that might make them unsuitable to have contact with vulnerable persons. People working in health care require an enhanced DBS check. These are applied for through a registered body or by a recruiting organisation who needs the applicant to be checked. This applies for England, Wales, the Channel Islands and the Isle of Man. This process was previously called Criminal Records Bureau Enhanced Disclosure (CRBED).

In Scotland, there is a separate but similar scheme called the Protecting Vulnerable Groups (PVGs) Scheme. This is managed and delivered by Disclosure Scotland.

Never Events
The NHS has a National Reporting and Learning System (NRLS) to report never events and advise on minimising their re-occurrence. A never events list is published annually by NHS Improvement, included in this list is the extraction of the wrong tooth. It is expected that this event should be reported to NRLS or the local health authority, unless it is a deciduous tooth removed under general anaesthesia. Currently, the only other never event listed that might possibly occur in a dental environment is the mis-selection of high strength midazolam for use in intravenous sedation.

Safeguarding
It is important to have safeguarding training for all staff, and, to this end, Public Health England has issued a booklet 'Safeguarding in General Dental Practice – A Toolkit for Dental Teams'. This recommends that:

- each dental practice have a named safeguarding practice lead
- all members of staff (clinical and non-clinical) undertake the appropriate level of safeguarding training
- there is a safeguarding reporting system in place and staff are familiar with this
- all members of staff know how to access the NHS Safeguarding app for local safeguarding contact details.

Similarly, the GDC in principle 8 of *Standards for the Dental Team* require that:

8.1. Always put patients' safety first.
8.2. Act promptly if patients or colleagues are at risk, and take measures to protect them.
8.3. Make sure if you employ, manage or lead a team that you encourage and support a culture where staff can raise concerns openly and without fear of reprisal.
8.4. Make sure if you employ, manage or lead a team that there is an effective procedure in place for raising concerns, that the procedure is readily available to all staff and that it is followed at all times.
8.5. Take appropriate action if you have concerns about the possible abuse of children or vulnerable adults.

Cases of neglect or abuse may be obvious to the practice staff and care is needed to confirm this. There will be a local Social Services Team who deal with these cases, and any concerns should be reported to that Team rather than pursuing the investigation in the practice.

Whistleblowing
The Public Interest Disclosure Act [1998] (PIDA) specifically protects whistleblowers, giving protection to employees who raise genuine concerns about potentially illegal or dangerous practices. It applies to everyone working in the NHS. A disclosure must be made in good faith which the reporter believes is true and is not making the disclosure for personal gain. This act applies to all dental professionals within the NHS whether employees or self-employed. Action is required if any of the following are seen:

- Attitudes or skills below expected levels.
- Poor clinical skills or lack of competence.
- Behavioural problems.
- Poor managerial or organisational skills in health care delivery.
- A high number of patient complaints.
- Inadequate induction or training of staff.
- A bullying culture.
- Financial irregularities.

Raising concerns is also endorsed by the GDC in its guidance within *Standards for the Dental Team* (Section 8.11).

If advice is needed before raising concern in the NHS, NHS Improvement has advice in its website and a whistleblowing helpline; also the charity *Protect* (formerly called *Public Concern at Work*) will offer advice.

There is a duty to raise any concern that you might have, it is a matter of highlighting a potential problem rather that proving the case. After that, it is up to the head or designated person in your organisation to investigate the measure.

Friends and Family Tests
There are two contexts in which this can be used:

Firstly, in gaining patient feedback, a questionnaire can ask, 'How likely are you to recommend us [our practice/our hospital/our clinic/etc.] to your friends and family?':

- Extremely likely
- Likely
- Neither likely or unlikely
- Extremely unlikely
- Don't know

Secondly, when deciding on a particular treatment for a patient, ask yourself, 'Would you do the same treatment for a friend or family member?'.

General Liability
Owners of property and/or land have a general liability concerning safety to the general public, and prudent owners take out insurance to cover this liability.

Discrimination
There have been several pieces of antidiscrimination legislation passed over the years. These have been brought together by the formation of the Commission for Equality and Human Rights (see previously mentioned details).

Legislation Involved in Dental Treatment
NATIONAL HEALTH SERVICE ACTS AND REGULATIONS. Naturally these only cover patients receiving NHS treatment. Copies of the appropriate rules and regulations should be issued to all independent practitioners undertaking treatment under Health Service regulations by the appropriate health authority. In the case of employees, the appropriate health authority or NHS trust has this responsibility.

DATA PROTECTION. See GDPR (already discussed).

The Consumer Protection Act 1987

The provision of dental treatment may be considered as the provision of goods or services under this Act. However, the vast majority of actions in dental and medical matters are dealt with via the negligence route.

Social Security Acts

Certain patients on low income are able to have the patient's contribution to NHS dental treatment paid for by the State. Employees applying for Statutory Sick Pay, Statutory Maternity Pay or various other allowances come within the umbrella of Social Security.

Agreements and Contracts of Employment

It would be expected, or considered essential, that there is a legal framework governing the interaction between an individual professional and an employing (contracting) organisation. In many cases, terms within the contract are likely to be structured around nationally negotiated terms and conditions of service. This is likely to be variable both within the United Kingdom (England, Scotland, Wales, Northern Ireland) and internationally. It is recommended that the individual reviews carefully all documentation and, if necessary, seeks advice and guidance by a relevant organisation. For example, in the United Kingdom, this may be the BDA as the trade union for dental practitioners.

Awareness of the Law

Individuals are subject to the law of the land whether international, national or regional. In addition, dental professionals must also appreciate how the law may interface with delivery of health care for patients and how changes in law may impact on their clinical practice, for example, the Mental Capacity Act in relation to patient choice. The impact of the law can have a profound effect on the delivery of health care, both for the individual and the professional; it is therefore essential to keep up-to-date and have a contemporary understanding.

The law is such a diverse field, which is ever changing. As such, it is beyond the scope of this book to explore, other than raising awareness. It is also important to be aware that there are also differences in the legal systems dependent on the jurisdiction involved. An example of this is that there are several differences between the Scottish legal system and the legal system applying to England and Wales as well as Northern Ireland: for instance, the category of cases seen in the various levels of courts and the naming of those levels. Whichever jurisdiction is involved, it is essential to obtain legal advice from someone trained in that jurisdiction.

Acronyms

There are many bodies and organisations that affect the practice of dentistry; these are often known by their initials. Also, there are several acronyms in general use within the healing professions, many of which are listed here for reference. Whilst every effort has been made to ensure these are contemporary, reorganisation of bodies, changes in structures and procedural updates mean that some of these will become less relevant as they are replaced over time.

ABDFT	Advisory Board for Dental Foundation Training
ABSTD	Advisory Board for Specialty Training in Dentistry
ACF	Academic Clinical Fellow
AccessNI	Equivalent to DBS in England
ADEE	Association for Dental Education in Europe
AGP	Aerosol Generating Procedure
ALARA/ ALARP	As Low As Reasonably Achievable/ Practicable (Radiation dose minimalisation)
ALB	Arm's Length Body
ARCP	Annual Review of Competence Progression
ARF	Annual Retention Fee (to stay on GDC Register)
ASA	Advertising Standards Agency
AT	Area Team (previously PCT)
BAOMS	British Association of Oral & Maxillofacial Surgeons
BASCD	British Association for the Study of Community Dentistry
BDA	British Dental Association
BDS (BChD)	Bachelor of Dental Surgery
BNF	British National Formulary [of medicines]
BOS	British Orthodontic Society
BSDH	British Society for Disability & Oral Health
BSDMFR	British Society of Dental & Maxillofacial Radiology
BSPD	British Society of Paediatric Dentistry
CBD	Case-Based Discussion
CCG	Clinical Commissioning Group
CCST	Certificate of Completion of Specialist Training (see also FTTA)
CDEC	Continuing Dental Education Committee (Wales)
CDO	Chief Dental Officer (of England, or Northern Ireland, or Scotland or Wales)
CDS	Community Dental Service
CDT	Clinical Dental Technician
CEX	Clinical Evaluation Exercises
CGDent	College of General Dentistry
COPDEND	Committee of Postgraduate Dental Deans & Directors
COPMeD	Conference of Postgraduate Medical Deans (UK)
CPD	Continuing Professional Development
CQC	Care Quality Commission
CQUIN	Commissioning for Quality & Innovation (Scheme)
CRB	Criminal Records Bureau (now DBS – Disclosure & Barring Service)
CRG	Clinical Reference Groups

CT	Computed Tomography
DBS	Disclosure & Barring Service (previously CRB)
DCS	Dental Complaints Service (of GDC for private patients)
DCT	Dental Core Trainee
DDRB	Doctors & Dentists Review Body (Advises Government on NHS pay rates)
DFT	Dental Foundation Training/Trainee
DFY1	Dental Foundation Year One
DFY2	Dental Foundation Year Two (previously SHO (Senior House Officer))
DGA	Dental (extractions under) General Anaesthetic
DHSC	Department of Health and Social Care
DOPS	Direct Observation of Procedural Skills
DSC	Dental Schools Council
DWSI	Dentist with Special Interest (in carrying out certain treatments)
EBP	Evidence-Based Practice
ES	Educational Supervisor
EWTD	European Working Time Directive
FOIA	Freedom of Information Act
FD	Foundation Dentist
FDI	(Federation Dentaire International) World Dental Federation
FDS [RCS]	Faculty of Dental Surgery (of a Royal Surgical College)
	Fellowship in Dental Surgery (of a Royal Surgical College)
FFGDP	Fellowship of the Faculty of General Dental Practice
FFT	Friends & Family Test
FGDP [UK]	Faculty of General Dental Practice
FSG	Freedom to Speak up Guardian
FtP	Fitness to Practise Investigation (by GDC)
FT	Foundation Trust (NHS organisation)
FTTA	(Orthodontic) Fixed Term Training Appointment (now Post CCST Trainee)
GDC	General Dental Council
GDS	General Dental Services (NHS dental practice services)
GDPC	General Dental Practice Committee (of the BDA)
GDPR	General Data Protection Regulations
GMC	General Medical Council
GPT	General Professional Training (now Foundation Training)
HCAIs	Health Care Associated Infections
HCP	Health Care Provider
HCW	Health Care Worker
HEE	Health Education England
HEFCE	Higher Education Funding Council for England

HEIW	Health Education and Improvement Wales
HIW	Health Care Inspectorate – Wales
HMRC	Her Majesty's Revenue & Customs
HSC	Department of Health and Social Care in Northern Ireland
HSCIC	Health & Social Care Information Centre
HTM 01-05	Health Technical Memorandum on Decontamination
IACSD	Intercollegiate Advisory Committee for Sedation in Dentistry
IADR	International Association for Dental Research
IAT	Integrated Academic Training (pathway)
IC	Investigating Committee (of the GDC)
ICO	Information Commissioners Office (Data Protection)
IDA	Irish Dental Association
IELTS	International English Language Testing System
IOC	Interim Orders Committee (of the GDC)
IQE	International Qualifying Examination (now replaced by ORE)
IR(ME)R	Ionising Radiation (Medical Exposures) Regulations
IRR	Ionising Radiations Regulations
IS	Inhalation Sedation
ISCP	Intercollegiate Surgical Curriculum Programme
ISFE	Intercollegiate Specialist Fellowship Examination
IOSN	Index (Indicator) of Sedation Need
ITF	International Training Fellow
JCPTD	Joint Committee for Postgraduate Training in Dentistry
JSCT	Joint Committee for Surgical Training
KPI	Key Performance Indicators (in NHS dental contracts and other clinical services)
LAT	Local Area (Health) Team
LDC	Local Dental Committee
LDN	Local Dental Network
LDS	Licence in Dental Surgery
LETB	Local Education & Training Board
LocSSIPs	Local Safety Standards for Invasive Procedures
LPN	Local Patient Network
MCN	Managed Clinical Network
MDT	Multi-Disciplinary Team
MFDS	Member of the Faculty of Dental Surgery (of a Royal Surgical College)
MFGDP	Member of the Faculty of General Dental Practice (of a Royal Surgical College)

MHRA	Medicines and Health Care Products Regulatory Agency
Mini-PAT	Mini Peer Assessment Tool
MJDF	Member of the Joint Dental Faculties (of the Royal College of Surgeons of England)
MMI	Multiple Mini Interviews
MRC	Medical Research Council
MSF	Multi-Source Feedback
NACPDE	National Advice Centre for Postgraduate Dental Education
NAO	National Audit Office
NatSSIPs	National Safety Standards for Invasive Procedures
NDPB	Non-Departmental Public Body
NES	NHS Education for Scotland
NHS	National Health Service
NHS FFT	NHS Friends & Family Test
NHS QIS	National Health Service Quality Improvement Scotland
NHSBSA	National Health Service Business Service Authority
NICE	National Institute for Health and Clinical Excellence
NIDPC	Northern Ireland Dental Practice Committee
NIHR	National Institute for Health Research
NIMDTA	Northern Ireland Medical & Dental Training Agency
NSF	National Service Framework
NTN	National Training Number
NTNa	Academic National Training Number
OMFS	Oral & Maxillofacial Surgery
ORE	Overseas Registration Examination (of GDC)
OSCE	Objective/Observed Structured Clinical Examination
PBA	Procedure-/Problem-Based Assessment
PCC	Professional Conduct Committee (of the GDC)
PCN	Primary Care Network
PCO	Primary Care Organisation
PCSE	Primary Care Support, England
PCT	Primary Care Trust (now disbanded)
PDS	Personal Dental Services
PECR	Private & Electronic Communication Regulation (GDPR)
PGMDE	Postgraduate Medical and Dental Education
PHE	Public Health England
PIDA	Public Interest Disclosure Act (protection for whistleblowers)
PIDO	Public Interest Disclosure Order (Northern Ireland) – as mentioned previously
PLAB	Professional & Linguistic Assessment Board

PLG	Patient Liaison Group
PPC	Professional Performance Committee (of the GDC)
PPE	Personal Protective Equipment
PPI	Patient & Public Involvement (in decision making)
PREMs	Patient-Reported Experience Measures
PROMs	Patient-Reported Outcome Measures
PSA	Professional Standards Authority for Health & Social Care
Pt	Patient
PVG	Protecting Vulnerable Groups Scheme (in Scotland)
QUANGO	Quasi-Autonomous Non-Governmental Organisation
QOF	Quality & Outcomes Framework
QoL	Quality of Life
RAG	Red–Amber–Green (to advise patients of their oral health risk)
RCPS[Glas]	Royal College of Physicians and Surgeons (of Glasgow)
RCS[Edin]	Royal College of Surgeons (of Edinburgh)
RCS[Eng]	Royal College of Surgeons (of England)
RCSI	Royal College of Surgeons in Ireland
REF	Research & Excellence Framework
RIDDOR	Reporting of Injuries, Diseases & Dangerous Occurrences Regulations (1995)
RITA	Record of In-Training Assessment
RQIA	Regulation & Quality Improvement Authority (Northern Ireland)
RTF	Research Training Fellowship
SAAD	Society for the Advancement of Anaesthesia in Dentistry
SAC	Specialist Advisory Committee
SAS	Staff & Associate Specialist (a non-consultant hospital career grade for Doctors & Dentists)
SCD	Special Care Dentistry
SDCEP	Scottish Dental Clinical Effectiveness Programme
SDPB	Scottish Dental Practice Board (NHS)
SEDENTEXCT	EU Guidelines on the use of CBCT in dental & maxillofacial radiology
SHA	Strategic Health Authority (now replaced)
SIGN	Scottish Intercollegiate Guidelines Network
SJT	Situation Judgement Test (used in interviews & examinations)
SMART[Goal-setting]	Specific, Measurable, Attainable, Relevant & Timebound (multiple variations)
SMC	Scottish Medicines Consortium

SPDCSs	Salaried Primary Dental Care Services	UOA	Unit of Orthodontic Activity (in NHS treatment)
SpR	Specialist Registrar (changed to StR in 2009)	VT	Vocational Training
StR	Specialty Registrar	VTE	Vocational Training Equivalence (a scheme for overseas dentists to allow them to undertake NHS practice in the United Kingdom)
STC	Specialty Training Committee		
TPD	Training Programme Director		
UCAT	University Clinical Aptitude Test	WBA	Work-Based Assessment
UDA	Unit of Dental Activity (in NHS dental treatment)	WHO	World Health Organisation (part of United Nations)
UK NARIC	National Recognition Information Centre for the UK	WPBA	Workplace-Based Assessment

Self-Assessment: Questions

MULTIPLE CHOICE QUESTIONS (TRUE/FALSE)

1. The following are eligible for full registration with the GDC:
   a. Dentists who qualified in the United States
   b. Dentists who qualified in India
   c. Dentists who qualified from a UK University
   d. Dentists who have not completed dental foundation training
   e. Dentists who only have a Licentiate of Dental Surgery from a Royal College, not a Bachelor of Dental Surgery from a UK university

2. The Overseas Registration Examination:
   a. Is in three parts
   b. Each part can only be attempted once
   c. Includes an English language test
   d. Has to be passed by UK qualified dentists for full registration
   e. Has to be passed by Israeli dentists for full registration

3. The following specialties are recognised by the GDC for specialist registration:
   a. Dental public health
   b. Maxillofacial surgery
   c. Endodontics
   d. Oral surgery
   e. Crown and bridge

4. Consent to treatment:
   a. Can be verbal
   b. Can be written
   c. Can be implied
   d. Is not required for patients under 16 years of age
   e. Can be withdrawn by the patient

5. A dentist referring a patient for general anaesthesia must:
   a. Fully justify why a general anaesthetic is required
   b. Take a full medical history
   c. Explain to the patient the risks involved
   d. Obtain consent from the patient or their guardian
   e. Offer alternative methods of pain control in order to complete treatment for the patient

6. When treating a patient under general anaesthesia, the dentist must:
   a. Repeat the history taking
   b. Repeat the explanations concerning risk, alternative treatments and pain control
   c. Obtain verbal consent
   d. Keep careful records of the treatment
   e. Give written pre- and postoperative instructions

7. Before undertaking treatment under sedation, the dentist must:
   a. Assess the patient
   b. Take a full medical history
   c. Obtain written informed consent
   d. Ensure that equipment and facilities are adequate
   e. Advise on alternative methods of completing treatment

8. When treating a patient under sedation:
   a. A chaperone must be present
   b. The patient should be monitored only during the sedation
   c. Drugs must be available for resuscitation
   d. The patient's recovery must be supervised
   e. The patient must be accompanied by a responsible adult

9. Complaints from patients:
   a. Every dental practice should have a complaints procedure
   b. Only dentists and doctors can deal with complaints from patients
   c. Should be managed by an outside body or organisation
   d. Only complaints in writing can be accepted

10. The following would not be considered negligent:
    a. Something going wrong when treating a friend out-of-hours
    b. Not treating a patient to the standard that would be expected of a specialist
    c. If the patient did not suffer harm or damage from a dentist's error
    d. If the dentist had a duty of care at the time
    e. If the dentist did not exercise reasonable skill and care

11. A claim for compensation for negligence against a dentist is unlikely to succeed:
    a. If the patient pleads 'res ipsa loquitur'
    b. If the dentist carried out reasonable treatment
    c. If the patient persuaded the dentist to undertake treatment that the dentist was doubtful would be successful

d. If the damage occurred as a result of the patient grabbing the dentist's working arm
e. If the negligent act or omission was carried out by an employee

12. The following laws affect the practice of dentistry:
    a. COSHH Regulations
    b. The Dentists Act
    c. Health and Safety at Work Acts
    d. General Data Protection Regulation
    e. Financial Services Act

13. It is illegal to discriminate against people because of their:
    a. Race
    b. Dietary habits
    c. Pregnancy
    d. Sex
    e. Age

SINGLE BEST ANSWER QUESTIONS

1. The UK General Dental Council is:
   A. A department of the government
   B. A higher education provider
   C. A health care regulator
   D. An indemnity organisation
   E. A trade union organisation

2. Which of the following registration types are included in the General Dental Council's Dental Care Professional register:
   A. Clinical Dental Technician
   B. Dental Practice Manager
   C. Dental Receptionist
   D. Maxillofacial Prosthetist and Technologist
   E. Oral Health Educator

3. A requirement when renewing registration with the General Dental Council includes declaration of:
   A. Income protection
   B. Membership of a trade union organisation
   C. Membership of one of the Royal Colleges
   D. NHS performer number
   E. Professional indemnity

4. According to the GDC in the United Kingdom, continuing professional development should be planned:
   A. As opportunities arise as long as all necessary topics are covered
   B. Based on local opportunities, availability and delivery
   C. In conjunction with scope of practice and a personal development plan
   D. On a 3-year rolling cycle
   E. To focus on topics a dental professional has interest in and is proficient at

5. The following is recognised on the General Dental Council Specialist list:
   A. Aesthetic dentistry
   B. Cosmetic dentistry
   C. Maxillofacial surgery
   D. Oral surgery
   E. Surgical dentistry

6. The following would not be within the Scope of Practice of a Dental Hygienist in the United Kingdom:
   A. Application of fissure sealant
   B. Periodontal examination and charting
   C. Restoration of a primary tooth
   D. Root surface debridement
   E. Smoking cessation advice

7. Which of the following options would be the most appropriate registrant for a dentist to refer a patient to for caries removal and restoration of a permanent tooth in a 12-year-old child?
   A. Dental Hygienist
   B. Dental Nurse
   C. Dental Technician
   D. Dental Therapist
   E. Orthodontic Therapist

ESSAY QUESTIONS

1. Whilst working as a Dentist in an Oral Surgery department, you see a patient and carry out multiple tooth extractions under local anaesthetic. When you complete the extractions you notice you have been working from an old dental pantomogram (DPT) taken several years ago, rather than the one taken at the patient's recent assessment visit. After re-checking your notes you realise you have extracted a tooth that was not included in the treatment plan. Describe how you would manage this situation.

2. How would you deal with a complaint from a patient whom you treated a few months earlier?

Self-Assessment: Answers

MULTIPLE CHOICE ANSWERS

1. a. False.
   b. False.
   c. True.
   d. True.
   e. True.
2. a. False.
   b. False.
   c. False.
   d. False.
   e. True.
3. a. True.
   b. False. It is a medical specialty.
   c. True.
   d. True.
   e. False.
4. a. True.
   b. True.
   c. True.
   d. False. Required for all patients, in loco parentis if necessary.
   e. True.
5. a. True.
   b. True.
   c. True.
   d. True.
   e. True.

6. a. True.
   b. True.
   c. False. Written informed consent is essential.
   d. True.
   e. True.
7. a. True.
   b. True.
   c. True.
   d. True.
   e. True.
8. a. True.
   b. False. The patient must also be monitored during recovery.
   c. True.
   d. True.
   e. True.
9. a. True.
   b. False. Every practice or health organisation should have someone nominated to deal with complaints, but they do not have to be a doctor or dentist.
   c. False. Complaints should be dealt with internally in the first instance.
   d. False. Complaints can be verbal or written.
10. a. False. Liability is present whenever treating any patient.
    b. False. Unless you are a specialist in the same or a related field.
    c. True.
    d. False.
    e. False.
11. a. False.
    b. True.
    c. False. A dentist should refuse to treat in this case.
    d. True.
    e. False. A dentist is liable for acts and omissions of employees.
12. a. True.
    b. True.
    c. True.
    d. True.
    e. False.
13. a. True.
    b. False.
    c. True.
    d. True.
    e. True.

SINGLE BEST ANSWER QUESTION ANSWERS

1. C
2. A
3. E
4. C
5. D
6. C
7. D

ESSAY QUESTIONS

1. Points to consider when structuring your answer:
   - Immediate management and patient care
   - Communication and informing the patient (Duty of candour)
   - Incident reporting (considered to be a 'never event') discussing whom you would inform and the process that would take place following this
   - Long-term care arrangements or follow-up
   - Reflection and avoiding similar incidences in the future (how: audit, clinical governance)
   - For completeness, sign-posting any complaints procedure a patient may wish to follow

2. Points to consider when structuring your answer:
   - All health care organisations must have a system for dealing with complaints. In the United Kingdom, in addition to this, the General Dental Council's 'Standards for the Dental Team' Principle 5 outlines the need to have a clear and effective complaints procedure
   - Respecting the patient's right to complain
   - Communication: Acknowledgement of complaint, listening to their complaint, keeping the patient informed of progress, prompt and constructive response
   - Flexibility of approach and responding appropriately to the complaint – how this may be achieved if the complaint was received by telephone, in person or in writing
   - Appropriate recording
   - Information gathering and investigating
   - Options for resolution
   - Involvement of Indemnity organisation
   - Local resolution if possible, options for escalation if complaint cannot be resolved
   - Future learning: personal or practice development and risk management (personal development planning for continuing professional development)

Index

Page numbers ending in 'b', 'f' and 't' refer to Boxes, Figures and Tables respectively. The letter 'Q' following a page number indicates a related question.